Huda A Kil

T5-ASR-543

CHARACTERISTICS AND FUNCTION OF OPIOIDS

Developments in Neuroscience

CHARACTERISTICS AND FUNCTION OF OPIOIDS

Proceedings of the International Narcotic Research
Conference, held in Noordwijkerhout, The Netherlands on
July 23-27, 1978

Edited by

JAN M. VAN REE   and   **LARS TERENIUS**

Rudolf Magnus Institute for
Pharmacology
State University of Utrecht
Utrecht
The Netherlands

Department of Pharmacology
University of Uppsala
Uppsala
Sweden

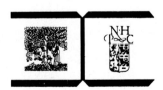

ELSEVIER/NORTH-HOLLAND BIOMEDICAL PRESS
AMSTERDAM · NEW YORK · OXFORD · 1978

© 1978 Elsevier/North-Holland Biomedical Press

All rights reserved. No part of this publication may be reproduced, stored in a retrieval system, or transmitted, in any form or by any means, electronic, mechanical, photocopying, recording or otherwise, without the prior permission of the copyright owner.

Published by:
Elsevier/North-Holland Biomedical Press
335 Jan van Galenstraat, P.O. Box 211
Amsterdam, The Netherlands

Sole distributors for the U.S.A. and Canada:
Elsevier North-Holland, Inc.
52 Vanderbilt Avenue
New York, N.Y. 10017

ISBN: 0-444-80028-X (series)
ISBN: 0-444-80076-X (Vol. 4)

PRINTED IN THE NETHERLANDS

David I. Macht   1915
Thus if we trace the history of opium
from its earliest beginnings to the
brilliant researches of recent years,
if we but compare the analytic and
synthetic, chemical, physiologic and
pharmacologic studies of the same old
drug with the fantastic and puerile
effusions on the subject of our
medical predecessors, we cannot help
being impressed with the long strides
forward which medicine has made; yet,
on the other hand, our very recent
studies on opium and its alkaloids
serve but to emphasize the more our
meager knowledge of the subject and
the still greater task before us.

JAMA 64 (1915) 481

Organizing Committee of the IRNC Meeting
"Characteristics and function of opioids"

Jan M. van Ree (general chairman)
Lars Terenius (program chairman)
Willem Hendrik Gispen
Dirk H.G. Versteeg
David de Wied

Executive Committee
International Narcotic Research Conference

Sydney Archer
Albert Herz
Joseph J.C. Jacob
Hiroshi Kaneto
Eric J. Simon
Lars Terenius
Eddy Leong Way

ACKNOWLEDGEMENTS

The congress has been arranged by the staff of the Rudolf Magnus Institute for Pharmacology, University of Utrecht, Vondellaan 6, Utrecht.

The congress has been made possible by the support of:
The Dutch Ministry of Education, The Netherlands,
The Dutch Ministry of Health and Environmental Protection, The Netherlands,
The Dr. Saal van Zwanenberg Foundation, Utrecht, The Netherlands.

The organizers gratefully acknowledge donations from:
ACF-Chemiefarma B.V., Maarssen, The Netherlands,
Algemene Bank Nederland N.V., Amsterdam, The Netherlands,
Bachem A.G., Bubendorf, Switzerland,
CIBA-Geigy B.V., Arnhem, The Netherlands,
Endo Laboratories Inc., New York, N.Y., USA,
Gist Brocades, Delft, The Netherlands
Hoechst A.G., Frankfurt/Main, Fed. Republic of Germany,
ICI Americas Inc., Wilmington, Del., USA,
Janssen Pharmaceutica, Beerse, Belgium,
Lily Research Laboratories, Indianapolis, Ind., USA,
Merck, Sharp and Dohme N.V., West Point, Penn., USA,
Miles Laboratories Ltd., Slough, U.K.,
Organon International B.V., Oss, The Netherlands,
Paul-Martini-Stiftung, Frankfurt/Main, Fed. Republic of Germany
Pfizer Inc, Groton, Conn., USA,
Pharmachemie B.V., Haarlem, The Netherlands,
Sandoz Ltd., Basel, Switzerland,
Schering A.G., Berlin, Fed. Republic of Germany,
Sterling-Winthrop Research Institute
Troponwerke, Köln, Fed. Republic of Germany,
UCB, Brussels, Belgium,
Upjohn Comp., Kalamazoo, Mich., USA,
The Wellcome Research Laboratories, Beckenham, U.K.

PREFACE

After the brain had been shown to contain specific binding sites for opioids, there followed successful attempts to isolate and to analyse the structure of endogenous ligands for opioid receptors. These endogenous morphine-like substances, endorphins, appeared to be neuropeptides structurally related to the pituitary hormone, β-lipotropin. The discovery of the endorphins has already led to a better understanding of brain function.

Since the International Narcotic Research Conference of 1976, the research concerning endorphins has broadened as is witnessed by the present Proceedings of the 1978 INRC meeting (The Netherlands, July 23 - 27). The general topic of this meeting was "Characteristics and Function of Opioids". From the contributions there emerged some insight into the functional significance of the endorphins and a dawning of the importance of their role in mental illness. Several other communications dealt with the classical opioids, their specific effects and their interference with biological functions.

On behalf of the International Narcotic Research Conference we thank all those who contributed to the success of the meeting, the chairmen, the speakers and the discussants. We wish to extend our special thanks to the various sponsors and to Dr. P. Siderius, from the Department of Health and Environmental Protection, for his opening address to the meeting. We would also like to mention the valuable assistance of the members of the Rudolf Magnus Institute for Pharmacology, and, in particular, of the secretarial and technical staff.

Lars Terenius
Department of Pharmacology
University of Uppsala
Sweden

Jan M. van Ree
Rudolf Magnus Institute for
Pharmacology
State University of Utrecht
The Netherlands

CONTENTS

SECTION V: BIOSYNTHESIS, RELEASE AND METABOLISM OF ENDORPHINS

SECTION VI: NEUROCHEMICAL AND ENDOCRINE EFFECTS OF OPIOIDS

Characteristics and Function of Opioids, editors Van Ree and Terenius
© *1978 Elsevier/North-Holland Biomedical Press*

NEUROPEPTIDES AND DRUG DEPENDENCE

JAN M. VAN REE*, DANIEL M. DORSA* & FRANCIS C. COLPAERT**
*Rudolf Magnus Institute for Pharmacology, Medical Faculty, University of
Utrecht, Vondellaan 6, Utrecht, the Netherlands.
** Janssen Pharmaceutica Research Laboratories, Beerse, Belgium.

INTRODUCTION

This survey deals with the ability of neuropeptides to modulate drug dependence and with the possible role of the recently isolated neuropeptides derived
from β-lipotropin (β-LPH) in drug dependence. The meaning of the concepts
'dependence' and related phenomena which result from drug use (e.g. tolerance
and physical dependence) varies with the discipline of the investigator involved; it thus seemed appropriate first to describe these phenomena as
referred to in the present survey and second to consider the validity of
animal experiments pertaining to them.

DRUG DEPENDENCE

Drug dependence can be defined as a state produced by repeated self-
administration of a psychoactive drug and such that the drug user will
engage in substantial amounts of behavior leading specifically to further
administration of the drug, or will continue to administer the drug even when
this requires the sacrifice of other reinforced behaviors[1]. A severe degree
of drug dependence is commonly designated as addiction. The drug concerned
is said to be reinforcing, since the drug user continues to show a particular
behavioral pattern resulting in a certain consequence (in this case, the drug).
Obviously, this reinforcing action is the common denominator for dependence
on various drugs[1], and can reliably be analysed in tests in which humans or
animals can self-administer the drugs under standard experimental conditions
[2,3]. In such experiments, subjects are given access to a device which, when
manipulated appropriately, results in the delivery of the drug. It has become
clear that this technique can be used to study both the reinforcing properties
of drugs and the variables which can influence drug-taking behavior and
consequently drug dependence, the state produced by this behavior[2,3,4]. The
significance of this test for drug dependence is based firstly on the technical
and theoretical similarities between experimental self-administering behavior
and human drug-seeking behavior; secondly, most drugs which appear to serve
as reinforcers in self-administering behavior have substantial dependence

potential [2,4]; thirdly, the behavioral and pharmacological characteristics of
drug self-administration seem similar to those found in drug dependence[2,3,5];
fourthly, variables influencing self-administering behavior may also be
important for drug dependence, though more research is needed in this respect[6];
finally, successful clinical programs have been developed which are based on
the outcome of experimental self-administration[7].

SUBJECTIVE EFFECTS OF DRUGS

In man, subjective effects of drugs may play a role in initiating and maintaining drug-seeking behavior[8]. Several classes of psychoactive drugs produce
highly characteristic subjective effects: this applies to the hallucinogens
and the minor tranquillizers[9]. The evaluation of these effects in man has
been used to ascertain the dependence potential of drugs[10]. The predictive
validity of this test rests on the assumption that drugs may be taken because
of their desirable subjective effects. The test procedure involves the re-
quest that subjects evaluate the ability of the drug tested to produce subjective effects similar to those induced by the presently or formerly taken drug.
This test proceeds as a discrimination procedure i.e., test substances are
being assayed for stimulus generalization with the reference drug. Such drug
discrimination procedures have also been shown to be applicable to experimental animals[11]. In a typical experiment, animals are trained to produce a
certain response in order to obtain food in a two-response device. Responding
to the devices is then linked to the administration of a drug or of a placebo
[12,13]. When the animals perform well in discriminating the stimulus effects
of the drug from those of the placebo (as shown by selection of the appropriate
device), they can then be "asked" whether a test drug produces stimulus effects
reminiscent of those of the training drug or of placebo. It has been
extensively shown that narcotics can act as discriminative stimuli[13,14].
This discriminative stimulus complex appears to be exclusively associated
with the specific central actions of narcotic analgesic drugs, and has been
designated as the narcotic cue[12]. This narcotic cue has been proposed as a
model for opiate-like subjective effects in man[12,14,15,16].

TOLERANCE AND PHYSICAL DEPENDENCE

Repeated administration of a drug can result in adaptive changes in the
organism such that tolerance develops, i.e., a given dose of the drug
produces less effect than it did on its first administration. These changes
may be due to alterations in drug availability or, more interesting for the

present survey, to adaptations in the nervous sytem subsequent to activation of the drug receptor complex. Physical dependence is characterized by a specific pattern of biological effects which occur when a chronically administered drug is withdrawn or displaced from its receptor complex. Both tolerance and physical dependence are characteristics of some dependence producing drugs and may contribute to the maintenance of drug-seeking behavior. It has been argued however that neither the induction of tolerance nor that of physical dependence is an essential condition for drug dependence[1,4,5]. Although both tolerance and physical dependence are induced by narcotic drugs, these phenomena are neither necessary nor sufficient to explain the reinforcing properties and subjective effects of these drugs[5].

As outlined above, the self-administration test is a reliable one for studying variables which influence drug dependence. Many experiments have been carried out to determine factors controlling drug-reinforced behavior, e.g. antecedent and current conditions, reinforcement variables, or conditional reinforcers[2,6]. However, the possible implication of endogenous principles in drug self-administering behavior has only recently been investigated. We have studied the influence of various neuropeptides related to neurohypophyseal hormones on acquisition and maintenance of heroin self-administration. These neuropeptides have been shown to affect memory processes in experimental animals[17,18] as well as in humans[19,20]. It has been postulated that neuro-hypophyseal hormones (i.c. vasopressin and oxytocin) and their fragments modulate brain processes selectively to consolidate, retrieve and repress recently acquired information[18]. The ring structure of the hormones may be important for the consolidating processes, the C-terminal part is more concerned with retrieval, while the intact oxytocin molecule represses the consolidation and reproduction of information[18]. Since learning and memory processes may be involved in self-administering behavior in that drug injections gain and maintain control over behavior, it seemed of interest to perform the studies now described.

Rats were allowed to self-administer heroin (0.03 µg dissolved in saline/ injection) via the intravenous route on a continuous reinforcement schedule. The animals were subjected to 6 hr experimental sessions for 5 consecutive days in sound attenuated chambers. One hr prior to the daily experimental session the animals were injected s.c. with placebo (saline) or peptide. Daily treatment with 1 or 5 µg of desglycinamide[9], arginine[8], vasopressin (DG-AVP) reduced self-administering behavior in a dose-dependent manner[21]. The inhibition was hardly detectable during the first two days of testing, but decreased gradually thereafter. Injections with DG-AVP on the first two days only resulted in a similar attenuation of the behavior, indicating that the effect of DG-AVP was long-lasting. From these data it was concluded that DG-AVP interfered with acquisition of heroin self-administration[21]. When the DG-AVP injections were started on day 3, a similar inhibition was observed, suggesting that DG-AVP may also interfere with the maintenance of heroin self-administration[21].

Structure-activity studies revealed that the effect of the vasopressin analog is mainly located in the covalent ring structure of vasopressin, since pressinamide had a similar effect although it was somewhat less potent. In contrast, oxytocin had an effect opposite to that of DG-AVP, in that self-administering behavior was slightly (n.s.) facilitated by this hormone. The covalent ring structure of oxytocin did not affect heroin self-administration, but 1 µg of the C-terminal tripeptide (PLG) markedly facilitated the behavior[21].

DG-AVP exerts its effect on heroin self-administration by interfering with processes in the central nervous system, since much lower amounts of this neuropeptide (50 ng) were required on intracerebroventricular (i.c.v.) injection than on subcutaneous (s.c.) injection to evoke the same attenuation of the behavior[22]. To investigate whether vasopressin was physiologically involved in the acquisition of heroin self-administration, antiserum against vasopressin was injected i.c.v. and the rats subsequently tested for self-administration. It appeared that in animals treated thus the behavior was markedly stimulated as compared to that of controls, indicating a physiological role for vasopressin in this behavior. Antiserum against oxytocin did not influence the acquisition of heroin self-administration[22].

The amount of heroin intake is considered a useful index of the reinforcing efficacy of the reinforcer (heroin injection)[5,23]. Thus, it may be concluded that the reinforcing efficacy of heroin was enhanced by PLG and attenuated by DG-AVP. Furthermore, it may be postulated that rewarding mechanisms triggered by heroin and involved in the acquisition and maintenance of drug seeking behavior, are under the control of neurohypophyseal hormones and their fragments.

NEUROHYPOPHYSEAL PRINCIPLES AND INTRACRANIAL SELF-STIMULATION

Electrical self-administration in animals is widely used to investigate the significance of certain brain structures with respect to reward[24]. This procedure involves placing electrodes in defined brain areas and giving the animals access to a device which, when activated, leads to electrical

stimulation of that particular brain structure. Because of similarities
between drug self-administering and brain self-stimulating behavior, it had
been hypothesized that neural processes which mediate the positively reinforcing characteristics of dependence producing drugs are also involved in self-
stimulation[25,26]. This idea is supported by recent findings that morphine
affected the excitability of neural systems which mediate self-stimulation
[25,27]. Interestingly, this effect of morphine seemed not to be susceptible
to tolerance[26], as may also hold for the reinforcing and subjective effects
of this drug. Thus, self-stimulating behavior may be used to analyse further
the presumed modulating effect of neurohypophyseal principles on rewarding
mechanisms triggered by heroin. Indeed, it was reported that hypothalamic
self-stimulation was enhanced following oxytocin treatment and attenuated
after injection with vasopressin[28]. There is evidence that the reinforcing
activity of various dependence producing drugs and of self-stimulation are
mediated by catecholamine (CA) containing neuronal systems[24]. As
Versteeg et al.[29] have shown that the most prominent effect of PLG on CA
metabolism was observed in the nigro striatal system, electrodes were implanted
in the substantia nigra of male rats. After self-stimulating behavior was
established, the effects of subcutaneously administered PLG (1 μg) were
determined. It appeared that PLG increased and DG-AVP attenuated responding,
especially when threshold currents were used[30]. These data fit rather well
with those obtained with heroin self-administration. Thus, the modulating
action of PLG and DG-AVP on heroin self-administration might be related to
their effectiveness to change the activity of the nigro striatal dopamine
(DA) system. Such a mode of action is readily conceivable for PLG. However,
with respect to DG-AVP. it has been shown that noradrenergic (NA) systems
are especially affected by vasopressin[32]. Furthermore, DG-AVP did not
have the long-term effect on self-stimulation of the substantia nigra, seen
in heroin self-administration. Thus it can not yet be excluded that an
interaction of vasopressin with other brain systems is responsible for its
interference with self-administering behavior.

NEUROHYPOPHYSEAL PRINCIPLES AND DEVELOPMENT OF TOLERANCE AND PHYSICAL
DEPENDENCE

The adaptive changes leading to the development of tolerance and physical
dependence can be regarded as learning or memory processes[32]. This postulate
is supported by the findings that both learning and memory, and the development of tolerance are reliably affected by similar agents or procedures
(e.g. protein synthesis inhibitors, electroconvulsive shock[33,34,35]).

Since vasopressin may be involved in memory processes[17,18], Krivoy et al. [36] studied the influence of DG-AVP on the development of tolerance in mice and found that this neuropeptide facilitated the development of resistance to the analgesic action of morphine. Subsequently, De Wied and Gispen[37] showed that the development of morphine tolerance was delayed in diabetes insipidus rats, which lack the ability to synthesize vasopressin. This impaired development could be restored by treatment with vasopressin and DG-AVP. Recently, it was observed that intracerebroventricular injection with anti-serum against vasopressin inhibited the development of tolerance to the analgesic action of morphine[38]. Both the consolidating and retrieval processes concerned in tolerance development were affected.

There is evidence that the development of tolerance to and physical dependence on morphine may co-vary[32]. The influence of vasopressin and related peptides on the development of physical dependence was studied and both DG-AVP and oxytocin were found to facilitate this development[39,40]. Oxytocin was approximately 5 times more potent than DG-AVP. The activity appeared to reside in the C-terminal part of the molecules, since the covalent ring-structures were inactive and the activity of both PAG (pro-arg-gly) and PLG was comparable to that of the parent hormones. Accordingly, PAG was 5-fold less active than PLG. Subsequent experiments showed that PLG was also active in facilitating the development of tolerance to the analgesic action of i.c.v. injected C-fragment (β-LPH$_{61-91}$)[41].

It is however not known whether the action of PLG on the development of opioid tolerance and physical dependence is related to the above mentioned effect of PLG on the activity of the nigro striatal DA pathway, although evidence has been presented that DA was implicated in the action of morphine [32,42,43]. Furthermore, it is not clear whether a common neural mechanism mediates the action of neurohypophyseal principles on both tolerance and physical dependence. It must be kept in mind that the ultimate degree of tolerance, as measured in the experimental situation, is the result of several neuronal processes[44]. One of these processes could be under the control of vasopressin as was suggested by the data obtained with the diabetes insipidus rats or with normal rats injected with antiserum against vasopressin and other processes could be preferentially affected by PLG.

ACTH NEUROPEPTIDES AND NARCOTIC CUE

The anterior pituitary hormone ACTH and its structural analogues affect brain functions, in particular those concerned with motivation and attention[17]. The latter function may play a critical role in discriminative behavior[45] and thus in evoking the narcotic cue. Since this narcotic cue is used as a model system to explore subjective effects of opioids, experiments were carried out to study the effects of the neuropeptide $ACTH_{4-10}$ in animals trained to discriminate fentanyl from saline[46]. After peptide treatment, there was a transient responding appropriate to the saline condition after fentanyl injection. This effect was selective in that no errors were seen after saline injections. It was also found that $ACTH_{4-10}$ caused up and down shifts in the apparent sensivity of trained rats to the cuing effects of fentanyl. These data suggest that $ACTH_{4-10}$ interfered with the subjective effects of narcotics and, in particular with the attentional mechanisms involved in the discriminative stimulus complex of narcotics. ACTH-like peptides have an affinity for brain opiate binding sites[47], for opiate receptors in the mouse vas deferens and for morphine antibodies[48], and antagonize morphine-induced analgesia in vivo[49]. However, since the response suppression induced by fentanyl appeared to be unaffected by peptide treatment[46], neither a direct agonist, nor a direct antagonist action by $ACTH_{4-10}$ of fentanyl at the receptor level can explain these effects of the neuropeptide in rats trained to evoke the narcotic cue.

DEPENDENCE AND ENDORPHINS

The presence of peptides with opiate-like activity in the pituitary and brain has raised the question of whether these entities are concerned in dependence. These endogenous substances may be involved in the functioning of physiological systems which are also susceptible to narcotic drugs. To test this hypothesis we have studied[50] the relative reinforcing efficacy of C-fragment (β-LPH_{61-91}), Met-enkephalin (β-LPH_{61-65}), and heroin, using an i.c.v. self-administration procedure. We also determined the discriminative stimulus properties of these peptides in rats trained to discriminate fentanyl from saline so as to investigate the narcotic cuing properties of the peptides. In the same procedure as outlined for i.v. self-administration, the rats on heroin (1 µg dissolved in artificial cerebrospinal fluid/ injection) showed i.c.v. self-administering behavior (approximately 16 injec- tions/6 hr). A similar pattern of responding was observed in animals on C-fragment (0.1 µg/injection) with a ceiling level at about 13 injections/ 6 hr. The behavior of the Met-enkephalin group was similar to that of the placebo group (table 1). These data indicated that at the dose levels used, C-fragment, but not Met-enkephalin, had reinforcing properties. The seeming discrepancy between our Met-enkephalin data and those of Belluzi and Stein[51] may be due to the fact that these authors used a Ringer's solution of pH 5.8

8

TABLE 1

PERFORMANCE OF ANIMALS TESTED FOR INTRACEREBROVENTRICULAR
SELF-ADMINISTERING BEHAVIOR ON TEST DAYS 3 - 5.

test substance	dose/injection	number of animals	mean number of self-injections ($+$ SEM)	$p^{1)}$
placebo[2]	2 µl	12	23 $\pm$ 5	
heroin	1 µg	12	50 $\pm$ 7	< 0.01
C-fragment	0.1 µg	9	39 $\pm$ 6	< 0.05
Met-enkephalin	2 µg	8	22 $\pm$ 4	> 0.05

[1] difference from placebo animals (P: level of statistical significance).

[2] artificial cerebrospinal fluid.

as vehicle for the peptide. This vehicle suppresses operant responding, and a peptide-induced counteraction of this suppression may have yielded a false-positive result.

After 5 days of self-administration, the animals were injected with naloxone and their behavior with respect to signs of abstinence was recorded in order to determine the degree of physical dependence. The degree of physical dependence appeared to be very low in animals which had experienced i.c.v. self-injections of heroin or C-fragment and was absent in rats on placebo or on Met-enkephalin[50]. The conclusion reached,that physical dependence did not contribute to the induction of self-administration, was consistent with conclusions from former experiments with heroin[5].

Since the nucleus raphe magnus (NRM) has been implicated in morphine analgesia[52] and the discriminative stimulus and analgesic potency of narcotics correlate very closely[53], the NRM was selected as the intracerebral injection site to establish the narcotic cuing properties of the peptides. All of the 7 animals, trained to discriminate s.c. injected fentanyl from saline, retained their ability to detect the discriminative stimuli associated with fentanyl when this drug was applied to the NRM in a dose of 2 µg. After injection of Met-enkephalin (40 µg) all animals selected the placebo lever, while after C-fragment (2 µg) the drug lever was chosen. These data[50] indicate that C-fragment, but not Met-enkephalin, possesses discriminative stimulus properties similar to those of narcotic drugs. Both the positive reinforcing and the discriminative stimulus properties of C-fragment substantiate the hypothesis that this peptide may exert powerful control on behavior. This action may be mimicked by narcotic drugs thus giving rise to similar internal stimuli which control behavior to such an extent that the functioning of the organism becomes conditional upon these substances. This control over behavior is characteristic for narcotic dependence. Thus, it might be postulated that the disturbances in brain processes, through which C-fragment exerts control over behavior, contribute to the development of drug dependence.

CONCLUDING REMARKS

The studies reviewed here strongly suggest that neuropeptides related to hypothalamic-hypophyseal hormones play a profound role in modulating the action of opioids in the central nervous system. These neuropeptides have been selectively implicated in brain mechanisms concerned with motivational, learning and memory processes[54]. A similar, selective mode of action can be described for the interference of neuropeptides with opioid action. $ACTH_{4-10}$ seems to affect attentional mechanisms involved in the subjective effects of narcotics. Vasopressin analogs attenuate the acquisition of heroin self-administering behavior and in particular the consolidation of this behavior[18]. PLG faciliates the development of tolerance to and physical dependence on opioids, and this may be related to the proposed role of this neuropeptide in retrieval[18]. Last but not least, endorphins, and in particular C-fragment, exert control over behavior in a way which is believed to be characteristic for narcotic dependence. The selective interference of neuropeptides with brain functions is not limited to narcotics as is seen from the modulating action of DG-AVP and PLG on intracranial self-stimulating behavior.

The pituitary-brain neuropeptide systems may contribute to the adaptation of the individual to his environment and it could be postulated that derangements in one or more of these systems lead to a state in which dependence can reliably develop.

REFERENCES

1. Kalant, H.,Engel, J.A., Goldberg, L., Griffiths, R.R., Jaffe, J.H., Krasnegor, N.A., Mello, N.K., Mendelson, J.H., Thompson, J.H. and Van Ree, J.M. (1978) in The Bases of Addiction of Fishman, J., ed. Dahlem Konferenzen, Berlin, pp. 463-496.

2. Schuster C.R. and Thompson, T. (1969), Ann. Rev. Pharmacol. 9, 483-502.

3. Thompson, T. and Pickens, R. (1975) Fed. Proc. 34, 1759-1770.

4. Van Ree, J.M., Slangen, J.L. and De Wied, D. (1974) in Neuropsychopharmacology: Proc. IX Congress of the Collegium Internationale Neuropsychopharmacologium Parijs, July 7-12, 1974, Excerpta Medica Congress Series no. 359, Amsterdam, pp. 231-239.

5. Van Ree, J.M., Slangen, J.L. and De Wied, D. (1978) J. Pharm. Exp. Ther. 204, 547-557.

6. Thompson, T. and Pickens, R. (1969) in Scientific Basis of Drug Dependence of Steinberg, H., ed., Churchill Ltd. London, pp. 177-198.

7. Mello, N.K. and Mendelson, J.H. (1978) in The Bases of Addiction of Fishman, E., ed., Dahlem Konferenzen, Berlin, pp. 133-158.

8. Martin, W.R. and Fraser, H.F. (1961) J. Pharmacol. Exp. Ther. 133, 388-399.

9. Fraser, H.F., Van Horn, G.D., Martin, W.R., Wolbach, A.B. and Isbell, H., (1961) J. Pharmacol. Exp. Ther. 133, 371-387.

10. Fraser, H.F. and Isbell, H. (1961) Bull. Narc. 13, 29-43.

11. Colpaert, F.C. (1977) Life Sci. 20, 1097-1108.

12. Colpaert, F.C., Lal, H., Niemegeers, C.J.E. and Janssen, P.S.J. (1975) Life Sci. 16, 705-716.

13. Shannon, H.E. and Holtzmann, S.G. (1976) J. Pharmacol. Exp. Ther. 198, 54-65.

14. Colpaert, F.C.,Niemegeers, C.J.E., Lal, H., and Janssen, P.S.J. (1976) Life Sci. 16, 705-716.

15. Colpaert, F.C., Niemegeers, C.J.E. and Janssen, P.A.J. (1976) J. Pharmacol. Exp. Ther. 197, 180-187.

16. Shannon, H.E. and Holtzmann, S.G. (1977) J. Pharmacol. Exp. Ther. 201, 55-66.

17. De Wied, D. (1977) Life Sci. 20, 195-204.

18. Van Ree, J.M., Bohus, B., Versteeg, D.H., De Wied, D. (1978) Biochem. Pharm. (in press)

19. Oliveros, J.C., Jandali, M.K., Timsit-Berthier, M., Remy, R., Benghezal, A., Audibert, A., Moeglen, J.M. (1978) The Lancet, January 7, 42.

20. Legros, J.J., Gilot, P., Seron, X, Claessens, J., Adam, A., Moeglen, J.M. Audibert, A. and Berchier, P. (1978) The Lancet, January 7, 41-42.

21. Van Ree, J.M. and De Wied, D. (1977) Europ. J. Pharmacol. 43, 199-202.

22. Van Ree, J.M. and De Wied, D. (1977) Life Sci. 21, 315-320.

23. Harrigan, S.E. and Downs, D.A. (1978) Life Sci. 22, 619-624.

24. Brain Stimulation Reward of Wauguier, A., and Eolls, E.T., eds. (1976) North Holland/American Elsevier.

25. Maroli, A.N., Tsang, W.K. and Stutz, R.M. (1978) Pharmacol. Biochem. & Behav. 8, 119-123.

26. Esposito, R. and Kornetsky, C. (1977) Science 195, 189-191.

27. Marcus, R. and Kornetsky, C. (1974) Psychopharmacol. 38, 1-13.

28. Schwarzberg, H., Hartmann, G., Kovacs, G.L. and Telegdy, G. (1976) Acta Physiol. Acad. Scient. Hung. 47, 127-131.

29. Versteeg, D.H.G., Tanaka, M., De Kloet, E.R.,Van Ree, J.M. and De Wied, D. (1978) Brain Res. 143, 561-566.

30. Dorsa, D. and Van Ree, J.M. (1978) in preparation.

31. Tanaka, M., De Kloet, E.R., De Wied, D. and Versteeg, D.H.G. (1977) Life Sci. 20, 1799-1808.

32. Clouet, D.H. and Iwatsubo, K. (1975) in Annual Review of Pharmacology of Elliott, H.W., George, R., and Okun, R., eds., Annual Review Inc. Palo Alto, Vol. 15, pp. 49-71.

33. Jarvik, M.E. (1972) Ann. Rev. Psychol. 23, 457-486.

34. Cox, B.M. and Osman, O.H. (1970) Brit. J. Pharmacol. 38, 157-170.

35. Kesner, R.P., Priano, D.J. and DeWitt, J.R. (1976) Science 194, 1079-1081.

36. Krivoy, W.A., Zimmermann, E. and Lande, S. (1974) Proc. Natl. Acad. Sci. USA 71, 1852-1856.

37. De Wied, D. and Gispen, W.H. (1976) Psychopharmacol. 46, 27-29.

38. Van Wimersma Greidanus, Tjon Kon Fat-Bronstein, H. and Van Ree, J.M. (1978) This Volume.

39. Van Ree, J.M. and De Wied, D. (1976) Life Sci. 1331-1340.

40. Van Ree, J.M. and De Wied, D. (1977) Psychoneuroendocrinol. 2, 35-41.

41. Van Ree, J.M., De Wied, D., Bradbury, A.F., Hulme, E.C., Smyth, D.G. and Snell, C.R. (1976) Nature 264, 792-794.

42. Takemori, A.E. (1975) Biochem. Pharmacol. 24, 2121-2126.

43. Lal, H. (1973) Life Sci. 17, 483-496.

44. Kalant, H. (1978) in The Bases of Addiction of Fishman, J., ed., Dahlem Konferenzen, Berlin, pp. 199-220.

45. Sutherland, N.S. and Mackintosh, N.J. (1971) Mechanisms of Animal Discrimination Learning, Academic Press, New York, p. 559

46. Colpaert, F.C., Niemegeers, C.J.E., Janssen, P.A.J., Van Ree, J.M. and De Wied, D. (1978) Psychoneuroendocrinol. in press.

47. Terenius, L., Gispen, W.H. and De Wied, D. (1975) Eur. J. Pharmacol. 33, 395-399.

48. Plomp, G.J.J. and Van Ree, J.M. (1978) Brit. J. Pharmacol. in press.

49. Gispen, W.H., Buitelaar, J., Wiegant, V.M., Terenius, T. and De Wied, D. (1976) Eur. J. Pharmacol. 39, 393-397.

50. Van Ree, J.M., Smyth, D.G. and Colpaert, F. (1978) submitted for publication

51. Belluzzi, J.D. and Stein, L. (1977) Nature 266, 556-558.

52. Basbaum, A.J., Marley, N.J.E., O'Keefe, J. and Clantan, C.H. (1977) Pain 3, 43-56.

53. Colpaert, F.C., Niemegeers, C.J.E. and Janssen, P.A.J. (1976) J. Pharm. Pharmacol. 28, 183-187.

54. De Wied, D. (1978) This Volume.

Characteristics and Function of Opioids, editors Van Ree and Terenius
© *1978 Elsevier/North-Holland Biomedical Press*

MULTIPLE MECHANISMS IN OPIATE TOLERANCE

BRIAN M. COX

Addiction Research Foundation, 701 Welch Road, Palo Alto, California 94304 U.S.A.

ABSTRACT

Many factors contribute to opiate tolerance. In this review, the characteristics of cellular tolerance in vivo and in vitro are discussed. Two phases are apparent. One component, apparently dependent on the presence of the tolerance inducing drug, decays rapidly after drug withdrawal. A second component long outlasts the presence of the drug, and is associated with changes in the properties of opiate sensitive neurons that are independent of the actions of opiate drugs. In neither phase is there evidence of a change in the binding properties of the opiate receptor for agonists.

INTRODUCTION

It is clear that there are many components of the phenomenon of tolerance to opiate drugs. I intend to concentrate on aspects that are commonly described as cellular tolerance; that is, tolerance manifest as a reduced sensitivity of neurons to a defined concentration of opiate drug. Although some minor changes in metabolism and distribution of drug may occur during chronic opiate administration, these are not of sufficient magnitude to account for the extent of tolerance that is achieved[1,2]. Drug-test interactions and associated environmental cues also contribute to opiate tolerance when behavioral responses of animals are measured. Behavioral tolerance may make a significant contribution to the total reduction in sensitivity to opiate drugs when low doses of drug are administered infrequently. Thus, Siegel[3] has provided evidence for a contribution by behavioral factors to the tolerance to morphine analgesia induced by a daily injection of 5 mg/kg morphine in rats, although the precise mechanisms responsible for this effect are in dispute[4,5].

OPIATE TOLERANCE IN VIVO

When opiate sensitive neurons are exposed to receptor saturating concentrations of opiate drug for periods of a few hours or more, the opiate becomes less effective. Behavioral adaptation is not essential to this phenomenon since the degree of tolerance is not reduced by minimizing exposure to the test apparatus[6]. A number of studies suggest that cellular tolerance is not mediated by a unitary mechanism. In experiments in which the rate of recovery of opiate analgesia in rats or mice was monitored, the time course of return of opiate sensitivity after termination of sustained exposure to high tolerance inducing doses of morphine indicated a biphasic recovery[7]. Over the first two days of the recovery period the analgesic response to a standard morphine treatment increased rapidly, but initial sensitivity did not return completely in this time. Further recovery occured much more slowly, with a half-time of about two weeks. During the first phase of the recovery process in rats, the dose-response curve for morphine analgesia showed a lower slope than that obtained with previously untreated animals. Other studies have documented this change in dose-response curve slope in more detail, demonstrating that the maximum analgesic response to opiate drug is depressed at this time[8,9]. This initial phase of tolerance lasts about two days in rats[7]. It is of interest that Tilson et al.[10] found significant hyperalgesia in rats from 12 to 36 hours after withdrawal of morphine, with return to normal threshold within 48 hours, when measuring reaction threshold by a modified flinch-jump technique. During the second phase of tolerance recovery, the morphine dose-response curve for analgesia is parallel to the curve obtained from control animals, but shifted to the right[7].

The biphasic nature of the recovery process is also apparent in studies of naloxone precipitated withdrawal jumping in morphine dependent mice. The ability of naloxone to induce withdrawal jumping decays rapidly within one or two days of opiate withdrawal[7,11,12]. However, sensitivity to naloxone induced jumping can be reinitiated in these animals by administration of a priming dose of morphine 0.5 to 2 hours prior to injection of the naloxone[12]. The time course for loss of sensitivity to naloxone parallels very closely the recovery of the analgesic response; the ability of naloxone to induce jumping in the absence of a priming dose of morphine declines within two days, while naloxone jumping after morphine priming was still detectable one month later. The half-life for loss of this effect was again about two weeks[12]. Two aspects of opiate tolerance with differing time courses are also seen in tolerance to morphine induced hyperthermia[13].

A biphasic recovery pattern is not seen with all actions of opiate drugs, however. Tolerance to the increase in locomotor activity induced by morphine in mice ("running fit") decays rapidly; after two days of recovery, opiates are as effective in inducing running as in previously untreated animals[14]. A similar rapid tolerance recovery is seen in the isolated mouse vas deferens preparation (see below). Thus, it seems likely that the characteristics of tolerance resulting from prolonged exposure to opiate agonists are in part dependent on the properties of the neural substrate or particular subclass of opiate receptor implicated in each effect.

OPIATE TOLERANCE IN ISOLATED TISSUES

Opiate tolerance can be studied in isolated tissues. Ileum preparations from morphine pretreated guinea pigs show reduced sensitivity to opiate drugs[15]. Again, two separate processes can be demonstrated. Schulz and Herz[16] found that if ileum preparations from pretreated guinea pigs were maintained in solutions containing morphine at a concentration similar to that in plasma in vivo immediately before sacrifice, a very high degree of tolerance was apparent. Exposure to naloxone induced a profound contracture followed by a series of waves of spasmogenic activity[16,17]. We have examined the dose-response curve for normorphine under these conditions (Fig 1). As in the intact animal, the maximum inhibition attainable by opiates is depressed in the maintained presence of opiate drug.

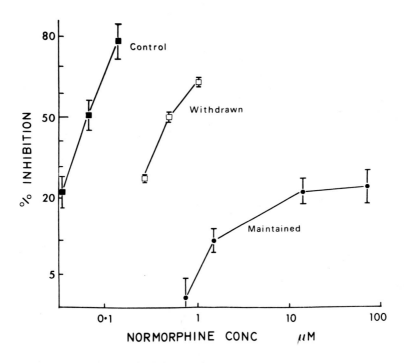

Fig. 1. Two aspects of opiate tolerance in isolated guinea pig ileum. Four ileum preparations from a morphine pretreated guinea pig were kept in Krebs solution containing normorphine 140 nM during preparation and for the initial part of the experiment (maintained condition). The tissues were stimulated with 80 V, 0.25 ms, 0.1 Hz square wave pulses, and inhibition of contractions induced by additional concentrations of normorphine was measured. The bathing fluid was then changed to opiate free Krebs, and after 2 hours of repeated washing, sensitivity to normorphine was re-examined (withdrawan condition). A normorphine dose-response curve in tissues from an untreated guinea pig (control) is included for comparison. Tension (above resting 1 g tension) induced by electrical stimulation was: control, 1.31 ± 0.23 g (mean ± s.e.m.); morphine pretreated preparations, maintained condition 1.11±0.24 g, withdrawn condition, 1.04±0.23 g. Ordinate presents (on a probit scale) the mean % inhibition (± s.e.m.) of the electrically stimulated increase in tension, for each concentration of normorphine.

When the opiate drug was washed from the tissue, tolerance decayed rapidly until a stable state was reached in which the preparation remained three to ten fold less sensitive to inhibition by opiates than untreated tissues[15,18]. There was now no evidence of a reduction in the maximum response. At this time, administration of naloxone did not induce a contracture[18], unless the tissue was again temporarily exposed to opiate drug[16].

Tolerance can also be induced in guinea pig ileum by prolonged exposure to opiate agonists in vitro[19,20]. The characteristics of this effect have not yet been completely analysed, but the phemonenon decays fairly rapidly[19], maximum opiate effects are much reduced[20], and naloxone provokes an acute withdrawal reaction[20]. Thus, in vitro tolerance

TABLE 1

EFFECT OF MORPHINE PRETREATMENT ON OPIATE SENSITIVITY OF ISOLATED MOUSE VAS DEFERENS

Pretreatment[a]	N[b]	IC_{50}(nM) (means s.e.m.)[c]	
		Normorphine	Leu[5]-enkephalin
None (controls)	20	581 ± 103	17.9 ± 3.9
Morphine, 1 pellet for 3 days	8	625 ± 174	12.9 ± 3.4
Morphine, 3 pellets for 5 days	4	413 ± 110	13.1 ± 1.9
Morphine, 3 pellets for 5 days, vas maintained in 500 nM normorphine	8	2419 ± 475[e]	23.7 ± 3.9

a Each morphine pellet contained 75 mg morphine base. When 3 pellets were used, 1 pellet was implanted s.c. on day 1, and 2 more on day 3.

b Number of preparations. Cox Standard mice, 30 - 42 g were used. Tissues were kept in Mg^{++}-free Krebs, except where indicated, under a 200 mg resting tension.

c Concentration of opioid reducing by 50% the response of the tissue to 80 V, 2 ms, 0.1 Hz stimuli, estimated from dose-response curves employing at least 4 concentrations of each opioid.

d Increase in tension induced by stimulation in these tissues was not significantly different from increase in control tissues.

e Significantly different from control value, $p < 0.01$.

shows many of the features of the initial phase of tolerance apparent in ileum preparations from morphine pretreated guinea pigs.

In the isolated mouse vas deferens preparation, tolerance induced by implantation of a morphine pellet in the mouse, declines rapidly and completely when the tissue is washed a few times, although significant tolerance is apparent when tissues from morphine pretreated mice are maintained in opiate containing solution[21]. Thus in this tissue, only one component of tolerance is apparent (Table 1).

The similarities and multiphasic character of opiate tolerance in vivo and in isolated tissues suggests that similar mechanisms are implicated. The features of each component of tolerance can be summarized as follows:

(1) One component, which for convenience I will call Type I tolerance, is associated with a depression of the maximum response to opiate drugs. This component decays rapidly, the decay apparently being associated with the removal of the tolerance inducing drug. Under this condition, opiate antagonists usually provoke acute withdrawal reactions.

(2) A second component, Type II tolerance, becomes apparent after withdrawal of the tolerance inducing drug, in some situations. The opiate dose-response curve is shifted to the right relative to control conditions but there is no depression of the maximum response. Antagonists do not provoke a withdrawal reaction unless opiate agonist is readministered. Type II tolerance decays slowly, with a half-life of about two weeks in vivo.

RECEPTOR MECHANISMS IN OPIATE TOLERANCE

The rapid decay of Type I tolerance, apparently related to the removal of opiate agonist from the system, together with the depression of the maximum response, suggest that the process is in some way akin to the phenomenon of receptor desensitization that occurs when a number of neurotransmitter or hormone receptors are exposed to agonists at high concentration for long periods of time. Desensitization has been most extensively studied in neurons at the cholinergic nicotinic receptor[22,23] and at the β-adrenocep-tor[24,25] although many other substances including insulin[26], glucagon[27], gonadotrophin[28], prolactin[29], prostaglandins[30], and muscarinic receptor agonists[31] produce similar effects. A characteristic feature of the desensitized state is a reduction in the availability of receptor sites for newly applied agonist ligands[23,25]. It is proposed that prolonged exposure to high concentration of agonist results in a transformation of agonist-receptor compleses from a functionally active state to an inactive conformation with much increased agonist affinity[25]. In any system where there is not a large excess of receptors, a change of this type will both reduce the number of functional receptors available to agonists and reduce the maximum attainable response. In some systems, however, loss of functional receptor sites does not provide a complete explanation for the reduced effectiveness of the activating ligand[27].

It is of interest to consider the possible role of receptor desensitization in opiate tolerance. If the mechanisms that apparently contribute to the reduced effectiveness of, for example, norepinephrine at β-adrenoceptors, are also relevant to opiate receptors, there should be a reduced availability of opiate receptors to newly applied labelled ligands in tolerant tissues. In general, however, no change in receptor binding characteristics has been observed in the tolerant state[32,33]. It could be argued that the washing procedures necessary for the removal of unbound morphine prior to the measurement of receptor availability in these studies also allowed the desensitized receptors to revert to their normal state (although washing of desensitized β-adrenoceptors in frog erythrocytes does not cause their immediate reversion to their initial state[25]).

We have therefore looked for evidence of opiate receptor conformational change in the tolerant state by methods which do not require repeated washing for removal of unbound drug. If there is an increase in receptor affinity for the tolerance inducing ligand, the rate of washout of morphine from brain membranes from morphine tolerant animals maintained in morphine solution should be slower than the rate of removal of morphine from control brain membranes briefly exposed to the same concentration. However, we could not detect such a change (unpublished observations). A second approach was to determine the sensitivity of opiate receptors in brain membranes from untreated guinea pigs briefly exposed to morphine, and in morphine pretreated guinea pig brain membranes maintained in morphine solution, to receptor degrading agents such as N-ethylmaleimide[34] and trypsin[35]. Again, no effect of the pretreatment on the sensitivity of the receptor to the perturbing agents was observed (unpublished results). Thus, there is as yet no evidence of a conformational change in the receptor in opiate tolerance.

However, a specific role for the receptor in Type I tolerance is suggested by some experiments in mouse vas deferens. Lord et al.[36] have proposed that two different subpopulations of opiate receptor are present in this tissue: δ-receptors, with high affinity for enkephalins (particularly Leu[5]-enkephalin) but relatively low affinity for alkaloid opiates such as morphine and naloxone; and μ-receptors, with much higher relative affinity for alkaloid opiates. The existence of these two subclasses of receptor in the mouse vas is supported by the observation that the apparent ratio of δ- to μ-receptors is not constant in different strains of mice; there appear to be few μ-receptors in C57/BL mice[37]. When tolerance was induced by morphine pretreatment of vasa subsequently maintained in normorphine solution, greater than four-fold tolerance to normorphine was apparent (the ratio of normorphine IC_{50}s in tolerant and control preparations was 4.2), but there was only a 40% increase in the Leu[5]-enkephalin IC_{50} (Table 1). It seems probable (although it has not yet been demonstrated) that the effects of activation of the two types of opiate receptor are similar in this preparation. The final result of activation of each type of receptor, depression of electrically stimulated contractions, is identical. Nevertheless, the extent of tolerance generated is related to the class of receptor activated. Some role for modified receptor function in this type of tolerance is therefore indicated. It should be noted, however, that Type I tolerance in this tissue is atypical in that depression of the maximum response does not occur, and naloxone does not provoke a contracture of the tissue, as seen in guinea pig ileum. (It is likely that changes in neuronal sensitivity associated with Type II tolerance are essential for the naloxone precipitated reaction.)

There is clear evidence that the opiate ligand binding properties of the receptor are not changed in Type II tolerance. Klee and Streaty[32] and Höllt et al[33] found no difference in the binding of ^{3}H-labelled opiates to well washed membranes from the brains of morphine tolerant and dependent rats relative to control animals. In isolated guinea pig ileum preparations where opiate binding and effect (inhibition of transmitter release) can be measured in the same tissue, no change in receptor affinity or number of receptors could be detected in morphine tolerant preparations[18]. Thus the reduced effectiveness of opiates in Type II tolerance is not a consequence of reduced ligand binding to the receptor.

NEURONAL SENSITIVITY CHANGES IN TOLERANCE

Accumulating evidence indicates that opiate tolerance is associated with changes in neuronal properties that can be demonstrated without the use of opiate drugs. Again, the guinea pig ileum has proved a useful experimental model. Schulz and Goldstein[38] showed that washed tolerant ileum preparations were supersensitive to stimulation by 5-hydroxytryptamine (5HT). Subsequent studies have demonstrated that the supersensitivity is not specific for 5HT but also seen with other neuronal stimulants such as prostaglandin E_1[39] and electrical stimulation[40,41]. The response of the muscle fibers to acetylcholine is not changed[15,18]. Concurrently, the tissue is subsensitive to agents depressing neuronal activity such as norepinephrine, dopamine[15], and clonidine[42]. Functionally, the observed changes in neuronal properties tend to compensate for the depression in transmitter release induced by the opiate drug, thus apparently promoting the restoration of normal function. Indirect evidence from in vivo experiments also implies changes in neuronal sensitivity to neurotransmitters in opiate tolerant dependent animals[43,44,45].

The mechanism by which supersensitivity to neuronal stimulants is achieved has not been elucidated completely. In tolerant, withdrawn ileum the increase in tension induced by electrical stimulation is greater than in non-tolerant tissues (Table 2). Since there is no change in the response of the muscle to acetylcholine[18], it is likely that a greater quantity of acetylcholine is released by each stimulus in tolerant preparations. Conceivably, such an effect might result if the neurons of the tolerant tissue maintained a lower membrane potential than neurons in untreated preparations. The increased sensitivity to stimulants, and reduced effectiveness of depressants would be explained. However, no change in threshold voltage for electrical stimulation could be detected in our experiments (Table 2).

TABLE 2

CHARACTERISTICS OF TOLERANCE IN ISOLATED GUINEA PIG ILEUM PREPARATIONS

Pretreatment[a]	Normorphine IC_{50}[b]	Total Response[c]		Opiate Insensitive Response[d]	
		Maximum Tension (g)	Threshold Voltage (V)	Maximum Tension (g)	Threshold Voltage (V)
None (controls)	235 ± 22	1.6 ± 0.2	8.5 ± 0.8	0.9 ± 0.1	14.8 ± 0.8
Morphine	679 ± 65[e]	3.2 ± 0.2[e]	8.5 ± 0.8	1.1 ± 0.2	16.1 ± 1.1

a   Morphine pretreated guinea pigs were implanted with 5 morphine pellets (each containing 75 mg morphine base) s.c., 3 days before the ileum was removed for estimation of opiate sensitivity. Tissues were mounted in Krebs solution with no added opiate, at 37^0, under 1 g resting tension.

b   Concentration giving 50% inhibiiton of contractions stimulated by 80 V, 0.25 ms, 0.1 Hz square wave pulses, estimated from dose-response curves with at least 4 concentrations of drug in each preparation. Mean values± s.e.m. from 20 control preparations and 28 morphine pretreated preparations.

c   Determined from stimulus voltage - response curves[41] in 12 preparations from each treatment group. All tissues were between 60 and 72 mm long under 1 g resting tension. Threshold voltage was arbitrarily defined as the stimulus voltage increasing the tension above resting tension by 1% of the maximum increase.

d   The opiate insensitive component of the response is the residual response of the tissue occuring in the presence of 1 μM or more normorphine (see text).

e   Significantly different from control values, p < 0.01.

An alternative mechanism perhaps related to the change in neuronal sensitivity may be an increase in the activity of adenylate cyclase in opiate sensitive neurons. Sharma et al.[46] have shown that prolonged exposure of neuroblastoma X glioma hybrid cells in culture to opiate agonists results in an increase in activity of this enzyme, with a concomitant reduction in sensitivity to opiates. It is of interest that more than one process appeared to be involved in the increase in adenylate cyclase activity; the increase could only partially be prevented by inhibition of protein synthesis, and only partially reversed by regulatory ligands such as NaF or a guanosine nucleotide analogue.

In the guinea pig ileum two components of the response to low frequency electrical stimulation can be demonstrated[41]. In both normal and morphine pretreated tissues, part of the response to electrical stimulation is not inhibited by high concentrations of opiate. This component can be blocked by tetrodotoxin or atropine[41], suggesting that it results from the stimulation of cholinergic neurons without functional opiate receptors. This part of the response of the tissue to electrical stimulation is not altered in the tolerant state (Table 2). Thus the changes in neuronal properties associated with opiate tolerance appear to be limited to neurons directly inhibited by opiates, at least in guinea pig myenteric plexus.

ACKNOWLEDGEMENTS

I am grateful to Mrs. P. Lowery for technical assistance, to Dr. Frances Leslie for advice on the mouse vas preparation, and to Drs. Avram Goldstein, and C. E. Dunlap III for comments on the manuscript. The work reported from this laboratory was supported by National Institute on Drug Abuse Grant DA-1199.

REFERENCES

1. Richter, J. A., and Goldstein, A. (1970) Proc. Nat. Acad. Sci. (USA), 66, 944-951.
2. Goldstein, A., Judson, B. A., and Sheehan, P. (1973) Brit. J. Pharmacol., 47, 138-140.
3. Siegel, S. (1976) Science, 193, 323-325.
4. Hayes, R. L., and Mayer, D. J. (1978) Science, 200, 343-344.
5. Siegel, S. (1978) Science, 200, 344-345.
6. Cox, B. M., Ginsburg, M., and Osman, O. H. (1968) Brit. J. Pharmacol., 33, 345-256.
7. Cox, B. M., Ginsburg, M., and Willis, J. (1975) Brit. J. Pharmacol., 53, 383-391.
8. Theiss, P., Papeschi, R., and Herz, A. (1975) Eur. J. Pharmacol., 34, 263-271.
9. Mucha, R. F., Niesink, R., and Kalant, H. (1978) Life Sci., (In press).
10. Tilson, H. A., Rech, R. H., and Stolman, S. (1973) Psychopharmacologia, 28, 287-300.
11. Cheney, D. L., and Goldstein, A. (1971) Nature, 232, 477-478.
12. Brase, D. A., Iwamoto, E. T., Loh, H. H., and Way, E. L. (1976) J. Pharmacol. Exp. Ther., 197, 317-325.

13. Rosenfeld, G. C. and Burks, T. F. (1977) J. Pharmacol. Exp. Ther., 202, 654-659.

14. Goldstein, A., and Sheehan, P. (1969) J. Pharmacol. Exp. Ther., 169, 175-184.

15. Goldstein, A., and Schulz, R. (1973) Brit. J. Pharmacol., 48, 655-666.

16. Schulz, R., and Herz, A. (1976) Life Sci., 19, 1117-1128.

17. Ehrenpreis, A., Greenberg, J., and Comaty, J. C. (1975) Life Sci., 17, 49-54.

18. Cox, B. M., and Padhya, R. (1977) Brit. J. Pharmacol., 61, 271-278.

19. Hammond, M. D., Schneider, C., and Collier, H. O. J. (1976) in Opiates and Endogenous Opioid Peptides, North-Holland, Amsterdam, pp. 169-176.

20. North, R. A., and Karras, P. J. (1978) Nature, 272, 73-80.

21. Waterfield, A. A., Hughes, J., and Kosterlitz, H. W. (1976) Nature, 260, 624-625.

22. Magazanik, L. G., and Vyskocil, F. (1973) in Drug Receptors, Univ. Park Press, Baltimore, pp. 105-119.

23. Heidmann, T., and Changeux, J.-P., (1978) Ann. Rev. Biochem., 47 (in press).

24. Mickey, J. V., Tate, R., Mullikin, D., and Lefkowitz, R. J. (1976) Mol. Pharmacol., 12, 409-419.

25. Mukherjee, C., and Lefkowitz, R. J. (1977) Mol. Pharmacol., 13, 291-303.

26. Gavin, J. R., Roth, J., Neville, D. M., and Buell, D. N. (1974) Proc. Nat. Acad. Sci. U.S.A., 71, 84-88.

27. Soman, V., and Felig, P. (1978) Nature, 272, 829-831.

28. Conti, M., Harwood, J. P., Hsueh, A. J. W., Dufau, M. L., and Catt, K. J. (1976) J. Biol. Chem., 251, 7729-7731.

29. Posner, B. I., Kelley, P. A., and Friesen, H. G. (1975) Science, 188, 57-59.

30. Raff, M. (1976) Nature, 259, 265-266.

31. Richelson, E. (1978) Nature, 272, 366-368.

32. Klee, W. A., and Streaty, R. A. (1974) Nature, 248, 61-63.

33. Höllt, V., Dum, J., Bläsig, J., Schubert, P., and Herz, A. (1975) Life Sci., 16, 1823 1828.

34. Simon, E. J., and Groth, J. (1975) Proc. Nat. Acad. Sci. U.S.A., 72, 2404-2407.

35. Pasternak, G. W., and Snyder, S. H. (1975) Mol. Pharmacol. 11, 478-484.

36. Lord, J. A. H., Waterfield, A. A., Hughes, J., and Kosterlitz, H. W. (1977) Nature, 267, 495-499.

37. Waterfield, A. A., Lord, J. A. H., Hughes, J., and Kosterlitz, H. W. (1978) Eur. J. Pharmacol., 47, 249-250.

38. Schulz, R., and Goldstein, A. (1973) Nature, 244, 168-170.

39. Schulz, R., and Cartwright, C. (1976) Arch. Pharmacol., 294, 257-260.

40. Schulz, R., and Cartwright, C. (1974) J. Pharmacol. Exp. Ther., 190, 420-430.

41. Cox, B. M. (1978) Brit. J. Pharmacol., 62, 387.

42. Hughes, J., Kosterlitz, H. W., Robson, L. E., and Waterfield, A. A. (1978) Brit. J. Pharmacol., 62, 388.

43. Vasquez, B. J., Overstreet, D. H., and Russel, R. W. (1974) Psychopharmacologia, 38, 287-302.
44. Lal, H. (1975) Life Sci., 17, 483-496.
45. Schulz, R., and Herz, A. (1977) Arch. Pharmacol., 299, 95-99.
46. Sharma, S. H., Klee, W. A., and Nirenberg, M. (1977) Proc. Nat. Acad. Sci. USA, 74, 3365-3369.

Characteristics and Function of Opioids, editors Van Ree and Terenius
© *1978 Elsevier/North-Holland Biomedical Press*

TOLERANCE AND DEPENDENCE IN VITRO

R ALAN NORTH and PETER J KARRAS
Neurophysiology Laboratory, Department of Pharmacology, Loyola University
Stritch School of Medicine, Maywood, Illinois 60153 (U.S.A.)

INTRODUCTION

When an animal is chronically exposed to morphine, tolerance develops to
many of the acute actions of the drug. If the morphine is withdrawn, a
characteristic withdrawal syndrome occurs in which many of the clinical mani-
festations are in a direction which opposes those seen when morphine is given
acutely to the naive animal. Because an injection of naloxone can precipitate an even more florid syndrome, this is often termed precipitated abstinence. The experiments reviewed here indicate that the tolerance can be
demonstrated in an isolated tissue removed from an animal so treated, and
that the tissues will exhibit a prominent effect when exposed in vitro to a
concentration of naloxone similar to the tissue levels required to precipitate abstinence in the whole animal.

The preparations which have been used to investigate opiate tolerance and
dependence in vitro are segments of the ileum of the guinea-pig, the myenteric
plexus/longitudinal muscle strip preparation made from the ileum, and single
neurones within the myenteric ganglia of the ileum. Two techniques of exposure
to opiates have been used. First, in vivo exposure was achieved by implanting
the guinea-pig with morphine-containing pellets, by a single injection of a
sustained release formulation of morphine, or by repeated subcutaneous injections of morphine sulphate. Second, in vitro exposure was made whereby the
ileum was left in contact with a known concentration of opiate for up to 24 h.
In both these cases, the testing in vitro allows a high degree of control over
the measurement of the extent of tolerance and the effects of naloxone.
The second group of experiments, in which the entire exposure to opiates and
the subsequent testing are all carried out in vitro, has a further important
advantage. This is that the effects of the opiates must be a direct action
on the morphine-sensitive neurones within the preparation, and can not be
effects secondary to other actions of opiates in the whole animal such as
elevation of circulating corticosteroid levels[1].

EXPOSURE TO OPIATES IN VIVO

In these experiments the ileum was removed from an animal which had been pretreated with morphine in the manner described and was set up for recording either the contractile response of the muscle or the firing of individual neurones. One experimental circumstance must be clearly defined - namely, whether the tissue is removed from an animal and placed in a normal physiological saline solution, or whether the tissue is removed and placed in a solution which is similar but which also contains morphine in a concentration close to that in the guinea-pig plasma at the time of tissue removal. In the first paradigm, the experiments are performed during a time in which the tissue might be considered to be undergoing withdrawal; the time during which the tissue has been in morphine-free solution will markedly influence the results obtained. In the second paradigm, in which the in vitro solution contains morphine, it might be expected that the changes which were induced in vivo by the morphine would be maintained after the tissue removal. Unfortunately, one does not know the plasma concentration of morphine of the individual animal from which the tissue is removed, and it is necessary to use a concentration in the solution which is near to the average plasma concentration for similarly treated animals.

Changes in the properties of the neurones. Most of the experiments have been carried out in the first circumstance; that is, placing the isolated tissue into a morphine-free solution. Such tissues appear to be more sensitive to electrical stimulation - the tension produced by given stimulation parameters is greater than that found in tissue taken from naive animals[2-4]. This means that the neurones are more excitable (perhaps by virtue of a slight membrane depolarisation), or that the neurones release more acetylcholine for each action potential which invades the nerve terminal, or that the longitudinal muscle has become more sensitive to acetylcholine. The third mechanism may be discounted in view of the numerous reports that the sensitivtiy of the muscle to acetylcholine is not changed in these conditions[4-11]. Increased excitability of myenteric neurones is compatible with the findings that the preparation becomes supersensitive to agents which excite neurones and release acetylcholine (5-hydroxytryptamine (5-HT)[4-7,12], potassium chloride and nicotine[4]) and subsensitive to agents which inhibit the release of acetylcholine (adrenaline, dopamine[6] and noradrenaline[12]).

Similar experiments have been carried out in which the tissue was placed in a solution which contained morphine and in these circumstances also the preparation was supersensitive to 5-HT and prostaglandin E_1[13] and subsensitive to the presynaptic α-receptor agonist clonidine[14]. Because morphine pretreatment leads to changes in the sensitivities to such a wide range of substances (including potassium chloride), it seems likely that the underlying change is relatively non-specific. It may be that the myenteric neurones become slightly depolarised during prolonged exposure to morphine and/or markedly depolarised during 'withdrawal' (see ref. 4), these being the opposite change from the acute action of morphine[15]. This would lead to an apparent increase in sensitivity to substances which depolarise and an apparent subsensitivity to substances which hyperpolarise. On the other hand, it may be that the various agents to which the sensitivity is changed all share a common intra-terminal site of action which is not related directly to membrane excitability but is involved primarily in transmitter release - one candidate for such a site is adenylate cyclase[14]. Further experiments are required to discriminate between these possibilities.

Extracellular recordings from single neurones which have been taken from morphine-dependent animals and placed in normal Krebs solution indicated that the neurones fire at a somewhat higher rate than neurones taken from naive animals[16]; the neurones were also ten times more sensitive to the excitatory effects of 5-HT. Extracellular recordings made from neurones which have been removed from a morphine-dependent animal and placed in a morphine-containing solution showed no obvious changes in their pattern of spontaneous firing[17] except an increase in the proportion of cells which fired spikes in bursts rather than at random intervals (Karras and North, unpublished). The actual firing rate also appeared to be somewhat less in these circumstances than when the neurones were removed from naive animals[17] but this was difficult to quantitate because the rate of firing is to some extent dependent upon the size of the recording electrode and the degree of suction which is applied to it[17-19].

Tolerance. The contractions of tissue which is removed from a morphine-dependent animal and placed in a morphine-free solution are still depressed by morphine and this action is reversed by naloxone. However, the concentrations of morphine which are required to inhibit the contractile response are considerably increased; the preparation can therefore be said to be tolerant. The ratio by which the concentration of morphine must be increased in order to produce a 50% depression of the contractile response has been reported to be 3[20], 4.5[4], 5[8], 7[11], 8-10[21], 9[22] and 18[12]. The wide range of values is presumably attributable to at least two factors. The first is the degree of

tolerance existing in vivo at the time of killing the animal, which depends
on the administration schedule. The degree of tolerance found in vitro
increases from three-fold to seven-fold to nine-fold on the first, third and
sixth days respectively after pellet implantation[11]. The development of tolerance measured in vitro parallels closely in its time course the development
of tolerance to other actions of opiates measured in vivo[6,11]. The second
factor is the time after removal from the animal which elapses before the
degree of tolerance is tested. The time course of the loss of tolerance after
placing the tissue in a morphine-free solution has not been studied systematically, although this information is obviously required to interpret correctly
all of the above studies. It is known that the 12-fold tolerance which is
present at the time of killing the animal (the determination carried out in
the presence of normorphine (200 nM)) is reduced to six-fold when the opiate
has been withdrawn for 3 h[13].

The degree of tolerance has not been precisely reported in those experiments
in which the tissue was placed in a morphine-containing solution; however, it
appears to be at least four-fold[23] or higher[24]. Cross tolerance between morphine and other opiates[23] and enkephalin[24] occurs. When recordings are made
from single neurones in analogous circumstances (that is, when the tissue is
taken from morphine-dependent animals and placed in a morphine-containing
solution), the firing rate is not inhibited by concentrations of morphine
10-30 times higher than those required for maximal inhibition of firing of
neurones taken from naive animals (ref. 17, and Karras and North, unpublished).

The effect of naloxone. The first observation that a narcotic antagonist
caused an effect on tissue from a morphine-dependent animal while having no
effect on the tissue from a naive animal was made using nalorphine in the rat
isolated ileum[25]. The ileum which is removed from a morphine-dependent guinea-
pig shows a marked contracture when it is challenged with a relatively modest
dose of naloxone[2,9,10,26-28]. Frederickson's group have studied this in
detail[9]. The time course of the development of the capacity of the tissue
to sustain a naloxone contracture follows closely the time course of the
development of the capacity of the whole animal to respond to naloxone with
a typical constellation of withdrawal signs. The longer the period of time
during which the animals are exposed to morphine, the greater is the contracture of the ileum elicited by a given dose of naloxone[9,10]. With given conditions of morphine pretreatment, the contracture is greater when a larger dose
of naloxone is used to induce it[9]. The contracture is the result of the

relatively synchronous release of acetylcholine from the neurones which
innervate the longitudinal muscle layer, for it is abolished by tetrodotoxin[9,26]
and atropine[10]. Chronic in vivo treatment with nalorphine does not sensitise
the ileum to naloxone[28] even though the nalorphine itself has a typical acute
morphine-like effect on the ileum of the naive animal[29]. This finding is of
considerable importance for it is evidence that the induction of the changes
necessary for the naloxone contracture ('dependence') can be separated from
the acute agonist effect.

In similar vein, an antibody to morphine which is highly effective in re-
versing the acute depression of the contractile response caused by morphine
was quite ineffective in inducing a contracture when it was applied to tissue
taken from morphine tolerant/dependent animals - even though the same tissue
gave a clear contracture with naloxone[27].

A study of the naloxone contracture has also been made on the strip preparation continuously exposed to normorphine from the time of its removal
from the animal[13,23]. Essentially similar changes were found - the contracture
was blocked by tetrodotoxin and atropine, and its amplitude was dependent on
the dose of naloxone used to induce it. The underlying changes in the neurones
which are responsible for the naloxone contracture apparently fade rapidly when
the agonist is removed, for the ability of naloxone to cause a contracture
declines quickly. Within 1 h after the removal of the normorphine, naloxone
has lost its ability to cause a contracture. Reintroduction of normorphine
or another agonist quite rapidly (within 1 h) reinstates the capacity of the
tissue to respond to naloxone. This contrasts with the situation in the tissue
taken from a naive animal in which the naloxone contracture is initially absent,
but very slowly develops over the first 5 h of incubation with normorphine;
even after 5 h exposure to normorphine in vitro the naloxone contracture amplitude is only about 10% of that evoked in tissue taken from morphine-dependent
animals and maintained in a morphine-containing solution[13,28].

Schulz and Herz supposed from these findings that the actual presence of the
agonist was obligatory for the appearance of the contracture - even though the
underlying changes (which are the basis for the greatly accelerated reinstate-
ment of naloxone's effect upon reincubation with an agonist) persist following
washout of the agonist. They supported this by showing that the ability of
naloxone to cause a contracture was strongly correlated with the half-time for
washing out the drug from the tissue[23]. The half-time of wash-out for the
various drugs was measured directly from the reversal of its effect on the
contractile responses of the naive preparation. For example, when tissue was

taken from a morphine-dependent animal and placed in a solution containing buprenorphine, the buprenorphine maintained a state of cross-tolerance to morphine; but naloxone gave no contracture. This correlated with the extremely long wash-out time for buprenorphine (several hours). Although the correlation is impressive between the wash-out time of an agonist and its propensity to maintain a state in which naloxone can induce a contracture, the quantitative agreement is not perfect. Normorphine washes from the tissue within 5 min (as shown by the complete recovery of the contractile response) - yet it takes 1 h of washing the tolerant/dependent preparation before the ability of naloxone to induce a contracture is completely lost.

Analogous studies have been made at the single neurone level. Extracellular recordings were made from myenteric neurones which had been taken from a morphine pretreated guinea-pig and then placed in a morphine-containing Krebs solution[17]. Exposure to naloxone caused a dramatic excitation of these neurones. Rates of discharge of action potentials were observed which were never seen in neurones from naive animals. The capacity of naloxone to cause this excitation was shared by the (-) but not the (+) isomer of the enantiomeric antagonists 5,9α-diethyl-2-(3-furylmethyl)-2'-hydroxy-6,7-benzomorphan; nor was it shared by (+)-naloxone (Karras and North, unpublished). Of particular interest was the observation that a single short exposure (2 min) to naloxone sometimes caused a long-lasting (20-30 min) excitation of the neurones; a similar observation has been made with the contractile response in some preparations[13].

Changes in receptors. Receptor affinity for naloxone can be determined in the guinea-pig ileum by the pA_2 method, and this has been reported to be decreased about ten-fold in tissue taken from morphine-pretreated guinea-pigs[21]. It is difficult to assess the real validity of these findings to the morphine-dependent state, for the introduction of naloxone in order to measure the pA_2 immediately precipitates a state of withdrawal. The pA_2 method depends heavily on the assumption that a given receptor occupancy always produces the same effect independent of the presence of the antagonist - this may be a substantial assumption in the opiate tolerant/dependent state. Direct measurements of [^{3}H]-etorphine binding indicate that there is no change in receptor affinity or number in the myenteric plexus strips made from morphine-dependent guinea-pigs and repeatedly washed in a morphine-free solution[30].

EXPOSURE TO OPIATES IN VITRO

The guinea-pig ileum, or preparations made therefrom, has been exposed to opiates in vitro for periods of up to 24 h. It is convenient to separate the experiments using shorter periods of exposure (less than 2 h) from those using longer periods of exposure (more than 2 h); the distinction is arbitrary.

Short exposures

Tachyphylaxis or 'acute tolerance'. In 1957 Paton described his experiments on the action of morphine on the guinea-pig isolated ileum. He found that the sensitivity of the preparation to the inhibitory effects of morphine diminished with repeated large doses, or with smaller doses repeated at intervals of less than 15 min. He called this 'acute tolerance'[31]. The observations have been confirmed by others[32-34] and have led to the widespread use of normorphine, which shows less tachyphylaxis[35]. The 'acute tolerance' is induced only by high concentrations of opiates and is most probably related to their antichol-inesterase properties[33].

When a lower concentration of morphine is left in contact with the tissue for longer periods of time (90 min), the depression of the contractile response slowly disappears[36,37]. However, the inhibition of the electrically evoked acetylcholine output remains throughout the 90 min period. It therefore follows that the muscle has increased its sensitivity to the reduced amount of acetylcholine, and this was shown directly. The authors concluded that this supersensitivity of the smooth muscle represented a form of denervation super-sensitivity following the acute and maintained reduction of acetylcholine re-lease. If this is the case, then it developed much more rapidly than is nor-mally seen in smooth muscle[38].

The effect of naloxone. Short exposures (up to 1 h) to morphine in vitro are generally insufficient to produce any contracture when naloxone is added to the incubation solution. As the time of exposure is increased, the ability of naloxone to cause a contracture rises (see below). Similarly, when the firing of a single myenteric neurone is depressed by morphine for as much as 1 h, the introduction of naloxone does not cause a marked increase in firing rate but only a simple reversal of the depression to the original firing rate (Karras and North, unpublished). Villareal has found that naloxone in higher concentrations (up to 3 μM) sometimes produces a very weak contracture in tissue taken from naive animals after only 5 min in morphine, but like others found that this effect was enormously enhanced if the tissue was taken from a dependent animal[28]. Levorphanol appears to have a greater capacity than mor-phine to induce the changes necessary for the expression of the naloxone con-tracture, for incubation with levorphanol for as little as 15 min will enable the demonstration of a substantial contracture (Villareal, personal communication).

Long exposures

Villareal[39] incubated tissue at 4°C for about 24 h. Control incubations were without effect on the sensitivity of the preparation to the inhibitory effects of opiates, but it was noticed that the incubated tissue usually generated a lesser tension than tissue taken from newly killed animals and set up without incubation. Likewise, recordings from single neurones which have been incubated in morphine-free Krebs solution for 24 h at 25°C showed no significant differences from recordings made from freshly removed tissue[40]. Neuronal firing was also strongly inhibited by morphine.

Tolerance. Collier's group have found that incubation with morphine (350 nM - 17.5 μM) for 20 h produced a state of tolerance as measured by the reduced ability of morphine to inhibit the contractile response of the ileum[40]. Tolerance was also induced by levorphanol, but not by dextrorphan, and the degree of tolerance was dependent upon the concentration of morphine used to induce it. It was also reported that the tolerance development was reduced when either naloxone or cycloheximide was in the incubation medium. Tolerance development has also been studied at a less quantitative level by single neurone recordings[40]. That tolerance has developed during 24 h incubation (25°C) was evidenced by the fact that neuronal firing could be readily recorded in the continuing presence of morphine (1 μM). Tolerance is probably not complete, because the firing rate was somewhat lower than in control incubated tissue; but increasing the concentration of morphine by 10 to 30 times led to no inhibition of firing in the morphine incubated preparations. Levorphanol incubation induced tolerance to both levorphanol and morphine; dextrorphan incubation induced tolerance to neither.

The effect of naloxone. Naloxone has no effect on control preparations incubated for 24 h, but it causes a marked contracture in preparations incubated in the presence of opiates[39,41,42]. This contracture occurred with incubations at 4°C[39] or 37°C[41]: both the concentration of naloxone required to induce it, and its magnitude and time course, were similar to those seen in tissues removed from morphine-dependent guinea-pigs. The duration of the period of incubation required for the manifestation of the naloxone contracture appears to vary markedly with the agonist used. Normorphine incubation progressively induces an effect, but even after 5 h it is very small[13]. Four h in morphine appears to be sufficient for a prominent contracture[42]. These important observations require further systematic study. Not only morphine produces the substrate for the naloxone contracture, but also levorphanol, meperidine[39] and enkephalin analogues[42]. Cyclazocine, pentazocine and nalorphine were much less effective in sensitising the preparation to naloxone, even though all were applied, as were morphine, levorphanol and meperidine, in concentrations which were six times their respective ED_{50}s for the depression of the contractile response in naive preparations. This finding is of considerable importance in view of the low dependence liability of the morphine-type which these compounds have in monkeys and man.

A marked excitation of single myenteric neurones is the substrate for the naloxone contracture of the incubated tissue. Following incubation with morphine (1 μM) or levorphanol (100 nM), exposure to naloxone causes a dramatic excitation. This action is shared by the (-) but not by the (+) isomers of substituted benzomorphan antagonists, and it can also be closely simulated by simply removing the morphine from the incubation solution; that is, it may be correctly described as a withdrawal sign. The ability of morphine to induce these changes requires more than 1 h (see above) but less that 24 h; intermediate periods have not yet been studied. However, the changes do not require any ongoing neuronal or synaptic activity, for they occur in the presence of blockade of cholinergic synaptic transmission[40] and also in the presence of sufficient lidocaine to inhibit completely all neuronal activity (Karras and North, unpublished).

CONCLUSIONS

Is the model a good one for the study of the changes underlying tolerance and dependence? The prominent changes of tolerance which can be observed in the isolated tissue - either after pretreating the animal or incubating the tissue - and the fact that the time course of the development of tolerance so closely mimicks the development of tolerance in vivo strongly support the validity of the model. The situation with dependence is less clear, because insufficiently few workers have evoked effects simply by removing the morphine, but have relied on the administration of naloxone to 'precipitate abstinence'. The ability of naloxone to induce a prominent contracture does seem to be a manifestation of such 'abstinence', although neither that word (which implies volition) nor 'withdrawal' (which implies removal of opiate) should be used to describe the phenomenon. Again, the time course over which the tissue develops and loses its ability to contract to naloxone closely follows the time course during which the whole animal responds to naloxone with the typical clinical picture of precipitated abstinence. The concentrations of naloxone are small and relevant, the drug action is stereospecific, and the nature of the effect itself is actually a grossly exaggerated response of the neurones in an opposite direction to that of the acute administration of morphine to a naive preparation.

What questions have the experiments answered? One interesting result to emerge is the fact that the development of tolerance and the prominent effect of naloxone are not dependent on the ongoing electrical activity of the neurones. This was not at all obvious in advance of the single neurone studies, for the myenteric plexus in the whole ileum is a relatively complex assembly of neurones which are normally interacting synaptically. But the fact that the changes of tolerance and 'dependence' occur in vitro in the presence of lidocaine indicates that spike activity and synaptic transmission are not involved. This is compatible with the observation that the changes occur even during incubation at 4oC[39]. The latter observation also implies presumably that new protein synthesis may not be involved - though the experiments with cycloheximide in vitro[41] and in vivo[43] need to be taken into account.

The experiments may help to understand the basic change in the properties of the neurones in the tolerant/dependent state. If the neurones adapt to the presence of morphine by an intraterminal mechanism related to transmitter release, then it might be expected that naloxone would cause an outpouring of acetylcholine in such adapted neurones (and hence the contracture) without marked change in the excitable properties of the neuronal membrane. The fact that the individual neurones are so strongly excited by naloxone argues that the outpouring of acetylcholine which occurs is a direct consequence of their enormously increased frequency of firing. This implies that the primary change underlying the tolerant/dependent state is an enhanced neuronal excitability. This is of course compatible with the increased sensitivity of the neurones to a wide range of excitatory substances, and their reduced sensitivity to inhibitory substances.

What questions do the experiments pose? The in vitro experiments are beginning to indicate that the acute agonist effects of the opiates may be separable from their dependence producing effects. Much work is needed in order to determine whether the one action is an inevitable corollary of the other. This will require a systematic study of different opiates whose in vivo pharmacology is well understood. It will require a careful study of the conditions which are necessary for the development of the long term changes. It will require a study of the changes themselves at the receptor binding level, the biochemical level and the intracellular electrophysiological level. Then "it is likely that fundamental progress in understanding tolerance and dependence will be made in this (or a similar) isolated tissue in which the affected neurones and synapses are amenable to direct observation and experimentation, free of the complicating influences of the nervous system as a whole"[44].

ACKNOWLEDGEMENTS

Work carried out in the authors' laboratory was supported by US PHS Grants NS06672, DA01730 and the Schweppe Foundation.

REFERENCES

1. Gibson, A. and Pollock, D. (1975) J. Pharmacol. exp. Therap., 192, 390-398.

2. Ehrenpreis, S., Light, I. and Schonbuch, G.H. (1973) in Drug Addiction: Experimental Pharmacology, Miller, L.H. and Lal, H. eds., Futura, New York, pp. 319-342.

3. Schulz, R. and Cartwright, C. (1974) J. Pharmacol. exp. Therap., 190, 420-430.

4. Johnson, S.M., Westfall, D.P., Howard, S.A. and Fleming, W.W. (1978) J. Pharmacol. exp. Therap., 204, 54-66.

5. Schulz, R. and Goldstein, A. (1973) Nature, 244, 168-170.

6. Schulz, R., Cartwright, C. and Goldstein, A. (1974) Nature 251, 329-331.

7. Takagi, K., Takayanagi, I., Irikura, T., Nishino, K., Ichinoseki, N. and Shishido, K. (1965) Arch. intern. Pharmacodyn. Therap., 158, 39-44.

8. Haycock, V.K. and Rees, J.M.H. (1972) J. Pharmacol. 24, 47-52.

9. Frederickson, R.C.A., Hewes, C.R. and Aiken, J.W. (1976) J. Pharmacol. exp. Therap. 199, 375-384.

10. Ehrenpreis, S., Greenberg, J. and Comaty, J.E. (1975) Life Sci. 17, 49-54.

11. Goldstein, A. and Schulz, R. (1973) Brit. J. Pharmacol. 48, 655-666.

12. Ward, A. and Takemori, A.E. (1976) J. Pharmacol. exp. Therap. 199, 117-123.

13. Schulz, R. and Herz, A. (1976) Life Sci. 19, 1117-1128.

14. Hughes, J., Kosterlitz, H.W., Robson, L.E. and Waterfield, A.A. (1978) Brit. J. Pharmacol. 62, 388P.

15. North, R.A. and Tonini, M. (1977) Brit. J. Pharmacol. 61, 541-549.

16. Takayanagi, I., Sato, T. and Takagi, K. (1974) Europ. J. Pharmacol. 27, 252-254.

17. North, R.A. and Zieglgänsberger, W. (1978) Brain Res. 144, 208-211.

18. Dingledine, R., Goldstein, A. and Kendig, J. (1974) Life Sci. 14, 2299-2309.

19. North, R.A. and Williams, J.T. (1977) Europ. J. Pharmacol. 45, 23-33.

20. Cox, B.M. (1978) Brit. J. Pharmacol. 62, 387-388P.

21. Ward, A. and Takemori, A.E. (1976) J. Pharmacol. exp. Therap. 199, 124-130.

22. Ward, A. and Takemori, A.E. (1974) Fedn. Proc. 33, 502.

23. Schulz, R. and Herz, A. (1976) in Opiates and Endogenous Opioid Peptides, Kosterlitz, H.W., ed., Elsevier, Amsterdam, pp. 319-326.

24. Waterfield, A.A., Hughes, J. and Kosterlitz, H.W. (1976) Nature 260, 624-625.

25. Kaymakcalan, S. (1964) Arch. intern. Pharmacodyn. Therap. 151, 136-141.

26. Frederickson, R.C.A. and Aiken, J.W. (1975) Absts. VI intern. Congr. Pharmacol., 267.

27. Killean, A., Lamb, R. and Wainer, B. (1978) Fedn. Proc. 37, 274.

28. Villareal, J.E. and Dummer, G.E. (1973) Fedn. Proc., 32, 688.

29. Kosterlitz, H.W. and Watt, A.J. (1968) Brit. J. Pharmacol. 33, 266-276.

30. Cox, B.M. and Padhya, R. (1977) Brit. J. Pharmacol. 61, 271-278.

31. Paton, W.D.M. (1957) Brit. J. Pharmacol. 11, 119-127.

32. Gyang, E.A. and Kosterlitz, H.W. (1966) Brit. J. Pharmacol. 27, 514-527.

33. Kosterlitz, H.W. and Waterfield, A.A. (1975) Brit. J. Pharmacol. 53, 131-138.

34. Fennessy, M.R., Heimans, R.L.H. and Rand, M.J. (1969) Brit. J. Pharmacol. 37, 436-449.

35. Kosterlitz, H.W., Lord, J.A.H. and Watt, A.J. (1973) in Agonist and Antagonist Actions of Narcotic Analgesic Drugs, Kosterlitz, H.W., Collier, H.O.J. and Villareal, J.E., eds., University Park, Baltimore, pp. 45-61.

36. Shoham, S. and Weinstock, M. (1974) Brit. J. Pharmacol. 52, 597-603.

37. Shoham-Moshonov, S.R. and Weinstock, M. (1977) Europ. J. Pharmacol. 43, 153-161.

38. Fleming, W.W., McPhillips, J.J. and Westfall, D.P. (1973) Ergeb. Physiol. 68, 55-119.

39. Villareal, J.E., Martinex, J.N. and Castro, A. (1977) reported to the Committee on Problems of Drug Dependence, June 1977.

40. North, R.A. and Karras, P.J. (1978) Nature, 272, 73-75.

41. Hammond, M.D., Schneider, C. and Collier, H.O.J. (1976) in Opiates and Endogenous Opioid Peptides, Kosterlitz, H.W., ed., Elsevier, Amsterdam, pp. 169-176.

42. Frederickson, R.C.A. and Aiken, J.W. (1977) Fedn. Proc. 36, 994.

43. Feinberg, M.P. and Cochin, J. (1977) J. Pharmacol. exp. Therap. 203, 332-339.

44. Goldstein, A., Aronow, L. and Kalman, S.M. (1974) Principles of Drug Action, Wiley, New York, pp. 603-604.

Characteristics and Function of Opioids, editors Van Ree and Terenius
© 1978 Elsevier/North-Holland Biomedical Press

MEANING OF QUASI-WITHDRAWAL PHENOMENA FOR THE CELLULAR MECHANISM OF ABSTINENCE

D.L. FRANCIS, N.J. CUTHBERT, S.A. SAEED, N.M. BUTT, AND H.O.J. COLLIER.
Miles Laboratories Limited, Stoke Poges, Slough, SL2 4LY, England.

ABSTRACT

Evidence from studies of quasi-morphine abstinence induced by methylxanthines in the rat demonstrates that this very closely resembles true
morphine abstinence and that it can be attributed to inhibition of brain
cyclic AMP phosphodiesterase. This evidence, coupled with that from other
sources, indicates that opiate abstinence effects express an increase in
amount and/or activity of cyclic AMP in opiate-sensitive neurones.

INTRODUCTION

One method of exploring the mechanism of opiate dependence is to create,
in opiate-naive animals, by use of a non-opioid drug, a pattern of behaviour
resembling that of opiate abstinence, and then to study the character and
cause of this quasi-abstinence phenomenon[1]. For this method to be valid,
several criteria should be fulfilled: (1) The behaviour pattern of quasi-
morphine-abstinence (QMA) should closely resemble that of true morphine-
abstinence (TMA); (2) the effects of opiates on QMA and TMA should be parallel;
(3) the effects of opiate antagonists on QMA and TMA should also be parallel;
(4) the effects of other drugs on QMA and TMA should be comparable; (5) it
should be possible, by use of a non-opiate drug that induces QMA behaviour,
together with an opiate, to produce a combined effect; (6) any deviations
from these criteria should be readily explicable.

It may be objected that by this method, the attempt to answer one question
--"What is the molecular mechanism of opiate dependence?" -- simply raises
another question -- "What is the molecular mechanism of quasi-abstinence?" --
without answering the original question. The advantage of this procedure is,
however, that it provides more stringent criteria for a correct answer, since
the molecular mechanisms of both true and quasi-abstinence should correspond.
Hence, if both mechanisms are consistent, the likelihood of a misinterpretation
is much diminished. Furthermore, quasi-abstinence has the practical and
theoretical advantage of being obtainable for study without the delay inherent
in true dependence induction.

At the outset of this approach, the main problem is to find a non-opiate drug able to induce QMA behaviour; but it was argued by one of us (HOJC) from a theoretical analysis of the mechanism of morphine dependence, that abstinence effects might arise from a raised level of neuronal cyclic AMP. Therefore methylxanthines, as phosphodiesterase (PDE) inhibitors, were tested for ability to produce QMA behaviour in opiate-naive rats, at first in association with naloxone. In these experiments, it was observed that the methylxanthines alone produced many of the signs of abstinence and that naloxone only intensified and extended the effect.

The studies that resulted from these observations now constitute a considerable body of work, some of which has been published[2,3,4,5,6,7,8], but requires interpretation and some of which requires to be published and interpreted consistently with that already published. The present paper reviews and interprets the published results and describes some further, unpublished work, aimed to clarify the molecular mechanism of quasi-morphine-abstinence induced by methylxanthines in the rat and hence to throw light on the cellular mechanism of true opiate abstinence.

In this paper we use the term quasi-morphine-abstinence (QMA) for the state of behavioural excitation, produced in opiate-naive rats by administering a methylxanthine or like-acting drug. Rats in QMA behave like dependent rats from which morphine has been withdrawn, that is like rats in a state of true morphine abstinence (TMA). We use the term quasi-morphine withdrawal syndrome (QMWS) for the state of more intense behavioural excitement produced by treating rats in a state of QMA with a small dose of naloxone. The QMWS very closely resembles the naloxone-precipitated withdrawal syndrome of morphine-dependent rats[4].

RECENT FINDINGS AND INTERPRETATION

Fulfilment of criteria

To what extent does QMA, induced by methylxanthines in the rat, fulfil the criteria for a valid quasi-abstinence phenomenon enumerated in the first paragraph of this paper?

QMA and TMA behaviour. Administration of theophylline[2] or IBMX[4] to opiate-naive rats produces a significantly higher incidence than in normal animals of the following behavioural signs, all of which can be observed in TMA: rearing on the hind legs, restlessness, head shakes, body shakes, squeak on being touched, diarrhoea and ptosis. The methylxanthines do not produce behavioural responses not seen in TMA.

Effects of opiates. Opiate agonists are well known to suppress TMA with a potency directly related to agonist potency. Likewise they suppress QMA[2,7]. Suppression of QMA is specific (Fig.1), in that it is antagonised by naloxone[2,7], and stereospecific[5]. In recent work, the stereospecificity of opiate suppression of QMA is confirmed with (−)- and (+)-morphine[9] (Fig.1). It is noteworthy that (+)-morphine, given i.c.v., has a just significant suppressive effect, although this is far less intense than that of (−)-morphine.

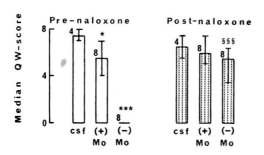

Fig.1. Stereospecificity and specificity of morphine inhibition of QMA. Rats given IBMX (15mg kg^{-1} s.c.) were treated immediately with the (+)- or (−)-enantiomer of morphine (10μg rat^{-1} i.c.v., (+)Mo or (−)Mo) in artificial csf (csf) or with csf. Thirty minutes later rats were placed in plastic cylinders and observed for 15 min (Pre-naloxone). They were then challenged with naloxone (1.0mg kg^{-1} s.c.) returned to the cylinders and observed for a further 10 min (Post-naloxone). The intracerebroventricular (i.c.v.) injections were given via a polythene cannula implanted in the left lateral cerebral ventricle at least 5 days previously. Vertical bars show the interquartile range about the median. The number of rats tested is shown above each histogram. The median QW-score was calculated using procedures described previously[4,7]. For statistical comparisons the Mann-Whitney U Test[11] was used; for comparison with rats given IBMX and csf; *, P <0.05; ***, P <0.001. For comparison between pre- and post-naloxone treatments; §§§, P <0.001.

How far does the suppression of QMA by opiates correspond with their known agonist and antagonist properties? Fourteen opioids -- agonists, partial agonists and antagonists -- were tested for effect on QMA, induced by IBMX (15mg kg^{-1}). Eleven of these drugs suppressed the QMWS, with the following order of potency; etorphine > buprenorphine > levorphanol > heroin > morphine > pentazocine > codeine > pethidine > dextropropoxyphene > normorphine > dextrorphan. All, except pentazocine, had similarly parallel dose/response lines. Nalorphine and cyclazocine had a non-significant effect on QMA. Diprenorphine, an oripavine with strong antagonist activity, potentiated QMA

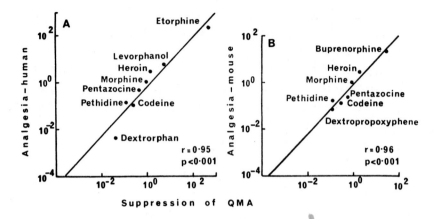

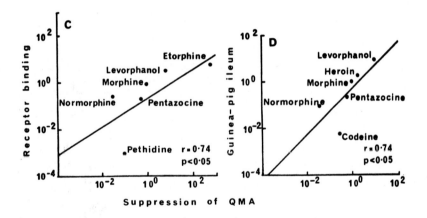

Fig.2. Correlations between the relative agonist potencies of opiates in
suppressing QMA with: A, analgesic activity in man[12,13]; B, antinociceptive
activity in the mouse[14,15,16,17]; C, inhibition of stereospecific naloxone
binding in rat brain homogenate with low sodium concentration[18]; and D[19]
inhibition of electrically evoked contractions of the guinea-pig ileum[19].
All potencies were calculated relative to that of morphine which was given a
value of unity. Slopes were calculated using a least squares linear regression
analysis.

in a dose-related manner. All agonists suppressed in a dose-related manner all individual signs of QMA except salivation, which was even increased by etorphine, buprenorphine, and levorphanol. The potencies of opiate agonists in suppressing the QMA correlate well with those for their analgesic actions in vivo and fairly well with corresponding potencies in vitro, for example for affinity to the opiate receptor and inhibition of neurally-evoked contractions of the guinea-pig ileum (Fig.2).

Effects of antagonists. Pure or nearly pure antagonists, such as naloxone and naltrexone, intensify QMA, with much the same potencies and relative potency as they intensify TMA[4]. That (-)-naloxone, but not its recently synthesized (+)-enantiomer[20] is effective in precipitating a QMWS shows that the intensification by naloxone of the QMA is stereospecific (Fig.3).

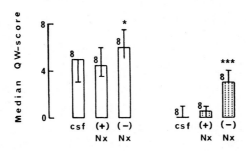

Fig.3. Stereospecificity of naloxone potentiation of QMA. Rats were given IBMX (10mg kg^{-1} s.c.), open columns; or IBMX (15mg kg^{-1} s.c.) plus heroin (3.0mg kg^{-1} s.c.), hatched columns. Rats were challenged 1h later with the (+)- or (-)-enantiomer of naloxone (3µg rat^{-1} i.c.v.-(+)Nx or (-)Nx) or csf; placed in plastic cylinders and observed for 15 min. For comparison with rats given IBMX and challenged with csf; *, P = 0.06; for comparison with rats given IBMX plus heroin and challenged with csf; ***, P <0.001. Other details as in Fig.1.

Effects of other drugs. Other drugs known to interact with opiate dependence have been tested on QMA. One of these, lanthanum, is an inhibitor of rat brain adenylate cyclase[21]. Lanthanum lessens the intensity of naloxone-precipitated withdrawal in morphine dependent mice[22]. In our experiments, lanthanum (0.3µmol rat^{-1} i.c.v.) significantly reduced the intensity of the QMWS induced by IBMX (P <0.004).

The other drug tested was cycloheximide which inhibits the induction of opiate dependence[23]. Cycloheximide (3 or 10mg kg^{-1} s.c.) given to opiate-naive rats 1h before treatment with IBMX to induce QMA, slightly but significantly intensified the QMWS ($\underline{P}$ <0.04). This constitutes a major difference between the induction of quasi- and of true dependence. It at least shows that the induction of QMA does not require protein synthesis and it suggests that the behavioural excitation of QMA would be greater, but for synthesis of a peptide that inhibits it. This finding, coupled with the finding that naloxone intensifies QMA, suggests that the inhibitory peptide is an endogenous opioid; but other explanations of the intensifying actions of cycloheximide are possible.

Sodium pentobarbitone (10mg kg^{-1}) significantly suppressed the incidence of paw tremors and diarrhoea and significantly reduced the QW score (P <0.05). These inhibitory effects of sodium pentobarbitone were not reversed by naloxone. Haloperidol (1.0mg kg^{-1}) significantly suppressed the incidence of chewing, rearing, restlessness, body shakes, paw tremors, head shakes and diarrhoea ($\underline{P}$ <0.05) and significantly reduced the QW score ($\underline{P}$ <0.001). Naloxone did not significantly reverse the effects of haloperidol on the incidence of individual signs although it just significantly ($\underline{P}$ <0.05) increased the QW score in rats treated with IBMX plus haloperidol. Diazepam (2.5mg kg^{-1}) significantly potentiated the incidence of jumping ($\underline{P}$ <0.01), decreased the incidence of salivation ($\underline{P}$ <0.05), but did not affect the overall score. Chlorpromazine (5mg kg^{-1}) produced a marked increase in the incidence and frequency of jumping ($\underline{P}$ <0.01) and significantly increased the incidence of teeth chattering, squeak on touch and squeak on handling ($\underline{P}$ <0.05), but decreased the incidence of head shakes, diarrhoea and salivation ($\underline{P}$ <0.05). Amphetamine (3.0mg kg^{-1}) significantly reduced the incidence of ptosis, chewing, and head shakes ($\underline{P}$ <0.05) and potentiated squeak on touch ($\underline{P}$ <0.05) but did not significantly affect the overall withdrawal score. The lack of effectiveness, in inhibiting QMA, of other drugs tested, when compared to the opioids, suggests that the QMA is mediated via opioid-sensitive neurones.

Combined effects of methylxanthines and opiates. When rats made quasi-abstinent with IBMX are given heroin, the quasi-abstinent state is suppressed; but, when they are shortly afterwards challenged with naloxone, a more intense behavioural excitation is seen[8]. This phenomenon may be attributed to a combination of quasi-and true-abstinence effects. Put another way, IBMX has the effect of enabling heroin more rapidly to induce responsiveness to naloxone. That this is indeed an acceleration of heroin dependence is indicated by the finding that cycloheximide inhibits the intensification revealed on naloxone challenge[8].

Another example of the combined action of the methylxanthines with naloxone is provided by experiments in which the non-opiate drug is given to morphine-dependent rats shortly before challenge with naloxone. When this is done, IBMX theophylline and caffeine each intensifies precipitated withdrawal[3]. Others[24] have shown that caffeine and IBMX precipitate withdrawal in morphine-dependent rhesus monkeys.

From this discussion it can be concluded that the state of quasi-morphine-abstinence induced by methylxanthines amply fulfils the criteria for a valid quasi-abstinence phenomenon.

Importance of studies with methylxanthines

Many studies have been reported, in which drugs that modify humoral trans-mitter mechanisms have been shown to interact with one or another aspect of withdrawal. As we pointed out in 1972, the results of these studies are usually paradoxical, in that the same drug modifies different withdrawal effects in different directions[25]. For example, atropine, given shortly before naloxone to dependent rats, significantly decreased withdrawal jumping, diarrhoea and chewing, but increased irritability and paw tremor.

Such observations not only call in question the idea that changes in extracellular messenger substances constitute the basic mechanism of depend-ence, but also indicate that, in attempting to analyse dependence through experiments in vivo, we should seek a drug that modifies all withdrawal effects in the same direction. The drugs that do this are few. So far three types of drug affecting all abstinence signs in the same direction have been identified: (1) opiates, which suppress withdrawal effects; (2) opiate anta-gonists, which intensify them; and (3) methylxanthines, which synergize with naloxone in intensifying withdrawal effects[3]. In this context, this finding with methylxanthines encourages us to suppose that, in our work with these drugs, we are reaching the intimate mechanism of opiate dependence.

Site of methylxanthine action.

Since heroin is far more effective in suppressing and naloxone in intensify-ing QMA, when each drug is given into a cerebral ventricle than systemically[7], we can conclude that the precipitated QMWS is largely central in origin. The question therefore arises: in what part of the CNS do methylxanthines produce the state of QMA? We do not have direct evidence on this, but the following considerations suggest that methylxanthines produce QMA by acting on opioid-sensitive neurones within the CNS.

It has recently been argued that opiate tolerance/dependence can occur within the opioid-sensitive neurone[26]. The evidence for this comes from studies of opiate tolerance/dependence in three preparations: (1) cultured neuroblastoma x glioma hybrid cells[27,28,29]; (2) isolated guinea-pig ileum[30,31,32]; and (3) single brain cells in situ[33,34].

If this argument is correct, theories of tolerance/dependence based on extracellular changes, such as changes in humoral messengers or neuronal pathways, are probably of secondary importance. If dependence occurs in opioid-sensitive neurones in vitro, it seems likely that the same molecular mechanism would also occur in vivo. If so, then the methylxanthines may be supposed to act on opioid-sensitive neurones in the rat brain to produce quasi-abstinence. This argument is supported by the only observation we have made on methylxanthines in tolerance/ dependence in vitro -- that the induction of tolerance in the isolated guinea-pig ileum is intensified by addition of caffeine to the incubation mixture[30].

Biochemical mechanism of QMA and TMA

Correlation of potencies. In a group of seven xanthines, we have correlated potencies in eliciting behavioural excitation with potencies in inhibiting low Km phosphodiesterase in rat brain homogenate in vitro (Fig.4). The correlation obtained has a value $r = 0.86$ ($\underline{P}$ <0.01).

Two non-xanthine phosphodiesterase inhibitors -- ICI63197 and RO201724 -- have also been found to produce a QMWS. The rank order of potency of the five compounds -- three xanthines and two non-xanthines -- so far found to produce an unmistakable QMWS (Table 1) is not significantly different from their rank order of potency in inhibiting low Km cyclic AMP phospho-diesterase $r = 0.87$; ($\underline{P}$ <0.05). These correlations strongly argue that the behavioural effects of the methylxanthines and like-acting drugs are due to their ability to inhibit brain phosphodiesterase, which would be expected to raise the level of a neuronal cyclic AMP.

The conclusion that QMA is due to a raised level of neuronal cyclic AMP is supported by the finding that, at doses effective in producing signs of quasi-abstinence, theophylline and ICI63197 significantly raise brain cyclic AMP[35].

One potent phosphodiesterase inhibitor, papaverine, does not produce QMA. Papaverine, however, unlike theophylline, when administered systemically, does not raise the cyclic AMP level of rat cerebrospinal fluid[36].

45

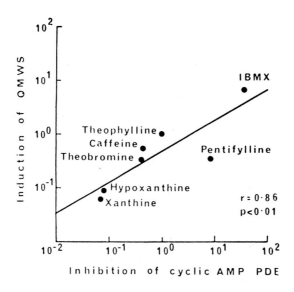

Fig.4. Correlations between the relative potencies of xanthines in inducing the QMWS in rats _in vivo_ and in inhibiting the activity of low Km cyclic AMP phosphodiesterase in rat brain homogenate. Potencies were calculated relative to that of theophylline, which was given a value of unity. The slope of the regression lines was determined using a least squares linear regression analysis.

Several other modes of action of the effective drugs are possible including the inhibition of cyclic GMP phosphodiesterase and mobilization of calcium. We have not specifically excluded these; but it seems unlikely that the fit, in all respects, would be as close as the fit with cyclic AMP phosphodiesterase.

Raised cyclic AMP level or activity. We have argued that quasi-abstinence is produced by raising the level of cyclic AMP and that this happens in opioid-sensitive neurones. Furthermore, the resemblance between quasi- and true morphine abstinence is so close that a comparable mechanism may be supposed to occur in true dependence; but, in this, an increased activity of adenylate cyclase, of protein kinase or of both enzymes might operate equally well as might a decreased activity of phosphodiesterase. Indeed, a decrease of phosphodiesterase activity has not been found in dependent cells, whereas increased adenylate cyclase activity has been reported in neuroblastoma x glioma cells[27,28,29], and in brain preparations[39,40]. Furthermore, an increase in protein kinase has also been observed in dependent brain homogenate[41,42].

TABLE 1

COMPARISON OF POTENCIES IN INDUCING THE QMWS IN RATS IN VIVO AND IN INHIBITING
LOW Km CYCLIC AMP PHOSPHODIESTERASE IN RAT BRAIN HOMOGENATE

	Induction of the QMWS			Inhibition of PDE	
Drug	Maximal QW score $\pm$ s.e.m.	QWD_{50} (mg kg^{-1})	Slope function $\pm$ s.e.m.	IC_{50} mM	Slope function $\pm$ s.e.m.
Saline	1.8 $\pm$ 0.3	-	-	-	-
ICI 63197	8.1 $\pm$ 0.6	5.1	2.9 $\pm$ 0.7***	0.02	7.8 $\pm$ 5.3
IBMX	8.6 $\pm$ 0.6	5.4	6.6 $\pm$ 1.2***	0.03	39.5 $\pm$ 2.4***
RO201724	6.6 $\pm$ 1.4	26.2	4.6 $\pm$ 1.7**	1.63	47.1 $\pm$ 5.3***
Theophylline	8.2 $\pm$ 0.6	35.4	8.1 $\pm$ 2.1***	1.0	41.1 $\pm$ 4.0***
Caffeine	6.4 $\pm$ 1.2	97.1	4.2 $\pm$ 1.5***	1.9	61.1 $\pm$ 3.2***

Cyclic AMP PDE activity was assayed using a modification of the two-stage
isotopic procedure first described by Thompson and Appleman[37] and later by
Boudreau and Drummond[38]. A substrate concentration of 1 µM cyclic AMP was
used. ICI63197, 2-amino-6-methyl-5-oxo-4-n-propyl-4,5-dihydro-5-triazolo
(1,5-a) pyrimidine; IBMX, 3-isobutyl-1-methylxanthine; RO201724, 4-(3-butoxy-
4-methoxybenzyl)-2-imidazolidone. QWD_{50}, dose required to produce a half-
maximal quasi-withdrawal score; IC_{50}, concentration required to inhibit
cyclic AMP phosphodiesterase of rat brain homogenate by 50%. For significance of slopes; **, $\underline{P}$ <0.01; ***, $\underline{P}$ <0.001.

The increase in protein kinase in dependence is consistent with two theories
of dependence put forward in the 1960's. Because protein kinase is an enzyme,
its increase in dependence is consistent with the enzyme expansion theory of
Goldstein & Goldstein[43,44] and of Shuster[45]. Because protein kinase can be
regarded as the receptor for cyclic AMP, its increase in dependence is
consistent with the theory of drug induced changes in number or efficiency of
receptors put forward by Collier[46,47].

SUMMARY

In summary, the evidence of quasi-morphine abstinence induced by methylxanthines and the related evidence that has been marshalled, indicate that
opiate abstinence effects express an increased level or activity of cyclic

AMP in opioid-sensitive neurones. This conclusion, which is substantially the same as that proposed in 1975[3], leads to a prediction with which to close this discussion. This prediction is that quasi-morphine abstinence signs should be inducible not only by inhibitors of phosphodiesterase, but also by stimulants of neuronal adenylate cyclase, if these were applied to appropriate morphine-sensitive neurones of the brain. In this effect, the stimulant of adenylate cyclase should be potentiated by a methylxanthine.

ACKNOWLEDGEMENTS

We thank Janet Cornall and Helen Hughes for help in observing animals, L.C. Dinneen for statistical advice, and Dr. K.C. Rice for (+)-morphine and (+)-naloxone. The following companies kindly supplied the substances indicated: I.C.I. Pharmaceuticals, ICI63197; Roche Products, RO201724, dextrorphan and levorphanol; Reckitt and Colman, buprenorphine and diprenorphine; Burroughs Wellcome, normorphine.

REFERENCES

1.   Collier, H.O.J. (1974) Pharmacology, 11, 58-61.

2.   Collier, H.O.J., Francis, D.L., Henderson, G. and Schneider, C. (1974) Nature, 249, 471-473.

3.   Collier, H.O.J. and Francis, D.L. (1975) Nature, 255, 159-162.

4.   Francis, D.L., Roy, A.C. and Collier, H.O.J. (1975) Life Sci., 16, 1901-1906.

5.   Collier, H.O.J. and Francis, D.L. (1976) Br.J.Pharmacol., 56, 382P.

6.   Cuthbert, N.J., Dinneen, L.C., Francis, D.L. and Schneider, C. (1976) Br.J.Pharmacol., 56, 386P.

7.   Collier, H.O.J., Butt, N.M., Francis, D.L., Roy, A.C. and Schneider, C. (1978) in Proc.10th Congress Collegium Internationale Neuropsychopharmacologicum, Deniker, P., Radouco-Thomas, C. and Villeneuve, A. eds., Pergamon, Oxford, pp 1331-1338.

8.   Francis, D.L., Cuthbert, N.J., Dinneen, L.C., Schneider, C. and Collier, H.O.J. (1976) in Opiates and Endogenous Opioid Peptides, Kosterlitz, H.W. ed., Elsevier/North Holland, Amsterdam, pp 177-184.

9.   Jacquet, Y.F., Klee, W.A., Rice, K.C., Iijima, I. and Minamikawa, J. (1977) Science, 198, 842-845.

10. Palaic, D., Page, I.H. and Khairallah, P.A. (1967) J.Neurochem., 14, 63-69.

11. Dinneen, L.C. and Blakesley, B.C. (1973) Applied Statistics, 22, 269-273.

12. Ehrenpreis, S. and Teller, D.N. (1972) in Chemical and Biological Aspects of Drug Dependence, Mulé, S.J. and Brill, H. eds., C.R.C. Press, Cleveland, pp 177-207.

48

13. Jacobson, A.E. (1972) in Chemical and Biological Aspects of Drug Dependence, Mulé, S.J. and Brill, H. eds., C.R.C. Press, Cleveland, pp 101-117.

14. Cho, T.M., Cho, J.S. and Loh, H.H. (1976) Life Sci, 18, 231-244.

15. Cowan, A. (1973) in Advances in Biochemical Pharmacology, Vol 8, Braude, M.C. Harris, L.S., May, E.L., Smith, J.P. and Villarreal, J.E. eds., Raven Press, New York, pp 427-438.

16. Eddy, N.B., Halbach, H. and Braenden, O.J. (1956) Bull. W.H.O., 14, 353-402.

17. Schneider, C. (1974) PhD Thesis University of London.

18. Creese, I. and Snyder, S.H. (1975) J.Pharmacol.Exp.Ther., 194, 205-219.

19. Kosterlitz, H.W. and Waterfield, A.A. (1975) Ann.Rev.Pharmacol., 15, 29-47.

20. Iijima, I., Minamikawa, J., Jacobson, A.E., Brossi, A., and Rice, K.C. (1978) J.Med.Chem., 21, 398-400.

21. Nathanson, J.A., Freedman, R., and Hoffer, B.J. (1976) Nature, 261, 330-332.

22. Harris, R.A., Loh, H.H., and Way, E.L. (1976) J.Pharmacol.Exp.Ther., 196, 288-297.

23. Ho, I.K., Loh, H.H., Bhargava, H.N. and Way, E.L. (1975). Life Sci., 16, 1895-1900.

24. Aceto, M.D. and Harris, L.S. (1978) Fedn.Proc., 37, 764.

25. Collier, H.O.J., Francis, D.L. and Schneider, C. (1972) Nature, 237, 220-223.

26. Collier, H.O.J. (1978). Paper presented at Second Meeting of European Soc. Neurochemistry, Gottingen, 28 August-1 September.

27. Sharma, S.K., Klee, W.A. and Nirenberg, M. (1975) Proc.Nat.Acad.Sci.USA, 72, 3092-3096.

28. Traber, J., Gullis, R. and Hamprecht, B. (1975) Life Sci., 16, 1863-1868.

29. Sharma, S.K., Klee, W.A. and Nirenberg, M. (1977) Proc.Nat.Acad.Sci. USA., 74, 3365-3369.

30. Hammond, M.D., Schneider, C., and Collier, H.O.J. (1976) in Opiates and Endogenous Opioid Peptides, Kosterlitz, H.W. ed., Elsevier/North Holland, Amsterdam, pp 169-176.

31. Villarreal, J.E., Martinez, J.N. and Castro, A. (1977) in Problems of Drug Dependence 1977, pp. 305-314. Committee on Problems of Drug Dependence.

32. North, R.A. and Karras, P.J. (1978) Nature, 272, 73-75.

33. Satoh, M., Zieglgänsberger, W. and Herz, A. (1976): Brain Res., 115, 99-110.

34. Fry, J.P., Zieglgänsberger, W. and Herz, A. (1978) in Iontophoresis and Transmitter Mechanisms in the Mammalian Central Nervous System, Ryall, R.W. and Kelly, J.S. eds., Elsevier/North Holland, Amsterdam.

35. Chiu, A., Eccleston, D. and Palomo, T. (1977) Br.J.Pharmacol., 61, 119P-120P.

36. Kiessling, M., Lindl, T. and Cramer, H. (1975) Arch.Psychiatr.Nervenkr., 220, 325-333.

37. Thompson, W.J. and Appleman, M.M. (1971) Biochemistry, 10, 311-316.

38. Boudreau, R.J. and Drummond, G.I. (1975) Analytical Biochemistry, 63, 388-399.

39. Collier, H.O.J., Francis, D.L., McDonald-Gibson, W.J., Roy, A.C. and Saeed, S.A. (1975) Life Sci., 17, 85-90.

40. Hosein, E.A. and Lau, A. (1977) Trans.Amer.Soc.Neurochem., 8, 83 (Abstr. No. 39).

41. Clark, A.G., Jovic, R., Ornellas, M.R. and Weller, M. (1972) Biochem. Pharmacol., 21, 1989-1990.

42. Kuriyama, K., Nakagawa, K., Naito, K. and Muramatsu, M. (1978) Japan J. Pharmacol., 28, 73-84.

43. Goldstein, D.B. and Goldstein, A. (1961) Biochem.Pharmacol., 8, 48.

44. Goldstein, A. and Goldstein, D.B. (1968) in The Addictive States, Wikler, A. ed. Williams & Wilkins, Baltimore, pp 265-267.

45. Shuster, L. (1961) Nature, 189, 314-315.

46. Collier, H.O.J. (1966) Advances in Drug Research, 3, 171-188.

47. Collier, H.O.J. (1972) Br.J.Addict., 67, 277-286.

Characteristics and Function of Opioids, editors Van Ree and Terenius
© *1978 Elsevier/North-Holland Biomedical Press*   51

INABILITY OF ACUTE OR CHRONIC THALAMIC, LIMBIC, OR CORTICAL LESIONS
TO ALTER NARCOTIC DEPENDENCE AND ABSTINENCE IN RATS

MARTIN W. ADLER, ELLEN B. GELLER, PHYLLIS B. BEETON and PHILIP L. GILDENBERG
Dept. of Pharmacology, Temple U. Med. Sch., Phila., Pa. 19140 U.S.A.

INTRODUCTION

Specific sites for the analgesic effects of narcotics have been identified, but little is known about the neuronal pathways mediating narcotic dependence and abstinence. Destruction of discrete areas of the brain is a useful means of investigating central sites of drug action, particularly if the chronicity of the lesion is taken into account and if simultaneous comparisons of multiple lesion sites are made[1]. The purpose of this study was to determine if acute or chronic lesions of several thalamic, limbic, or cortical loci would modify morphine dependence or abstinence in rats.

MATERIALS AND METHODS

Two series of studies were conducted in male Sprague-Dawley (Zivic-Miller) rats, using bilateral anodal d.c. lesions for subcortical damage, and tissue aspiration for cortical areas. For chronic studies, rats (270-310 g) were lesioned and then group-housed for 3 months prior to s.c. implantation of 2 morphine pellets, each containing 75 mg of the base. Naloxone (1.0 mg/kg s.c. or i.p.) was injected 72 hr later and the abstinence syndrome assessed. For acute studies, rats (260-290 g) were implanted with pellets and lesioned 72 hr later. The naloxone-precipitated withdrawal syndrome was assessed 4-6 hr after lesioning.
Histological verification of all lesion sites was carried out using paraffin-embedded serial sections stained with luxol blue and cresyl violet.

RESULTS

Histology. Thalamic lesions were in the centre median, parafascicularis, or ventral and dorsomedial thalamus. Limbic lesions were in the amygdala (primarily the cortical amygdaloid nucleus), lateral septum, or dorsal hippocampus. Cortical ablations were in the frontal cortex (primarily area 10) or posterior cortex (primarily area 17).

Acute Lesions. In rats made dependent on morphine, lesioned, and subsequently injected with naloxone 4-6 hours postop, weight loss, teeth chattering, and wet-shakes were not significantly altered by any of the lesions. Jumping, however, was dramatically reduced following damage to the hippocampus. Lesions of the parafascicularis, ventral and dorsomedial thalamus, and lateral septal nuclei resulted in a markedly decreased incidence of this sign. Writhing was diminished by several of the lesions. Other signs of abstinence (e.g., chromo-dacryorrhea, diarrhea, ptosis) were generally unaffected, although small changes in the incidence of individual signs were noted.

Chronic Lesions. In the case of animals lesioned and then housed for 3 months prior to pellet implantation, none of the lesions modified the weight loss seen during morphine withdrawal. With respect to jumping, lesions of the parafascicularis, lateral septal nuclei, and hippocampus again decreased the incidence of this sign, but the effect with hippocampal damage was less drama-tic than that seen after acute lesions. Little difference was seen in the in-cidence of teeth chattering or wet shakes with any of the lesions. In regard to other signs of abstinence, the only marked changes noted were a decrease in the incidence of diarrhea with lateral septal lesions, a decrease in ptosis with centre median and ventral and dorsomedial thalamus lesions, and a de-creased incidence of salivation with centre median and frontal cortex damage.

DISCUSSION AND CONCLUSIONS

Based on the results from these studies, it appears that, although indivi-dual signs of abstinence are altered by lesions in specific brain loci, none of the lesions affected the production of narcotic dependence or the overall ab-stinence syndrome. Wikler[2] reached a similar conclusion after lesioning the dorsomedial thalamus and some limbic areas. In view of the large number of signs that characterize abstinence and the probability that different neuronal pathways subserve the various signs, we do not believe that there is a single anatomical locus or pathway solely responsible for the development of depen-dence or the abstinence syndrome.

Future research utilizing brain lesions to investigate actions of narcotics should probably be directed towards exploring neuroanatomical and/or neurochem-ical pathways involved with specific actions of the drug rather than attempting to find a single locus for dependence or abstinence.

ACKNOWLEDGEMENTS

This work was supported by grants DA 00049 and DA 00376 from the National Institute on Drug Abuse.

REFERENCES

1. Adler, M.W. and Geller, E.B. (1978) in Factors Affecting the Action of Nar-cotics, Adler, M.W., Manara, L. and Samanin, R. eds., Raven Press, N.Y., pp. 93-101.
2. Wikler, A., Norrell, H. and Miller, D. (1972) Exp. Neurol., 34, 543-557.

Characteristics and Function of Opioids, editors Van Ree and Terenius
© *1978 Elsevier/North-Holland Biomedical Press*

THE EFFECTS OF NATURALLY OCCURRING AND D-AMINO ACID CONTAINING ENKEPHALINS ON MORPHINE ABSTINENCE AND LOCOMOTOR ACTIVITY.

HEMENDRA N. BHARGAVA

Department of Pharmacognosy and Pharmacology, College of Pharmacy, University of Illinois at the Medical Center, Chicago, Illinois 60612, U.S.A.

ABSTRACT

Intracerebral administration of methionine-enkephalin (MEK), leucine-enkephalin (LEK), D-Met^2-Pro^5-enkephalinamide, D-Ala^2-Met^5-enkephalinamide and morphine inhibited the naloxone-induced abstinence syndrome in morphine-dependent mice. The most potent compound was D-Met^2-Pro^5-enkephalinamide and the least potent was MEK. Dose and time dependent effects on locomotor activity were produced by enkephalins and morphine. No correlation was found between the effects of the drugs on locomotor activity and their ability to inhibit morphine abstinence.

INTRODUCTION

Considerable *in vivo* and *in vitro* evidence has been presented for the existence of peptides, MEK, LEK, and endorphin, which act as endogenous ligands for the opiate receptors[1]. The enkephalins, however, do not cross the blood brain barrier and show pharmacologic activity only when administered directly into the brain. Although the ability of MEK and β-endorphin to produce some withdrawal signs when perfused into the periaqueductal gray-fourth ventricular spaces of the rat brain has been demonstrated[2], the relative addiction liability of these peptides appears to be lower than morphine. More recently, attempts have been made to synthesize, orally active[3], longer lasting peptides which are devoid of abuse potential. Our continued effort to find such agents has led us to explore,on morphine abstinence signs,the effects of naturally occurring as well as some D-amino acid containing peptides which are presumably resistant to enzymatic degradation. An attempt was also made to see if a relationship existed between the effects on morphine abstinence and locomotor activity.

MATERIAL AND METHODS

Male Swiss-Webster mice, 25-30g (Scientific Small Laboratories, Arlington Heights, Ill.) were maintained on food and water *ad libitum* in a room maintained on 12 hr light-dark cycles. Mice were rendered dependent by the subcutaneous implantation[4] of a morphine pellet, containing 75 mg of morphine base. Three days after implantation, the pellets were removed and after an additional 6 hr period, either saline or various doses of enkephalins and morphine in saline were injected intracerebroventricularly[6] in volumes such that each mouse received 0.5 µl/g. Withdrawal was precipitated by s.c. injections of naloxone HCl, which was administered immediately after the administration of saline or the test drug, and the withdrawal signs were monitored as described before[5]. At least eight mice were used for each of the three doses of naloxone to calculate the naloxone ED$_{50}$, the potency ratio, their 95% confindence limits, and the statistical significance[7].

Locomotor activity was measured by means of three sets of circular activity cages (35 cm in diameter and 20 cm in height) equipped with six light sources and six photocells placed just above the floor level. The lights were placed orthogonally to each other so that the light beams crossed in the center of the cages. The measure of activity was the number of times the light beam was broken within a specified period of time and was recorded automatically on a counter. The experiments were carried out only with MEK since other compounds were available only in small amounts. The drug was injected ICV as described previously. Immediately after the injection the mice were put in the activity cages and their activity recorded at various time intervals for a period of 30 min. The experiments were repeated four times using three mice per determination. Activity was measured at the same time of the day to minimize the diurnal variations. The data were analyzed by two way ANOVA upon the untransformed scores using a split-plot design[8] and for significant F ratios, Scheffe's S method[9] was used to make all possible comparisons among means.

RESULTS AND DISCUSSION

Administration of either enkephalins or morphine inhibited the stereotyped jumping syndrome, a characteristic sign of morphine abstinence in morphine-dependent rodents[10,11]. As shown in Table 1, both MEK and LEK were equiactive in increasing the naloxone ED_{50} by 2-to 3-fold compared to saline controls. A dose related increase in naloxone ED_{50} was seen with both the D-amino acid containing pentapeptides, D-Met[2]-Pro[5]-enkephalinamide and D-Ala[2]-Met[5]-enkephalinamide. In a dose range of 0.875 to 3.5 μmole/kg, D-Met[2]-Pro[5]-enkephalinamide produced 8 to 217-fold increase in naloxone ED_{50}, while D-Ala[2]-Met[5]-enkephalinamide produced a 10 to 85-fold increase over the corresponding saline controls. All the enkephalins, however, failed to affect other abstinence signs such as defecation, diarrhea, micturition etc.

The effect on the cumulative locomotor activity of MEK and morphine for a 30 min period is presented in Fig. 1. A dose of 1.75 μmole/kg of MEK decreased the motor activity which was evident only at 30 min after its administration; however, at other time intervals no change in activity was observed. Morphine, at the same dose (1.75 μmole/kg) was without any effect during the 30-min observation period (Fig. 1A). It must be noted that at this dose both MEK and morphine significantly inhibited the naloxone-induced withdrawal when the observations were made within the first 15-min of their administration. The motor activity was significantly depressed by 7.0 μmole/kg dose of MEK and morphine compared with saline at all time intervals beginning with 6 min after their administration (Fig. 1B). MEK in doses of 0.2 and 0.4 μmole/kg had no effect on motor activity during 1 hr observation period (Fig. 1C), whereas, morphine in the same doses increased the motor activity which was evident only at 45 and 60 min after its administration (Fig. 1D).

The present studies indicate that like morphine, ICV administration of naturally occurring pentapeptides, LEK and MEK and their analogs containing D-aminoacids can inhibit the withdrawal jumping observed during morphine abstinence. It appears that the stereotyped jumping response observed following naloxone administration, a highly characteristic sign of morphine dependence is centrally mediated, while the other signs such as defecation, diarrhea, micturition are not. This observation is supported by other studies[2,12] which showed the absence of profuse diarrhea during precipitated withdrawal in animals made dependent by intracerebral infusion of morphine. Thus, ICV injections of narcotic agonists do not seem to affect some peripheral signs of withdrawal. Furthermore, the potency of the peptides is enhanced when D-amino

TABLE 1

Effects of intracerebrally administered enkephalins and morphine on the naloxone ED_{50} in morphine-dependent mice.

Treatment	Dose μmole/kg	Naloxone ED_{50} μg/kg (95% C.L.)[a]	Potency Ratio (95% C.L.)[a]
Saline	-	166(109-255)	-
Morphine Sulfate	0.875	200(117-341)	1.20(0.62-2.34)
	1.75	729(476-1117)	4.39(2.47-7.81)[b]
Leucine-enkephalin	1.75	366(239-561)	2.20(1.20-3.96)[b]
	3.50	387(242-620)	2.33(1.23-4.31)[b]
	7.00	410(261-643)	2.46(1.37-4.43)[b]
Methionine-enkephalin	1.75	172(85 -348)	1.03(0.46-2.30)
	3.50	364(238-558)	2.19(1.22-3.94)[b]
	7.00	490(303-795)	2.95(1.44-6.02)[b]
Saline	-	43(28 -66)	-
D-Met[2]-Pro[5]-enkephalinamide	0.875	331(225-487)	7.72(4.36-13.66)[b]
	1.75	3905(1842-8279)	91.12(38.77-214.13)[b]
	3.50	9283(5592-15410)	216.59(112.22-418.02)[b]
Saline	-	25(15 -43)	-
D-Ala[2]-Met[5]-enkephalinamide	0.875	242(144-410)	9.60(4.60-20.20)[b]
	1.75	278(111-697)	11.10(3.82-32.19)[b]
	3.50	2130(928-4891)	85.20(31.56-230.04)[b]

[a] = confidence limits

[b] = $p<0.05$ vs. saline controls

acids are substituted in position 2 of the naturally occurring petapeptides, the methionine analog being more potent than the alanine analog. There appears to be a lack of correlation between the effect of the agonists on withdrawal symptoms and their effect on motor activity since they were able to inhibit withdrawal jumping response at a time when they did not alter motor activity. Finally, some of the orally active peptides may be useful in managing narcotic withdrawal signs both central and peripheral in nature.

56

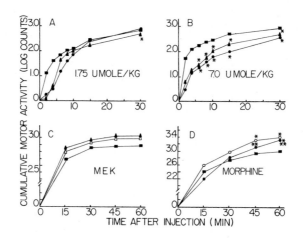

Fig. 1. Effect of drugs on motor activity ■—■ saline (A and B) ●—● morphine; ▲—▲ MEK; (C)△—△(0.2 μmole/kg); ▲—▲ (0.4 μmole/kg) (D)○—○ (0.2 μmole/kg); ●—● (0.4 μmole/kg). *p<0.05 vs. the saline controls

REFERENCES

1. Kosterlitz, H.W. ed., Opiates and Endogenous Opioid Peptides, Elsevier/North Holland Biomedical Press, Amsterdam, 1976.

2. Wei, E. and Loh, H. (1976) Science, 193, 1262-1263.

3. Roemer, D. et. al., (1977) Nature, 268, 547-548.

4. Bhargava, H.N. (1978) Pharmacol. Biochem. Behav. 8, 7-11.

5. Bhargava, H.N. (1977) Europ. J. Pharmacol. 41, 81-84.

6. Haley, T.J. and McCormick, W.G. (1957) Brit. J. Pharmacol 12, 12-15.

7. Litchfield, J.T. and Wilcoxon, F. (1949) J. Pharmacol. Exp. Ther. 96, 99-113.

8. Kirk, R.E. (1968) Experimental Design: Procedures for the Behavior Sciences. Brooks/Cole Publishing Co., California, p. 245.

9. Scheffe, H. (1953) Biometrika 40, 87-104.

10. Bhargava, H.N. (1977) Psychopharmacology 52, 55-62.

11 Way, E.L., Loh, H.H. and Shen, F.H. (1969) J. Pharmacol. Exp. Ther. 167, 1-8.

12. Lascka, E., Herz, A. and Blasig, J. (1976) Psychopharmacologia 46, 133-139.

Characteristics and Function of Opioids, editors Van Ree and Terenius
© *1978 Elsevier/North-Holland Biomedical Press*

CARBACHOL-INDUCED THERMOREGULATORY TOLERANCE TO MORPHINE

THOMAS F. BURKS and GARY C. ROSENFELD
Departments of Pharmacology, University of Arizona College of Medicine,
Tucson, Arizona 85724 and The University of Texas Medical School at
Houston, Houston, Texas 77030 (USA)

ABSTRACT

Intracerebral injections of carbachol inhibited subsequent hypothermic
responses to peripherally injected morphine in rats. Carbachol enhanced
hypothermic responses to dopamine. The antimorphine effect of carbachol
was inhibited by atropine and by haloperidol.

INTRODUCTION

Thermoregulatory tolerance to morphine, which can occur after a single
dose of the drug, is characterized in rats by attenuation or reversal of
the usual hypothermic response [1,2] and by increased sensitivity to dopamine[3,4]. Intracerebral injections of acetylcholine are known to produce
morphine-like antinociceptive effects[5]. We have found that carbachol also
induces a condition which closely resembles thermoregulatory tolerance to
morphine.

MATERIALS AND METHODS

Rectal temperature was monitored in male Sprague-Dawley rats which had
been implanted previously with polyethylene cannulae for intracerebroventricular (icv) injections.

RESULTS

Rats which were pretreated with carbachol (5 μg, icv) showed attenuated
hypothermic responses to morphine (30 mg/kg, sc) in comparison with rats
which received saline pretreatment. The antimorphine effect of carbachol
persisted for 24 hr but was not evident at 72 hr.

Atropine (50 μg, icv) had no effect on responses to morphine, but antagonized the antimorphine effect of carbachol (Table 1). Naloxone did not
prevent the carbachol inhibition of responses to morphine.

Carbachol did not affect hypothermic responses to icv 5-hydroxytrypta-
mine or norepinephrine, but enhanced hypothermic responses to dopamine

58

from 0.6 ± 0.1 to 1.3 ± 0.2 °C. The antimorphine effect of carbachol was partially reversed by haloperidol (25 µg, icv) from a fall of only 0.4 ± 0.1 °C to 1.0 ± 0.3 °C.

TABLE 1

ATROPINE BLOCKADE OF CARBACHOL ANTIMORPHINE EFFECT

Pretreatments[a] (icv injections)		Temperature response (°C) to morphine (30 mg/kg sc)	N
Saline	Saline	-2.2 ± 0.4	10
Carbachol	Saline	-0.4 ± 0.2	9
Carbachol	Atropine	-1.2 ± 0.5	8
Saline	Atropine	-1.7 ± 0.3	10

[a]Saline 10 µl, carbachol 5 µg, atropine 50 µg; injections 2 hr apart.

SUMMARY

The thermoregulatory tolerance induced by carbachol was specific for morphine, persisted for at least 24 hr, and was associated with exaggerated responses to icv dopamine. The antimorphine effect of carbachol was inhibited by atropine and by haloperidol, but not by naloxone. The results suggest that the neurochemical alterations associated with thermoregulatory tolerance to morphine may be mimicked by carbachol through actions on mechanisms distal to the opiate receptor.

ACKNOWLEDGEMENTS

Supported by USPHS Grant DA00926. The technical assistance of Mrs. Peggy Gerba is gratefully acknowledged.

REFERENCES

1. Lotti, V.J., Lomax, P. and George, R. (1966) Neuropharmacology, 5, 35-42.

2. Rosenfeld, G.C. and Burks, T.F. (1977) J. Pharmacol. Exp. Ther., 202, 654-659.

3. Ary, M., Cox, B. and Lomax, P. (1977) J. Pharmacol. Exp. Ther., 200, 271-276.

4. Ary, M., Lomax, P. and Cox, B. (1977) Proc. West Pharmacol. Soc., 20, 375-380.

5. Pedigo, N.W., Dewey, W.L. and Harris, L.S. (1975) J. Pharmacol. Exp. Ther., 193, 845-852.

Characteristics and Function of Opioids, editors Van Ree and Terenius
© *1978 Elsevier/North-Holland Biomedical Press*

INHIBITION BY DICLOFENAC OF MORPHINE WITHDRAWAL DIARRHOEA IN THE RAT

D.L. FRANCIS, N.J. CUTHBERT AND H.O.J. COLLIER

Miles Laboratories Ltd., Stoke Poges, Slough, SL2 4LY, England.

We reported previously that prostaglandin (PG) E_2 inhibits the induction of morphine tolerance/dependence, when the isolated guinea-pig ileum is incubated overnight with morphine[1]. This observation, coupled with that of the supersensitivity of morphine-dependent ileum to PGE_1 and PGE_2[2], indicates an intimate relationship between PGE's and morphine dependence in the guinea-pig ileum. That a similar relationship might exist in the rat is suggested by the recent observation[3] -- that opioids specifically antagonise the secretion of fluid into the lumen of the jejunum in vivo, induced by intra-arterial infusion of PGE_1. We have now extended the exploration of the relationship of PG's to morphine dependence, by testing how far inhibitors of PG synthesis affect withdrawal signs, particularly diarrhoea, precipitated by naloxone in the dependent rat. For this purpose we chose diclofenac, because, of several non-steroidal anti-inflammatory drugs administered subcutaneously (s.c.) to rats and tested for ability to inhibit PG synthesis in brain ex vivo, diclofenac was outstandingly effective[4]. We also tested the effects of indomethacin.

Table 1 shows the effects of the lowest active doses of diclofenac or indomethacin on precipitated withdrawal. At $3.0 mg\ kg^{-1}$ both drugs significantly reduced the incidence of diarrhoea ($p < 0.05$) and at $30 mg\ kg^{-1}$ the difference was highly significant ($p < 0.001$). Over the dose range tested ($1-100 mg\ kg^{-1}$) the ED_{50} for inhibition of diarrhoea was $14.2 mg\ kg^{-1}$ for diclofenac and $13.1 mg\ kg^{-1}$ for indomethacin. At these doses no other signs of withdrawal were significantly affected although at high doses both drugs reduced the overall withdrawal score. Diclofenac at $100 mg\ kg^{-1}$ s.c. also reduced jumping. Given i.c.v. diclofenac did not affect any signs of withdrawal except ptosis, the incidence of which it reduced ($p < 0.01$).

That diclofenac, when given s.c. in fairly low doses, but not when given i.c.v. at the highest practicable dose, inhibited withdrawal diarrhoea suggests that PG's are involved in the peripheral mediation of this sign, i.e. in the gut. That indomethacin given s.c. is also effective supports this conclusion. This does not imply that withdrawal diarrhoea is without a central component, and, indeed, it has been shown that naloxone given i.c.v. precipitates all signs of withdrawal including diarrhoea[5]. We have confirmed this observation (Cuthbert & Francis, unpublished).

TABLE 1 EFFECTS OF DICLOFENAC OR INDOMETHACIN ON MORPHINE WITHDRAWAL

Drug	Dose mg kg^{-1} s.c.	Incidence of diarrhoea	Median No. jumps	Median withdrawal score
Vehicle[a]	–	94	–	3(2.5-4)
Diclofenac[a]	3.0	50**	–	3(2-4)
Indomethacin[a]	3.0	50**	–	3.5(2-4)
Saline[b]	–	92	2(1-6)	8(7.5-10)
Diclofenac[b]	100	25***	1.5(0-3)*	7(5-8)***

Rats made dependent on morphine (150mg kg^{-1}) in a slow-release preparation, were challenged 24h later with s.c. naloxone to precipitate withdrawal. a,- Diclofenac, indomethacin or vehicle was given s.c. 1h before naloxone (0.3mg kg^{-1}) and each rat was observed 0.5h after challenge, for 2 min. b,-Diclofenac or saline was given s.c. 1h before naloxone (1.0mg kg^{-1}) and immediately after challenge each rat was observed for 15 min. Numbers in brackets show the interquartile range. For significance of difference from controls, *, $p=0.06$; **, $p<0.05$; ***$p<0.001$.

Given i.c.v. (30 + 30μg rat^{-1}), diclofenac was without significant effect on any sign except ptosis. The failure of i.c.v. diclofenac to affect withdrawal might be interpreted in two ways: either that PG's are not involved in central withdrawal mechanisms or that diclofenac, given in this way, did not reach the appropriate site(s) of action.

Although acute experiments have shown an antagonism in the brain between PG's and opioids[6,7], the only evidence as yet of their involvement centrally in dependence is that of Weeks and Collins[8]. That a high systemic dose of diclofenac did reduce jumping, supports the view that there may be some antagonism between PG's and opioids centrally in the expression of abstinence. To pursue these studies further, it would seem necessary to inject diclofenac directly into these brain areas mediating withdrawal.

REFERENCES

1. Hammond, M.D., Schneider, C. and Collier, H.O.J. (1976) in Opiates and Endogenous Opioid Peptides, Kosterlitz, H.W. ed., Elsevier/North Holland, Amsterdam, pp.169-176.

2. Schulz, R. and Herz, A. (1976) Life Sci., 19, 1117-1128.

3. Coupar, I.M. (1978) Br.J.Pharmacol., 63, 57-63.

4. Halim, S.A., Sjöquist, B. and Anggard, E. (1976) Acta Physiol.Scand., Suppl. 440, 109.

5. Laschka, E., Herz, A. and Blasig, J. (1976) Psychopharmacologia,46,133-139.

6. Oltmans, G.A., Comaty, J.E. and Ehrenpreis, S. (1977) Abstracts, 7th Meeting, Society for Neuroscience, Anaheim, 3:299 (Abstr.No.957).

7. Ferreira, S.H., Lorenzetti, B.B. and Correa, F.M.A. (1978) Prostaglandins, 15, 703-704.

8. Weeks, J.R. and Collins, R.J. (1976) Prostaglandins, 12, 11-19.

Characteristics and Function of Opioids, editors Van Ree and Terenius
© *1978 Elsevier/North-Holland Biomedical Press*

STUDIES ON TOLERANCE DEVELOPMENT TO β-ENDORPHIN

J. P. HUIDOBRO-TORO AND E. LEONG WAY
Department of Pharmacology, University of California, San Francisco, USA

ABSTRACT
Tolerance to the analgetic effect of β-endorphin in mice develops within five hours after a single administration. Pretreatment with naloxone, dactinomycin or cycloheximide blocks tolerance development. An antinociceptive response can be elicited in β-endorphin-tolerant mice shortly after the animals recover from an analgetic dose of β-endorphin.

INTRODUCTION
β-Endorphin, an unitriakontapeptide with opiate-like activity, was isolated from the pituitary.[1] It has been found to be more potent than morphine as an analgetic.[2] After sustained β-endorphin administration, both primary tolerance[3] and physical dependence develop;[4] cross-tolerance and cross-dependence to morphine are also exhibited.[3,4] Since we previously noted that tolerance is demonstrable after a single dose of morphine,[5] it was of interest to perform similar studies with β-endorphin and to extend an earlier study reporting that the tolerance, which develops to the analgetic action of β-endorphin in the cat is reversible by 5-hydroxytryptophan (5-HTP).[6]

EXPERIMENTAL PROCEDURES
Adult male ICR mice were given an intracranial injection of β-endorphin and the analgetic response was determined by the tail-flick procedure. Percent analgesia was determined at repeated intervals until a return of the tail-flick latency to baseline. The results were plotted on coordinate paper and the area given by the curve (AA in cm^2) used as a quantitative measure of the degree of analgesia. After recovery (5 hours later) a second dose of β-endorphin was administered and the AA was redetermined. A significant decrease in the AA was considered to be evidence of tolerance development. The effect of several pharmacologic agents on the AA produced by the two doses of β-endorphin was then investigated.

RESULTS

A dose of 0.6 µg β-endorphin produced marked analgesia lasting about 5 hours. At this time of recovery, the administration of a second dose of β-endorphin resulted in a decreased antinociceptive response, the AA being decreased approximately 50 percent. Pretreatment with naloxone, 2 mg/kg s.c., antagonized the antinociception produced by β-endorphin and blocked the development of tolerance to β-endorphin. The administration of either dactinomycin (0.35 mg/kg i/p.) or cycloheximide (30 mg/kg i.p.) 30 minutes prior to the first dose of β-endorphin also reduced the development of tolerance to β-endorphin. In mice rendered tolerant to β-endorphin and just recovered from a dose of β-endorphin, 5-HTP, 80mg/ kgm i.p. produced transient antinociception. The latter effect could be elicited in animals only after tolerance had developed to β-endorphin and was not reversed by naloxone. Effects similar to those of 5-HTP were also produced by 5-hydroxytryptamine but to a lesser degree. It appears that the responsivity of pain pathways is altered by β-endorphin and 5-hydroxytryptamine may be involved. It also seems that the biochemical processes involved in the development of tolerance to β-endorphin resemble those of morphine.

ACKNOWLEDGEMENTS

The study was funded in part by The National Institute on Drug Abuse.

REFERENCES

1. Li, Citti and Chung, D., 1976, Proc. Nat'l. Acad. Sci., 73, 1145.

2. Loh, H.H., Tseng, L.F., Wei, E. and Li, C.H., 1976, Proc. Nat'l. Acad. Sci., 73, 2895.

3. Tseng, L.F., Loh, H.H., and Li, C.H. 1976, Proc. Nat'l. Acad. Sci., 73, 4187.

4. Wei, E., and Loh, H.H. 1976, Science, 193, 1262.

5. Huidobro, F., Huidobro-Toro, J.P. and Way, E.L., 1976, J. Pharmacol. Exptl. Therap., 198, 318.

6. Hosobuchi, Y., Meglio, M., Adams, J.E. and Li, C.H., 1976, Nature, 74, 4017.

Characteristics and Function of Opioids, editors Van Ree and Terenius
© *1978 Elsevier/North-Holland Biomedical Press*

INDUCTION OF MORPHINE TOLERANCE IN ISOLATED GUINEA PIG ILEUM

FRED A. OPMEER AND JAN M. VAN REE

Rudolf Magnus Institute for Pharmacology, University of Utrecht, Vondellaan 6, Utrecht (The Netherlands)

ABSTRACT

Tolerance developed when guinea pig ileum segments were exposed in vitro to morphine; this could be inferred from the diminished inhibition of electrically evoked contractions of strips prepared from these segments to a test dose of morphine. The inhibition of contractions after high frequency stimulation (HFS) was increased in these tolerant strips. Detailed experiments showed that the response to HFS could be used to quantitate the degree of in vitro-induced tolerance.

INTRODUCTION

The guinea pig ileum (GPI) has been shown to be a useful peripheral system for the study of acute and chronic effects of opioids. Morphine, by inhibiting the release of acetyl choline from myenteric neurones, diminishes the contractions evoked by electric field stimulation of the tissue. After being exposed to morphine in vitro[1], or in vivo[2] for longer periods, GPI preparations show signs of opiate tolerance and dependence. The present study deals with a quantitative assay for in vitro-induced tolerance and may contribute to elucidate the underlying mechanisms of tolerance development.

METHODS

GPI segments were exposed overnight to graded doses of morphine (0.08-80 µM) for 18-22h (20°C). GPI strips prepared from the segments were mounted in organ baths containing Krebs solution (37°C) with morphine at the same dose level as used for the overnight exposure. After 30 min equilibration, electric field stimulation (0.1 Hz, 0.7 msec) at a voltage giving submaximal twitch tension, was applied and the contractions were registered with a polygraph. The strips were then washed extensively. At various time intervals after the withdrawal of morphine, the inhibition of contraction was tested after a test dose of morphine (400nM) or after 10 Hz stimulation for 1 min (HFS). The inhibitory response (IR) was calculated by measuring the 1 min area of contractions preceding and following HFS or the addition of the test dose of morphine.

RESULTS AND DISCUSSION

The response of control strips to the test dose of morphine was constant for 2h (about 40% IR). The time course, starting after withdrawal, for the effect of this test dose on contractions of strips from GPI segments exposed overnight to 0.08, 0.8, 8 or 80 μM of morphine showed that the IR to morphine was less in these strips than in control strips and that it was gradually normalized. The reduced IR (tolerance) was related to the incubating dose, i.e.: the higher the incubating dose, the higher the tolerance level and the longer tolerance lasted. With a test dose of 500nM methionine enkephalin (ME) and tolerant strips (exposing dose: 80 μM of morphine) the IR did not differ significantly from the IR to the morphine test dose, indicating that cross-tolerance was present. The basal contractions were markedly inhibited after HFS. Puig et al[3] demonstrated the opiate-like nature of the electrically evoked inhibition by showing that naloxone substantially reversed the inhibition upon HFS. Accordingly, evidence is presented[4,5] for the presence of enkephalins in GPI and the release of opioid-like material from this tissue by HFS[6]. The IR of control strips following HFS remained constant for at least 2h (about 55%) and could be blocked partly (to about 70%) by adding naloxone (50nM) to the bath fluid prior to HFS. A substantially stronger inhibition upon HFS was observed in strips exposed overnight to morphine as outlined above. The increased IR was completely antagonised by naloxone, was related to the dose of morphine to which the GPI had been exposed and gradually disappeared. Whether the increased inhibition in tolerant strips was due to an increased release of opioid-like material or to a supersensitivity of the strip to endogenously released material or to other mechanisms is not yet understood. Furthermore, it is not clear whether tolerant strips are cross-tolerant to exogenously applied ME and whether ileum strips from guinea pigs made tolerant by morphine pellet implantation have a reduced IR to HFS[7]. The response to HFS is nevertheless reliable for quantifying the degree of in vitro-induced tolerance.

REFERENCES

1. Hammond, M.D., Schneider, C. and Collier, H.O.J. (1976) in Opiates and Endogenous Opioid Peptides, Kosterlitz, H.W. ed., Elsevier:North-Holland Biomedical Press, pp. 169-176.

2. Schulz, R. and Herz, A. (1976) Life Sci., 19, 1117-1128.

3. Puig, M.M., Gascon, P., Cravisio, G.L. and Musacchio, J.M. (1977) Science, 195, 419-420.

4. Elde, R., Hökfeldt, T., Johansson, D. and Terenius, L. (1976) Neuroscience, 1, 349.

5. Schulz, R., Wüster, M., Simantov, R., Snyder, S. and Herz, A. (1977) Eur. J. Pharmacol., 41, 347-348.

6. Hughes, J., Kosterlitz, H.W. and Sosa, R.P. (1978) Br. J. Pharmacol., 63, 397P.

7. Puig, M.M., Gascon, P. and Musacchio, J.M. (1977) Eur. J. Pharmacol., 45, 205-206.

Characteristics and Function of Opioids, editors Van Ree and Terenius
© *1978 Elsevier/North-Holland Biomedical Press*

THE INFLUENCE OF DRUG-RECEPTOR KINETICS ON THE PHARMACOLOGICAL AND PHARMACO-
KINETIC PROFILES OF BUPRENORPHINE

MICHAEL J. RANCE, AND JEAN M. DICKENS

Reckitt and Colman Pharmaceutical Division, Dansom Lane, Hull, HU8 7DS, U.K.

INTRODUCTION

We have previously reported[1] that the dissociation of buprenorphine from
stereo-specific binding sites in rat brain is slow, a result consistent with
the length of action of the highly lipophilic drug in animals[2] and man[3], and
with the relative difficulty with which the established effects of the drug
are reversed in vitro[4] and in vivo[2]. The present study was designed to
evaluate the influence of   in vivo drug-receptor interactions on the
pharmacokinetics of buprenorphine in rat with the objective of relating these
data to the unusual pharmacological profile of the drug.

MATERIALS AND METHODS

$[15,16 \text{ (n)} - ^3H]$ Buprenorphine (28 or 50 Ci/mmol   ) was prepared by the
Radiochemical Centre, Amersham. Brain levels of ^3H-buprenorphine (BUP) were
determined in male Sprague-Dawley rats (160-240g). Drugs were given intravenously into the tail vein in 0.9% saline $(1.0cm^3$ per 200g body weight). The
dose of BUP used was 20 $\mu g/kg^{-1}$, material of maximum specific radioactivity
being utilised. The effect of diprenorphine hydrochloride (DIP, 0.3mg kg^{-1}) on
brain levels of BUP was also investigated. For measurement of total and
stereospecifically bound ^3H-BUP, whole brains were removed following cervical
dislocation, the cerebella separated and both portions homogenised (10% w/v) in
ice-cold Tris buffer $(0.01\underline{M}$, pH 7.4) containing sucrose $(0.32\underline{M})$ and NaCl $(0.1\underline{M})$.
Total radioactivity was determined by combustion (Packard 306 oxidiser). After
dilution (x 5) with the same buffer, stereospecific binding was determined as
previously described[1]. Non specific binding was estimated by inclusion of
Triton X-100 (0.02%) in the diluted homogenate. Binding to cerebellum was used
as a check on this parameter.

RESULTS AND DISCUSSION

DIP significantly $(p < 0.001)$ reduced the level of stereospecific binding of
BUP when administered 15 min before, concurrently with or 15 min after ^3H-BUP
though the effect of the antagonist when administered after the ^3H-drug was
significantly reduced $(p < 0.001)$(Fig.1). A similar dependency on time of
administration of the antagonist was not seen 4 hr after ^3H-BUP administration.

66

The effect of DIP on rate of efflux of BUP from brain was determined by administration of the antagonist 2 hr after the labelled drug (Fig.2). The results
show that the high dose of DIP promoted a dissociation rate from the receptors
similar to that seen <u>in vitro</u> ($t_{\frac{1}{2}} \approx 60$ min). Total radioactivity ($> 90\%$ accounted
for as unchanged BUP) declined at a similar rate in the presence of the antagon-
ist indicating that, in this situation, drug-receptor dissociation appears to be
the rate limiting pharmacokinetic parameter.

It is interesting to speculate that such behaviour may result in the controlled elimination of BUP from receptors on cessation of chronic therapy with
the result that biochemical imbalances (e.g. increase in c-AMP[5]) produced as a
result of the removal of the inhibitory effects of the opiate will be minimised.
The separation of tolerance and dependence demonstrated in animals[2] and the
delayed, mild withdrawal syndrome seen in man[6] with BUP would be consistent
with the hypothesis.

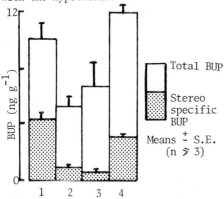

Fig.1 Effect of DIP (0.3mgkg^{-1}) on
brain levels of BUP: 1,No antagonist;
2, DIP at -15 min; 3, DIP at 0 min;
4, DIP at +15 min. BUP (20μgkg^{-1}) at
0 min. Brain levels measured at + 30
min.

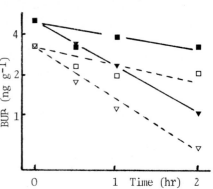

Fig.2 Effect of DIP on rate of
efflux of BUP from stereospecific
sites and from brain:BUP (20μgkg^{-1})
at -2 hr., DIP (0.3mgkg^{-1}) at 0 hr.
■, Total BUP; □, Stereospecific
BUP (no antagonist).▼,Total BUP;
▽, Stereospecific BUP(following
DIP). Results are means (n ⩾ 3).

REFERENCES

1. Hambrook, J.M., & Rance,M.J. (1976) in Opioids & Endogenous Opioid Peptides,
   H. W. Kosterlitz, ed., North Holland, Amsterdam, pp. 295-301.
2. Cowan,A., Lewis, J.W. and Macfarlane, I. R., (1977) <u>Br. J. Pharmac.,</u>
   60, 537-545.
3. Kay, B., (1978), <u>Br. J. Anaesth.</u>, 50, 599-603.
4. Shulz, R and Herz, A., (1976) in Opioids and Endogenous Opioid Peptides,
   H.W.Kosterlitz, ed. North Holland, Amsterdam, pp.319-326.
5. Sharma,S.K., Klee,W.A., and Nirenberg,M. (1975),<u>Proc.Natl.Acad.Sci.U.S.,</u>
   72, 3092-3096.
6. Jasinski,D.R.,Pevnick,J.S. and Griffith,J.D. (1978),<u>Arch.Gen.Psychiat.</u>,35,
   501-516.

Characteristics and Function of Opioids, editors Van Ree and Terenius
© *1978 Elsevier/North-Holland Biomedical Press*

THE INHIBITORY EFFECTS OF PRESYNAPTIC α-ADRENOCEPTOR AGONISTS ON THE
CONTRACTIONS OF THE GUINEA-PIG ILEUM AND MOUSE VAS DEFERENS IN THE
MORPHINE-DEPENDENT AND WITHDRAWN STATES

L.E. ROBSON, M.G.C. GILLAN, A.A. WATERFIELD and H.W. KOSTERLITZ
Unit for Research on Addictive Drugs, University of Aberdeen, Scotland

INTRODUCTION

   The inhibitory effects of adrenaline and dopamine, on the contractions of
the longitudinal muscle of the isolated ilea from guinea-pigs previously implanted with morphine pellets and suspended in morphine-free Krebs solution,
are smaller than those observed in preparations from control animals[1].   This
paper investigates possible interactions between the inhibitory effects due to
stimulation of presynaptic α-adrenoceptors and opiate receptors.

MATERIALS AND METHODS

   Guinea-pigs were implanted with 2 or 4 pellets of morphine base (150-300 mg).
After 3 days the ilea were mounted for coaxial stimulation (0.1 Hz, 0.5 ms,
maximal voltage) in Krebs solution containing 0.5-2 µM morphine.   The vasa
deferentia of mice implanted with 2 pellets were tested by field stimulation
under the same conditions.   The sensitivity to the inhibitory actions of clonidine, oxymetazoline or adrenaline on the evoked longitudinal contractions, was
tested before and after morphine was removed from the bath fluid.   0.4 µM (-)-
propranolol was added to the Krebs solution when adrenaline was used.

RESULTS

   In ilea from morphine-dependent guinea-pigs the IC_{50} values for clonidine,
tested in the presence of 1 µM morphine, (16.3 ± 1.0 nM; n = 14) did not differ from those obtained from non-implanted animals and tested in the absence of
morphine (16.8 ± 1.4 nM; n = 14).   When abstinence was mimicked by removal of
morphine from the Krebs solution, the effect of clonidine was almost abolished.
In the presence of 1 µM morphine the maximum reduction in the twitch tension by
clonidine was 1.66 ± 0.11 g (n = 14), in contrast to 0.66 ± 0.04 g (n = 14) in
the absence of morphine.   In preparations from non-implanted guinea-pigs, depression of 15-50% of the twitch by morphine did not alter the IC_{50} values for
clonidine.   Similar results were obtained with oxymetazoline.
   Replacement of morphine restored the effect of clonidine to its original

level. This effect was stereospecific because levorphanol, but not its inactive (+)-isomer dextrorphan, restored sensitivity to clonidine. The endogenous opioid peptides met- and leu-enkephalin could not be tested because of their instability but the analogues, Tyr-D-Ala-Gly-Phe-D-Leu[2] and Tyr-D-Ala-Gly-MePhe-Met(O)-ol[3], restored the sensitivity to clonidine.

The effect of removal of morphine from the bath fluid on the inhibitory effects of adrenaline was not so clear cut. In preparations from dependent guinea-pigs the IC_{50} value for adrenaline was about twice as high in the absence as in the presence of morphine, but in contrast to the flat curves obtained for clonidine and oxymetazoline after withdrawal of morphine, maximum inhibition was obtainable in the absence of morphine. The reduction in the effectiveness of adrenaline was more pronounced at low than at high concentrations.

This change in the effectiveness of clonidine was absent in vasa deferentia from implanted mice, even when withdrawal was effected by addition of naloxone.

CONCLUSIONS

Since the presynaptic opiate receptors and α-adrenoceptors are independently stimulated by their respective agonists[4], the observed interaction is probably beyond their recognition sites. This is possibly due to an increase in adenylate cyclase activity during the development of tolerance and dependence, as has been shown for mouse neuroblastoma X glioma hybrid cells[5]. In the presence of opiates this increased activity would be depressed and clonidine could exert its normal effect, but since in the withdrawn state opiate receptors are not activated, stimulation of the α-adrenoceptors would be much less effective. In this context, the recent observation that clonidine reduces the severity of the withdrawal syndrome in man[6], is of particular interest.

Supported by grants from the Medical Research Council, the U.S. National Institute on Drug Abuse and the U.S. Committee on Problems of Drug Dependence.

REFERENCES

1. Goldstein, A. and Schulz, R. (1973) Br. J. Pharmac., 48, 655-666.
2. Baxter, M.G., Goff, D., Miller, A.A. and Saunders, I.A. (1977) Br. J. Pharmac., 59, 455-456P.
3. Roemer, D., Buescher, H.H., Hill, R.C., Pless, J., Bauer, W., Cardinaux, F., Closse, A., Hauser, D. and Huguenin, R. (1977) Nature, 268, 547-549.
4. Kosterlitz, H.W. and Watt, A.J. (1968) Br. J. Pharmac., 33, 266-276.
5. Sharma, S.K., Klee, W.A. and Nirenberg, M. (1975) Proc. natn. Acad. Sci. U.S.A., 72, 3092-3096.
6. Gold, M.S., Redmond, Jr., D.E. and Kleber, H.D. (1978) Lancet, 1, 929-930.

Characteristics and Function of Opioids, editors Van Ree and Terenius
© *1978 Elsevier/North-Holland Biomedical Press*

MODE OF ANTAGONISTIC ACTION OF LEVALLORPHAN IN RATS DEPENDENT ON OPIOIDS

E. Tagashira, T. Izumi and S. Yanaura
Department of Pharmacology, Hoshi College of Pharmacy, Tokyo 142, Japan

INTRODUCTION

Hosoya[1], Wei et al.[2] and Yanaura et al.[3] have reported the dose-response relationship between the severity of abstinence signs and morphine antagonists when mice or rats in which was developed morphine (M) dependence were challenged with narcotic antagonists. This study was made to investigate the antagonistic action of levallorphan (Lev), or the Lev-challenged abstinence signs in the rats made dependent on M-type drugs by the drug-admixed food method (DAF method) developed in our department[3,4] from the standpoint of the dose of M and the lengths of its application and further from the timing for challenging with Lev following withdrawal of M; and furthermore, the role of the Lev-test in the physical dependence liability test and its limitations have been discussed.

MATERIALS AND METHODS

Male Sprague-Dawley rats (5 to 6 weeks old) were used in groups each of 6 animals. M and codeine (Cod) were applied by the DAF method. Exp. I: Two groups of animals were provided for each drug: one on M 0.5 and 1 mg/g food (average M intake: 60 mg/kg/day; M-L) and the other on M 1 and 2 mg/g food (average M intake: 100 mg/kg/day; M-H), and also one on Cod 0.5 and 1 mg/g food (Cod-L) and the other on Cod 1 and 2 mg/g food (Cod-H). The rats made M-dependent by application of M-L and M-H and those made Cod-dependent by application of Cod-L and Cod-H, both for 3 and 6 weeks, were challenged with Lev (2 and 5 mg/kg, s.c.) only once without withdrawal of the drugs, respectively. Exp. II: Of the four groups of M-dependent rats, one was left for natural withdrawal, but the other three received the application of Lev only once 6, 12 or 24 hours after withdrawal of M by replacing the DAF with normal food. Exp. III: The same animals received the application of Lev 3 times 0, 5 and 10 hours after withdrawal of M.

RESULTS

The alterations with Lev challenge (2 mg/kg, s.c.) in body weight of M-and Cod-dependent rats varying in the severity of drug dependence as the result of application of M-L, M-H, Cod-L and Cod-H for 3 or 6 consecutive weeks showed that both in the M- and Cod-dependent animals the maximum ratio of loss in body weight was elevated in dependence on the applied *amounts* of drug, but that no responses parallel with the *lengths* of drug application period occurred. Exp. II: Challenging with Lev after withdrawal of M was followed by the abstinence signs becoming weaker with the passage of time after the withdrawal. In other words, the abstinence sign induced by Lev challenge tended to be reduced with the disappearance of the *in vivo* M amount. When Lev challenge was made 24 hours after withdrawal of M, the abstinence signs were hardly intensified with Lev, despite the persistent severe abstinence signs in the group of natural withdrawal. Exp. III: When the same rats received the application of Lev 3 times, 0, 5 and 10 hours after withdrawal of M, the first challenge caused a 7% loss in body weight, but the second and the third application no longer caused a weight loss. Moreover, the animals showed gains in body weight from about 14 hours after withdrawal of M onwards despite the M withdrawal, and recovered already 24 hours after the withdrawal, which was very contrasting to the control rats in natural withdrawal.

SUMMARY

The results of the experiments may be summarized below:

(a) The antagonism between M or Cod and Lev which was seen in the rats receiving M or Cod continuously was rather intimately correlated with the dose of the agonist than with the length of its application period.

(b) The abstinence sign induced by Lev challenge in the physical dependence test was severest when the challenge with Lev was made without withdrawal of M or Cod (0 hour of withdrawal), which most facilitated the evaluation of dependence liability.

(c) The fact that the application of an antagonist to M-dependent rats at proper intervals to allow the antagonistic action to persist expedited the recovery of the animals from abstinence signs suggested the possibility of therapeutic effects of long acting antagonists on opioid addicts.

REFERENCES

1. Hosoya, E. (1975) in Methods in Narcotic Research, Ehrenpreis, S. and Neidle, A. eds., Marcel Dekker, pp. 261-291.
2. Wei, E., Loh, H.H. and Way, E.L. (1973) J. Pharmacol. Exp. Ther. 184, 398-403.
3. Yanaura, S., Tagashira, E. and Suzuki, T. (1975) Japan. J. Pharmacol. 25, 453-463.
4. Yanaura, S., Tagashira, E., Suzuki, T. and Izumi, T. (1975). Sixth Int. Cong. on Pharmacol., Helsinki, July 20-25, Abstract 1365.

Characteristics and Function of Opioids, editors Van Ree and Terenius
© 1978 Elsevier/North-Holland Biomedical Press

THE UPTAKE AND NALOXONE-SPECIFIC RELEASE OF MORPHINE FROM CORPUS STRIATAL
SLICES OF MORPHINE-DEPENDENT MICE

A. E. Takemori and Takafumi Kitano
Department of Pharmacology, University of Minnesota, Health Sciences Center,
Medical School, Minneapolis, Minnesota 55455 U.S.A.

INTRODUCTION

We recently reported that a specific portion of the morphine which had been
accumulated by corpus striatal slices of mice was released by superfusion with
solutions containing naloxone. Furthermore slices from morphine-dependent mice
were more sensitive to the naloxone-induced release of morphine than those of
control mice[1]. We proposed that the affinity of the opioid receptor in the
corpus striatum for naloxone is increased in morphine-dependent mice.

We now report herein additional evidence for an enhanced opioid receptor
affinity for naloxone which is associated with the development of tolerance and
dependence.

MATERIALS AND METHODS

Male, Swiss-Webster mice weighing 22-30 g were used. Accumulation of morphine by corpus striatal slices[2], the superfusion technic for the release of
^{3}H-morphine[1], the assessment of analgesia[3] and physical dependence[4] were described earlier.

RESULTS

Striatal slices in the presence of 10 nM ^{3}H-morphine accumulated morphine
and maximum T/M ratio of about 2 was reached after 30 min incubation. T/M ratio
decreased with increasing concentration of morphine up to 50 nM suggesting that
the uptake process was saturable below this concentration. During superfusion
of these slices with Krebs-Ringer bicarbonate solution, the introduction of
naloxone in the superfusion fluid, produced an immediate, transient increase
in the release of morphine from the slices. Preincubation of the slices with
levorphanol together with morphine decreased the subsequent amount of morphine
released by superfusion with naloxone but preincubation with dextrorphan had no
effect. The slices from morphine-dependent mice were more sensitive to this
naloxone-induced release of morphine than those from control animals. Using a
concentration range of 0.1 pM to 1 nM of naloxone in the superfusion, the half-

72

maximal release of morphine from slices of naive mice was observed at 7.5 pM while that of dependent animals occurred at 0.8 pM. Although the maximum amount of morphine released did not differ between slices from control and dependent mice, maximum release of morphine from slices of control mice was seen at naloxone concentrations of 10 nM while that of dependent mice was seen at 7.5 pM. The enhanced naloxone-induced release of morphine from striatal slices was evident in mice that had been implanted with morphine pellets for 24 hr. The enhancement was maximal 72 hr after morphine implantation, a time course similar to that of the development of tolerance and dependence. The enhancement was also observed in slices of acutely dependent mice which had received a single 100 mg/kg dose of morphine. The enhancement was no longer evident 5 days after morphine implantation. At this time substantial tolerance and dependence were lost but the mice still exhibited an appreciable amount of residual tolerance and dependence.

DISCUSSION

The confirmation of previous results strengthen the conclusion that the affinity for naloxone of striatal opioid binding sites is enhanced in morphine-dependent mice. There appeared to be a good temporal relationship between the development of tolerance and dependence and the enhanced affinity of naloxone by striatal slices but the relationship was not exact in the withdrawal phase. Perhaps this is related to the fact that striatal areas of brain are less sensitive than other areas e.g. medial thalamus, to the naloxone-precipitated withdrawal[5].

ACKNOWLEDGEMENT

This investigation was supported by U.S. Public Health Service Grant DA 00289.

REFERENCES
1. Kitano, T. and Takemori, A. E. (1977) Res. Comm. Chem. Path. Pharmacol. 18, 341-351.
2. Huang, J. T. and Takemori, A. E. (1976) Biochem. Pharmacol. 25, 47-51.
3. Hayashi, G. and Takemori, A. E. (1971) Eur. J. Pharmacol. 16, 63-66.
4. Way, E. L., Loh, H. H. and Shen, F. H. (1969) J. Pharmacol. Exp. Ther. 167, 1-8.
5. Wei, E., Loh, H. H. and Way, E. L. (1973) J. Pharmacol. Exp. Ther. 185, 108-115.

Characteristics and Function of Opioids, editors Van Ree and Terenius
© 1978 Elsevier/North-Holland Biomedical Press

ANTISERA TO PITUITARY HORMONES MODULATE DEVELOPMENT OF TOLERANCE TO MORPHINE

TJEERD B. VAN WIMERSMA GREIDANUS, HAIDI TJON KON FAT-BRONSTEIN AND JAN M.
VAN REE
Rudolf Magnus Institute for Pharmacology, Vondellaan 6, Utrecht (The Nether-
lands)

Various peptides of pituitary and/or hypothalamic origin affect avoidance
behaviour of rats by a direct action on the brain[1,2]. Evidence exists that some
of the peptides modulate behaviour by interference with memory processes[2,3]. In
this respect much attention has been paid to vasopressin and it has been argued
that vasopressin affects memory function by improvement of the storage of information in the brain (memory consolidation) as well as the retrieval of
stored information[4,5]. In addition, it has been shown that endogenous vasopressin is physiologically involved in these memory processes[3,5].

Development of tolerance can be regarded as a process related to learning
and memory or at least both development of tolerance and learning and memory
can be interpreted as similar adaptive phenomena. Krivoy et al. reported that
desglycinamide-lysine-8-vasopressin facilitates the development of resistance
to the analgesic action of morphine in mice[6] and it has been found that desgly-
cinamide-arginine-8-vasopressin facilitates the development of physical depen-
dance on morphine[7]. In addition De Wied and Gispen[8] observed a delayed development of tolerance in homozygous diabetes insipidus rats which lack the ability to synthesize vasopressin.

Therefore it was of interest to study the role of endogenous vasopressin
on development of tolerance to morphine in rats by intracerebroventricular
(icv) administration of antisera to vasopressin, which neutralize centrally
available vasopressin. Since not only antisera to vasopressin, but also antisera to prolactin enhance heroin-selfadministration behaviour in rats[9], this
latter antiserum was included in part of the present study as well.

The development of tolerance to morphine was studied in rats in an electric
footshock (EFS) test paradigm. Animals were tested for their responsiveness to
EFS by scoring the percentages of jerks, flinches or no responses, displayed
by the animal during a 8 min. session of 20 EFS's of different shock levels.
Two different ways of treatment schedules were used.

At first, rats received an initial intraperitoneal (ip) injection of either
saline or morphine (40 mg/kg), followed by a second injection of morphine

(10 mg/kg) 17 hr later. Thirty min. after the latter injection animals were tested for their responsiveness to EFS. Antisera to vasopressin or to prolactin, or normal rabbit serum as control, were icv injected (2 μl), either 1 hr after the first morphine injection (storage processes), or 30 min. prior to the second one (retrieval). Control animals showed ca. 30% no responses, 10% flinches and 60% jerks. An acute injection of morphine changed this pattern significantly, into ca. 30% no responses, 30% flinches and 40% jerks. After two morphine injections tolerance had been developed: the percentages no responses, flinches and jerks were similar to that in the controls. Administration of anti-vasopressin serum or anti-prolactin serum either after the first morphine injection or prior to the second one inhibited the development of tolerance to morphine; the rats displayed a similar responsiveness to EFS as after acute morphine treatment.

Secondly, morphine (30 mg/kg) or saline was injected once daily for 3 consecutive days, 20 min. prior to testing for the responsiveness to EFS. Anti-vasopressin serum or control serum (2 μl) was icv injected immediately after the EFS test on day 1 and 2. In controls development of tolerance to morphine was observed on day 2 and 3. However, animals treated with anti-vasopressin serum showed on day 2 and 3 a similar responsiveness to EFS as on day 1, indicating that tolerance did not develop in thus treated animals.

In summary neutralization of centrally available vasopressin or prolactin by specific antisera results in inhibition of development of tolerance to morphine. From these data it is concluded that endogenous vasopressin and prolactin are physiologically involved in the development of tolerance to morphine at the level of storage as well as retrieval of information.

REFERENCES
1. Wied, D. de (1977) Life Sci., 20, 195-204.
2. Wied, D. de and Gispen, W.H. (1977) in Peptides in Neurobiology, Gainer, H. ed., Plenum Press, New York, pp. 397-448.
3. Wimersma Greidanus, Tj.B. van and Wied, D. de (1977) in Biochemical Correlates of Brain Structure and Function, Davison, A.N. ed., Acad. Press, London, pp. 215-248.
4. Rigter, H., Riezen, H. van and Wied, D. de (1974) Physiol. Beh., 13, 381-388
5. Wimersma Greidanus, Tj.B. van and Wied, D. de (1976) Behav. Biol., 18, 325-333.
6. Krivoy, W.A., Zimmermann, E. and Lande, S. (1974) Proc. Nat. Ac. Sci., 71, 1852-1856.
7. Ree, J.M. van and Wied, D. de (1976) Life Sci., 19, 1331-1340.
8. Wied, D. de and Gispen, W.H. (1976) Psychopharmacologia, 46, 27-29.
9. Ree, J.M. van and Wied, D. de (1977) Life Sci., 21, 315-320.

Characteristics and Function of Opioids, editors Van Ree and Terenius
© 1978 Elsevier/North-Holland Biomedical Press

EFFECTS OF OPIOIDS ON SINGLE UNIT ACTIVITY

Walter Zieglgänsberger[*], George Siggins, Edward French, Floyd Bloom.   The Salk
Institute, La Jolla, CA 92037, U.S.A.

INTRODUCTION

Electrophysiologic research on opiates and opioid peptides has been primarily
extracellular, and more recently also intracellular, single unit recordings
directed at CNS areas with a high density of opiate receptors or involved with
nociception[1]. The interpretation of drug effects on neurones with systemic
injections can be partially avoided by employing the microiontophoretic technique. To document that responses of single neurones to opioids involve stereospecific opiate binding sites two tests have been relied upon: 1) blockade of
effects with an antagonist like naloxone; and 2) mimicry of actions by agonists
like levorphanol but not by its inactive D+ enantiomer, dextrorphan.

Most researchers employing microiontophoretic application of the opiate
alkaloids have also reported unspecific opiate actions. Such "local anesthetic-
like" effects are scarcely observed with the opioid peptides, but the latter
exhibit still other "non-specific" (i.e. naloxone-resistant) responses, especially in structures with low density of opiate receptors (e.g. cerebellum,
hippocampus[41,42]). In the following survey, special emphasis will be given
to stereospecific actions of opiates and opioids in the CNS.

Most of these stereospecific, naloxone-antagonisable actions are inhibitions
of single unit discharge which are qualitatively similar throughout the mammalian central and peripheral nervous system. However, some major exceptions
exist: naloxone-reversible excitatory responses were seen with pyramidal cells
in the hippocampus[2,3], Renshaw cells in the spinal cord and some less well
identified cells in various parts of the CNS[2,4-7]. The excitatory responses
of hippocampal neurones may now be viewed as a primary inhibitory effect resulting in excitation by disinhibition (see below).

CEREBRAL CORTEX: Only the frontal parts of the cortex contain relatively high
concentrations of opiate binding sites[8] and modest amounts of enkephalin-
immunoreactivity[9,10]. Neurones in this area are depressed by opiate agonists

[*]permanent address: Max Planck Institut für Psychiatrie, München, G.F.R.

via stereospecific opiate receptors[11-13]. Both spontaneous and chemically-
or synaptically-evoked activity were depressed. Like opiate alkaloids,
phoretically applied met- and leu-enkephalin depress spontaneous and l-glutamate
induced discharge of most units tested in this part of the cortex[14]. Prior
application of naloxone antagonized this depressant effect in the majority of
tests. The effects of the opiate alkaloid and the opioid peptide are qualitatively the same in most neurones (although some exceptions are described[4]).
Other parts of the cortex[6,15-17] may show lesser responsivity to opiates and
opioids because of the even lower density of opiate receptors.

STRIATUM: Besides some limbic structures, the striatum contains the highest
concentration of opiate binding sites[18], see also[19]. Its role in the pharmacological or physiological actions of opiates and opioid peptides remains
unclear. Striatal neurones are depressed by opioid and opiate agonists applied
microiontophoretically[2,15,20-22] or systemically[23,24]. The speeding of some
neurones in substantia nigra by systemic applications[25] would be in accord
with neurochemical evidence that opiates increase the synthesis and release
of dopamine at striatal nerve terminals, see[19]. Iontophoretic studies indicate
that the inhibitions produced by opioids or by dopamine are mediated by separate
receptors[20,21].

THALAMUS: Noxious thermal and mechanical stimulation excites cells in the
ventrobasal complex and the nucleus lateralis anterior of the thalamus. These
responses are depressed by phoretically or systemically administered opiates
or opioids[26-31]. Some of these effects were antagonized by systemic naloxone;
phoretically-applied antagonists gave strong spike blocking side-effects[32].
In contrast to the results in the rat[29], Duggan et al.[6] found that morphine
caused a naloxone-reversible enhancement of spontaneous and acetylcholine-
induced discharge activity of neurones in the cat ventro-basal thalamus (but
see data from medial thalamus[32]).

HIPPOCAMPUS: · The hippocampus of the rat contains a relatively low, patchy
density of opiate receptors[33]. Radioimmunoassay has shown low amounts of
enkephalin[34-36], whereas histochemical studies have displayed discrete fibers
containing enkephalin in this part of the limbic system[10]. It is not clear,
however, whether these fibers are intrinsic or project from other limbic
regions.

In contrast to most neurones in other regions of the rat's brain hippocampal pyramidal neurones are predominantly excited by phoretically and systemically applied opiate agonists and opioid peptides[2,3]. This excitatory effect is in accord with the excitatory[37] and seizure-inducing properties of systemically, topically and intraventricularly applied endorphines[38,39]. The excitation is clearly not due to an interaction with the muscarinic cholinergic input to pyramidal cells[40]. This type of hippocampal unit is the most frequently en-countered species when conventional multibarrelled electrodes were employed[2]. However, all hippocampus studies report both excitations and inhibitions to opioids. Because some authors were unable to antagonize these excitations with phoretically applied naloxone, the specificity of the opiate-related effects, and other unspecific actions remained uncertain[41,42]. Interestingly, on some hippocampal neurons, inhibitory effects were stereospecific, and toler-ance developed to the excitatory effect of opiate agonists in morphine tolerant/dependent animals[41].

Recent experiments employing single and simultaneous double unit recordings from hippocampal pyramidal and basket cells have revealed that some of the excitatory responses were brought about by naloxone-sensitive inhibitory actions of opiate agonists (morphine, met-enkephalin, D-ala^2-enkephalin, β-endorphin) on nearby basket cells leading to disinhibition of pyramidal cells. The exci-tatory responses were readily antagonized when naloxone was applied by a micro-pressure ejection system. The GABA-antagonist bicuculline speeded pyramidal cells, indicating that gaba-ergic, spontaneously activity interneurons may tonically depress pyramidal cell discharge activity. To test this hypothesis Mg^{2+} was applied phoretically to block synaptic transmission. Such applica-tions slightly decreased pyramidal cell spontaneous activity and also partly or completely blocked excitatory effects of opioid peptides. Sometimes, Mg^{2+} application converted excitatory responses of pyramidal cells into weak in-hibitions. Pyramidal cells give biphasic responses to stimulation of the contralateral hippocampus: a primary response consisting of a few spikes, fol-lowed by a discharge free interval due to basket cell mediated inhibition. This inhibitory phase can be overridden by phoretically applied met-enkephalin. This overriding action was not due to the excitatory effect, because acetyl-choline, which also excites pyramidal cells only shortens the duration of the inhibitions. These results indicate that the effects of a phoretically applied drug depend not only on the receptors involved but also on the circuitry in a given brain region (Figure 1). Results obtained by various groups in different sites in the brainstem have recently been extensively reviewed[1].

SPINAL CORD: a) Extracellular recordings. Although most neurones located in the dorsal horn of the spinal cord are involved in somatosensory perception or in processing nociception, neurones in lamina 1 and 5 are considered to play the major role in nociceptive processes, see[43,44]. There exists a close anatomical correlation of opiate binding sites in the dorsal horn of the spinal cord[8,33] and the enkephalin-containing small neurones in lamina 2 and 3[10,45-47]. The reports conflict as to the specificity of the observed effects, and whether opiate agonists selectively depress nociceptive responses and involve stereospecific opiate receptors in all cases[4,6,48-53]. Some but not all inhibitory responses to phoretically and systemically applied opiates and opioid peptides were antagonized by naloxone, whereas some – but not all – excitatory responses and other effects were obviously not mediated via stereospecific opiate receptors.

The dorsal horn neurones are particularly sensitive to inhibition when the opiate agonists are applied to the lamina 2 and 3 (corresponding to the substantia gelatinosa of Rolandi[4,6,51]). The mechanism of these inhibitory effects is unknown. The data would support a primary distal dendritic action of opiates, although an excitatory action on inhibitory interneurons in this layer or an effect directly on primary afferent terminals cannot now be excluded. A hypothetical scheme (Fig. 2) summarizing the findings of systemic and phoretic studies obtained by different groups (see[1]) on dorsal cord proposes that enkephalinergic cells in this structure may modulate all cells subserving somatosensory perception, not simply those subserving pain responses.

The first published data on actions of microiontophoretically applied opiates on single units was that on Renshaw cells in the ventral horn of the spinal cord[54-56]. These cells which mediate the recurrent inhibition of motoneurones are most likely not involved directly in nociception but might play a role in the expression of nociceptive responses. Recent studies showed that excitations induced by opiate alkaloids[5] are mimicked by opiate peptides and are stereospecific[4,6,7]. This excitatory effect seems to be a unique property of these specialized interneurones because here naloxone also antagonizes the excitatory (nicotinic) actions of acetylcholine.

b) Intracellular studies on dorsal horn neurones: Early studies of morphine agonists in the spinal cord showed that intravenous administration depressed polysynaptic EPSPs (excitatory postsynaptic potential). This effect was re- duced by opiate antagonists[57,58]. More recent studies employing intracellular recording and simultaneous extracellular microiontophoretic application re- vealed that morphine and opioid peptides do not change membrane potential or resting membrane resistance[22,52]. Nevertheless, opiates still decrease the rate of rise of the postsynaptic excitatory potential in motoneurones, inter- neurones and neurones in the dorsal horn involved in somatosensory perception. Antagonism by naloxone and inactivity of dextrorphan in these tests indicate stereospecificity.

Some clarification of these various opiate actions may be gained from a consideration of the mechanisms by which dorsal horn neurones are activated by sensory stimuli[22,52]. The synaptic pattern of noxious versus non-noxious activation is usually different: moving hairs in the restricted peripheral fields of lamina 4 type neurones causes a fast rising EPSP with a high synaptic safety margin, whereas activation brought about by heating this area causes a slowly increasing depolarization consisting of slow-rising EPSPs[52]. Opiates cause a naloxone-reversible decrease of the rate of rise of EPSPs in spinal neurones[52]. Such an effect would certainly influence the heat-induced response in the same neurone more readily than the excitation evoked by the fast rising EPSP. This hypothesis is supported by the finding that the primary response following dorsal root stimulation is much less readily affected by phoretically applied opiates than the late response. The inhibitory effects of opiate agonists upon certain sensory stimuli might, therefore, depend on the rate at which EPSPs rise towards the threshold rather than on the membrane potential.

In addition to synaptic activation, opiates and opioids also depress the l-glutamate induced depolarization[52]. As far as cat spinal neurones are con- cerned microiontophoretically applied l-glutamate is considered to cause an increase of the permeability of the postsynaptic membrane to sodium ions[59]. It is postulated therefore that the opiates interfere with the chemically excitable sodium channel comparable to those also operated by synaptically released excitatory transmitters. The fact that these depolarizing responses are clearly antagonized by opiate agonists indicates that the opiate receptors involved in this effect are located on the postsynaptic membrane.

The in vivo antiglutamate actions have recently been confirmed with spinal neurones grown in tissue culture[60]. The analysis of the kinetics of the action indicates that the inhibitory action of the opiate peptides are brought about by a "non-competitive mechanism" on the postsynaptically located sodium-ionophore. A similar interpretation was also suggested by effects of opiates upon the depolarizing response to DA seen in neuroblastoma/glioma hybrid cells[61].

Concerning the topographic location of the opiate receptor there are few data. In a study in murine neuronal cell cultures employing the statistical analysis of the synaptic responses it was shown that etorphine, a powerful opiate agonist,depresses monosynaptic EPSPs via presynaptic opiate receptors[62]. Rhizotomy at the spinal cord level reduces the opiate binding in the spinal cord to about 50%[63]. Although transsynaptic changes cannot be excluded, these data suggest presynaptic opiate receptive sites. Recent studies employing electrophysiological techniques in the spinal cord of cats (Calvillo et al., personal communication) and dorsal root ganglia explants also seem to involve presynaptically located receptors[64]. In the latter study the primary location of opiate receptive sites was demonstrated in the processes of the dorsal root ganglia cells. It remains totally obscure as to how the sodium ionophore in the postsynaptic membrane is linked to the opiate receptor. Possibly the pre- and the postsynaptic receptive mechanisms involve similar ionic processes, which may be more easily detected in tissue culture preparations with their lower degree of differentiation. In a most recent study, systemically applied morphine was found to produce a weak but rather selective decrease of the antidromic excitability of C-fibers (Zieglgänsberger et al., in preparation).

MYENTERIC PLEXUS: The analgesic potency of opiates correlates with their depressant effect upon the electrically induced twitch of the guinea-pig ileum and is accurately reflected in single unit studies[65-71]. The stereospecific depressant effect can be seen also in Ca^{++}-free/high Mg^{++} solution, indicating a postsynaptic effect[72,73]. Gut is relatively rich in enkephalins, and the peptide produces actions identical to opiates: hyperpolarizing actions occasionally associated with decreased input resistance[74]. This effect is superficially at variance to the data obtained in central neurones[22,52]. Although a different ionic mechanism cannot be excluded, two reasons speak in favour of a common mechanism. First, the hyperpolarizing response to enkephalin becomes smaller as the basal membrane potential of myenteric plexus cells becomes more negative (the central neurones had initial membrane potentials in the range -60 to -70 mV) and second, non-linearity in the current/voltage characteristic (anomalous rectification) may then account for the fall in membrane input resistance seen in a few neurones.

TOLERANT AND DEPENDENT ANIMALS: When animals are pretreated with increasing doses of morphine for several days, the primarily inhibitory responses[11-13] of cortical and striatal[14,22] neurones are either absent or are inverted into naloxone insensitive excitatory responses. Increased sensitivity to the excitatory effects of opiates also occurs in Renshaw cells[7]. Cross tolerance seems likely between morphine and the opioid peptides, while the sensitivity to phoretically administered l-glutamate and acetylcholine was markedly increased in these animals[75].

CONCLUDING REMARKS

The most frequently observed response of single unit activity to phoretic application of opiate agonists is a naloxone-reversible depression of the firing rate mediated by postsynaptically located opiate receptors. There are a few important exceptions: e.g. the hippocampus, where the behaviorally significant excitatory effect is the result of the intrinsic specific circuitry and yet the basic primary cellular mechanism is most likely the same (inhibition) as in other brain areas. The excitatory responses in Renshaw cells seem stereospecific and even more unique in that acetylcholine induced excitations are also antagonized by naloxone. The possible involvement of additional presynaptic opiate receptors in the dorsal spinal cord, interfering with the release of transmitters, is suggested by histochemical and biochemical studies[8,33,63,64,76] but this part of the nervous system still resists more elaborate electrophysiological exploration.

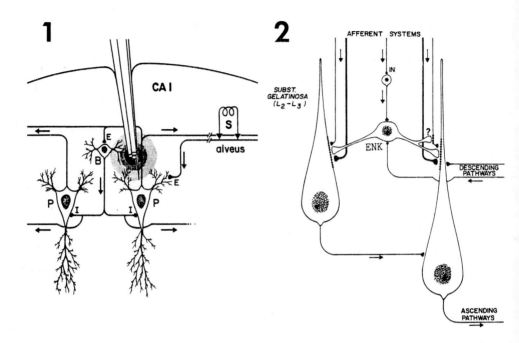

Figure 1: Schematic illustration of the circuitry most likely responsible for the excitatory response of the hippocampal neurones to opiate agonists. Tonically active gaba-ergic interneurones (basket cells, B-cells) are postulated to inhibit pyramidal cells (P-cells). B-cells are synaptically activated by recurrent collaterals of P-cells. Phoretically applied opiate agonists reach both P-cells and B-cells. A depressant effect of these compounds on B-cells results in an excitatory response of P-cells due to disinhibition. Evidence in favor of this hypothetical scheme is presented in text.

Figure 2: Hypothetical scheme of an enkephalinergic mechanism in which neurones in the substantia gelatinosa Rolandi (L_2–L_3) control neurones involved in somatosensory perception (L_4–L_5). The small bipolar, enkephalinergic (ENK) neurone impinges together with large and small diameter excitatory fibers (afferent systems) on dendrites of L_4 and L_5 cells. Inhibitory interneurones (IN) have to be postulated to make the C-fiber input to subst. gel. Rolandi neurones inhibitory[77]. Descending pathways can act directly on L_4 and L_5 cells or on ENK-containing cells. Evidence in favor of such a model: Systemical-ly[78–80] and microiontophoretically applied opiate agonists decrease firing of L_4 and L_5 neurones[1]. Assuming that these enkephalinergic neurones were in the sample recorded by Cervero et al.[77], cells in L_4 and L_5 would be under a tonic inhibitory influence, which could be modulated by pathways involving partial naloxone-sensitive mechanisms. The question mark indicates the possibility that systemically applied opiates can decrease antidromic excitability through a selective mechanism on C-fiber afferents.

REFERENCES

1. Zieglgänsberger, W. and Fry, J. (1978) in Development in Opiate Research, Herz, A. ed., Marcel Dekker, New York.

2. Nicoll, R.A., Siggins, G.R., Ling, N., Bloom, F.E. and Guillemin, R. (1977) Proc. Natl. Acad. Sci. U.S.A., 75, 1591.

3. Hill, R.G., Mitchell, J.F., Pepper, C.M. (1976) J. Physiol. (Lond.) 272, 50-51.

4. Davies, J. and Dray, A. (1978) Brit. J. Pharmacol. 63, 87-96.

5. Davies, J. and Duggan, A.W. (1974) Nature New Biol. 250, 70-71.

6. Duggan, A.W., Davies, J. and Hall, J.G. (1976) J. Pharmacol. exp. Ther. 196, 107-120.

7. Davies, J. (1976) Brain Res. 112, 311-326.

8. Pert, C.B., Kuhar, J.J. and Snyder, S.H. (1974) in: The Opiate Narcotics, Pergamon Press, New York, pp. 97-101.

9. Uhl, G.R., Kuhar, M.J. and Snyder, S.H. (1977) Proc. Natl. Acad. Sci. (U.S.A.) 74, 4059-4063.

10. Hökfelt, T., Elde, R., Johansson, O., Terenius, L. and Stein, L. (1977) Neuroscience Letters 5, 25-31.

11. Satoh, M., Zieglgänsberger, W., Fries, W. and Herz, A. (1974) Brain Res. 82, 378-382.

12. Satoh, M., Zieglgänsberger, W. and Herz, A. (1975) Life Sic. 17, 75-80.

13. Satoh, M., Zieglgänsberger, W. and Herz, A. (1976) Brain Res. 115, 99-110.

14. Zieglgänsberger, W., Fry, J.P., Herz, A., Moroder, L. and Wünsch, E. (1976) Brain Res., 115, 160-164.

15. Frederickson, R.C.A. and Norris, F.H. (1976) Science, 194, 440-442.

16. Stone, T.W. (1973) Life Sci., 13, 123-133.

17. Biscoe, T.J., Duggan, A.W. and Lodge, D. (1972) Brit. J. Pharmacol., 46, 201-212.

18. Kuhar, M.J., Pert, C.B. and Snyder, S.H. (1973) Nature (Lond.), 245, 447-450.

19. Herz, A. (1978) Development in Opiate Research, Marcel Dekker, New York.

20. Bradley, P.B. and Gayton, R.J. (1976) Brit. J. Pharmacol., 57, 425-426.

21. Gayton, R.J. and Bradley, P.B. (1976) in: Opiates and Endogenous Opioid Peptides, Kosterlitz, H.W. ed., Elsevier/North-Holland Biomedical Press, Amsterdam, pp. 213-219.

22. Zieglgänsberger, W. and Fry, J.P. (1976) in: Opiates and Endogenous Opioid Peptides, Kosterlitz, H.W. ed., Elsevier/North-Holland, Biomedical Press, Amsterdam, The Netherlands, pp. 213-238.

23. Bigler, E.D. and Eidelberg, E. (1976) Life Sci., 19, 1399-1406.

24. Chan, S.H.H., Lee, C.M. and Wong, P.C.L. (1977) Fed. Proc., 36, 668.

25. Iwatsuto, K. and Clouet, D.H. (1977) J. Pharm. exp. Ther., 202, 429.

26. Frederickson, R.C.A., Norris, F.H. and Hewes, C.R. (1975) Life Sci., 17, 81-82.

84

27. Hill, R.G., Pepper, C.M. and Mitchell, J.F. (1976) Nature (Lond.) 262, 604-606.

28. Hill, R.G., Pepper, C.M. and Mitchell, J.F. (1976) in: Opiates and Endogenous Opioid Peptides, Kosterlitz, H.W. ed., Elsevier/North-Holland Biomedical Press, Amsterdam, pp. 225-230.

29. Hill, R.G. and Pepper, C.M. (1976) Brit. J. Pharmacol., 58, 459-460.

30. Hill, R.G. and Pepper, C.M. (1977) J. Physiol. (Lond.), 269, 378.

31. Hill, R.G. and Pepper, C.M. (1977) in: Microiontophoresis and Transmitter Mechanisms in the Mammalian Central Nervous System, Ryall, R.W. and Kelly, J.S. eds., Elsevier/North-Holland Biomedical Press, Amsterdam.

32. Duggan, A.W. and Hall, J.G. (1977) Brain Res., 122, 49-57.

33. Atweh, S.F. and Kuhar, M.J. (1977) Brain Res., 129, 1-12.

34. Simantov, R. and Snyder, S.H. (1976) in: Opiates and Endogenous Opioid Peptides, Kosterlitz, H.W. ed., Elsevier/North-Holland Biomedical Press, Amsterdam, The Netherlands, pp. 41-48.

35. Hong, J.S., Yang, H.-Y., Fratta, W. and Costa, E. (1977) Brain Res., 134, 383-386.

36. Wesche, D., Höllt, V. and Herz, A. (1977) Naunyn-Schmiedeberg's Arch. Pharm., 301, 79-82.

37. Chou, T. and Wang, S.C. (1976) Fed. Proc., 35, 357.

38. Henriksen, S.J., Bloom, F.E., Ling, N. and Guillemin, R. (1977) Abstract, Society for Neurosciences, p. 293.

39. Teitelbaum, H., Blosser, J. and Catravas, G. (1976) Nature (Lond.), 260, 158-169.

40. French, E.D., Siggins, G.R., Henriksen, S.J. and Ling, N. (1977) Abstract, Society for Neurosciences, p. 291.

41. Fry, J., Zieglgänsberger, W. and Herz, A. (1978) J. Physiol., p. 21.

42. Segal, M. (1977) Neuropharmacology, 16, 587-592.

43. Yaksh, T.L. and Rudy, T.A. (1977) J. Pharm. Exp. Ther., 202, 411-428.

44. Yaksh, T.L. and Rudy, T.A. (1978) Pain, 4.

45. Elde, R., Hökfelt, T., Johansson, O. and Terenius, L. (1976) Neuroscience, 1, 349-351.

46. Simantov, R., Kuhar, M.J., Uhl, G.R. and Snyder, S.H. (1977) Proc. Natl. Acad. Sci. (U.S.A.), 74, 2167-2171.

47. Watson, S.J., Akil, H., Sullivan, S. and Barchas, J.D. (1977) Life Sci., 21, 733-738.

48. Calvillo, O., Henry, J.L. and Neuman, R.S. (1974) Canad. J. Physiol. Pharmacol., 52, 1207-1211.

49. Henry, J.L. and Neuman, R.S. (1974) Proc. Canad. Fed. Biol. Soc., 17, 158.

50. Neuman, R.S., Calvillo, O. and Henry, J.L. (1974) Pharmacologist, 26, 203-208.

51. Duggan, A.W., Hall, J.G. and Headley, P.M. (1976) Nature (Lond.), 264, 456-458.

52. Zieglgänsberger, W. and Bayerl, J. (1976) Brain Res., 115, 111-128.

53. Belcher, G. and Ryall, R.W. (1977) in: Microiontophoresis and Transmitter Mechanisms in The Mammalian Nervous System, Ryall, R.W. and Kelly, J.S. eds., Elsevier/North-Holland Biomedical Press, Amsterdam.

54. Curtis, D.R. and Duggan, A.W. (1969) Agents and actions, 1, 14-19.

55. Duggan, A.W. and Curtis, D.R. (1972) Neuropharmacology, 11, 189-196.

56. Felpel, L.P., Sinclair, J.G. and Yim, G.K.W. (1970) Neuropharmacology, 9, 203-210.

57. Jurna, I. (1966) Int. J. Neuropharmacol., 5, 117-123.

58. Jurna, I., Grossmann, W. and Theres, C. (1973) Neuropharmacology, 12, 983-993.

59. Zieglgänsberger, W. and Puil, E.A. (1972) Exp. Brain Res., 17, 35-49.

60. Barker, J.L., Neale, J.H., Smith, T.G., Jr. and Macdonald, R.L. (1978) Science, 199, 1451-1453.

61. Myers, P.R., Livengood, D.R. and Shain, W. (1975) Nature (Lond.), 257, 238-240.

62. Macdonald, R.L. and Nelson, P.G. (1978) Science, 199, 1449-1451.

63. LaMotte, C., Pert, C.B. and Snyder, S.H. (1976) Brain Res., 112, 407-412.

64. Hiller, J.M., Simon, E.J., Crain, S.H. and Peterson, E.R. (1978) Brain Res., 145, 396-400.

65. Dingledine, R., Goldstein, A. and Kendig, J. (1974) Life Sci., 14, 2299-2309.

66. Dingledine, R. and Goldstein, A. (1975) Life Sci., 17, 57-62.

67. Dingledine, R. and Goldstein, A. (1976) J. Pharmacol. exp. Ther., 196, 97-106.

68. Sato, T., Takayanagi, I. and Takagi, T. (1973) Jap. J. Pharmacol., 23, 665-671.

69. North, R.A. and Henderson, G. (1975) Life Sci., 17, 63-66.

70. North, R.A. (1976) Neuropharmacology, 15, 1-9.

71. North, R.A. and Tonini, M. (1976) in: Opiates and Endogenous Opioid Peptides, Kosterlitz, H.W. ed., Elsevier/North-Holland Biomedical Press, Amsterdam, pp. 205-212.

72. North, R.A. and Williams, J.T. (1976) Nature (Lond.), 264, 460-461.

73. North, R.A. and Williams, J.T. (1977) Fed. Proc., 36, 3667.

74. Smith, T.W., Hughes, J., Kosterlitz, H.W. and Sasa, R.P. (1976) in: Opiates and Endogenous Opioid Peptides, Kosterlitz, H.W. ed., Elsevier/North-Holland Biomedical Press, Amsterdam, pp. 57-62.

75. Satoh, M., Zieglgänsberger, W. and Herz, A. (1976) Naunyn-Schmiedeberg's Arch. Pharmak. exp. Path., 293, 101-103.

76. Jessel, T.M. and Iversen, L.L. (1977) Nature, 268, 549-551.

77. Cervero, F., Molony, V. and Iggo, A. (1977) Brain Res., 136, 565-569.

78. Besson, J.M., Wyon-Maillard, M.C., Benoist, J.M., Conseiller C. and Hamann, K.F. (1973) J. Pharmacol. exp. Ther., 187, 239-245.

79. Le Bars, D., Menetrey, D., Conseiller, C. and Besson, J.M. (1973) Brain Res., 98, 261-277.

80. Le Bars, D., Guilbaud, G., Jurna, I. and Besson, J.M. (1976) Brain Res., 115, 518-524.

Characteristics and Function of Opioids, editors Van Ree and Terenius
© *1978 Elsevier/North-Holland Biomedical Press*

ENKEPHALIN: PHARMACOLOGIC EVIDENCE FOR DIVERSE FUNCTIONAL ROLES IN THE
NERVOUS SYSTEM USING PRIMARY CULTURES OF DISSOCIATED SPINAL NEURONS

J.L. Barker, D.L. Gruol, L.M. Huang, J.H. Neale and T.G. Smith

Laboratory of Neurophysiology, NINCDS, NIH, Bethesda, Maryland and

Department of Biology, Georgetown University, Washington, D.C., U.S.A.

INTRODUCTION

The effects of opiate alkaloids and opioid peptides on neuronal function
have been studied by many investigators using a variety of preparations and
techniques. Pharmacologic actions in various bioassays have been highly
correlated with binding constants to stereospecific receptor sites in the
same tissues, suggesting that opiate and opioid actions are mediated
through engagement of specific receptors.[1,2] . Those who have examined the
effects of the opiates and opioids on neuronal physiology at the cellular
level have used intact central or peripheral nervous system preparations.
The experiments have generated an initial level of phenomenology, demonstrating
effects in a variety of regions in the nervous system.[3] Study of the mechanisms of opiate or opioid action in the nervous system at the cellular or
membrane level using electrophysiological techniques in vivo is difficult
owing to the inherent complexity and heterogeneity of the CNS and to technical difficulties. Thus, the level of resolution attained has not
allowed complete characterization of the mechanisms of action. We have
utilized mammalian spinal neurons grown in tissue culture as an in vitro
model to study the mechanisms of opioid peptide action at the membrane
level. The preparation consists of growing dissociated spinal neurons
derived from mouse embryos for more than four weeks under tissue culture
conditions, after which time the cells are large enough to permit hours-
long, stable intracellular recordings. Such stability not only allows
fine control over experimental manipulations but also provides relatively
high resolution of membrane events. Since primary cultures grow as virtual
monolayers, they represent definite, but unknown departures from the
normal organization of the nervous system and thus their appropriateness as
"models" of CNS physiology naturally invites doubt. These cultures do
not appear useful in elucidating mechanisms requiring a physiologically
organized population of neurons. At present, the preparation's major
attraction is for studying mechanisms at membrane and monosynaptic levels.
The preparation exhibits excitability[4], spontaneous synaptic activity[5]

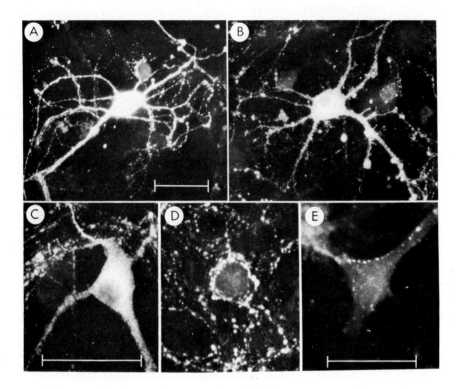

Fig. 1. Dissociated spinal neurons grown in tissue culture which exhibit
fluorescence, reflecting reactivity to anti-met[5]-enkephalin antibody. Both
cell bodies and processes show fluorescence (A and B) with reactivity likely
being intracellular, since nuclear regions are only weakly fluorescent
(B and C). Closer inspection reveals a granular nature to the fluorescence
(C). Fluorescent processes often invest the cell body and proximal processes of unreactive neurons in an intimate manner (D and E). From reference
10. Copyright, The American Association for the Advancement of Science,
1978.

and paroxysmal depolarizing events when convulsants are added[6]. All of the
spinal cord cells thus far studied show sensitivity to putative inhibitory
and excitatory amino acids and individual cells possess a definite topography of chemosensitivity[5,7]. These observations do not appear to differ
from those using intact CNS preparations[8]. Furthermore, a variety of
clinically important anesthetics, anticonvulsants and convulsants can modulate specific amino acid responses,[6,9] results consistent with those obtained
using intact preparations. These observations suggest that neuronal physiology
at the single cell level has been preserved in culture and that certain
classes of receptors for endogenous and exogenous ligands are present.

We have further examined the cultures for their suitability in studying the cellular mechanisms of opioid peptide effects by searching for evidence of 1) opioid peptide receptors, 2) opioid peptide-containing neurons and 3) opioid peptide synthesis. We have found binding of labeled D-ala-methionine enkephalinamide in a stereospecific manner, the specific binding accounting for about 80% of the total peptide bound and increasing some 20-fold over the four week developmental period in culture (J.H. Neale, K. Blank and J.L. Barker, unpublished observations). Using immunohistochemical techniques we have observed that 1-3% of spinal neurons in a given culture stain positively for either leucine- or methionine-enkephalin (Fig. 1).[10] These enkephalinergic neurons do not appear to show any distinctive morphological characteristics. The cultures also exhibit viability in biochemical terms as demonstrated by their ability to incorporate labeled methionine into met^5-enkephalin. The results show labeling of met^5-enkephalin in nanomole quantities, as well as secretion of met^5-enkephalin into the medium (J.F. McKelvy, J.H. Neale and J.L. Barker, unpublished observations). These observations indicate that primary cultures of dissociated spinal neurons possess both opioid peptides and receptors and thus would appear to be appropriate to study what roles these peptides and their receptors play in neuronal function.

MATERIALS AND METHODS

Neurons were dissociated from spinal cords dissected from 13 day-old mouse embryos and grown in tissue culture according to methods previously described[4,7]. Intracellular recordings using one or two microelectrodes were made from spinal neurons with somata 20-30 μ in diameter on the modified stage of an inverted phase microscope at 250X magnification. Leucine^5-enkephalin (ENK) (obtained from Pierce Chemical or generously supplied by Dr. B.A. Morgan of Reckitt and Colman), naloxone (from Dr. W.A. Klee), γ-aminobutyric acid (GABA), glutamate, and glycine (all from Sigma Chemical) were iontophoresed from extracellular pipettes closely positioned at the surface of the cell under study. The peptide and naloxone were iontophoresed with cationic current from 10 mM solutions at pH 4, while the amino acids were applied with current of the appropriate polarity from 1 M solutions. $MgCl_2$ was added to the recording media to suppress spontaneous synaptic activity and allow clearer examination of post-synaptic pharmacology.

RESULTS

A variety of opioid peptide effects on membrane properties have been observed and studied using cultured spinal cord neurons. It should be emphasized that none of the observations to be discussed has been characterized completely. For convenience, the peptide actions will be divided into those which directly alter membrane excitability and those which indirectly affect membrane excitability through modulation of neurotransmitter responses.

Direct Effects on Membrane Properties

Transmitter-like Effects. We have observed two actions of ENK which appear to be neurotransmitter-like. An excitatory response, observed in about 10% of the cells studied, was characterized by a dose-dependent, rapid depolarization which triggered action potentials (Fig. 2A). The time course of the response appeared to be considerably faster than that of the putative amino acid neurotransmitter glutamate, which elicited excitatory responses on 100% of the spinal cord neurons tested.[7] Iontophoretic pulses of glutamate and ENK applied to different areas of the cell surface revealed a non-uniform topography of sensitivity for both, with glutamate responses observed on the cell body and processes[7] and ENK responses apparently restricted to the cell body. The ENK response rapidly desensitized during sustained application, unlike that evoked by glutamate which did not desensitize. The extrapolated inversion potentials of the ENK and glutamate responses were similar, averaging about -4 mV, which suggests a role for Na^+ ions in both responses. Another ENK response, inhibitory in nature, was observed in about one-third of the cells studied. It consisted of a slowly developing membrane hyperpolarization which took several seconds to plateau and which was associated with an increase in membrane conductance (ca. 20%) (Fig. 2B). The response was depolarizing when recording with KCl electrodes, suggesting a role for Cl^- ions in the responses. Both the excitatory and inhibitory responses were depressed by naloxone on a number of occasions, suggesting that specific receptors mediate the responses. The results indicate that two actions of ENK on cultured CNS neurons appear to be similar to those of putative neurotransmitters in that they involve activation of a receptor-coupled conductance which is independent of membrane potential.

Abrupt Depolarizations. An unusual effect of ENK, observed in about 10% of cells studied, consisted of a dose-dependent, reversible abrupt depolarization[11] (Fig. 3A1). In some cells these events triggered action potentials. Under voltage clamp an abrupt increase in inward current associated with a

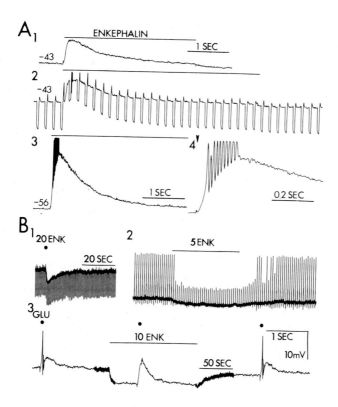

Fig. 2. Transmitter-like effects of enkephalin on cultured spinal neurons. KAc recordings from two different cells. A. Depolarizing responses to ionto- phoresis of 50 nA leu-enkephalin (marked by bar above traces or downward arrowhead) develop rapidly and desensitize almost completely during sustained application. At -56 mV the response is <u>excitatory</u>, eliciting a brief burst of spikes, while at -43 mV, with spikes inactivated, the response is simply depolarizing. The increase in membrane conductance, manifested by the decrease in voltage response to -0.8 nA-50 msec current stimuli, which is evident at the peak of the response, partly reflects the voltage-dependent nature of membrane conductance. B. Hyperpolarizing responses to iontophoretic pulses (B1) or steps (B2,3) of leu-enkephalin develop slowly and are maintained during the application period. The potential change is accompanied by a 10-15% increase in membrane conductance. The response is <u>inhibitory</u>, suppressing spikes evoked both by suprathreshold, 0.1 nA-50 msec current stimuli (B2) and by 30 nA-100 msec pulses of glutamate (B3). Resting potential: -48 mV.

large conductance increase was seen (Fig. 3B) which did not fade during

sustained peptide application. These events were sometimes preceded either

by a slowly developing, low amplitude depolarization associated with a

decrease in membrane conductance (Fig. 3) or by the neurotransmitter-like

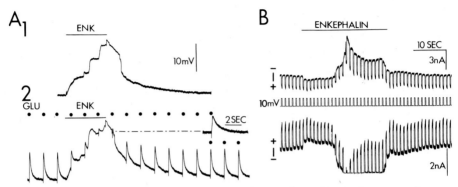

Fig. 3. Abrupt depolarizing events induced on cultured spinal neurons by enkephalin. KCl recordings from two different neurons. A1. Iontophoresis of 50 nA leu-enkephalin leads to a gradual, low-amplitude depolarization which is abruptly followed by membrane depolarization in discrete steps. The membrane repolarizes both slowly and abruptly following cessation of peptide iontophoresis. A2. Superimposition of 40 nA-50 msec glutamate pulses (black dots) before, during and after ENK iontophoresis show a marked, reversible attenuation of depolarizing glutamate responses during the peptide-induced depolarization. The depression cannot be accounted for by the depolarization per se since the glutamate response at the depolarized potential under control conditions is considerably larger than that evoked during the peptide iontophoresis (see inset). Membrane potential: -80 mV. B. Under voltage clamp, 100 nA ENK, sufficient to produce an abrupt depolarizing event under unclamped conditions, causes an initial decrease in both inward holding current and membrane conductance, followed by an abrupt increase in inward current and conductance. Membrane current is shown at low (upper trace) and high gain (bottom trace), with upper trace inverted. Middle trace shows holding potential of -80 mV with superimposed 10 mV-100 msec depolarizing commands.

effects described above. The abrupt depolarizations were not reversed by naloxone on three occasions tested. They effectively attenuated responses to putative inhibitory and excitatory neurotransmitters[11] (Figs. 3A2). Thus, the peptide appears to change qualitatively the membrane properties of some neurons.

Elevation of Spike Threshold. In a number of cells studied the peptide directly depressed excitability by elevating threshold for action potential generation in a dose-dependent, reversible manner with little, if any detectable effects on resting membrane properties (Fig. 4). Excitability was assessed by stimulating with brief, constant-current depolarizing pulses sufficient to evoke action potentials. The observed alteration in threshold occurred within seconds of peptide iontophoresis, did not fade and disappeared within 5-10 seconds following cessation of iontophoresis. On several cells tested the depressant effect of the peptide was reversed with

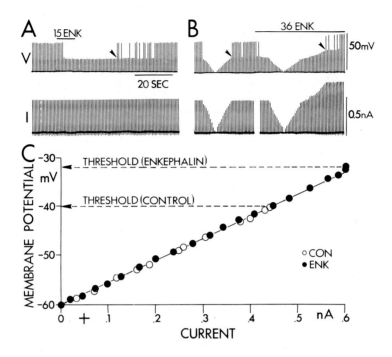

Fig. 4. Enkephalin elevates threshold for action potential generation in
a cultured spinal neuron. KAc recording. Cell excitability assessed using
suprathreshold 0.4 nA-50 msec depolarizing current pulses. Voltage traces
above current traces. A. Iontophoresis of 15 nA ENK (marked by bar above
voltage trace) rapidly blocks action potential generation evoked by current
pulses without detectable change in resting membrane potential. The
depression clearly outlasts the iontophoretic application. Arrowhead del-
ineates suprathreshold (spike) from subthreshold responses. B. Iontophoresis of 36 nA ENK blocks current-evoked excitation. Increasing amplitude of current pulse reveals elevation in spike threshold without change
in the current-voltage relations of the membrane. C. Plot of voltage
response to depolarizing currents of increasing amplitude demonstrates
similar current-voltage relations and membrane slope conductance in control
and during ENK iontophoresis.

co-iontophoresis of naloxone. In contrast, the putative inhibitory amino
acids GABA and glycine did not alter spike threshold, but rather depressed
excitability indirectly by hyperpolarizing the membrane potential and moment-
arily increasing the membrane's conductance to Cl$^-$ ions. Peptide-induced
elevation of spike threshold would provide a subtle yet effective means of
depressing excitability.

94

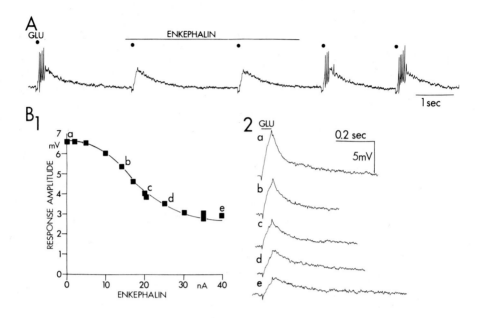

Fig. 5. Enkephalin depresses glutamate voltage responses on cultured spinal neurons. KAc recordings from two different cells. A. Continuous trace of membrane potential showing depolarizing responses to 40 nA-50 msec pulses of glutamate (black dots) which evoke spikes. Frequency responses of pen-writer attenuates spike amplitude. Iontophoresis of 20 nA ENK (marked by bar above trace) rapidly and reversibly blocks excitatory effect of glutamate without affecting resting membrane properties. Resting potential: -54 mV. B. ENK depression of depolarizing response to 25 nA-50 msec glutamate pulse is dose-dependent but incomplete with maximal depression being about 50%. Data plotted in B1, specimen records in B2. A slowing of the response time course is evident at higher ENK currents. Membrane potential: -80 mV. From reference 12. Copyright, The American Association for the Advancement of Science, 1978.

Indirect Effects on Membrane Properties

Modulation of Amino Acid Responses. ENK depressed the excitatory effects of putative amino acid neurotransmitter glutamate in a dose-dependent, reversible manner, independent of any other effects on membrane properties (Fig. 5A)[12]. Although this depression was observed in the majority of the cells studied, glutamate responses insensitive to the peptide were also seen (see Fig. 7A). When present, the peptide effect was evident within seconds of the beginning of the iontophoretic application. Glutamate responses were never completely abolished by the peptide, maximal depression averaging close to 50% of control amplitude (Fig. 5B). Peptide-depressed glutamate responses usually exhibited slower time courses relative to control responses

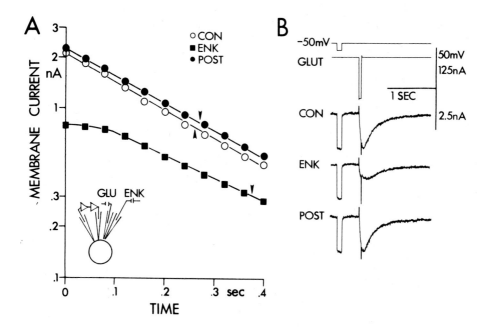

Fig. 6. Enkephalin depresses glutamate-evoked membrane current response and slows its time course without changing resting membrane conductance. Cell impaled with two KCl microelectrodes and membrane potential voltage-clamped; glutamate and leu-enkephalin iontophoresed from extracellular microelectrodes (schematic insert in A). B shows experimental paradigm with potential clamped to -50 mV and a 10 mV-100 msec hyperpolarizing command superimposed, followed by a 100 nA-100 msec glutamate pulse. Membrane current responses to voltage command and glutamate pulse are illustrated before (CON), during (ENK) and after (POST) iontophoresis of 20 nA ENK. ENK depresses the glutamate-evoked current response without changing the amplitude of current response to the voltage command. Current from peak of response is plotted semi-logarithmically in A. Time constant of glutamate current response decay (marked by arrowhead) increases during ENK iontophoresis. Modified from references 11 and 12. Reproduced with permission of the American Association for the Advancement of Science and of the Elsevier Publishing Company.

(Figs. 5B,6). The depressant effects were partially reversible with co-iontophoresis of naloxone.[12] Pharmacological analysis of the effects of ENK on glutamate dose-response curves revealed a complex interaction which does not appear to involve the glutamate binding site. The depression was not due to a change in the driving force underlying the glutamate responses nor was the depression voltage-dependent. Although the physiology of enkephal-inergic neurons is unknown, it is clear from these pharmacologic experiments

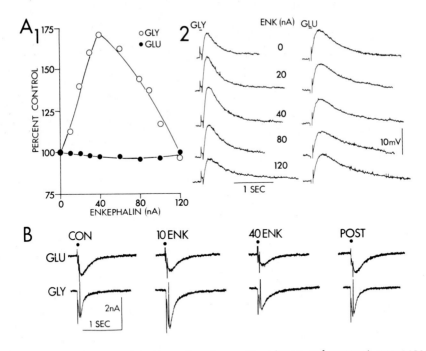

Fig. 7. Enkephalin modulation of amino acid voltage and current responses on cultured spinal neurons. KCl recordings from two different cells. A. Modulation of voltage response to 20 nA-50 msec glycine pulse is dependent on ENK iontophoretic current with enhancement at low and moderate ENK current. ENK has little effect on response to 30 nA-50 msec glutamate pulse. Normalized data plotted in A1 with specimen records in A2. Glycine response is depolarizing when recording with KCl microelectrodes. Membrane potential: -65 mV. B. Potential clamped to -70 mV and membrane current responses to 25 nA-50 msec glutamate and 40 nA-50 msec glycine pulses examined before (CON), during iontophoresis of 10 and 40 nA ENK and following recovery (POST). The response to glutamate is depressed in a dose-dependent manner by ENK, while the response to glycine is enhanced at the lower, and depressed at the higher ENK current, relative to control.

that ENK can modulate the subsynaptic actions of a neurotransmitter-coupled event without itself activating ionic conductances like a transmitter.

ENK also altered membrane responses to the two putative inhibitory amino acid neurotransmitters, GABA and glycine[11]. GABA responses were usually depressed by ENK in a dose-dependent, reversible manner. Glycine responses were either enhanced by ENK in a dose-dependent, reversible manner or enhanced at low, and depressed at high iontophoretic current applications of the peptide. The effects were seen independent of direct peptide actions on membrane properties (Fig. 7). The time course of the modulatory effects and the apparent lack of desensitization were similar to those described for the ENK-glutamate interaction. On a few occasions where ENK had both direct and indirect effects, the GABA or glycine inversion potential was shifted approximately 5 mV. Thus, some of the peptide "modulation" of GABA and glycine responses may be indirectly mediated through an alteration in the Cl⁻ ion gradient. Since we have seen direct depressant effects of naloxone on the GABA and glycine responses, the question of naloxone reversibility is difficult to answer.

DISCUSSION

   The pharmacological evidence presented in this paper indicates that ENK can alter the membrane properties of spinal neurons in a variety of ways. Of the three types of direct effects described the first type -- membrane receptor-coupled conductance increases associated with excitatory or inhibitory responses which occur largely independent of membrane potential and are reversed by a specific antagonist, naloxone -- appears to fall within the classical definition of neurotransmitter action[13]. Thus, the peptide may mediate excitatory or inhibitory transmission at specific synapses in the CNS. The fast time course and rapidly desensitizing nature of the excitatory response contrasts with that observed with the putative amino acid neurotransmitter glutamate, suggesting that ENK-mediated transmission would be short-lived relative to glutamate-mediated events. The second type of direct effect consisted of an unusual membrane depolarization we have labeled an "abrupt depolarization." It is unclear whether this effect falls within the definition of neurotransmitter action and, if such an event occurs physiologically, exactly how it would act to alter excitability. Perhaps such an event is involved in the epileptic activity evoked by ENK[14]. The third direct effect -- depression of excitability through elevation of spike threshold which is reversed by naloxone -- indicates that ENK can change the voltage at which activation of the voltage-dependent conductances underlying the spike occurs. Direct effects of peptides on voltage-dependent pacemaker and spike conductances in invertebrate nervous systems have been reported and previously characterized as neurohormonal to distinguish them from neurotransmitter actions[15]. ENK effects on spike threshold may fall into this neurohormonal category. Other examples of neurohormonal-like actions on voltage-dependent conductances not mediated by peptides include epinephrine[16] and acetylcholine[17] regulation of pacemaker and spike conductances of cardiac muscle, and norepinephrine and acetylcholine depression of spike conductances of sympathetic neurons[18,19]. Thus, substances which serve as neurotransmitters at one site may also act as neurohormones at other sites. The indirect effects of ENK on the amino acid responses fall outside the definitions of neurotransmitter and neurohormone actions since they involve modulation of neurotransmitter-activated conductances and occur irrespective of any direct effects on resting membrane conductance. We have chosen to call this type of effect neuromodulation[12]. ENK modulation of glutamate responses was reversed with naloxone[12]. However, naloxone depression of glycine and GABA responses prevented simple interpretation of the naloxone-sensitivity of this type of modulation by ENK. Neuromodulation would allow fine control of synaptic efficacy at specific synapses in the CNS.

In conclusion, the data presented show that an opioid peptide is potentially capable of acting as either a neurotransmitter, neurohormone or neuromodulator. Whether the same or different receptors are associated with the three different functions and whether met[5]-enkephalin also acts in multiple ways remains to be determined.

REFERENCES

1. Kosterlitz, H.W. (1976) Opiates and Endogenous Opioid Peptides, Elsevier, Amsterdam, pp. 1-380.

2. Costa, E. and Trabucchi, M. (1978) The Endorphins, Raven Press, New York, pp. 1-367.

3. Frederickson, R.C.A. (1977) Life Sci., 21, 23-42.

4. Ransom, B.R. et al. (1977) J. Neurophysiol. 40, 1132-1150.

5. Ransom, B.R. et al. (1977) J. Neurophysiol. 40, 1151-1162.

6. Macdonald, R.L. and Barker, J.L. (1978) Neurology, 28, 325-330.

7. Barker, J.L. and Ransom, B.R. (1978) J. Physiol. (in press).

8. Krnjevic, K. (1974) Physiol. Rev. 54, 418-530.

9. Macdonald, R.L. and Barker, J.L. (1978) Science, 200, 775-777.

10. Neale, J.H. et al. (1978) Science, (in press).

11. Barker, J.L. et al. (1978) Brain Res., (in press).

12. Barker, J.L. et al. (1978) Science, 199, 1451-1453.

13. Katz, B. (1966) McGraw-Hill, New York.

14. Urca, G. et al. (1977) Science, 197, 83-86.

15. Barker, J.L. and Smith, T.G. (1977) in Biological Approaches to Neurons, Neuroscience Symposia Vol. II, Cowan, W.M. and Ferendelli, J.A., eds., Society for Neuroscience, Bethesda, Md. pp. 340-373.

16. Tsien, R.W. (1974) J. gen. Physiol., 64, 293-305.

17. Giles, W. and Noble, S.J. (1976) J. Physiol., 261, 103-123.

18. Horn, G. and Macafee, J. (1978) Soc. Neurosci. Abst., (in press).

19. Kuba, K. and Koketsu, K. (1976) Jap. J. Physiol., 26, 703-716.

Characteristics and Function of Opioids, editors Van Ree and Terenius
© *1978 Elsevier/North-Holland Biomedical Press*

SINGLE NEURONE STUDIES OF OPIOID TOLERANCE AND DEPENDENCE

J.P. FRY, W. ZIEGLGÄNSBERGER AND A. HERZ
Department of Neuropharmacology, Max-Planck-Institut für Psychiatrie, Kraepelinstrasse 2, D-8000 München 40 (F.R.G.)

INTRODUCTION

Opiates and opioid peptides have been shown to decrease the sensitivity of neurones to putative excitatory transmitter substances
in several regions of the vertebrate nervous system. Tolerance
appears to develop to these inhibitory actions, whether the opioids
are administered systemically[1,2] or in the immediate vicinity of
the neurone through a microelectrophoretic pipette[3]. An attempt
has been made to investigate the mechanisms underlying such homeostatic adjustments in the neurone, by studying the changes in
chemical sensitivity that occur upon withdrawal of the opioid. Specificity of the effects observed has been checked by employing
stereoisomers of the opiate antagonist naloxone.

MATERIALS AND METHODS

Male Sprague-Dawley rats (250-350 g) were anaesthetised with a
mixture of α-chloralose and urethane (90 and 300 mg/kg respectively, i.p.), and prepared[2] for recording from the frontal cerebral
cortex and rostral striatum. For some experiments, the animals were
made highly tolerant/dependent to morphine by the s.c. implantation
of 6 pellets, each containing 75 mg morphine base[2]. They were used
on the 10-12th days after the start of implantation.

RESULTS AND DISCUSSION

In morphine tolerant/dependent rats, as compared to naive animals, a higher proportion of frontal cortical and striatal neurones
responded to microelectrophoretic application of naloxone: excitatory responses, associated with increases in the activity evoked
by L-glutamate and acetylcholine, occured more frequently during
application of the drug with low phoretic currents of up to 40 nA/
1-2 min and were elicited only by the (-)-isomer, whereas the application of naloxone with higher currents (40-160 nA) and for
longer periods often resulted in depressant actions, shared by both
(+)- and (-)-enantiomers.

100

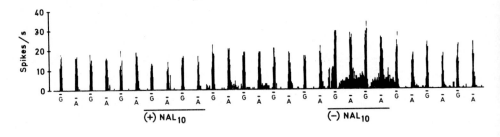

Fig. 1 Local withdrawal of a striatal neurone in a morphine toler-
ant/dependent rat by the microelectrophoretic application of (-)-
naloxone (current in nA) during which the spontaneous activity of
the neurone increases, as does that evoked by L-glutamate (G:30 nA)
and acetylcholine (A:20 nA). Application of (+)-naloxone has a
slight depressant effect.

The reason for the higher incidence of non-specific depressant
effects of naloxone in morphine tolerant/dependent rats remains unclear. Naloxone induced increases in spontaneous and/or L-gluta-
mate- and acetylcholine-induced activity, however, appear to represent specific withdrawal effects at the single neurone level. The
present results, therefore, indicate that the development of tolerance and dependence to opioids involves homeostatic adjustments in
the chemical excitability of the postsynaptic membrane and that
such changes are revealed as supersensitivity to excitatory transmitters upon withdrawal of the opioid.

REFERENCES

1. Zieglgänsberger, W. and Fry, J.P. (1978) in Developments in
   Opiate Research, A. Herz ed., Marcel Dekker, New York, pp.
   193-239.

2. Satoh, M., Zieglgänsberger, W. and Herz, A. (1976) Brain
   Research, 115, 99-110.

3. Fry, J.P., Zieglgänsberger, W. and Herz, A. (1978) in Micro-
   iontophoresis and Transmitter Mechanisms in the Mammalian
   Central Nervous System, Ryall, R.W. and Kelly, J.S. eds.,
   Elsevier/North-Holland Biomedical press, Amsterdam, pp. 323-325.

Characteristics and Function of Opioids, editors Van Ree and Terenius
© *1978 Elsevier/North-Holland Biomedical Press*

MET-ENKEPHALIN AND D-ALA^2-MET-ENKEPHALINAMIDE EFFECTS ON DORSAL HORN UNITS IN THE CAT

JAMES L. HENRY

Department of Research in Anaesthesia, McGill University, Montreal (Canada)

INTRODUCTION

The recent discovery of endogenous peptides with opiate-like properties, the first being termed "Met-enkephalin"[1], and the resemblance of their distribution in the spinal cord to that of opiate receptors[2] prompted the suggestion that these peptides functioned perhaps as part of a descending modulatory pathway to inhibit transmission early in nociceptive afferent pathways, ie: in the spinal dorsal horn. As part of an examination of this possibility, an earlier study[3] was extended to determine the effects of Met-enkephalin on single dorsal horn units in the lumbar spinal cord of chloralose-anaesthetised cats.

METHODS

Details of the preparation of cats, the type of electrodes and the classification of units are found elsewhere[4]. Solutions for iontophoresis included Met-enkephalin (ME, 5mM in 165mM NaCl, pH 5.5, Peninsula Labs), D-Ala^2-Met-enkephalinamide (DAME, 5mM in 165mM NaCl, pH 5.5, Lilly Research Labs), 165mM NaCl acidified to pH 5.5 (to detect artifacts due to changes in current or pH at the electrode tip), Na-L-glutamate (1M, pH 7.4, Sigma) and Morphine HCl (25mM, pH 4.8, BDH). Some sites of recording were marked with Pontamine Sky Blue, and histological sections were checked for dye marks.

RESULTS

The iontophoretic application of ME and DAME induced a current-related and reproducible depression of the on-going discharge rate of 17/46 and 12/17 units, respectively (figs 1&2). Characteristically, depression began within 20 sec and reached its maximum at 30-60 sec. With both peptides, this depression occurred only with units classified as nociceptive, non-nociceptive units remaining unaffected. Each peptide also depressed the responses of nociceptive units to noxious stimuli applied to the skin. Generally, the units depressed by these peptides were also depressed by morphine, although often greater current was required through the morphine barrel to induce the same magnitude of depression. While the two peptides had effects which were generally similar, there were also differences. ME caused excitation of 3 units, while this was not seen with DAME. Comparison of the typical responses of the two peptides (figs 1 & 2) shows a difference in the patterns of the depressant effects: ME induced a depression which in most cases was reversed before the end of the application; DAME induced a depression which was not readily reversible in time, but rather persisted for periods sometimes exceeding one hour. Naloxone, administered i.v. (0.1 mg/kg), antagonized the responses of 4/4 units depressed by ME and 2/4 units depressed by DAME. In the two cases where DAME-induced depression was not antagonized, the depressant effect persisted even after additional naloxone, to 0.3 mg/kg.

DISCUSSION

The similarity of the depressant effects of ME and DAME to those of morphine[3], especially the specificity of effects on nociceptive units and the reduction of their responses to noxious cutaneous stimuli, and the reversibility of some of these responses by naloxone suggest an action by ME and DAME on an "opiate receptor". The difference in the persistence of the effects of the two peptides may be due to a more rapid catabolism of ME. The irreversibility of the effects of DAME in two cases suggests a stronger binding of this peptide than either morphine or ME. The evidence from this study provides further evidence that ME may be involved in endogenous mechanisms reducing transmission of nociceptive information and that central modulation of nociception occurs in the spinal cord.

ACKNOWLEDGMENTS

Supported by the Canadian MRC, the Québec MRC and Lilly Research Laboratories. The author is a Chercheur-Boursier of the Québec MRC.

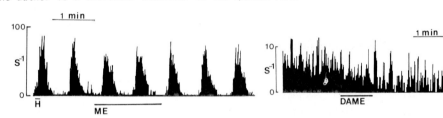

Fig. 1. Ratemeter record in impulses/sec of single nociceptive unit responding to periodic applications of noxious radiant heat to the skin. Unit was depressed by application of ME with 100 nA of current.

Fig. 2. Ratemeter record of single nociceptive unit depressed by 100 nA of DAME.

REFERENCES
1. Hughes,J., Smith,T., Morgan,B. & Fothergill,L.(1975) Life Sci. 16:1753-1758.
2. Hokfelt,T., Ljundahl,A., Terenius,L., Elde,R. & Nilsson,G. (1977) Proc. Nat. Acad. Sci., USA 74:3081-3085.
3. Calvillo,O., Henry,J.L. & Neuman,R.S. (1974) Can. J. Physiol. Pharmacol. 52: 1207-1211.
4. Henry,J.L. (1976) Brain Res. 114:439-451.

Characteristics and Function of Opioids, editors Van Ree and Terenius
© *1978 Elsevier/North-Holland Biomedical Press*

MORPHINE AND NALOXONE EFFECTS ON SUBSTANCE P EXCITATION
IN CAT SPINAL DORSAL HORN

JAMES L. HENRY

Department of Research in Anaesthesia, McGill University, Montréal (Canada)

INTRODUCTION

Iontophoretic application of substance P[1] and of morphine[2] to single units in cat spinal dorsal horn have both been shown to have effects specifically associated with units classified as nociceptive on the basis of their responses to natural cutaneous stimulation. Substance P causes excitation of these units[1], morphine causes depression[2]. In addition, responses of these units to noxious stimuli applied to the skin are facilitated by substance P[1] and depressed by morphine[2]. In view of the parallel in the specificity of these agents and the fact that "opiate receptors" are found in the dorsal horn[3], the present study was done to investigate the possibility that the substance P effects might be due to an action on these opiate receptors: the effects on substance P excitation of the i.v. administration of morphine or naloxone were studied.

METHODS

Cats were anaesthetized with alpha-chloralose (60 mg/kg i.v.). The spinal cords, from L_5-L_7, were exposed for recording and iontophoresis, and were transected at the L_1 level to eliminate influences from supraspinal structures. Details of recording extracellular single unit spikes and classification of units are found elsewhere[1]. The experimental protocol was basically that substance P was applied by iontophoresis in the lumbar dorsal horn; when a unit was found which was excited by this application, morphine (2.8-3.2 mg/kg) or naloxone (0.1 mg/kg) was given i.v. Substance P was then applied again to determine whether the response persisted.

RESULTS

The iontophoretic application of substance P had a delayed, slow and prolonged excitatory effect specifically on nociceptive units, as has been reported previously[1]. Morphine reduced the on-going discharge rate of 4/4 units but failed to abolish the substance P-induced excitation. An example of responses to substance P before and after the administration of morphine is given in Fig. 1. Naloxone also failed to abolish the excitatory response to substance P (5/5). A typical response is shown in Fig. 2. In three cases the response to substance P appeared greater after naloxone was given than before.

DISCUSSION

The failure of either morphine or naloxone to abolish the excitatory response to substance P suggests that the peptide is unlikely to be acting on an "opiate receptor", for which both morphine and naloxone would be competing. The depressant effect of morphine on the on-going activity of the nociceptive units is consistent with earlier observations[4], and suggests that substance P and the opiates were acting ultimately on the same units, but that their actions were via different mechanisms. In fact, the evidence from the present study is not inconsistent with the suggestion of Jessell and Iversen[5] that the opiates may be having an inhibitory effect presynaptically on substance P terminals. Interpretation of the facilitation of substance P excitation is difficult on the basis of iontophoretic studies but it may suggest an additional action of naloxone in the spinal cord independent of opiate receptors.

ACKNOWLEDGMENTS

Supported by grants from the Canadian MRC and the Québec MRC. The author is a Chercheur-Boursier of the Québec MRC.

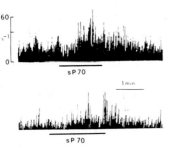

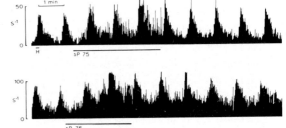

Fig. 1. Ratemeter record (impulses/sec) of single nociceptive unit excited by substance P (sP, 70 nA) both before (upper record) and after 2.4mg/kg morphine i.v.

Fig. 2. Ratemeter record of single unit responding to periodic applications of heat (H) to the skin. Substance P caused excitation of this unit before (upper record) and after (lower record) 0.1 mg/kg naloxone i.v.

REFERENCES

1. Henry,J.L. (1976) Brain Res. 114:439-451.
2. Calvillo,O., Henry,J.L. & Neuman,R.S. (1974) Can. J. Physiol. Pharmacol. 52: 1207-1211.
3. Lamotte,C., Pert,C.B. & Snyder,S.H. (1976) Brain Res. 112:407-412.
4. Calvillo,O., Henry,J.L. & Neuman,R.S. (1976) in Advances in Pain Research and Therapy, Vol; 1, Bonica,J.J. & Albe-Fessard,D; eds., Raven, pp.629-633.
5. Jessell,T. & Iversen,L.L. (1977) Nature 268:549-551.

Characteristics and Function of Opioids, editors Van Ree and Terenius
© *1978 Elsevier/North-Holland Biomedical Press*

NON-SOMATIC SITE OF ACTION OF ENKEPHALIN ON SINGLE MYENTERIC NEURONES

YOSHIFUMI KATAYAMA and ALAN NORTH

Neurophysiology Laboratory, Department of Pharmacology, Loyola University
Stritch School of Medicine, Maywood, Illinois 60153 (U.S.A.)

Intracellular recordings were made from the somata of neurones in the
myenteric plexus of the guinea-pig ileum. The experiments were carried out
in vitro at 37^{0}C. Methionine- and leucine-enkephalin were applied to the
neurones either by addition to the perfusion solution or by iontophoresis.

Enkephalin (1 nM - 1 μM) in the perfusing solution caused a concentration
dependent hyperpolarisation of the soma membrane of about 50% of neurones.
This was of rapid onset and reversed fully when the enkephalin was washed
out; in about 25% of affected cells the hyperpolarisation was associated
with a fall in neuronal input resistance. The hyperpolarisation was reversed
or prevented by naloxone (10-300 nM).

Enkephalin was applied by iontophoresis from an electrode whose tip could
be positioned directly on the cell soma membrane or at other places on the
surface of the ganglion. Iontophoretic application of enkephalin to the cell
soma never hyperpolarised myenteric neurones. In some electrode tip positions
application of enkephalin caused dose-related depolarisations (Fig. 1A).
These depolarisations were not current effects; they were not affected by
adding naloxone (1 μM) to the perfusing solution.

The effect of application of similar amounts of enkephalin (10-200 nA;
1-20 s) to the surface of the ganglion away from the soma of the impaled cell
depended critically on the position of the electrode tip. In most positions
enkephalin caused no effect; in some positions enkephalin caused hyperpolarisation of the soma membrane (Fig.1A). The hyperpolarisations disappeared
with small movements of the electrode tip, were dependent on the amount of
enkephalin ejected, and were reversibly abolished by adding naloxone (1 μM)
to the perfusing solution. In no positions away from the cell soma did
application of enkephalin ever cause depolarising responses.

The observations suggest that the site of action at which enkephalin
hyperpolarises myenteric neurones is not the soma membrane, but that effects
recorded in the soma are the result of electrotonic spread from enkephalin-
sensitive sites on the cell processes. It is possible that these are also
the sites of acetylcholine release. If this is the case, then the

inhibition of acetylcholine release by enkephalin might be brought about by a hyperpolarising block of propagation or by the shunting effect of a conductance increase.

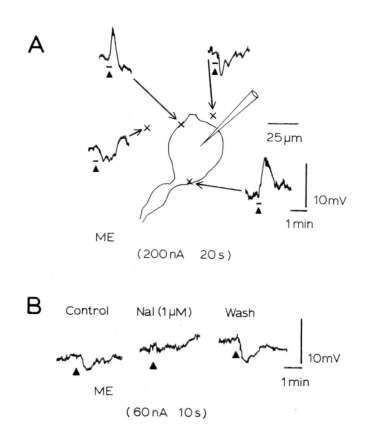

Fig. 1. A. Responses of a single myenteric neurone to iontophoretic application of met-enkephalin. The crosses indicate the positions of the tip of the iontophoresis electrode on the surface of the ganglion, with respect to the outline of the impaled cell. When enkephalin was applied directly onto the soma (upper left and lower right responses) a depolarisation was observed; application of enkephalin to sites slightly removed from the soma usually had no effect but in the two sites indicated (upper right and lower left) caused hyperpolarising responses.

   B. Hyperpolarising response to iontophoretic application of met-enkephalin to a site away from the soma of the impaled cell (not the same cell as depicted in A). The response was eliminated by perfusing the preparation for 4 min by a solution which contained naloxone (1 μM).

ARE ENDORPHINS INHIBITORY NEUROTRANSMITTERS ACTING ON NOCICEPTIVE NEURONES IN THE RAT BRAIN?

C.M. PEPPER & R.G. HILL

Department of Pharmacology, Medical School, Bristol BS8 1TD, U.K.

INTRODUCTION

The most attractive role proposed for the endogenous opiate-like peptides is the modulation of transmission in nociceptive pathways. We have investigated this possibility on single nociceptive neurones located in nucleus lateralis of the rat thalamus[1]. The noxious evoked excitation of these neurones is readily depressed by opiates and the enkephalins or their enzymically stable analogues[2,3]. After antagonism of such depressions by naloxone the noxious evoked response was occasionally more pronounced, ·suggesting a possible tonic inhibitory effect of an endogenous opioid and, indeed, the enkephalins are present in rat thalamus[4]. However, unlike most other sensory neurones, synaptic inhibition following evoked excitation, or produced by sensory stimulation outside the receptive field was only rarely seen in nucleus lateralis. We therefore decided to investigate the possibility that electrical stimulation of the periaqueductal gray (PAG) which is reported to produce naloxone-sensitive analgesia[5], would produce inhibition of thalamic nociceptive neurones.

METHODS

Adult male rats were anaesthetised with chloral hydrate (300 mg/kg i.p.) and guide cannulae stereotaxically implanted above target sites in PAG. Electro-physiological experiments were performed under halothane anaesthesia (1 to $1\frac{1}{2}$% in O_2) at least one week later. Conventional single unit recording techniques were used, and general experimental procedures were similar to those previously described[7,2,3]. A concentric bipolar electrode was used to electrically stimulate PAG (40 Hz, 0.1 mS, 2 to 10V, for up to 40 s). After each experiment correct positioning of stimulating and recording electrodes was confirmed histologically.

RESULTS

Twenty four neurones located within nucleus lateralis were studied in 5 animals. In the majority of cases (18/24 neurones) the spontaneous firing of these neurones was unaffected by PAG stimulation, as was the noxious evoked excitation of 4 neurones. 5 neurones were clearly excited by PAG stimulation, 4 of these also being excited by noxious thermal peripheral stimulation. In only one case was inhibition seen, and this is illustrated in the figure. The inhibition of the spontaneous firing of this neurone by PAG stimulation was not blocked by intravenous naloxone (total dose 1.35 mg). After intravenous bicuculline (0.05 mg), however, PAG stimulation then caused excitation. Recovery of the inhibition was seen 14 min after bicuculline injection.

DISCUSSION

Other studies have shown that central stimulation of sites such as the PAG produces inhibition of nociceptive neurones in the spinal cord[6] and reticular formation[7]. In the present study, however, not only was inhibition rarely seen but excitation of nociceptive neurones was observed. It seems possible that this apparent discrepancy could be attributed to a functional heterogeneity within the PAG but this must await confirmation by a detailed electrophysiological study of neurones in this region.

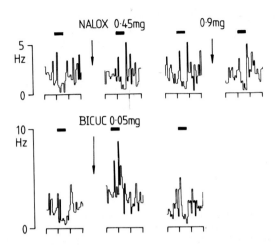

Fig. 1. Stimulation of PAG (40 Hz, 0.1 mS, 5V; filled bars) produces inhibition of spontaneous firing of nucleus lateralis neurone. Records making up each row show responses to consecutive stimuli, the interval between records in each row being approximately 10 minutes. The interval between upper and lower rows is 35 min. Time scales are marked in min. Upper row: i.v. naloxone (0.45 mg, 8 min before 2nd record; 0.9 mg, 1.5 min before last record) does not block inhibition. Lower row: after i.v. bicuculline (0.5 mg, 1.5 min before middle record) PAG stimulation now produces excitation.

Our observation that the single instance of inhibition by PAG stimulation was blocked by bicuculline but not naloxone suggests that this inhibition was mediated by the release of GABA. Inhibition of a nucleus lateralis neurone produced by noxious stimulation was also resistant to naloxone but was blocked by bicuculline. Thus, although studies in this and other laboratories[6,8,9] have suggested that synaptic inhibition of nociceptive neurones in other brain areas may be mediated by an endogenous opiate or 5HT, in the thalamus at least, GABA may also play an important role.

REFERENCES

1. Hill, R.G. & Pepper, C.M. (1977) J. Physiol., (Lond.), 269, 37-38P.
2. Hill, R.G. & Pepper, C.M. (1976) Br. J. Pharmac. 58, 459P.
3. Hill, R.G. & Pepper, C.M. (1978) Eur. J. Pharmacol. 47, 223-225.
4. Snyder, S.H., Uhl, G.R. & Kuhar, M.J. (1978) in Centrally Acting Peptides, Hughes, J. ed., Macmillan, London, pp 85-97.
5. Akil, H., Mayer, D.J. & Liebeskind, J.C. (1976) Science, 191, 961-962.
6. Oliveras, J.L., Besson, J.M., Guilbaud, G. & Liebeskind, J.C. (1974) Exp. Brain Res. 20, 32-44.
7. Morrow, T.J. & Casey, K. (1976) in Advances in Pain Research & Therapy, Bonica, J.J. & Albe-Fessard, D. eds., Raven Press, N.Y. pp 503-510.
8. Mayer, M.L. & Hill, R.G. (1978) Neuropharmacology, in press.
9. Frederickson, R.C.A. & Norris, F.H. (1978) in Iontophoresis and Transmitter Mechanisms in the Mammalian Central Nervous System, Ryall, R.W. & Kelly, J.S. eds. Elsevier/North Holland, Amsterdam, pp 320-322.

Characteristics and Function of Opioids, editors Van Ree and Terenius
© 1978 Elsevier/North-Holland Biomedical Press

EFFECTS OF ENKEPHALIN AND MORPHINE ON SINGLE NEURONS OF NUCLEUS RETICULARIS PARAGIGANTOCELLULARIS IN RATS

HIROSHI TAKAGI, MASAMICHI SATOH AND AKINORI AKAIKE

Department of Pharmacology, Faculty of Pharmaceutical Sciences,

Kyoto University, Kyoto 606, Japan

ABSTRACT

The effects of microelectrophoretically applied leucine-enkephalin (L-E) and morphine (M) on the activity of single neurons in the nucleus reticularis para-gigantocellularis (NRPG), located immediately ventral to the nucleus reticularis gigantocellularis (NRGC), of the rat were investigated. L-E as well as M increased the spontaneous firing rate in almost all of the NRPG neurons which were excited by intra-arterial injection of bradykinin (BK). The excitatory action of L-E and M was antagonized by naloxone (0.5 mg/kg) injected intravenously. These results indicate that L-E and M have at least a direct excitatory action on the NRPG neurons mediated through specific opiate receptors.

Recently Takagi et al.[1,2] found by means of a microinjection technique that the NRGC and NRPG of the medulla oblongata of the rat are highly sensitive sites in the production of analgesia by M and enkephalins. Moreover, Akaike et al.[3] noted that the NRPG is much more sensitive in such a sense than the NRGC and that electrical stimulation of the NRPG but not the NRGC produces a definite analgesia. Takagi et al.[4] reported that electrical stimulation of the bulbar reticular formation of the rabbit corresponding to the NRPG of the rat inhibits the neuronal response in lamina V cells of the spinal dorsal horn following intra-arterial injection of BK. In order to evaluate local actions of enkephalin and M on unitary activities of the NRPG neurons, the present experiments were performed using a microelectrophoretic method.

Male Sprague-Dawley rats (300 - 500 g) were anesthetized with α-chloralose (90 mg/kg i.p.) and immobilized by gallamine and artificially respired. Micro-electrophoresis and recording unitary discharge were done according to the method described by Satoh et al.[5] The NRPG cells under study were physiologically characterized in terms of the responses to BK (2 - 5 µg in 0.2 ml saline) which was injected into the right common iliac artery through a polyethylene cannula inserted in a retrograde manner into the left common iliac artery. At the termination of each experiment the recording sites were lesioned by anodal current and determined histologically.

The results were obtained from 24 neurons in the NRPG which were spontaneously active and excitable by phoretically applied L-glutamate.

110

BK-injection into the common iliac artery evoked an excitatory response in 11 out of 24 neurons tested in the NRPG, inhibitory response in only 1 and no clear effect in the other 12, indicating that the main response induced by BK is excitatory in the NRPG neurons. L-E phoretically applied (100 - 200 nA, 2 - 3 min) increased spontaneous discharge activity in 5 out of 11 neurons examined in the NRPG, decreased it in 2 and had no clear effect in the other 4. M (100 - 200 nA, 2 - 3 min) accelerated spontaneous firing in 12 out of 19 neurons tested, and produced no clear effect in the other 7. In 5 out of 6 NRPG neurons in which the effects of L-E and M on the same neuron were examined, these compounds had a similar effect (excitation:3 and no clear effect:2). The facilitatory action appeared within 30 sec after start of the phoresis of both substances but disappeared within 30 and 300 sec after termination of ejection of L-E and M, respectively. Almost all the neurons excited by BK-injection were also stimulated by L-E and/or M and such a stimulatory action of L-E and M was antagonized by intravenous injection of naloxone (0.5 mg/kg), indicating that the action was mediated by specific opiate receptors. If the results of this study are considered together with the findings of Akaike et al.[3] and Takagi et al.[4], enkephalin and M, at least in part, may directly excite the NRPG neurons, leading to inhibition of nociceptive inputs at the spinal dorsal horn through a descending inhibitory system originating from the NRPG.

On the other hand, about half the number of NRGC neurons affected by L-E and/or M were depressed by these compounds. Our results correspond to the observation of Sun and Gatipon[6] that M (1 - 2 mg/kg i.v.) had a predominantly depressant action on NRGC neurons. Physiological and pharmacological relationships between the NRPG and NRGC are under investigation by our group.

REFERENCES

1. Takagi, H., Satoh, M., Akaike, A., Shibata, T. and Kuraishi, Y. (1977) Eur. J. Pharmacol., 45, 91-92.
2. Takagi, H., Satoh, M., Akaike, A., Shibata, T., Yajima, H. and Ogawa, H. (1978) Eur. J. Pharmacol., 49, 113-116.
3. Akaike, A., Shibata, T., Satoh, M. and Takagi, H. (1978) Neuropharmacology, 17, in press.
4. Takagi, H., Doi, T. and Kawasaki, K. (1975) Life Sci., 17, 67-72.
5. Satoh, M., Zieglgansberger, W. and Herz, A. (1976) Brain Res., 115, 99-110.
6. Sun, C.-L. and Gatipon, G.B. (1976) Exp. Neurol., 52, 1-12.

Thanks are due to M. Ohara, Kyoto University, for assistance with the manuscript.

Characteristics and Function of Opioids, editors Van Ree and Terenius
© *1978 Elsevier/North-Holland Biomedical Press*

DEPRESSION OF s-IPSP AND HYPERPOLARIZATION BY MET-ENKEPHALIN IN FROG SYMPATHETIC GANGLION

WOUT WOUTERS and JOEP VAN DEN BERCKEN
University of Utrecht, Institute of Veterinary Pharmacology and Toxicology,
Biltstraat 172, 3572 BP Utrecht, The Netherlands

Since the finding of the enkephalins much evidence is accumulating that these pentapeptides act as neuromodulators or neurotransmitters[1]. In the central nervous system postsynaptic as well as presynaptic effects are described for enkephalins. In the myenteric plexus the firing of neurons is depressed by opiates and opioid peptides. A possible mechanism could be the hyperpolarization of the myenteric neurons as described for normorphine[2].

To explore the enkephalinic involvement in neuronal transmission, we studied the effect of met-enkephalin on the slow inhibitory postsynaptic potential (s-IPSP) in frog sympathetic ganglion. The results show that met-enkephalin exerts a dual effect: a depression of the s-IPSP, probably mainly due to a presynaptic action, and a hyperpolarization of the postsynaptic membrane. Both these effects were antagonized by naloxone.

The experiments were performed on the ninth or tenth sympathetic ganglion of the frog, R. esculenta, using the sucrose gap technique. s-IPSP's are evoked in these ganglia by electrical stimulation of the ramus to the eighth ganglion. The simultaneously evoked fast excitatory postsynaptic potential was selectively suppressed by 30 µM nicotine sulphate which was present in all superfusion liquids. Drugs were applied to the ganglion by changing the continuous superfusion from normal ringer to one containing the desired concentrations of drugs. To be able to detect small changes in the membrane potential, which is reflected by the voltage across the gap, much care was taken to maintain the stability of the gap.

Application of met-enkephalin or D-ala-met-enkephalin in a concentration of 1 µM caused a hyperpolarization of the membrane potential within one minute after the peptide reached the ganglion (see figure). This hyperpolarization although small in amplitude was consistently observed because of the gap's stability (better than 1 mV/hr). Simultaneously with the hyperpolarization, the s-IPSP was depressed by 39.3±6.5% (n=6) (see figure). The enkephalin induced hyperpolarization and s-IPSP depression were fully reversed and prevented by 1 µM naloxone. Morphine (5 µM) also caused this hyperpolarization and depression of the s-IPSP.

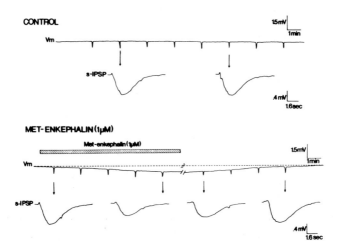

Fig. 1. Effects of met-enkephalin upon membrane potential and s-IPSP.
Traces denoted Vm represent continuous recording of the voltage across the
gap. The small downward deflections are the s-IPSP's. Traces denoted s-IPSP
represent the enlarged s-IPSP's.

To determine whether the enkephalin induced s-IPSP depression was due to the
induced hyperpolarization, experiments were performed in which the driving force
for the s-IPSP (E_K-Vm) was changed by varying the external potassium concentration. From these experiments it can be concluded that the enkephalin induced
hyperpolarization is too small to account for the s-IPSP depression of 39.3%.

To test the sensitivity of the ganglion for dopamine, the putative transmitter for the s-IPSP, small amounts of dopamine were applied just over the
preparation by means of a motor driven syringe. The postsynaptic hyperpolarizing
response evoked in this way was only depressed 13.8+6.1% (n=5) by met-enkephalin.
Thus the s-IPSP depression is largely not due to a decreased postsynaptic
sensitivity. In these experiments the enkephalin induced hyperpolarization was
equally as large as in the s-IPSP experiments. This further indicates that the
s-IPSP depression is not due to the hyperpolarization itself.

In conclusion, met-enkephalin modulates neuronal transmission in frog
sympathetic.ganglion by means of a specific opiate receptor system. The hyperpolarization is probably due to a direct action of the enkephalins on the postsynaptic membrane, while the s-IPSP depression seems to be due to a presynaptic
action, possibly by decreased transmitter release.

REFERENCES

1. Fredericson, R.C.A. (1977) Life Sciences, 21, 23.
2. North, R.A. (1976) Neuropharmacology, 15, 719.

Characteristics and Function of Opioids, editors Van Ree and Terenius
© 1978 Elsevier/North-Holland Biomedical Press

PSYCHOPATHOLOGY AS A NEUROPEPTIDE DYSFUNCTION

DAVID DE WIED

Rudolf Magnus Institute for Pharmacology, Medical Faculty, University of
Utrecht, Vondellaan 6, Utrecht (The Netherlands).

ABSTRACT

Neuropeptides derived from ACTH, MSH and the neurohypophyseal hormones vasopressin and oxytocin are instrumental in adaptive processes by affecting motivational, learning and memory processes. Disturbances in the formation of these
neuropeptides may be an underlying cause in cognitive dysfunction. Non-opiate-
like neuropeptides such as the [des-Tyr] endorphins related to α- and γ-endorphin
which may be generated from β-endorphin in the brain, have opposite effects on
extinction of avoidance behavior. In this respect α-type endorphins on avoidance
behavior resemble amphetamine and other psychostimulants, while γ-type endorphins resemble haloperidol and other neuroleptic drugs. An inborn error in the
generation of these endorphin fragments from β-endorphin may lead to a dys-
balance in these two types of endorphins in the brain. This may be an etiological factor in schizophrenia. This hypothesis is supported by the marked beneficial effects of treatment with the non-opiate-like neuropeptide [des-Tyr]-
γ-endorphin in schizophrenic patients.

The implication of the anterior pituitary hormone adrenocorticotrophic hormone (ACTH), the intermediate pituitary hormone, melanocyte stimulating hormone
(α-MSH) and the neurohypophyseal hormones, vasopressin and oxytocin on behavior
has been derived from studies using classical endocrine approach. This involved the removal of the endocrine gland, in this case parts of the pituitary
or the whole gland, the subsequent demonstration of a deficiency syndrome and
the correction of this deficiency by substitution with hormones produced by
the extirpated gland[1]. Partial or complete hypophysectomy resulted in a serious
impairment in avoidance acquisition which could be corrected by treatment with
pituitary hormones such as ACTH, α-MSH, or vasopressin. It subsequently appeared that fragments of these hormones which are practically devoid of the
classical endocrine activities of the precursor hormones such as the production
of steroids by the adrenal cortex in the case of ACTH or the influence on
water metabolism in the case of vasopressin could remove the behavioral impairment of the hypophysectomized rat as effectively as the parent molecules. Thus

the sequence $ACTH_{4-10}$ which is present in ACTH and α-MSH as well as in lipotropin (β-LPH) as part of β-MSH is behaviorally as active as the whole ACTH
molecule. The same was found for various fragments of vasopressin.

The studies suggested that behavioral and endocrine effects of pituitary
and hypothalamic hormones are dissociated and that these hormones may act as
precursor molecules from which neuropeptides may be enzymatically generated.
Extensive studies in hypophysectomized as well as in intact rats revealed
that neuropeptides derived from ACTH, α- and β-MSH and β-LPH, vasopressin
and oxytocin are involved in acquisition and maintenance of new behavioral
patterns. These neuropeptides are instrumental in adaptive processes by
affecting motivational, learning and memory processes. In addition, neuropeptides of neurohypophyseal origin are involved in the development of
tolerance to and physical dependence on opiates[2] and in the modulation of
the reinforcing properties of addictive drugs[3]. The motivational effects of
$ACTH_{4-10}$ were also demonstrated in studies in man[4]. Others found that in
humans this heptapeptide affected concentration and selective visual attention
[5,6]. In addition, the memory effects of vasopressin as predicted from animal
studies were recently demonstrated in patients with severe amnesia[7] and in a
group of elderly people[8]. These observations point to an important role of
neuropeptides in mental performance and suggest that disturbances in the
hormonal climate of the brain as a result of a reduced formation or release
of these neuropeptides may be the underlying causes of cognitive dysfunctions.

The marked behavioral effects of ACTH and related peptides prompted
the hypothesis that the pituitary might manufacture other more
potent and specific neuropeptides. In view of this, a programme
was set up around 1970 to isolate peptides
related to ACTH/MSH from hog pituitary material. Fractions were tested on
avoidance acquisition of hypophysectomized rats in a shuttle box, or on
extinction of pole-jumping avoidance behavior or retention of passive
avoidance behavior in intact rats[9,10]. These studies demonstrated the presence
of potent behavioral peptides in the pituitary. One of the peptides which
was obtained in pure form, yielded three oligopeptides after tryptic digestion.
The amino acid composition of two of these appeared to be similar to that
of β-LPH$_{61-69}$ and β-LPH$_{70-79}$ respectively. Unfortunately, the amount of
material available at the time was insufficient to allow structure analysis
studies. Meanwhile several studies had demonstrated the presence of opioid
binding sites in the brain[11,12,13] and suggested the existence of an endogenous ligand for these sites. Hughes[14] using a bioassay for opiates provided evidence for opiate-like substances in the brain which appeared to

be of peptide character. A number of amino acids were identical to the ones found in $ACTH_{4-10}$. Indeed, $ACTH_{4-10}$ and several other sequences including $ACTH_{1-28}$ appeared to possess some affinity for opiate binding sites in the brain[15,16]. Analysis of the binding revealed low selectivity of these peptides for agonist and antagonist binding sites comparable to that of the partial agonist nalorphine[17]. However, in view of the relatively low affinity $ACTH_{4-10}$ could not be regarded as a physiological ligand for opiate receptors in the brain. Hughes et al[18] identified the active principles as two pentapeptides, Met-enkephalin and Leu-enkephalin. It was noted that the peptide sequence of Met-enkephalin corresponded to the positions 61 to 65 of the pituitary hormone β-LPH. Teschemacher et al.[19] found an endogenous opioid with a larger molecular weight in the pituitary. Subsequently Li and Chung isolated $\beta\text{-LPH}_{61-91}$ from camel pituitaries and the opiate-like properties of the C-fragment of β-LPH was demonstrated[20,21]. Another endorphin, α-endorphin which is $\beta\text{-LPH}_{61-76}$ was isolated by Guillemin et al[22]. In view of the above it is of interest to note that Mains et al.[23] and Roberts and Herbert[24] recently found evidence for a single precursor molecule with a molecular weight of about 31000 for β-LPH and ACTH.

After the various enkephalins and endorphins became available we verified our previous findings on the behavioral effect of peptides related to the C-terminal β-LPH fragments. Extinction of pole-jumping avoidance behavior was used to assay the behavioral effect of Met-enkephalin, $\beta\text{-LPH}_{61-69}$, α-endorphin, β-endorphin and a number of related peptides. $\beta\text{-LPH}_{61-69}$ indeed was found much more potent than $ACTH_{4-10}$ but α-endorphin was the most potent peptide in the series that were tested. On a molar basis it appeared to be 30 times more active than $ACTH_{4-10}$ following systemic injection[25]. Peptides were active following systemic as well as intracerebroventricular administration in relatively low doses. Interestingly, the effect of the endorphins and that of ACTH fragments on avoidance behavior could not be prevented by specific opiate antagonists. This in contrast to excessive grooming in the rat which occurs following intracerebroventricularly administered ACTH or β-endorphin. This effect can be readily blocked by pretreatment with opiate antagonists[26,27]. Thus, the influence of the endorphins and of ACTH and related peptides on avoidance behavior takes place independently of opiate receptor sites in the brain.

Unlike the analgesic effect of β-endorphin which decreases when the peptide chain is shortened, the influence of several β-endorphin fragments on avoidance behavior is more marked than that of the parent molecule. Could it be that β-endorphin possessed moieties with opposite behavioral effects and that the eventual activity would depend on the fragmentation of this peptide ? In view of this we explored the influence of other β-endorphin fragments such as γ-endorphin (β-LPH$_{61-77}$) and β-LPH$_{78-91}$ on active and passive avoidance behavior[28]. It was found that γ-endorphin in the amounts in which α-endorphin delayed extinction tended to facilitate it. γ-Endorphin seemed to have an effect opposite to that of α-endorphin. When tested in rats made more resistant to extinction, γ-endorphin indeed facilitated extinction of pole-jumping avoidance behavior. A significant effect was found following subcutaneous injection of 30 nanograms.

The opiate-like activity of the endorphins is lost by the removal of the N-terminal amino acid residue tyrosine[29] and some studies suggested that the tyrosine residue is removed from γ-endorphin in the brain[30]. We found that [des-Tyr^1]-γ-endorphin (DTγE) was without opiate-like activity on the guinea pig ileum preparation of Hughes et al[18]. However, it was even more potent than γ-endorphin in facilitating extinction of pole-jumping avoidance behavior. In addition it had a marked attenuating effect on passive avoidance responding.

Since the introduction of neuroleptics, we know from the classical studies by Courvoisier et al.[31] that acquisition and extinction of conditioned behavior are extremely sensitive substrates for neuroleptic activity. Further studies designed to explore other activities of DTγE revealed that it possessed neuroleptic activities. DTγE given either subcutaneously or intraventricularly was active in various "grip tests" which are characteristic for neuroleptic drugs such as haloperidol. However, DTγE had no sedative effects and failed to affect gross behavior in an open field. No effects on the corneal reflex, the righting reflex or on rigidity (bridge test[32]) were found but it slightly decreased the mobility of the rats in the observation cage.

The most striking results that were obtained were that α- and γ-endorphin and DTγE had opposite effects on active and passive avoidance behavior. The presence or absence of the amino acid residue leucine (β-LPH-77) or β-endorphin apparently determines the influence of β-endorphin fragments on adaptive behavior. The effects of α- and γ-endorphin on avoidance behavior resemble those of amphetamine and haloperidol respectively. Amphetamine delays extinction of pole-jumping avoidance behavior and facilitates passive avoidance responding. Conversely, haloperidol facilitates extinction of pole-jumping avoidance behavior and attenuates passive avoidance responding[33]. The effect of amphetamine and haloperidol are partly due to sedative influences and to

effects on locomotor activity[34,35]. In fact, amphetamine in a dose of 90 µg
per rat given subcutaneously which delayed extinction of pole-jumping
avoidance behavior markedly increased the rate of ambulation as well as
rearing in an open field. Haloperidol in a dose of 0.1 µg per rat which
facilitated extinction of pole-jumping avoidance behavior significantly decreased ambulation and grooming in an open field. However, at lower doses,
amphetamine and haloperidol significantly affect extinction of pole-jumping
avoidance behavior without effects on ambulation, rearing and grooming in
the open field. The endorphins even in amounts many times the effective dose
on extinction of pole-jumping avoidance behavior do not affect gross behavior
in an open field. Nevertheless one might postulate that α-endorphin or a related neuropeptide such as DTαE represent a psychostimulant type of ligand
while γ-endorphin and in particular DTγE represent a neuroleptic type of ligand (endoleptic).

Are the fragments of β-endorphin such as DTαE and DTγE normal constituents
in the brain ? Endorphins are present in the highest concentration in the
pituitary but are also present in the brain[36,37,38,39]. Pituitary and brain
endorphins are synthetized independently. Enkephalins are present mainly in
the brain. An enkephalin system has been found in the brain with various
cell groups throughout the spinal cord and brain stem and a β-endorphin system has been detected in the brain as well but with a single cell group in
the hypothalamus which innervates midbrain and limbic structures through
long axons[40,41]. Immunocytochemical studies indicate that these axons contain
β-LPH, β-endorphin and ACTH suggesting that the precursor of these molecules
is present in brain like in the pituitary[36,41,42]. Behaviorally active endorphins might originate either from the pituitary or from the brain since
both tissues contain β-LPH inactivating enzymes. Several authors found evidence
that β-endorphin might be cleaved in brain tissue around the residues
67-69, 77-80, 82-84 and 86-88 indicating endopeptidase activity[43,44,45].
Aminopeptidase activity is responsible for the release of the N-terminal
amino acid residue tyrosine. Smyth and associates[46,30,47,48] investigated the
conversion of $[^{125}I\text{-tyrosine}]$-β-endorphin by brain synaptosomal preparations
and striatal slices. Protecting the release of tyrosine by bacitracin they
found that incubation at pH 7.4 with synaptosomal membranes yielded γ-
endorphin, small amounts of enkephalin and tyrosine. At pH 5.0 the main products were α-endorphin and enkephalin, small amounts of β-LPH$_{61-73}$ and β-
LPH$_{61-68}$. On incubation with striatal slices in physiological conditions the
major product was γ-endorphin, but prolonged incubation yielded α-endorphin

as well in addition to small amounts of β-LPH$_{61-67}$ and β-LPH$_{61-66}$. From these
experiments they concluded that the conversion of β-endorphin takes place
extracellularly at the synaptosomal membrane. Additionally they suggested
that the initial step involved attack by an endopeptidase since the half
life of β-endorphin in striatal slices is unchanged in the presence of bacitracin while that of γ-endorphin is markedly prolonged. Their observations
suggest that β-endorphin in the brain is degraded into γ-endorphin followed
by the formation of DTγE then of DTαE and smaller fragments.

In view of the neuroleptic-like effects of DTγE we have postulated that
an inborn error in the generation or metabolism of this neuropeptide is an
etiological factor in psychopathological processes for which neuroleptic drugs
are beneficial[49]. The dramatic antipsychotic action of DTγE in schizophrenic
patients supports this assumption[50,51]. The implication of the endorphins
in schizophrenia originated from a number of observations in man. The
endorphin concentration in the cerebrospinal fluid is altered in some
psychiatric disorders[52] and the specific opiate antagonist naloxone may temporarily decrease psychotic symptoms[53,54] although these findings are still
equivocal[55,56,57]. It has been reported that β-endorphin had therapeutic
effects in a number of psychotic patients[58]. Finally, [leucine[5]]-β-endorphin
was found in great quantities in the dialysate of chronic schizophrenics[59,60].
However, our studies indicate that the neuroleptic effects of DTγE are independent of the typical morphine-like action of the endorphins.

Acquisition and extinction of a new behavior is an illustration of an
adaptive process. Acquisition is a forced readjustment in behavior due to
an environmental change, while extinction of that particular behavior takes
place when the behavior is no longer relevant. Adequate interpretation of
the environmental situation is thereby essential. In this context it is not
difficult to visualize the role of the endorphins of the α- and γ-type in
behavioral adaptation. Derangements in the formation of these neuropeptides,
lack or excess of either of the β-endorphin fragments, must lead to misinterpretation of environmental cues, resulting in abnormal behavior which may
become manifest as a psychopathological syndrome.

The schizophrenic syndrome includes abnormal motor behavior which ranges
from total immobilization (catatonia) to purposeless activity and stereotypy,
perceptual distorsions including hallucinations which can be of any sensory
modality, disturbed thinking, bizarre speech and illogical thoughts, paranoid
delusions etc. Expressions of emotions are often absent, blunted or inappropriate. Intense anxiety or deep rage unrelated to environmental stimuli are

found. Accordingly, schizophrenia encompasses a range of different behaviors. Our hypothesis which suggests a disturbance in the balance between α- and γ-type endorphins might give an explanation for the variability in which the schizophrenic syndrome manifests itself.

If we assume that DTγE or a related neuropeptide is the rate limiting step in the degradation of β-endorphin, a deficiency in this compound would lead to a derangement in β-endorphin homeostasis. Due to a disturbed feed back regulation excess amounts of β-endorphin would accumulate in the brain. This may lead to schizophrenia of the catatonic type since animal experiments have shown that excess β-endorphin in the brain induces catatonia[32]. If the disturbance is not located in the generation of γ-endorphin but in the release of the N-terminal amino acid tyrosine, the generated fragments still contain opiate-like activity in addition to their behavioral effects; this would cause an excess of β-endorphin, γ-endorphin and even α-endorphin and this might give rise to a mixed symptomatology. Likewise if the cleavage of β-endorphin would take place outside the region 77-78 due to abnormalities in the amino acid sequence of β-endorphin, or if DTγE is degraded more rapidly due to abnormal enzyme activity, excess of endorphins of the β- and in particular of the α-types might induce effects which in several aspects are similar to those of amphetamine. This and related compounds might elicit stereotypies, aggressive or paranoid forms of the schizophrenic syndrome, because drugs such as amphetamine in high doses are known to induce schizophrenic (paranoid) psychosis (see for review Meltzer and Stahl[61]). It has been postulated that schizophrenia results from excess dopaminergic transmission in specific structures in the brain. This hypothesis borrowed support among others from the fact that the antipsychotic agents block dopamine receptors and that the amphetamines which enhance dopaminergic activity can exacerbate psychotic symptoms in schizophrenics and induce psychotic symptoms in normal individuals. However, no direct evidence is available for an altered dopamine metabolism or activity in schizophrenia[62]. For further arguments in favour of the dopamine hypothesis see the review by Berger[63].

It is possible that the endorphins of the α- and γ-type modulate neurotransmitter activity in specific limbic midbrain structures. Few data are available concerning the interaction of endorphins with catecholaminergic transmission in the brain. Versteeg et al.[64] studied the effect of β-endorphin, α-endorphin and DTγE administered intraventricularly on catecholamine disappearance in α-MPT treated rats in discrete regions of the forebrain. Relatively low doses of these neuropeptides already exerted pronounced effects in various regions of the brain. Dopamine disappearance was decreased following α-endorphin in 7 out of 20 regions that were investigated, among these were the caudate nucleus and the globus pallidus. The effects of β-endorphin and DTγE were not as widespread. Moreover these neuropeptides caused an enhancement in catecholamine disappearance. Interestingly, DTγE affected the dopamine disappearance in the paraventricular nucleus and the zona incerta in a direction opposite to that caused by α-endorphin. No clear effects of this neuropeptide were found on striatal dopamine. It is possible therefore that the main effects of DTγE are the results of an interaction with dopaminergic systems other than the nigrostriatal system. However, Gispen and Bohus[65] showed that DTγE implanted in the striatal area or in the nucleus accumbens inhibits ACTH induced excessive grooming. Haloperidol, the antagonist of DA_e receptors[66] in the striatal area which contains predominantly DA_e receptors but not in the nucleus accumbens which contains mainly DA_i receptors has a similar effect on ACTH-induced grooming. Ergometrine an antagonist of DA_i receptors has a similar inhibitory action when implanted in the nucleus accumbens but not in the striatum[67]. Accordingly, DTγE may interfere with dopaminergic neurotransmission in the nigrostriatal system as well. Such an effect may not be picked up in studies on the disappearance rate due to limitations of the techniques used. These preliminary findings relate the hypothesis based on an inborn error in the generation of DTγE to the dopamine hypothesis of schizophrenia.

Much work has to be done to substantiate our views. This would include studies on the metabolism of β-endorphin in schizophrenic patients. These studies may not be easy to perform particularly since one may have to use cerebrospinal fluid or even brain tissue. The radioimmunoassay and chemical analysis of the various β-endorphin fragments in the CSF may be intermediate steps to obtain evidence for an abnormal metabolism of β-endorphin. The beneficial effects of DTγE we have found in severe schizophrenics demand intensive investigations in this respect.

REFERENCES

1. De Wied, D. (1969) in Frontiers in Neuroendorcrinology of Ganong, W.F. and Martini, L., Oxford University Press, London/New York, pp. 97-140.

2. Van Ree, J.M. and De Wied, D. (1976) Life Sci. 19, 1331-1340.

3. Van Ree, J.M., Dorsa, D.M. and Colpaert, F.L. (1978) This volume.

4. Gaillard, A.W.K. and Sanders, A.F. (1975) Psychofarmacologia (Berl.) 42, 201-208.

5. Kastin, A.J., Sandman, C.A., Stratton, L.O., Schally, A.V. and Miller, L.H.

(1975) in Hormones, Homeostasis and the Brain, Progress in Brain Research 42 of Gispen, W.H., Van Wimersma Greidanus, Tj.B., Bohus, B. and De Wied, D., eds., Elsevier, Amsterdam, pp. 143-150.

6. Van Riezen, H., Rigter, H. and De Wied, D. (1977) Behav. Biol. 20, 311-324.
7. Oliveros, J.C., Jandali, M.K., Timsit-Berthier, M., Remy, R., Benghezal, A., Audibert, A. and Moeglen, J.M. (1978) The Lancet, January 7, 42.
8. Legros, J.J., Gilot, P., Seron, X., Claessens, J., Adam, A., Moeglen, J.M., Audibert, A. and Berchier, P. (1978) The Lancet, January 7, 41-42.
9. Lande, S., Witter, A. and De Wied, D. (1971) J. Biol. Chem. 246, 2058-2062.
10. Lande, S., De Wied, D. and Witter, A. (1973) in Drug Effects on Neuro-endocrine Regulation of Zimmermann, E., Gispen, W.H., Marks, B.H. and De Wied, D., eds., Elsevier, Amsterdam, Progress in Brain Research 39, pp. 421-427.
11. Pert, C.B. and Snyder, S.H. (1973) Science 179, 1011-1014.
12. Simon, E.J., Hiller, J.M. and Edelman, J. (1973) Proc. Natl. Acad. Sci. USA, 70, 1947-1949.
13. Terenius, L. (1973) Acta Pharmacol. Toxicol. 33, 377-384.
14. Hughes, J. (1975) Brain Res. 88, 295-308.
15. Terenius, L. (1975) J. Pharm. Pharmacol. 27, 450-452.
16. Terenius, L., Gispen, W.H. and De Wied, D. (1975) Europ. J. Pharmacol. 33, 395-399.
17. Terenius, L. (1976) Europ. J. Pharmacol. 38, 211-213.
18. Hughes, J., Smith, T.W., Kosterlitz, H.W., Fothergill, L.A., Morgan, B.A. and Morris, H.R. (1975) Nature 258, 577-579.
19. Teschemacher, H., Opheim, K.E., Cox, B.M. and Goldstein, A. (1975) Life Sci. 16, 1771-1776.
20. Li, Ch.H. and Chung, D. (1976) Proc. Natl. Acad. Sci. USA 73, 1145-1148.
21. Bradbury, A.F., Feldberg, W.F., Smyth, D.G. and Snell, C.R. (1976) in Opiates and Endogenous Opioid Peptides of Kosterlitz, H.W., ed., North Holland, Amsterdam, pp. 9-17.
22. Guillemin, R., Ling, N. and Burgus, R. (1976) C.R. Acad. Sci. (Paris), Ser. D 282, 783-785.
23. Mains, R., Eipper, B.A. and Ling, N. (1977) Proc. Natl. Acad. Sci. USA 74, 3014-3018.
24. Roberts, J.L. and Herbert, E. (1977) Proc. Natl. Acad. Sci. USA 74, 5300.
25. De Wied, D., Bohus, B., Van Ree, J.M. and Urban, I. (1978)J. Pharmacol. exp. Ther. 204, 570-580.
26. Gispen, W.H. and Wiegant, V.M. (1976) Neuroscience Lett. 2, 159-164.
27. Gispen, W.H., Wiegant, V.M., Bradbury, A.F., Hulme, E.C., Smyth, D.G., Snell, C.R. and De Wied, D. (1976) Nature 264, 794-795.
28. De Wied, D., Kovacs, G.L., Bohus, B., Van Ree, J.M. and Greven, H.M. (1978) Eur. J. Pharmacol. 49, 427-436.
29. Frederickson, R.C.A. (1977) Life Sci. 21, 23-42.
30. Austen, B.M., Smyth, D.G. and Snell, C.R. (1977) Nature 269, 619-621.
31. Courvoisier, S., Fournel, J., Ducrot, R., Kolsky, M. and Koetschet, P. (1952) Arch. Intern. Pharmacodyn. Therap. 92, 305.
32. Bloom, F., Segal, D., Ling, N. and Guillemin, R. (1976) Science 194, 630-632.
33. Kovacs, G.L. and De Wied, D. (1978) submitted to Eur. J. Pharmacol.
34. Kelly, P.H., Seviour, P.V. and Iversen, S.D. (1975) Brain Res. 94, 507-522.
35. Ahlenius, S., Engel, J. and Zöller, M. (1977) Physiol. Psychol. 5, 290.
36. Watson, S.J., Barchas, J.D. and Li, C.H. (1977) Proc. Natl. Acad. Sci. USA 74, 5155-5158.
37. Akil, H., Watson, S.J., Berger, P.A. and Barchas, J.D. (1978) Adv. Biochem. Psychopharmacol. 18, 125-139.
38. Cheung, A.L. and Goldstein, A. (1976) Life Sciences 19, 1005-1008.
39. Bloom, F., Battenberg, E., Rossier, J., Ling, N., Leppaluoto, J., Vargo,

122

T.M. and Guillemin, R. (1977) Life Sci. 20, 43-47.
40. Rossier, J., Vargo, T.M., Mirick, S., Ling, N., Bloom, F.E. and Guillemin, R. (1977) Proc. Natl. Acad. Sci. USA 74, 5162-5165.
41. Barchas, J.D., Akil, H., Elliott, G.R., Holman, R.B. and Watson, S.J. (1978) Science 200, 964-973.
42. Watson, S.J., Richard III, C.W. and Barchas, J.D. (1978) Science 200, 1180-1182.
43. Marks, N., Grynbaum, A. and Neidle, A. (1977) Biochem. Biophys. Res. Comm. 74, 1552-1559.
44. Grynbaum, A., Kastin, A.J., Coy, D.H. and Marks, N. (1977) Brain Res. Bull. 2, 479.
45. Patthy, A., Graf, L., Kenessey, A., Székely, J.I and Bajusz, S. (1977) Bioch. Biophys. Res. Comm. 79, 254.
46. Austen, B.M. and Smyth, D.G. (1977) Biochem. Biophys. Res. Comm. 77, 86.
47. Austen, B.M. and Smyth, D.G. (1977) Biochem. Soc. Transact. 5, 1394-1397.
48. Smyth, D.G. and Snell, C.R. (1977) Biochem. Soc. Transact. 5, 1397-1399.
49. De Wied, D., Bohus, B., Van Ree, J.M., Kovacs, G.L. and Greven, H.M. (1978) The Lancet I, 1046, May 1978.
50. Verhoeven, W.M.A.,Van Praag,H.M., Botter, P.A., Sunier, A., Van Ree, J.M. and De Wied, D. (1978) The Lancet I, 1046-1047, May 1978.
51. Van Ree, J.M., Verhoeven, W.M.A., Van Praag, H.M. and De Wied, D. (1978) This volume.
52. Terenius, L., Wahlström, A., Lindström, L. and Widerlov, E. (1976) Neurosci. Lett. 3, 157.
53. Gunne, L.-M., Lindström,L. and Terenius, L. (1977) J. Neural Transm. 40, 13-19.
54. Emrich, H.M., Cording, C., Piree, S., Kolling, A., Uzerssen, D. and Herz, A. (1977) Pharmakopsychiatrie und Neuropharmakologie 10, 265.
55. Volavka, J., Mallya, A., Baig, S. and Perez-Cruet, J. (1977) 196, 1227-1228.
56. Davis, G.C., Bunney Jr., W.E., DeFraites, E.G., Kleinmann, J.E., Van Kammen, D.P., Post, R.M. and Wyatt, R.J. (1977) 197, 74.
57. Janowski, D.S., Segal, D.S., Bloom, F., Abrams, A. and Guillemin, R. (1977) Am. J. Psychiat. 134, 926.
58. Kline, N.S., Li, C.H., Lehman, H.E., Lajtha, A., Laski, E. and Cooper, T. (1977) Arch. Gen. Psychiat. 34, 1111-1113.
59. Wagemaker, H., and Cade, R. (1977) Am. J. Psychiat. 134, 684.
60. Palmour, R.M., Ervin, F.R., Wagemaker, H. and Cade, R. (1977) Abstr. Soc. Neurosci. p. 320.
61. Meltzer, H.I.Y. and Stahl, S.M. (1976) Schizophrenia Bull. 2, 19-75.
62. Barchas, J.D., Berger, P.A., Elliott, G.R., Erdelyi, E. and Wyatt, R.J. (1977) in Biochemistry and Function of Monoamine Enzymes of Usdin, E., Weiner, M. and Youdin, M.B.H., eds., Dekker, New York, p. 863.
63. Berger, P.A. (1978) Science 200, 974-981.
64. Versteeg, D.H.G., De Kloet, E.R. and De Wied, D. (1978) submitted to Brain Res.
65. Gispen, W.H. and Bohus, B. (1978) This volume.
66. Cools, A.R. (1977) in Adv. Biochem. Psychopharmacol. Vol. 16, Nonstriatal Dopaminergic Neurons of Costa, E. and Gessa, G.L., eds., Raven Press, New York, pp. 215-225.
67. Wiegant, V.M., Cools, A.R. and Gispen, W.H. (1977) Eur. J. Pharmacol. 41, 343-345.

Characteristics and Function of Opioids, editors Van Ree and Terenius
© *1978 Elsevier/North-Holland Biomedical Press*

β-ENDORPHIN AND OTHER 31K FRAGMENTS: PITUITARY AND BRAIN SYSTEMS

HUDA AKIL, STANLEY J. WATSON, ROBERT M. LEVY and JACK D. BARCHAS
Nancy Pritzker Laboratory of Behavioral Neurochemistry, Department of
Psychiatry and Behavioral Sciences, Stanford University School of Medicine,
Stanford, California 94305, U.S.A.

ABSTRACT

We have studied β-lipotropin (β-LPH) and β-endorphin (β-END) systems in the
pituitary and brain. Our work indicates that the 31K precursor of these substances appears to be present in brain as well as in intermediate and anterior
pituitary lobe. It is hypothesized that within pituitary, β-END may be preferentially synthesized in the intermediate lobe, its release leading to higher
circulating blood levels in animals possessing this structure in contrast to
man. Pituitary β-END/β-LPH appear susceptible to the same treatments which
alter β-MSH, and brain β-END/β-LPH shares some of these same susceptibilities,
although it can be altered differentially by some pharmacological manipulations. Finally, our results indicate that brain β-END, or some structurally
similar material, is releasable into the CSF upon electrical stimulation in
man.

INTRODUCTION

During the past year, we have focused our efforts on the study of
β-lipotropin (β-LPH) and β-endorphin (β-END) in pituitary and brain. The systems that contain these substances offer several challenging questions. The
relationship between the brain and pituitary systems remains to be determined,
although there is ample evidence suggesting that one is not directly derived
from the other[1-4]. The target organ for pituitary endorphin is unknown and
its potential for CNS effects has not been determined. While brain β-END
appears to be stored like a neurotransmitter[2,5,6], other requirements for
characterizing a putative transmitter have yet to be established. Finally,
β-LPH and β-END have been shown to share a common 31K precursor with
ACTH[7,8]. This work was carried out primarily in pituitary systems and the
existence of 31K in brain remained to be determined. The possibility that
ACTH and β-END could be manufactured in the same neuron was particularly
intriguing, since both substances are known to be active in brain, bringing
about numerous behavioral changes ranging from motor disruptions to addiction[9-12]. The potential for interactions between ACTH and β-END is further

124

reinforced by the finding that ACTH fragments in relatively high concentrations can interact with opiate binding[13], and that some of the ACTH effects are reversible by naloxone[14].

In this report we describe our attempts to further characterize the β-END systems in pituitary and brain. We have carried out immunocytochemical studies confirming the existence of the 31K precursor in 2 pituitary systems (anterior and intermediate lobes) and strongly suggesting the same synthetic route in the hypothalamic β-END neurons. We have measured β-END immunoreactivity in human and rat blood and derived some hypotheses as to the regulation of β-END in intermediate vs. anterior lobes of pituitary. We have attempted to examine the potential role of β-END as a putative transmitter in brain, and obtained evidence of release of endorphin-like material in human CSF. Finally, we have searched for studies in the literature where ACTH or β-MSH (both 31K fragments) were altered by a given treatment, and tested the effects of such treatments on brain and pituitary β-END. These investigations are part of our search for useful models for studying the physiological functions of β-END and ACTH.

BLOOD LEVELS OF β-ENDORPHIN-LIKE IMMUNOREACTIVITY IN RAT AND MAN

β-LPH/β-END immunoreactivities have been demonstrated in 3 structures in mammalian encephalon: the intermediate lobe of the pituitary where they exist in every cell; the anterior lobe of the pituitary where the immunoreactivity coincides with ACTH immunoreactivity; and the periarcuate region of the hypothalamus, where scattered neurons give rise to multiple long projections which travel to numerous brain regions, including amygdala, medial thalamus and central grey[2-6,15-17].

While both pituitary structures exhibit both β-LPH and β-END immunoreactivities, the relative concentration of these peptides appears different across the two areas. There are several recent reports suggesting a relatively high β-END/β-LPH ratio in the intermediate lobe and a relatively low ratio in the anterior lobe[18-20]. This discrepancy may be due to the differential conversion of β-LPH into β-END in the two structures. Alternatively, it could be due to more rapid release of β-END from anterior lobe than from intermediate lobe. Since humans do not have an intermediate lobe, circulating β-END levels should reflect anterior lobe release. In rat, on the other hand, blood β-END could be derived from either or both lobes. We therefore set out to measure blood levels of β-END-like immunoreactivity in rat and human blood.

The antiserum employed was obtained from Dr. C. H. Li at U.C. San Francisco. It does cross react with β-LPH, but that cross reactivity is only partial, with β-LPH being 6-10 fold less potent than β-END in displacing

^{125}I-β-END. The assay sensitivity is 1.5-2 fmoles/tube, allowing us to detect 7.5-10 fmoles of β-END-like material per ml of plasma. In order to avoid nonspecific effects of serum, we carried out the measurement by comparing normal plasma from a given species to a pool of plasma from hypophysectomized subjects from the same species. The control values and standard curves were all carried out in either human or hypophysectomized plasma to allow the comparison. In the case of human subjects, an endocrine profile including GH, prolactin and TSH levels was obtained to determine the completeness of the hypophysectomy, prior to using that plasma as "blank."

Table 1 shows the levels of β-END-like immunoreactivity under these conditions. As can be seen, the levels in normal human subjects are at the limit of the assay sensitivity. With these low levels, we are unable to ascertain, by using chromatographic procedures, that the immunoreactivity is in fact due to β-END. The only condition where we have obtained a significant reading from human plasma is from a patient who had received metapyrone (Table 1)--a substance known to increase ACTH levels (in collaboration with Drs. Schteingart and Stockman, Univ. of Michigan). The levels in normal rat, on the other hand, are significantly higher than in hypophysectomized rats. Those levels exhibit a further dramatic rise with adrenalectomy. The dilution curve of material derived from rat plasma is parallel to the standard curve. Nonetheless, some of the immunoreactivity measured in rat blood could be due to circulating β-LPH or other cross-reacting material. Preliminary studies with other β-LPH and β-END sera with differing antigenic determinants suggest that β-LPH cross reactivity is not likely to account for the full activity being measured in rat, and that a significant portion of the immunoreactivity is likely to be due to β-END.

TABLE 1

BLOOD LEVELS OF β-ENDORPHIN-LIKE IMMUNOREACTIVITY IN RAT AND MAN (fmoles/ml plasma)

Normal Rat	75 ± 15
Adrenalectomized Rat (4 days post)	288 ± 32
Normal Humans	< 12 fmoles/ml
1 Subject post-metapyrone	31.2 fmoles/ml

The finding that β-END-like immunoreactivity exists in higher levels in rat than in human blood suggests that the intermediate lobe may be an important source of circulating β-END. It is not consistent with the hypothesis that anterior lobe β-END is more readily released, unless one makes the further assumption that in man, β-END is degraded much more rapidly than in rat. We are currently carrying out studies on the half-life of β-END in human blood, which permits a comparison with half-life in rat. The results from the first subject indicate a half-life of 20 minutes in human blood, as opposed to the 9.2 minutes half-life in rat blood reported by Chang et al.[21]. This renders the hypothesis of increased release coupled with active breakdown in human blood more unlikely. It suggests that β-END synthesis is more active in the intermediate lobe and that blood endorphin in rat may be derived from that structure.

THE BRAIN β-ENDORPHIN/ACTH SYSTEM

Both our laboratory and that of Drs. Bloom and Guillemin have shown that the brain β-END system is separate from the brain enkephalin system[6,22] and that specific lesions can lead to the selective depletion of β-END/β-LPH or enkephalin[6]. We have further shown that this system contains β-LPH[3] and ACTH[6,23] immunoreactivites, suggesting the presence of 31K precursor in these neurons. In these anatomical studies, we could not conclusively determine whether the precursor or its individual fragments are stored within the neuron. In a further series of anatomical experiments, we have explored the possible existence of specific fragments of the 31K precursor within these neurons, as well as in pituitary. Furthermore, since there are reports of differential levels[4] or localization[24] of ACTH and β-END in brain, we have studied the possibility that there are multiple ACTH systems containing different portions of the ACTH molecule. In a series of studies employing a number of antibodies obtained from Dr. C. H. Li and Drs. Mains and Eipper (cf. Table 2), we have addressed the following questions:

1. Is the β-LPH immunoreactivity we have previously described due primarily to β-END, or is β-LPH stored in the periarcuate system? Any antibody directed against the C-terminus of β-LPH would be likely to recognize both β-END and β-LPH. The β-LPH antibody previously employed is directed against the N-terminus, but showed some cross-reactivity with β-END (< 1%). In the present studies we employed Dr. C. H. Li's β-LPH affinity-purified antibody. The purification step eliminates any cross-reactivity with β-END.

2. Are we visualizing all of ACTH 1-39 in the periarcuate system?
Multiple antisera directed against various framents (from Drs. Mains & Eipper)
were necessary for these experiments (cf. Table 2).

3. Is ACTH-like immunoreactivity present in nonendorphinergic neurons?
Here again the multiple ACTH antisera were critical.

4. Is ACTH stored as a separate peptide or are we visualizing it as part
of the 31K precursor? For this, we needed an antibody which bound free ACTH
but not the 31K precursor. The ACTH 34-39 antibody from Drs. Mains & Eipper
provided a partial solution in that it only reacts with the free C-terminus of
ACTH, i.e., after it has been cleaved from the 31K precursor.

5. Can we identify the existence of 31K independently of the existence of
β-LPH, β-END, or ACTH? This necessitated the use of an antibody to the 16K
fragment of the 31K precursor which is neither ACTH nor β-LPH (Table 2).

These studies were carried out employing standard immunohistochemical procedures as described elsewhere[3,6]. Both normal and colchicine-treated rats
were studied. All antisera showed immunoreactivity in the same periarcuate
system previously shown to contain β-END, β-LPH, and ACTH (Figure 1). There
was no evidence of cellular immunoreactivity outside this system. These
results suggest that β-LPH and ACTH are stored in these neurons as separate
entities and that the same neurons can be visualized by all of the β-END,
β-LPH, ACTH, and 16K antisera described in Table 2. β-END immunoreactivity
could be attributable to β-LPH. However, β-LPH immunoreactivity does not seem
due to β-END, as both the original β-LPH antiserum and the affinity purified
β-LPH antibody demonstrated the same neuronal system. The full ACTH structure
appears represented in these neurons, either as a single peptide or in fragments. Furthermore, ACTH appears to be cleaved away from 31K since the ACTH
34-39 antiserum was also positive. Finally, the reactivity with the 16K antibody further reinforces the notion that the full 31K synthetic machinery exists
in these neurons, although we cannot determine whether 31K per se (as opposed
to its individual components) is stored. Thus there is immunocytochemical
support for similarity of pituitary and brain β-END/ACTH biosynthetic systems
and for the possible existence of ACTH as a free peptide. Colchicine-treated
animals revealed the same neurons and immunoreactivity with the exception that
perikarya were more easily visualized. In untreated rats, the ACTH 34-39
antiserum showed faint cell bodies and bright axons and terminals, suggesting
less free peptide in cells of origin and relatively more in axonal areas.

To date, we have been unable to visualize any ACTH-like immunoreactivity
outside this 31K brain system. None of these antisera demonstrated cells or
fibers in enkephalin positive structures.

TABLE 2

SUMMARY OF ANTISERA AND CROSSREACTIVITY

Antisera and Titer for Immunocytochemistry	Crossreactivity
β-LPH (1/800) (C. H. Li - UCSF)	Not blocked by leu-enkephalin, met-enkephalin, ACTH, β-MSH (< 1% cross-reactive with β-END by RIA)
β-LPH (1/500) (C. H. Li - UCSF)	Same as above, except for being affinity purified to eliminate β-END cross-reactivity.
β-END (1/800) (Mains & Eipper, U. Colo)	Not blocked by met-enkephalin, leu-enkephalin, ACTH, β-MSH (100 % cross-reactive β_hLPH)
β-END (1/500) (C. H. Li - UCSF)	Not blocked by met- or leu-enkephalin, β-MSH, ACTH (partially cross-reactive with β_hLPH)
ACTH 11-24 (1/1500) (Mains & Eipper, U. Colo)	Not blocked by β-END, β-LPH, met-enkephalin, leu-enkephalin, β-MSH
ACTH 1-16 (1/500) (Mains & Eipper, U. Colo)	Not blocked by β-END, β-LPH, met-enkephalin, leu-enkephalin, β-MSH (as above). Non-parallel with alpha-MSH and $ACTH_{1-13}$
ACTH 34-39 (1/500) (Mains & Eipper, U. Colo)	Not blocked by β-END, β-LPH, met-enkephalin, leu-enkephalin, β-MSH. Only recognizes "free" C-terminus ACTH.
"16K" (1/500) (Mains & Eipper, U. Colo)	Precipitates 16K fragment of precursor 99% and β_{rat}LPH 1%. Noncross-reactive with β-END, enkephalins or ACTH, β-MSH.

PEPTIDES WHICH ALTER BRAIN AND PITUITARY β-END

While there are few studies demonstrating significant effects of hormonal manipulations on β-END, particularly in brain[25,26], there are a number of lines of evidence showing such effects on other 31K-derived peptides, such as β-MSH and ACTH. One such line of work is of particular interest since a peptide in very low concentrations has led to significant and differential effects on β-MSH and ACTH in pituitary. Pavel[27] injected arginine-vasotocin (AVT) intracerebroventricularly and inhibited compensatory adrenal hypertrophy and, by inference, ACTH release. Yet, the same treatment resulted in decrease in pituitary β-MSH, suggesting increased MSH release[28]. Another peptide, melanocyte stimulating hormone release inhibiting factor (MIF) has been shown upon intraperitoneal systemic injections to lead to significant elevations in β-MSH gland levels and a significant decrease in β-MSH release[29]. The effect of MIF injection intracerebroventricularly has not--to our knowledge--been reported.

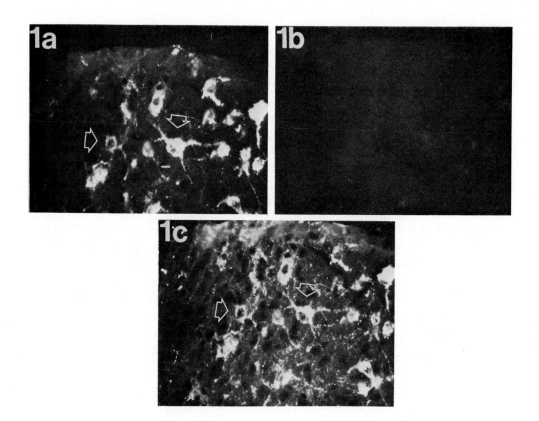

Fig. 1. Demonstration of ACTH 11-24 and β-END 1-9 in colchicine pretreated
rat. Cells are in the periarcuate region of rat hypothalamus.
1A: ACTH antiserum demonstrates these hypothalamic cells in the arcuate
region. After a wash with 6M guanidine HCl, exposure to UV light, and
incubation with goat-antirabbit antiserum, control photo 1B was taken. Note
the lack of residual activity. 1C: reexposure of the same section to
anti-β-END antiserum and then FITC tagged goat-antirabbit IgG resulted in the
visualization of the same cells (arrows). In other sections β-LPH was also
visualized in the same cells. Normal rats were studied with the same result.
All visualization could be blocked by the appropriate peptide (i.e., ACTH
1-24, 1 μM etc). X 100.

The potential effect of the two peptides AVT and MIF on pituitary and brain β-LPH/β-END was of interest since it might allow us to uncover general effects on 31K-containing cells, or, alternatively, lead us to find differential effects on various 31K fragments. We therefore undertook a study of the effect of icv injection of MIF and AVT in varying doses, and intraperitoneal injection of MIF on both brain and pituitary β-END/β-LPH.

For icv injection, the peptides were dissolved in saline at the appropriate concentration such that the varying doses could be administered in 10 μl volume. Both the experimental and control animals were injected into the lateral ventricle under light ether anesthesia. All animals were sacrificed 20 minutes after injection. The brains were rapidly removed from the skull and the hypothalami and pituitaries dissected and immediately frozen on Dry Ice. The tissue was extracted using the method of Rossier et al.[22]. β-END-like immunoreactivity was measured by means of the radioimmunoassay described above.

Tables 3a,b,c,d summarize some of the results of these studies. The peripheral injection of MIF (Table 3a) led to a significant increase in levels of β-END/β-LPH in the pituitary gland, suggesting an effect parallel with β-MSH changes. However, hypothalamic content remained unaltered. The central injection of MIF, on the other hand, led to little change in pituitary level. Yet, a dose of 5.6 pg icv resulted in a significant reduction in hypothalamic levels (Table 3b). However, a consistent dose response relation between icv MIF and levels of β-END immunoreactivity was not obtained.

Arginine vasotocin, when injected intracerebroventricularly, led to a decrease in β-END/β-LPH hypothalamic levels. Only the 20 pg dose produced a significant change (Table 3c). In pituitary, no significant changes with icv AVT were observed, although a 22% drop was obtained at the highest dose (Table 3d).

The above studies lead to two conclusions. It appears likely that substances which affect other 31K fragments, such as β-MSH and ACTH, may also affect pituitary β-END. The parallel to β-MSH appears rather striking. This is particularly intriguing if, in fact, a large proportion of pituitary β-END is derived from the intermediate lobe.

The second conclusion concerns the relationship between hypothalamic and pituitary β-END. It is apparent that the same manipulation in a given animal can lead to differential effects on hypothalamic and pituitary systems. While it is clear that the three systems are not regulated in an identical fashion, they may share some of the same neurochemical and pharmacological susceptibilities.

TABLE 3

(a) MIF ip: EFFECT ON PITUITARY β-END/β-LPH (n=5)

(pmoles/mg tissue)

Dose	Control	Experimental	%C
200 μg	29.7 ± 4.13	44.82 ± 5.25	151 %**

[handwritten: ~ 300 pmols/gland]

(b) MIF icv: EFFECT ON HYPOTHALAMIC β-END/β-LPH (n=4)

(pmoles/g tissue)

Dose	Control	Experimental	%C
5.6 pg	82.6 ± 14.6	30.6 ± 9.2	37 %**

(c) AVT icv: EFFECT ON HYPOTHALAMIC β-END/β-LPH (n=5)

(pmoles/g tissue)

Dose	Control	Experimental	%C
10 pg	64.53 ± 3.3	52.07 ± 4.8	81 %
20 pg	82.6 ± 14.6[†]	29.6 ± 3.8[†]	36 % ***
200 pg	75.9 ± 6.9	63.8 ± 3.6	84 %

[handwritten: 2.5 ~ 3 pmol/ HT]

(d) ACT icv: EFFECT ON PITUITARY β-END/β-LPH (n=5)

(pmoles/mg tissue)

Dose	Control	Experimental	%C
10 pg	42.63 ± 2.8	44.00 ± 2.8	103 %
20 pg	37.40 ± 7.5	44.00 ± 8.8	118 %
200 pg	39.05 ± 2.2[†]	27.50 ± 4.7	78 %*

[handwritten: ~ 10 ng / HT]

$^{*}p = .07$

$^{**}p < .05$

$^{***}p < .02$

$^{†}n = 4$

β-ENDORPHIN-LIKE IMMUNOREACTIVITY IN CSF: APPEARANCE UPON ANALGETIC STIMULATION

If brain β-END functions as a neurotransmitter, then it would be released upon activation of its pathways. We are currently studying this possibility in rat. Simultaneously, we have examined the occurrence of stimulated release in humans. The subjects were patients suffering from chronic intractable pain. They were undergoing a procedure for pain relief involving the implantation of a fine electrode in the periventricular region of the medial thalamus[30]. The

homologous site in rat is known to contain β-END/β-LPH fibers[2,5,6]. During
the surgical procedure, the patients were under local anesthesia. A catheter
was introduced into the third ventricle as a standard part of the surgical
procedure. It was employed to withdraw a sample of ventricular cerebrospinal
fluid prior to stimulation (baseline control) and at several time points during
stimulation. All samples studied were derived from subjects who reported
significant relief of pain upon stimulation during and after the surgical
procedure.

The samples were assayed unextracted using the β-END RIA described above.
All controls and the standard curve were carried out in artificial CSF to
permit the comparison. Table 4 summarizes the results. None of the baseline
samples exhibited any β-END-like immunoreactivity, suggesting levels below 25
fmoles. On the other hand, every sample obtained during stimulation exhibited
β-END-like immunoreactivity. This reactivity could be due, at least in part,
to other cross-reacting substances such as β-LPH. Nonetheless, it suggests
that β-END or some structurally related compound could be released upon
electrical stimulation. The magnitude of the change observed here is much
larger than the elevation observed with enkephalin-like immunoreactivity[31].

This finding, aside from pointing to the possible release of β-END from
brain into CSF, supports the hypothesis that stimulation-produced analgesia
may involve the activation of endogenous opioids[32].

TABLE 4

EFFECT OF ELECTRICAL STIMULATION ON β-ENDORPHIN-LIKE IMMUNOREACTIVITY IN
VENTRICULAR CSF

(in fmoles/ml of β-END equivalents)

Patient	Baseline Pre- Stimulation	0-5 min Post- Stimulation	5-10 min Post- Stimulation	10-15 min Post- Stimulation	15-20 min Post- Stimulation
Nm	< 25	250	450	500	
B	< 25	750	300	250	325
S	< 25	Not collected	250	400	
Ns	< 25	575	270	270	
LB	< 25	350	325	350	
Mean	< 25	481.25	319.0	354.0	
± SEM		± 112.44	± 35.16	± 45.45	

CONCLUSIONS

The work we have summarized here is in its preliminary stages and does not yield firm conclusions. Yet, it has allowed us to formulate a few working hypotheses:

1. The 31K precursor appears to be present in brain as well as in intermediate and anterior pituitary lobe.

2. Within pituitary, β-END may be more readily synthesized in (and released from) the intermediate lobe, leading to higher circulating blood levels in animals possessing this structure in contrast to man.

3. Pituitary β-END/β-LPH appear susceptible to the same treatments which alter β-MSH--another 31K fragment synthesized in intermediate lobe.

4. Brain β-END/β-LPH share some of the same susceptibilities as pituitary--although it can be altered differentially by some pharmacological manipulations.

5. Brain β-END (or structurally similar material) is releasable into the CSF upon electrical stimulation in man.

ACKNOWLEDGEMENTS

Our research has been supported by MH 23861, DA 01207, and the ONR. HA is recipient of a Sloan Foundation Fellowship in Neurophysiology, BR 16091. SJW is recipinet of an NIMH Fellowship, MH 11028, and a Bank of American Giannini Foundation Fellowship. RML is supported by the Medical Scientist Training Program. JDB holds Research Scientist Development Award, MH 24161. We express our gratitude to Sue Poage for typing and editorial guidance. We are especially indebted to Drs. Mains and Eipper (Univ. of Colorado) and Dr. C. H. Li (UCSF) for their generous gifts of antisera and peptides.

REFERENCES

1. Guillemin, R., Vargo, T., Rossier, J., Minick, S., Ling, N., Rivier, C., Vale, W. and Bloom, F. (1977) Science 197, 1367-1369.

2. Bloom, F. E., Battenberg, E., Rossier, J., Ling, N. and Guillemin, R. (1978) Proc. Natl. Acad. Sci. USA 75, 1591-1595.

3. Watson, S. J., Barchas, J. D. and Li, C. H. (1977) Proc. Natl. Acad. Sci. USA 74, 5155-5158.

4. Krieger, D. T., Liotta, A., Suda, T., Palkovits, M. and Brownstein, M. J. (1977) Biochem. Biophys. Res. Communica. 73, 930-936.

5. Watson, S. J., Akil, H. and Barchas, J. D. (in press) in Endorphins in Mental Health Research, Usdin, E., Bunney, W. E. and Kline, N. S. eds., MacMillan Press, New York.

6. Watson, S. J., Akil, H., Richard, C. W. and Barchas, J. D. (in press) Nature.

134

7. Mains, R. E., Eipper, B. A. and Ling, N. (1977) Proc. Natl. Acad. Sci. USA 74, 3014-3018.

8. Roberts, J. L. and Herbert, E. (1977) Proc. Natl. Acad. Sci. USA 74, 5300-5304.

9. Bloom, F. E., Segal, D., Ling, N. and Guillemin, R. (1976) Science 194, 630-632.

10. Loh, H. H., Tseng, L. F., Wei, E. and Li, C. H. (1976) Proc. Natl. Acad. Sci. USA 73, 2895-2896.

11. Wei, E. T., Tseng, L. F., Loh, H. H. and Li, C. H. (1977) Life Sci. 21, 321-327.

12. Wei, E. and Loh, H. (1976) Science 1262-1263.

13. Terenius, L., Gispen, W. H. and DeWied, D. (1975) Eur. J. Pharmacol. 33, 395-399.

14. Wiegant, V. M., Gispen, W. H., Terenius, L. and DeWied, D. (1977) Neuroendocrinology 2, 63-69.

15. Bloom, F. E., Battenberg, E., Rossier, J., Ling, N., Leppaluoto, J., Vargo, T. M. and Guillemin, R. (1977) Life Sci. 20, 43-48.

16. Zimmerman, E. A., Liotta, A. and Krieger, D. T. (1978) 186, 393-398.

17. Pelletier, G., De'sy, L., Lissitszky, J. C., Labrie, F. and Li, C. H. (1978) Life Sci. 22, 1799-1804.

18. Rubinstein, M., Stein, S., Gerber, L. D. and Udenfriend, S. (1977) Proc. Natl. Acad. Sci. USA 74, 3052-3055.

19. Liotta, A. S., Suda, T. and Krieger, D. T. (in press) Proc. Natl. Acad. Sci. USA.

20. Eipper, B. and Mains, R. (in press) J. Supramolec. Structure.

21. Chang, W-C., Rao, A. J. and Li, C. H. (1978) Int. J. Pept. Prot. Res. 11, 93-94.

22. Rossier, J., Vargo, T. M., Minick, S., Ling, N., Bloom, F. E. and Guillemin, R. (1977) Proc. Natl. Acad. Sci. USA 74, 5162-5165.

23. Watson, S. J., Richard, C. W. and Barchas, J. D. (1978) Science 200, 1180-1182.

24. Tramu, G., Leonardelli, J. and Dubois, M. P. (1977) Neurosci. Let. 6, 305-309.

25. Mata, M-M., Gainer, H. and Klee, W. A. (1977) Life Sci. 21, 1159-1162.

26. Cox, B. M., Baizman, E. R., Su, T. P., Osman, O. H. and Goldstein, A. (1978) in The Endorphins. Advances in Biochemical Psychopharmacology, Vol. 18, Costa, E. and Trabucchi, M. eds., Raven, New York.

27. Pavel, S. (1975) Experentia 31, 1469-1470.

28. Pavel, S., Gheorghiu, C., Colb, M. and Petrescu, M. (1975) Endocrinology 97, 674-676.

29. Schally, A. V. and Kastin, A. J. (1966) Endocrinology 79, 768-772.

30. Richardson, D. E. and Akil, H. (1977) J. Neurosurg. 47, 178-183.

31. Akil, H., Richardson, D. F., Hughes, J. and Barchas, J. D. (in press) Science.

32. Akil, H., Mayer, D. J. and Liebeskind, J. C. (1976) Science 191, 961-962.

Characteristics and Function of Opioids, editors Van Ree and Terenius
© *1978 Elsevier/North-Holland Biomedical Press*   135

SIGNIFICANCE OF ENDOGENOUS OPIOIDS FOR REGULATION OF NOCICEPTIVE SENSITIVITY IN THE
NORMAL AND STRESSED CONDITIONS.

R.C.A. Frederickson

The Lilly Research Laboratories, Eli Lilly and Co., Indianapolis, Ind., 46206 (USA)

INTRODUCTION

The analgesia produced by acupuncture or electrical brain stimulation [1-3] provided
important functional clues to the existence of endogenous substances modulating reaction to pain. The development of simple in vitro systems for studying the interaction of opiates with receptors [4] provided a detailed understanding of the structure
activity relationships and pharmacology of these interesting drugs and provided
important tools for the search for endogenous ligands. The demonstration of stereospecific opioid receptors in brain [5-7] had a catalytic effect on this search. Within
1-2 years of the demonstration of the receptors evidence for the existence of opioid
peptides in brain was reported [8,9] and was rapidly confirmed and extended. The
apparent lack of marked direct pharmacologic effects of the opioid antagonists, which
had discouraged hopes of finding endogenous ligands, apparently indicates that the
tonic activity of the endorphins in the normal condition is very low and/or that the
behaviors they mediate or modulate may be very subtle and difficult to measure under
normal conditions. Narcotic antagonists have been reported to have very little direct
effects except possibly to cause a slight increase in anxiety [11,12]. Opiates are reported to be more effective on pain tolerance than pain threshold, that is to affect
more the emotional or psychosomatic reaction to pain than its detection [13]. If this is
indeed true it would be expected to be very difficult to detect antagonism by naloxone
of an opioid peptidergic system modulating such feelings in an individual not
experiencing pain.

The subtlety of the effects of blocking endogenous opioid systems is emphasized by
the conflicting reports on the effects of the narcotic antagonist naloxone on pain
models utilizing normal animal or man. This indicates the importance in attempting
to study the results of interfering with the endogenous opioid systems of measuring
the appropriate parameters and under the appropriate conditions to increase their activity. The use of appropriate pathological models may also be very useful in these
studies. Work undertaken along these lines and its implication for the functions of
opioid peptides is the subject of discussion here.

HYPERALGESIC ACTIVITY OF NARCOTIC ANTAGONISTS
RODENT

Jacob et al [14] in 1974, before the discovery of the endogenous ligands was published, reported a hyperalgesic effect of naloxone in mice and rats using a hot plate
technique. They suggested that positive effects were contingent upon utilizing control

reaction times that were 'sufficiently long' and interpreted the activity of relatively low doses of naloxone (0.1 - 1,0 mg/kg sc) to indicate that specific opioid receptors were involved in the effect. These results were confirmed by Frederickson et al [15] although a slightly higher range of naloxone doses (0.5 - 4 mg/kg sc) was used by the latter group. Both groups found the effects to be specific to the jump response, the paw lick response being rather insensitive to naloxone. Goldstein et al [16], however, using a different paradigm in rats, had failed to observe a hyperalgesic effect of naloxone. These authors recognized that the lack of an effect in their test (shock escape) may have been due to measurement of pain threshold rather than pain 'tolerance' but, concluded that their data offered no support to the hypothesis that an endogenous opioid modulates responsiveness to pain.

Subsequently, Grevert and Goldstein [17] utilized the mouse hot plate test and provided a second confirmation of the results of Jacob et al [14]. Apparently the latency to jump from the hot plate provides a measure of pain tolerance. The latency to paw lick on the hot plate may be more a measure of pain threshold and is therefore not lowered by naloxone. There has since been further confirmation of the hyperalgesic effect of naloxone in rodent with several different test systems [18-20]. One group [20] used acetic acid-induced writhing and reiterated the importance of prolonged nociceptive stimulation for obtaining positive results with naloxone. Another group observed hyperalgesic effects of naloxone on tail flick (thermal) but not tail pinch (mechanical) and suggested the opiate systems may have differential actions on different pain stimuli [19].

MAN

The initial studies in humans, like several of the earlier studies in rodent, failed to demonstrate the 'hyperalgesic' activity of naloxone. The lack of effect in the studies of El-Sobky et al [10] could have been predicted from what has been learned from the animal studies. This group postulated and tested for changes in threshold for perception of painful electric shock stimulus. The perception of such a stimulus was also not altered by naloxone in the rat [16]. Studies with naloxone in animal models and experience with opiates in the clinic indicate it is more likely pain tolerance than pain threshold which is regulated by endorphims. The latter authors concluded that it is unlikely that there is a tonic release of an endogenous opioid which interacts with pain perception in normal conditions and suggested that such a material may be released only under special conditions. Using a different method for administering pain (ischemic) Grevert and Goldstein [12] also found no effect of naloxone on pain ratings in humans. They reported an increase in anxiety but were unable to repeat the effect on tension-anxiety in a subsequent study [21].

The above studies indicated that naloxone has little if any effect on the threshold to experimentally - induced pain in humans. However, in 1965 Lazagna [22] reported a "curious hyperalgesic effect" of naloxone in patients with postoperative pain. Levine

et al [23] assumed from this that clinical pain might be a more appropriate model than
experimental pain to study the actions of endorphins and naloxone and tested this in
oral surgery patients. They observed an increase in pain ratings after naloxone
treatment (9mg) and concluded that the stress and prolonged duration associated with
clinical pain may make it particularly effective for activating the endogenous analgesia system. These studies were, however, confounded by premedication with diazepam
and the administration of nitrous oxide during surgery. Buchsbaum et al [24] were able to
demonstrate a hyperalgesic effect of naloxone on sensitivity of human subjects to experimentally-induced pain. They divided their subjects into 'pain sensitive' and 'pain
insensitive' groups and analyzed ratings of severity of pain from various levels of
shock rather than determining specific thresholds for pain. There was no effect on the
pain sensitive group but the pain insensitive subjects rated more of the stimuli as
unpleasant or worse on naloxone than on placebo. The latency of evoked potentials in
cortical EEG recording was also decreased by naloxone in the pain insensitive individ-
usals.

   In summary, when thresholds to experimentally-induced pain in unselected individuals was examined naloxone appeared to have little effect, while to the contrary, when
reaction to rather than threshold for perception of clincial pain, or experimental
pain in selected pain-insensitive subjects, was examined naloxone produced a hyperalgesic effect. Hence, under the proper conditions behavior suggestive of the activity of
an endogenous opioid system modulating reactivity to pain can be observed.

EFFECTS OF STRESS ON NOCICEPTION AND ENDOGENOUS OPIOIDS
   Several studies have been performed to examine the effects of stress on various
measures of endogenous opioid systems. Madden et al [25] thought it reasonable to consider that 'the opioid peptides may normally function to modulate pain responsiveness'
and undertook to examine stress-induced changes in central opioid levels and pain
responsiveness in the rat. They found that the whole brain total opioid activity was
increased after foot-shock stress and this rise was accompanied by significant analgesia. The effect on pain responsiveness confirms other reports of the analgesic effect
of acute stress which has been reported to be partially or completely prevented by
naloxone administration [26-28]. Chronic exposure to pain-induced stress (hot plate)
during early postnatal life has also been reported to result in an increase in endogenous opioid ligands as measured by radioreceptor assay. Another group [30] used chronic exposure to electric shock to condition fear to the tail flick apparatus in rats.
They then tested these animals for nociceptive response and immediately sacrificed
them in order to measure enkephalin binding. They observed an antinociceptive effect
from this treatment correlated with decreased binding of labelled Leu-enkephalin which
they interpreted to reflect increased occupancy by endogenous ligands.

   In contrast to the above studies which provide evidence for stress-induced increases in total opioid activity, when RIA techniques were utilized to measure levels of
specified opioid peptides decreases were seen after stress. Fratta et al [31] observed

138

a decrease in met-enkephalin immunoreactivity after foot-shock stress but the effect was not significant. Rossier et al [32,33] observed decreases in B-endorphin and Leu-enkephalin immunoreactivity after 30 min. or 1 hour of inescapable foot-shock stress. The apparent discrepancies between the above results are not surprising. The antinociceptive effect of stress and its antagonism by naloxone would be most understandable in terms of an increase in the activity of an endogenous opioid system. This could provide increases, decreases or no change in levels of the peptides depending on the specific conditions of the experiments. This will be discussed in more detail later in the next section.

EVIDENCE FOR TONIC ACTIVITY OF OPIOIDS VARYING IN A DIURNAL FASHION

The studies discussed above revealed considerable controversy concerning the hyperalgesic effect of the narcotic antagonist naloxone. Some results were positive and some were negative in the studies with animal tests and this situation was similar for the studies in man. These differences were clearly due to differences in experimental conditions but nevertheless tonic activity of endogenous opioids in the normal condition seemed not clearly established.

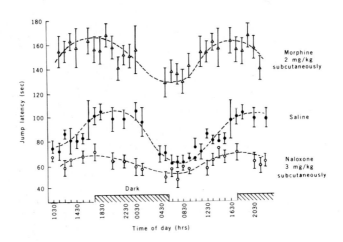

Fig.1. Diurnal rhythm in latencies to the jump response on the mouse hot plate maintained at 52°C. Closed circles refer to animals treated with saline, subcutaneously, 15 minutes before testing. Open circles refer to animals treated with naloxone at 3 mg/kg, subcutaneously, 15 minutes before testing. Open triangles refer to animals treated with morphine at 2 mg/kg, subcutaneously, 30 minutes before testing. The latencies (mean $\pm$ S.E., N = 10 to 100) in seconds are plotted as a function of the time of day. The datum points at each $\frac{1}{2}$ hour are the means of values collected over a 1-hour period. For example, the points plotted at 0930 hours are the means of measurements made from 0900 to 1000 hours. Lights were off during the time period marked by the hatched bars. Several points are repeated beyond 24 hours in order to better illustrate the rhythm. (Reproduced from Frederickson et al.[34]).

Recent studies, however, have provided evidence for tonic activity of endogenous opioids which varies in a diurnal fashion. Frederickson et al [34] observed a diurnal rhythm in responsivity of mice to noxious stimuli (as measured by jump latencies on a hot plate) and corresponding diurnal changes in the degree of naloxone-induced hyperalgesia (fig.1.). The rhythm and the hyperalgesic activity of naloxone are only demostrable for the jump response but not the paw lick response on the hot plate. Similar findings of a rhythm in the hyperalgesic activity of naloxone in a mouse AChBr-induced writing test has been recently reported[35]. This rhythm is not specific to rodents but in fact a very similar rhythm in nociceptive sensitivity to that reported in the mouse [34], has been reported for man[36,37]. It is, as would be expected, 180° out of phase with the rhythm detected in nocturnal rodent. Interestingly it has been recently observed that in man as in the rat the hyperalgesic activity of naloxone follows the diurnal rhythm in pain sensitivity, being more effective in the early morning hours than later in the afternoon[38]. Lack of consideration for this factor as well as the choice of inappropriate parameters to measure may explain many of the failures to demonstrate naloxone hyperalgesia.

But of course the significance of these observations goes beyond explaining the various conflicting reports in the literature. The rhythmic variations in reactivity to painful stimuli and the alteration of the peaks by naloxone suggests rhythmic activity of an endogenous opioid system(s) providing physiological modulation of nociceptive behavior. This in fact provides evidence for tonic activity in the normal condition since the changes occur naturally in a diurnal fashion without need to be activated by unnatural stressful stimuli.

Elsewhere in this volume Frederickson et al[39] report studies performed to test the above hypothesis. The longer latencies to jump in the afternoon compared to morning and the ability of naloxone to reduce the afternoon latencies was still apparent in hypophysectomized mice suggesting a mediation by an opioid system in brain rather than pituitary. This result must be considered with caution at this time however, since loss of the hyperalgesic activity of naloxone after hypophysectomy has been reported by another laboratory[40]. Nevertheless total opioid levels in whole brain were higher in the afternoon than in the morning. When levels of Met and Leu-enkephalin were measured by RIA higher levels of met-enkephalin were observed in the afternoon compared to morning but the difference was not significant. When the mice were stressed by exposure to a noxious stimulus (left on 52°C hot plate until jump) before sacrifice by focussed microwave, however, there was a significant increase compared to unstressed mice in met-enkephalin levels in the p.m. but not in the a.m. To what extent this diurnal difference may explain the controversy between previous studies [25-33] of the effects is not clear since there were many other methodological differences between the studies such as different species, different means of inducing stress, different durations of stress, different times and different means of sacrifice and different methods for extraction and purification of the opioid materials.

For example, in the studies of Frederickson et al[39] the mice were exposed to the noxious stimulus (hot plate) just long enough to express a stressful reaction (jump) and then were immediately sacrificed by microwave while in the studies of Rossier et al[33], who observed a decrease rather than increase in endorphin levels, the rats were exposed to the noxious stimulus (electric shock) for 30 or 60 minutes and then sacrificed either immediately or 15 minutes later by decapitation.

An adequate resolution of this question will not be forthcoming until it becomes possible to measure _turnover_ of specific endorphins or enkephalins with and without exposure to stress and with careful consideration of diurnal differences.

CONCLUSIONS

It seems clear at this time that the narcotic antagonist naloxone will produce hyperalgesic effects under the proper conditions. The many failures to demonstrate such activity in rodent or man were most likely due to measurement of inappropriate phenomena (threshold for detection of, rather than tolerance to, pain) and inadequate attention to diurnal variations. This activity can be most simply explained by assuming that the antagonist acts by blocking the modulation by an endogenous opioid system(s) of nociceptive reactivity. This system(s) can apparently be activated by appropriate stress since such stress produces antinociceptive effects which can be antagonized by naloxone. Evidence for tonic activity of this system(s) in the normal condition also has been provided by the demonstration of a diurnal rhythm in pain responsivity and in the hyperalgesic effect of naloxone in rodents and man. Various studies have provided evidence for diurnal variations and stress-induced changes in steady-state levels of various brain opioid materials. However, studies on the turnover of these materials under various conditions, necessary to establish that changing activity in an endogenous opioid system(s) regulates nociception, have not yet been reported.

While this paper has concentrated on studies dealing with the possible role of endogenous opioids in nociception it is likely that these materials mediate or modulate other behaviors as well. For example, there have been several reports, some conflicting, relating effects of opioid agonists and antagonists on mental disorders, notably schizophrenia (see for example reports by L.Terenius in this volume). Very recently De Wied et al[41,42] have reported on the neuroleptic-like activity of (Des-Tyr')-γ-endorphin in rats and man. The suggestion was made that this material may be an endogenous neuroleptic formed from β-endorphin in brain. Indeed there may be an important balance between these substances and their interconversion essential for maintenance of the normal condition. In this regard it would be interesting to know whether there is a diurnal rhythm in the susceptability of schizophrenics to psychotic episodes.

REFERENCES

1. Chiang, C.Y., Chang, C.T., Chu, H.L. and Yang, L.F. (1973) Sci. Sin. 16:210-217.
2. Reynolds, D.V. (1969) Science 164:444-445.
3. Mayer, D.J. and Price, D.D. (1976) Pain 2:379-404.
4. Kosterlitz, H.W. and Waterfield, A.A. (   ) Ann. Rev. Pharmacol.
5. Pert, C.B. and Snyder, S.H. (1973) Science 179:1011-1014.
6. Terenius, L. (1973) Acta Pharmacol. Tox. 32:397-320.
7. Simon, E.J. Hiller, J.M. and Edelman, I. (1973) Proc. Natl. Acad. Sci. USA 70:1947-1949.
8. Hughes, J. (1975) Brain Res. 88:295-308.
9. Terenius, L. and Wahlström, A. (1975) Acta Physiol. Scand. 94:74-81.
10. El-Sobky, A., Dostrovsky, J.O. and Wall, P.D. (1976) Nature 263: 783-784.
11. Jasinski, D.R., Martin, W.R. and Haertzen, C.A. (1967) J. Pharmacol. Exp. Ther. 157:420-426.
12. Grevert, P. and Goldstein, A. (1977) Proc. Natl. Acad. Sci. USA 74:1291-1294.
13. Jaffe, J.H. and Martin, W.R. (1975) pp. 245-283 in The Harmacological Basis of Therapeutics, L.S. Goodman and A. Gilman, Eds. MacMillan, New York.
14. Jacob, J.J., Tremblay, E.C. and Colombel, M.C. (1974) Psychopharmacol 37:217-223.
15. Frederickson, R.C.A., Nickander, R., Smithurick, E.L., Shuman, R. and Norris, F. H. (1976) pp. 239-246 in Opiates and Endogenous Opioid Ligands, H.W. Kosterlitz, Ed., Elsevier, Amsterdam.
16. Goldstein, A., Pryor, G.T., Otis, L.S. and Larsen, F. (1976) Life Sciences 18:599-604
17. Grevert, P. and Goldstein, A. (1977) Psychopharmacol. 53:111-113.
18. Walker, J.M., Berntson, G.G., Sandman, C.A., Coy, D.H., Schally, A.V. and Kastin, A.J. (1977) Science 196:85-87.
19. Berntson, G.G. and Walker, J.M. (1977) Brain Res. Bull 2:157-159.
20. Kokka, N. and Fairhurst, A.S. (1977) Life Sciences 21:975-980.
21. Grevert, P. and Goldstein, A. (1978) Science 199:1093-1095.
22. Lasagna, L. (1965) Proc. R. Soc. Med. 58:978-983.
23. Levine, J.D., Gordon, N.C., Jones, R.T. and Fields, H.L. (1978) Nature 272:826-827.
24. Buchsbaum, M.S., Davis, G.C. and Bunney, W.E.,Jr. (1977) Nature 270:620-622.
25. Madden, J.IV, Akil, H., Patrick, R.L. and Barchas, J.D. (1977) Nature 265:358-260.
26. Hayes, R.L., Bennett, G.J., Newlon, P. and Mayer, D.J. (1976) Soc. Neurosá, Abstr. No. 1350.
27. Akil, H., Madden, J., Patrick, R. and Barchas, J.D. (1976) in Opiates and Endogenous Opioid Peptides, H.W. Kosterlitz, Ed., Elsevier, Amsterdam.
28. Chesher, G.B. and Chan, B. (1977) Life Sci. 21:1569-1574.
29. Torda, C. (1978) Psychoneuroendocrinol. 3:85-91
30. Chance, W.T., White, A.C., Krynock, G.M. and Rosecrans, J.A. (1978) Brain. Res. 141:371-374.
31. Fratta, W., Yang, H-Y.T., Hong, J. and Costa, E. (1977) Nature 268:452.
32. Rossier, J., French, E., Rivier, C., Ling,N., Guillemin, R. and Bloom, F. (1977) Nature 270:618.
33. Rossier, J., Guillemin, R. and Bloom, F. (1978) Europ. J. Pharmacol. 48:465-466.
34. Frederickson, R.C.A., Burgis, V. and Edwards, J.D. (1977) Science 198:756-758.
35. Cuenca, E., Serrano, M.I., Gibert, J., Alamo, C. and Esteban, J. (1978) 7th International Congress of Pharmacology, Paris, abstr. no. 282.
36. Procacci, P., Byzelli, G., Passeir, I., Sassi, R., Voegelin, M.R. and Zoppi, M. (1972) Ros. Clin. Stud. Headache 3:260-278.
37. Rogers, E.J. and Vilkin, B. (1978) J.Clin. Psychiatry 39:431-432, 438.
38. Davis, G.C., Buchsbaum, M.S. and Bunney, W.E.,Jr. (in press) Life Sciences.
39. Frederickson, R.C.A., Wesche, D. and Richter, J. (1978) this volume.
40. Goldstein, A. (1978) presented at the 7th International Congress of Pharmacology, Paris.
41. De Wied, D., Bohus, B., Van Ree, J.M., Kovács, G.L. and Greven, H.M. (1978) The Lancet, May 13, p. 1046.
42. Verhoeven, W.M.A., van Praag, H.M., Botter, P.A., Sumer, A., Van Ree, J.M. and De Wied, D. (1978) The Lancet, May 13, pp 1046-1047.

Characteristics and Function of Opioids, editors Van Ree and Terenius
© *1978 Elsevier/North-Holland Biomedical Press*

THE IMPLICATIONS OF ENDORPHINS IN PATHOLOGICAL STATES

LARS TERENIUS

Department of Pharmacology, University of Uppsala, Box 573,

S-751 23 Uppsala, Sweden

INTRODUCTION

The recent discovery of endogenous morphine-like agents, the
endorphins, gives rise to several critical questions regarding
their functions under physiological conditions. It has so far been
found to be difficult to define these functions although several
possibilities have been suggested[1,2,3,4,5]. One reason for these
difficulties is the multiplicity and wide-spread distribution of
endorphin systems (cf. Table 1). In the CNS, for instance, enkephalin-containing neurons are found over a large number of nuclei
and form synapses with fibers containing several different transmitters[6,7,8,9]. In brain and periphery, there also seem to be two
separate endorphin systems, one with enkephalins as the active
species, the other with β-endorphin as the active species. This
difference is not trivial since the enkephalins are highly un-
stable both in brain and body fluids whereas β-endorphin at least
in the brain produces sustained effects[1-5,10]. Thus it may be proposed that enkephalins are neurotransmitter candidates in the
nervous system and have very transient effects in general, while
β-endorphin may have a more protracted (neuro)modulatory activity.

The importance of the brain-pituitary-adrenal endorphin axis
remains elusive at present. It seems possible that during stress
for instance, there are concomitant activation and release of
endorphins at all levels. It is important to keep in mind that
the endorphin systems show this complexity, and consequently, it
is quite difficult to define which endorphin system, if any, is
activated.

The possible involvement of endorphins in human pathology has
been investigated intensively ever since the endorphins were first
discovered[4,5]. These studies have utilized essentially two approaches, viz. studies of the effects of narcotic antagonists like
naloxone, and measurement of endorphins in body fluids, mainly
the cerebrospinal fluid (CSF). The naloxone approach, like any

TABLE 1
MULTIPLE OPIOID SYSTEMS (TENTATIVE LISTING)

SITE	PRINCIPAL PEPTIDE
CNS	ENKEPHALINS
	β-ENDORPHIN
GANGLIA	ENKEPHALINS
ADENOHYPOPHYSIS	β-ENDORPHIN
ADRENAL MEDULLA	ENKEPHALINS
GASTROINTESTINAL TRACT	ENKEPHALINS

pharmacologic approach, will be dependent on how perfect as a tool the drug is. In most studies it would seem to be a relatively pure antagonist, but there are reports to the contrary. For instance, naloxone seems to affect GABA-ergic transmission[11]. The second approach, to measure endorphins in body fluids, presents interpretative problems for several reasons. With regard to the body fluid analyzed, measurements in CSF will give the best information possible on CNS endorphin activity while blood, plasma, or urine measurements would rather give information on the peripheral systems. Most clinical studies have been performed on CSF with a radioreceptor assay developed by Terenius and Wahlström[12]. This is a bioassay and measures receptor-active material. The structure of the most significant component, Fraction I, has not yet been determined[13]. The assay was developed at a time when the structures of the endorphins were not yet established and was used as an entirely empirical tool. Since it has provided some quite interesting clinical information[14,15,16] it has been maintained in its original form.

This review covers the two most extensively studied areas, clinical pain and psychiatric disorders.

CLINICAL PAIN

In the first place it has been investigated whether or not endorphins are involved in clinical pain. An early observation by Lasagna[17] that naloxone worsens postoperative pain has recently been confirmed by Levine and collaborators[18]. In the latter study, effects of naloxone were compared with those produced by placebo on a double-blind basis. Naloxone produced a greater increase in reported pain levels within the 2-4 hour period after a standardized surgical procedure (removal of 2-4 teeth). The picture is somewhat complicated by the fact that the authors used diazepam as premedication and N_2O anaesthesia. It cannot be completely ruled out that these agents released endorphins. In healthy volunteers, on the other hand, it has been difficult to observe any effect of naloxone on pain sensitivity in an experimental situation[19,20]. Recent data, however, suggest that there may exist interindividual differences, some individuals reacting to naloxone with increased pain sensitivity[21]. The results discussed above strongly indicate that endorphins are released in the clinical pain situation whereas resting activity is individual but at any rate quite low.

The studies referred to deal with acute pain, and it is not difficult to understand that during the evolution of the species, mechanisms for reducing severe pain have been of considerable survival value. When pain lasts or becomes chronic this might also affect the endorphin homeostasis. Because of the permanent character of the chronic pain syndrome, it may be assumed that endorphin activity would be at a pathological steady-state level. From a clinical point of view, it is known that there is an adaptation phase during which the patient gradually adjusts to living with the pain and, after a period of about 6 months, the symptoms will be rather stable[22,23,24,25]. The patient with chronic pain is difficult to assess and hard to treat. Methods for the objective assessment of pain and its etiology are badly needed.

In an early investigation, we observed that the CSF levels of endorphin-like activity, measured in the radioreceptor assay, were very low in patients with neuralgic pain[12]. Since this very early study, CSF analyses have been carried out in this laboratory on several hundred patients with various diseases. We have also measured levels in healthy volunteers. These studies have confirmed our early observation, that patients with neurogenic pain have very low endorphin levels (Table 2). While collecting

TABLE 2

CSF ENDORPHIN LEVELS IN PATIENTS WITH CHRONIC NEUROGENIC PAIN
AND IN HEALTHY VOLUNTEERS (From refs. 12,16,26).

Subjects	Endorphin Fraction I (pmole/ml)*		
	< 0.6	0.6-1.2	> 1.2
Neurogenic pain patients	28	5	
Healthy volunteers	3	12	4

* calculated as if due to methionine-enkephalin

TABLE 3

CSF ENDORPHIN FRACTION I IN PATIENTS WITH CHRONIC PAIN
(n = 37). (From ref. 16).

Patient category	Endorphin Fraction I		
	$\leq$ 0.6	> 0.6 (pmole/ml)	Difference
Organic pain	13	7	$\chi^2 = 11.3$
Psychogenic pain	1	16	(p < 0.001)
Positive neurology	12	2	$\chi^2 = 18.1$
No positive neurology	2	21	(p < 0.001)

these data we decided to use the CSF analysis in a series of
chronic pain patients. This investigation is still running and
only some selected data will be reported here. The purpose of the
investigation is to define a patient with chronic pain by using
objective methods.

The patients were consecutive cases admitted to a University
Neurological clinic. The inclusion criterion was a chronic pain
syndrome (duration > 6 months). Exclusion criteria were old age,
organic brain syndrome, alcohol or drug abuse, or previous expo-

sure to strong analgesics. Every patient was subjected to extensive neurologic and psychiatric evaluation. Furthermore, a CSF sample was withdrawn for endorphin and monoamine metabolite measurements, and experimental pain thresholds as well as average evoked responses (AER) were recorded.

In the first examination, the possible use of CSF endorphin measurement for the differential diagnosis of chronic pain patients was investigated. From a clinical point of view, the chronic pain syndromes may be divided into the somatogenic, "organic pain" category and the diffuse type which is better described in psychologic terms, so-called psychogenic pain[23,25]. At a first level, the discrimination between organic and psychogenic pain syndromes was made from the general clinical impression and the patient's own description of his pain syndrome. At a second level, the patient was subjected to extensive neurologic analysis to evaluate if the pain syndrome was of neurogenic origin. The results can be seen from Table 3 which shows the highly significant differences in CSF endorphin levels between these two categories. The very low endorphin levels are particularly characteristic of the neurogenic pain patient whereas the patient with non-neurogenic, but still presumably organic, pain may have levels in the normal range. The low levels in neurogenic pain may indicate low, subthreshold endorphin activity. Contrary to the traditional view that pain is exclusively generated via pain fibers the hypothesis can be advanced that it might just as well derive from lack of activation of pain inhibitory systems. In fact, it has recently been proposed that phantom body pain and related pain syndromes may be due to decreased activity in central inhibitory systems[27]. These systems would be activated via peripheral fibers and rendered silent by a loss in sensory input. Probably the mechanism behind transcutaneous nerve stimulation (TNS) analgesia[28,29,30,31] is an increase in the sensory input activating central inhibitory systems. It is an attractive hypothesis that the central inhibitory systems should be endorphin-mediated.

The arguments advanced here depend very much on the validity of endorphin measurements with the present methodology. Some experimental findings support such validity. Firstly, there is a statistically significant relation between endorphin levels and the experimentally derived pain threshold as well as tolerance level[32]. Secondly, the endorphin levels rise on electroacupuncture[26], a treatment giving pain relief in certain chronic pain cases. This hypothesis becomes even more convincing as pain will return in such cases on naloxone injection[33]. We may therefore conclude that often a pain syndrome of neurogenic origin is probably related to a loss of endogenous central pain control. From a practical point of view it can also be concluded that CSF endorphin measurements can serve as a tool for differential diagnosis of neurogenic versus non-neurogenic pain syndromes.

Similar arguments have recently been put forward to explain background factors in essential headache[34]. The affected pain-prone patient is supposed to suffer from a dysfunctioning central antinociceptive system. In support of this hypothesis are findings that CSF endorphin levels, measured by the method of Terenius and Wahlström[12], are subnormal in the cases with headache[35]. A cornerstone in contemporary psychophysical theories is the individual capacity of adjusting to sensory input or stimulation in general. For instance in Pavlov's typology[36], individuals may have a "weak" or "strong" nervous system. An individual with a weak nervous system would have low stimulatory thresholds and with increasing stimulation intensity he would show a "defensive reduction" to cope with the excessive stimuli. Such an individual is considered lacking an internal inhibitory system. The individual with a "strong" nervous system shows high thresholds and would tolerate sensory loading much better. Reaction to sensory stimuli is also used in personality inventories. In Eysenk's typology[37], for instance, extraverts will show a tendency to attenuate sensory input. Specifically, such a personality would be connected with high pain endurance as indeed observed[38].

An experimental approach to the studies of the neurophysiological response to stimuli of different intensities was introduced by Petrie[39]. She also introduced the terms "augmenters" and "reducers" to classify the individual differences in reaction to increasing sensory stimuli. The augmenters would tend to enlarge the increases in the stimulus intensity they receive whereas the reducers would tend to diminish it. This distinction has been found to be of considerable conceptual value. At present, a common experimental approach is to use average evoked response (AER)

amplitudes recorded from the scalp[40,41,42]. The augmenting/reducing
tendency seems independent of sensory modality. Most studies have
been carried out with visual AER or somatosensory AER. The reducing
tendency is thought to act, at least partly, via descending inhibitory systems[41]. Could this inhibition be mediated via endorphins?
Two studies would suggest so. In the study of Buchsbaum and collaborators[21], a series of healthy volunteers was tested for pain
thresholds and for pain stimulus-response relationships measured
via AER. As predicted, the pain insensitive individuals tended to
be reducers. Interestingly, these individuals reacted to an injection of the narcotic antagonist naloxone with an increase in
pain sensitivity, which strongly suggests that endogenous production of endorphins increased pain thresholds and rendered the
individuals unresponsive to increases in stimulus intensity. The
picture is somewhat complicated by the fact that naloxone decreased
pain sensitivity in pain-sensitive augmenters - a paradoxical
finding with no explanation. In our study of the earlier discussed
series of 45 chronic pain patients, the visual AER amplitudes were
recorded. Thirty patients could be classified as augmenters and
15 as reducers[42]. This proportion is similar to that found in
healthy volunteers[43]. The results were compared with CSF endorphin
levels. There was a significant (p < 0.01) difference between
reducers and augmenters with regard to endorphin levels, the
former having the higher levels[42].

The close association between the mental state and pain has
been emphasized many times. Psychogenic abdominal pain or pains
associated with anxiety induced heart symptoms are familiar examples[23,25]. Probably less well-known is the association of pain
symptoms with disorders of neurotic or psychotic dimension. Particularly in depression, pain is a common complaint[25,44]. A recent
investigation of several hundred consecutive psychiatric hospital
admissions reveals that about 40% had pain, and about 20% mentioned
that spontaneously[45]. The pain cases were found proportionately
more frequently in conditions such as neurotic or mixed depression,
personality disorders or alcohol addiction. An evaluation of the
depth of depressive symptomatology in the previously described
series[16] of chronic pain patients further stresses the relation
between pain and psychic disorders. As expected, cases with

"psychogenic pain" showed higher ratings although not to a statistically significant extent in the items depressed mood, anxiety, and retardation. Incidentally, none of the patients had been found to have a psychiatric disorder and only a few had earlier consulted a psychiatrist. Interestingly, there was a statistically significant correlation between the depth of depression and CSF endorphin levels, whereas there was no correlation to retardation or anxiety. The correlations exist also within the subgroups "organic pain" and "psychogenic pain". This would indicate that CNS endorphin activity, as reflected in the CSF levels, is a very important factor in the mental homeostasis and influences our general sense of well-being. It will be recalled that enkephalins are postulated reward transmitters and, for instance, rats are willing to work for enkephalin injections[46].

In conclusion, the study of patients with chronic pain indicates that CNS endorphin activity may be associated not only with the type of pain syndrome and the response to pain or stress but also in a much broader sense with CNS activity (Table 4). Whether this association is a direct one or a secondary phenomenon is not known. It serves to stress, however, that unitary explanations of complex CNS phenomena are possible and should be looked for.

TABLE 4

SUMMARY OF CORRELATIONS BETWEEN CSF ENDORPHIN
FRACTION I LEVELS AND DIAGNOSTIC VARIABLES IN
CHRONIC PAIN (From refs. 16,32,42)

Variable	Direction of change with increasing CSF endorphins
Detection threshold	0
Pain threshold	+
Pain tolerance	+
Perceptual reactance	-
Depression	+
Anxiety	0
Retardation	0

PSYCHIATRIC DISORDERS

From what has been inferred above it may seem logical to explore the possibility that endorphins could also be involved in psychosis. This approach was not so obvious at the time our work in this field was started[47]. The first evidence came from CSF endorphin measurements[14,48]. Grossly abnormal levels were found in several cases of the classical disorders unipolar or bipolar depression and schizophrenia. In some cases the levels were spectacularly high. Furthermore, there was evidence that in schizophrenia CSF endorphin levels were affected by antipsychotic therapy. In general, as regards Fraction I endorphins, changes were towards normalization during therapy[14,15]. These observations suggested that, in psychotic disorders, the endorphin systems might be attacked directly. This could either be done by giving narcotic antagonists to block hyperfunction or by giving narcotic agonists, preferably endorphins, in hypofunction. Here, it may be recalled that morphine has a long history as antidepressant[49,50]. With the exception of one study on naloxone administration to depressed patients with essentially negative results[48] the interest has been focussed on schizophrenia. There are several reasons for this.

The starting point for the work on the possible role of endorphins in schizophrenia was the above-mentioned observation that CSF levels might be markedly elevated[14]. Secondly, it has been known for several years that certain morphine relatives having mixed agonist/antagonist properties show psychotomimetic effects, such as dysreality reactions, delusion and, characteristically, auditory hallucinations[51,52,53]. Although these effects have been known for long, they have never been associated with mental disorders since no possible links between these opiates and endogenous mechanisms were known at the time. For instance, these drugs, unlike LSD and others, have not been used to induce model psychosis. The third indication that endorphins might be associated with mental disorders comes from animal experiments showing that β-endorphin produces a catatonia-like syndrome in rats[54,55].

A logical way to test "the endorphin hypothesis of schizophrenia"[56] would be to explore the activity of naloxone in schizophrenic patients. A pilot study was initiated[56]. Considering the fact that auditory hallucinations are induced by certain opiates (see above) this was selected as the characteristic symptom.

The investigation was partially positive since 4 of 6 patients reported an almost immediate reversal of hallucinations after naloxone injection. This study has been replicated in several clinical centers. On the average, 30% of the patients have responded to naloxone (Table 5)[56-65].

TABLE 5

TRIALS OF NALOXONE IN CHRONIC SCHIZOPHRENIA

A response is characterized by a temporary extinction or reduction of hallucinosis.

Series	Dose (mg)	No. on neuro-leptics	No. of responders/ No. of patients	Ref.
1	0.4	All	4/6	56
2	0.4	All	0/7	57
3	0.4-10	5	0/14	58
4	1.2	All	0/8	59
5	0.4-1.2	All	0/12	60
6	4.0	2	12/20	61
7	10	?	6/9	62
8	25	?	7/12	63
9	0.8	All	1/10	64
10	0.4	All	1/1	65
			Total 31/99	

Although these results may not seem fully conclusive, it should be emphasized that most of the patients were treated with neuroleptics under presumably optimal conditions. It would be of great interest to repeat these studies in untreated patients or in patients whose dosage of neuroleptics had been reduced. It is also possible that only some schizophrenics have a hyperactive endorphin system as suggested by the highly variable CSF levels of endorphins[15]. Finally, the diagnosis schizophrenia is not so uniform and the variable results from different studies may depend on the grounds for patient selection.

The possible connection between endorphins and psychiatric disorders led Kline and colleagues to test β-endorphin in various

psychiatric patients. A total of 15 subjects with different diagnoses received one or more injections. Particularly interesting
were late "therapeutic" responses in 2 schizophrenics and 3 patients with neurosis[66,67]. Although preliminary, these results
would be supportive of the hypothesis that changes in endorphin
homeostasis are related to mental disorders. A very recent finding
by de Wied and co-workers[68,69] suggests that the therapeutic effect
of β-endorphin might have been due to the neuroleptic activity
of a β-endorphin fragment. They found that des-Tyr-γ-endorphin[1],
a compound which lacks opioid activity, produces neuroleptic-like
behavioral activity in rats[68]. This suggests that it may be an
endogenous neuroleptic (it should be recalled that Jacquet and
Marks[55] put forward the hypothesis that β-endorphin itself might
have this property). The substance has already been subjected to
clinical trials. It was given to schizophrenic subjects who were
not symptom-free on neuroleptics. All 6 subjects showed some response although it was of short duration in 3 of them[69].

Until now there is no evidence that the des-Tyr-γ-endorphin
compound is actually formed endogenously. The importance of the
observation lies in the fact that it emphasizes that the β-
endorphin molecule or its fragments may have other messages and
interact with other receptors than the opioid ones. This would
not be a unique case since de Wied's group has found many other
examples that one peptide chain may have several active sequences,
"messages"[70]. It is tempting to offer a unitary explanation of
all these observations in relation to schizophrenia. If we postulate a block in the break-down of β-endorphin in the CNS, there
will be an accumulation of β-endorphin and a concomitant decrease
in the formation of the "neuroleptic" peptide. This change in
balance could be restored by naloxone or neuroleptics.

Pharmacologic studies have strongly emphasized the role of
dopamine hyperactivity in schizophrenia[71]. All kinds of drugs
reducing dopaminergic activity seem to be equally effective. The
endorphin hypothesis and the dopamine hypothesis may actually be
related since it is well-known that opiates and dopamine show a
variety of interactions. For instance, enkephalinergic neurons

---

[1]β-Endorphin is equal to the sequence 61-91 in β-lipotropin whereas
des-Tyr-γ-endorphin is equivalent to the sequence 62-77.

probably terminate presynaptically on dopamine neurons in rat striatum[72] where morphine has been found to depress dopamine release[73]. Long-term blockade of dopamine receptors by neuroleptics has been found to increase enkephalin levels[74]. β-Endorphin is present in distinct fibers projecting through hypothalamic areas into the diencephalon and pons[9]. Fibers with β-endorphin and its possible precursor, β-lipotropin, may form contacts with the dopaminergic system[8,9]. The functional implications of these observations are not fully understood at the moment.

As we have seen the number of observations relating endorphins to psychiatric disorders is already considerable. However, the knowledge of basic mechanisms is still quite limited and further studies into this problem are in great need. The complex integration of the CNS makes it hard to determine whether a certain observed deviation in level or activity is a secondary phenomenon or at the core of the illness. The case of endorphins in schizophrenia or other mental disorders is no exception.

CONCLUDING REMARKS

In the clinical context, dysfunction may be one of decreased endorphin activity (hypofunction) or increased activity (hyperfunction). It is suggested that hypofunction, which may or may not relate to deafferentation, increases the proneness to pain. This seems to be a situation characteristic of the patient with chronic neurogenic pain. In hyperfunction there is indifference to pain and other sensory stimuli and in a broader sense it may relate to depression and personality disorders. Hyperfunction could be a common factor in "psychogenic pain" and depression which shows many similarities in the psychophysical sense. Evidence relating endorphin dysfunction to schizophrenia is accumulating. The disease may be a consequence of an error of metabolism which would lead to the loss of control and integration. The close anatomical and probably functional association with the dopamine system, offers a possibility to consider the well-known therapeutic effects of dopamine receptor blockers in a new context.

Endorphin research in the clinical area is still in its infancy. This review is intentionally selective. If it will stimulate to further work it has fulfilled its mission.

ACKNOWLEDGEMENTS

Work by the author is supported by the Swedish Medical Research
Council.

REFERENCES

1. Goldstein, A. (1976) Science, 193, 1081-1086.

2. Hughes, J. and Kosterlitz, H.W. (1977) Br. Med. Bull., 33,
   157-161.

3. Snyder, S.H. and Simantov, R. (1977) J. Neurochem., 28, 13-20.

4. Terenius, L. (1978) Ann. Rev. Pharmacol. Toxicol., 18, 189-204.

5. Terenius, L. (1978) in Endorphins, Bell, R.M.S. and Malick, J.
   eds., Marcel Dekker, New York, in press.

6. Hökfelt, T., Elde, R., Johansson, O., Terenius, L. and Stein,
   L. (1977) Neurosci. Lett., 5, 23-31.

7. Simantov, R., Kuhar, M.J., Uhl, G.R. and Snyder, S.H. (1977)
   Proc. Natl. Acad. Sci., 74, 2167-2171.

8. Watson, S.J., Barchas, J.D. and Li, C.H. (1977) Proc. Natl.
   Acad. Sci., 74, 5155-5158.

9. Bloom, F., Battenberg, E., Rossier, J., Ling, N. and Guillemin,
   R. (1978) Proc. Natl. Acad. Sci., 75, 1591-1595.

10. Bloom, F.E., Rossier, J., Battenberg, E.L.F., Bayon, A., French,
    E., Henriksen, J., Siggins, G.R., Segal, D., Browne, R., Ling,
    N. and Guillemin, R. (1978) in Advances in Biochemical Psycho-
    pharmacology, vol. 18, Costa, E. and Trabucchi, M. eds.,
    Raven Press, New York, pp. 89-109.

11. Dingledine, R., Iversen, L.L. and Breuker, E. (1978) Eur. J.
    Pharmacol., 47, 19-27.

12. Terenius, L. and Wahlström, A. (1975) Life Sci., 16, 1759-1764.

13. Wahlström, A., Johansson, L. and Terenius, L. (1978) Life Sci.,
    submitted.

14. Terenius, L., Wahlström, A., Lindström, L. and Widerlöv, E.
    (1976) Neurosci. Lett., 3, 157-162.

15. Lindström, L.H., Widerlöv, E., Gunne, L.-M., Wahlström, A. and
    Terenius, L. (1978) Acta Psychiat. Scand. 57, 153-164..

16. Almay, B.G.L., Johansson, F., von Knorring, L., Terenius, L.
    and Wahlström, A. (1978) Pain, in press.

17. Lasagna, L. (1965) Proc. R. Soc. Med., 58, 978-983.

18. Levine, J.D., Gordon, N.C., Jones, R.T. and Fields, H.L. (1978)
    Nature, 272, 826-827.

19. El-Sobky, A., Dostrovsky, J.O. and Wall, P.D. (1976) Nature,
    263, 783-784.

20. Grevert, P. and Goldstein, A. (1977) Proc. Natl. Acad. Sci.,
    74, 1291-1294.

21. Buchsbaum, M.S., Davis, G.C. and Bunney, W.E. (1977) Nature,
    270, 620-622.

22. Livingston, W.K. (1943) Pain Mechanisms, Macmillan, New York.

23. Merskey, H. and Spear, F.G. (1967) Pain: Psychological and Psychiatric Aspects, Ballière, Tindall and Cassell, London.

24. Melzack, R. (1973) The Puzzle of Pain, Basic Books/Harper Torchbooks, New York.

25. Sternbach, R.A. (1974) Pain Patients, Acad. Press, New York.

26. Sjölund, B., Terenius, L. and Eriksson, M. (1977) Acta Physiol. Scand., 100, 382-384.

27. Melzack, R. and Loeser, J.D. (1978) Pain, 4, 195-210.

28. Meyer, G.A. and Fields, H.L. (1972) Brain, 95, 163-168.

29. Shealy, C.N. and Maurer, D. (1974) Surg. Neurol., 2, 45-47.

30. Long, D.M. and Hagfors, N. (1975) Pain, 1, 109-123.

31. Melzack, R. (1975) Pain, 1, 357-373.

32. von Knorring, L., Almay, B.G.L. and Terenius, L. (1978) Neuropsychobiology, in press.

33. Sjölund, B. and Eriksson, M. (1976) Lancet, ii, 1085.

34. Sicuteri, F. (1976) Headache, 16, 145-159.

35. Sicuteri, F., Anselmi, B., Curradi, C., Michelacci, S. and Sassi, A. (1978) Adv. Biochem. Psychopharmacol, 18, 363-366.

36. Gray, J.A. (1964) Pavlov's Typology, Macmillan, New York.

37. Eysenck, H.J. (1967) The Biological Basis of Personality, Charles C. Thomas, Springfield, Ill.

38. Schalling, D. and Levander, S. (1964) Scand. J. Psychol., 5, 1-9.

39. Petrie, A. (1967) Individuality in Pain and Suffering, University of Chicago Press, Chicago.

40. Buchsbaum, M. and Silverman, J. (1968) Psychosom. Med., 30, 12-22.

41. Buchsbaum, M. (1976) in Consciousness and Self-Regulation, vol. 1, Schwartz, G.E. and Shapiro, D. eds., Plenum Press, New York, pp. 101-135.

42. von Knorring, L., Almay, B.G.L. and Terenius, L. (1978) Neuropsychobiology, in press.

43. von Knorring, L., Monakhov, K. and Perris, C. (1978) Neuropsychobiology, 4, 150-179.

44. von Knorring, L. (1975) The Experience of Pain in Patients with Depressive Disorders. A Clinical and Experimental Study, Umeå University Medical Dissertations, New series, 2, Umeå.

45. Delaplaine, R., Ifabumuyi, O.I., Merskey, H. and Zarfas, J. (1978) Pain, 4, 361-366.

46. Belluzzi, J.D. and Stein, L. (1977) Nature, 266, 556-558.

47. Terenius, L. and Wahlström, A. (1978) in Centrally Acting Peptides, Hughes, J. ed., McMillan, London, pp. 161-178.

48. Terenius, L., Wahlström, A. and Ågren, H. (1977) Psychopharmacology, 54, 31-33.

49. Kraepelin, E. (1905) Die Psychiatrische Klinik, Barth., Leipzig.

50. Comfort, A. (1977) Lancet, ii, 448-449.

51. Lasagna, L. and Beecher, H.K. (1954) J. Pharmacol. Exp. Ther., 112, 356-363.

52. Jasinski, D.R., Martin, W.R. and Hoeldtke, R.D. (1968) Clin. Pharm. Ther., 9, 215-222.

53. Forrest, W.H., Jr., Beer, E.G., Bellville, J.W., Ciliberti, B.J., Miller, E.V. and Paddock, R. (1969) Clin. Pharm. Ther., 10, 468-476.

54. Bloom, R., Segal, D., Ling, N. and Guillemin, R. (1976) Science, 194, 630-632.

55. Jacquet, Y.F. and Marks, N. (1976) Science, 194, 632-634.

56. Gunne, L.-M., Lindström, L. and Terenius, L. (1977) J. Neural Transm., 40, 13-19..

57. Volavka, J., Mallya, A., Baig, S. and Perez-Cruet, J. (1977) 196, 1227-1228.

58. Davis, G.C., Bunney, W.E., Jr. and de Fraites, E.G. (1977) Science, 197, 74-77.

59. Janowsky, D.R., Segal, D.S., Abrams, A., Bloom, F. and Guillemin, R. (1977) Psychopharmacology, 53, 295-297.

60. Kurland, A.A., McCabe, L., Hanlon, T.E. and Sullivan, D. (1977) Am. J. Psychiatry, 134, 1408-1410.

61. Emrich, H.M., Cording, C., Pirée, S., Kölling, A., v. Zerssen, D. and Herz, A. (1977) Pharmakopsychiatr. Neuropsychopharmakol., 10, 265-270.

62. Berger, P., Watson, S.J., Akil, H. and Barchas, J.D. (1978) in Endorphins in Mental Illness, Usdin, E. and Bunney, W.E. eds., McMillan, London, in press.

63. Emrich, H.M., Cording, C., Pirée, S., Kölling, A., Möller, H.-J., v. Zerssen, D. and Herz, A. (1978) in Endorphins in Mental Illness, Usdin, E. and Bunney, W.E. eds., McMillan, London, in press.

64. Gunne, L.-M., Lindström, L. and Widerlöv, E. (1978) in Endorphins in Mental Illness, Usdin, E. and Bunney, W.E. eds., McMillan, London, in press.

65. Orr, M. and Oppenheimer, C. (1978) Br. Med. J., 1, 481.

66. Kline, N.S., Li, C.H., Lehmann, H.E., Lajtha, A., Laski, E. and Cooper, T. (1977) Arch. Gen. Psychiatry, 34, 1111-1113.

67. Kline, N.S. and Lehmann, H.E. (1978) in Endorphins in Mental Illness, Usdin, E. and Bunney, W.E. eds., McMillan, London, in press.

68. de Wied, D., Bohus, B., van Ree, J.M., Kovács, G.L. and Greven, H. (1978) Lancet, i, 1046.

69. Verhoeven, W.M.A., van Praag, H.M., Botter, P.A., Sunier, A., van Ree, J.M. and de Wied, D. (1978) Lancet, i, 1046-1047.

158

70. de Wied, D., Bohus, B., Gispen, W.H., Urban, I. and van Wimersma Greidanus, Tj.B. (1975) Proc. Sixth International Congress of Pharmacology, Helsinki, vol. 3, 19-30.

71. Carlsson, A. (1978) Biol. Psychiatry, 13, 3-21.

72. Pollard, H., Llorens-Cortes, C. and Schwartz, J.C. (1977) Nature, 268, 745-747.

73. Loh, H.H., Brase, D.A., Sampath-Khanna, S., Mar, J.B. and Way, E.L. (1976) Nature, 264, 567-568.

74. Hong, J., Yang, H.-Y. T., Fratta, W. and Costa, E. (1978) in Endorphins in Mental Illness, Usdin, E. and Bunney, W.E. eds., McMillan, London, in press.

Characteristics and Function of Opioids, editors Van Ree and Terenius
© 1978 Elsevier/North-Holland Biomedical Press

NARCOTIC ANTAGONISTS INCREASE PAIN SENSITIVITY IN RATS

K.A. BONNET, P. ALPERT AND S. KLINEROCK
Department of Psychiatry, New York University School of Medicine,
550 First Avenue, New York, New York 10016

The demonstration of stereospecific, saturable receptors for opiates in vertebrate brain promoted the subsequent isolation of endogenous opiate-like peptides from brain[1,2]. The pharmacological effects of the endogenous endorphin peptides are reversible by treatment with the narcotic antagonists naloxone or naltrexone. The "pure" antagonists afford powerful tools for the study of the physiological roles for the endorphins. Naloxone has frequently been reported to have no effect on pain sensitivity in animals or in man although the role for the endorphins would seem to require that the antagonists would exert effects of increased pain sensitivity in opiate-naive subjects[3,4]. Nonetheless, naloxone has been reported to reduce the hot-plate latency in mice[5], to antagonize electrical anesthesia in rat[6], to block acupuncture anesthesia in man[7], and to block stress-induced analgesia that is related to stress-induced release of endorphins[8]. We report the lowering of footshock thresholds by naloxone or naltrexone in low doses in a time dependent manner in opiate-naive rats.

Male rats were 60 days of age. Animals were injected with sterile saline (1ml/Kg), naloxone-HCl or naltrexone-HCl i.p. and tested at various postinjection times by trained observers unaware of the nature of the drug or the purpose of the experiment. All effects were replicated at least twice with different observers. Fifty percent footshock thresholds were determined as described elsewhere[9].

Naloxone at 2mg/Kg significantly lowered the footshock threshold at one and five minutes postinjection (p<.05;Figure 1). By twenty minutes this effect was no longer evident. The decreased shock threshold was accompanied was accompanied by significant increases in rearing and in escape attempts during the shock session. The decreased shock threshold was most evident in a low intensity response type that is most sensitive to morphine-induced analgesia. Naltrexone at 2mg/Kg also showed a time-dependent reduction in thresholds that peaked at 20 minutes postinjection and persisted for at least 60 minutes. The naltrexone effects were most evident at higher shock intensities and hence in more complex response types than were naloxone effects.

160

Since the naloxone-induced decrease in thresholds exhibited a short
latency and duration we tested another set of animals by a discrete
procedure using five repititions of only two shock intensities per
animal, with a total test time of only one minute. Response category
records were treated as intensity ratings. Mean total intensity scores
for saline animals did not change even with repeated testing. Naloxone
at 2mg/Kg produced significantly greater response intensities at each
shock level above 100µA that persisted for only five minutes postinj-
ection(Figure 2). At 10mg/Kg, naloxone effected a slower onset of
increased response intensity and a duration of ten minutes.

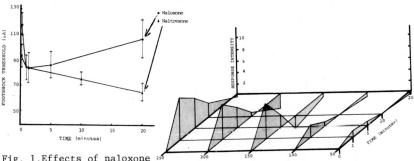

Fig. 1.Effects of naloxone
and naltrexone on footshock
thresholds in rats at
postinjection times.

Fig. 2. Net increases in response intensity
to footshock at various intensities at
times following naloxone injection(2mg/Kg).

The contribution of stress-induced analgesia may develop too late
to be a significant factor in these rapid phenomena. It seems clear,
though, that the effects are attributable to blocking of endogenous
endorphins in brain regions mediating pain perception. These effects
were highly reproducible and seen at various times throughout the day[10].

REFERENCES

1. Simon, E.J., Hiller,J. and Edelman,I.(1973)Proc.Nat.Acad.Sci.70,1947.

2. Hughes,J. et al., (1975) Nature,258, 577-579.

3. Goldstein,A., Pryor,G.,Otis,L.,Larsen,F.(1976) Life Sci.,18, 599.

4. El-Sobky,A., Dostrovsky,J. and Wall,P.(1976) Nature, 263,783.

5. Jacob,J.,Tremblay,E.,and Colombel,M.(1974)Psychopharm.,37, 217.

6. Akil,H., Mayer,D.,and Liebeskind,J.(1976) Science, 191, 961.

7. Mayer,D.J., Price,D. and Rabi,A.(1977) Brain Res,121, 368.

8. Madden,J., Akil,H., Patrick,J.,Barchas,J.(1977)Nature, 265, 359.

9. Bonnet,K. and Peterson,K.(1975) Pharm.Bioch.Behav. 3, 47.

10. Frederickson,R.,Burgis,V. and Edwards,J. (1978)Science, 198, 756.

ACKNOWLEDGEMENT

Supported by NIDA grant DA 01113.

Characteristics and Function of Opioids, editors Van Ree and Terenius
© *1978 Elsevier/North-Holland Biomedical Press*

PHARMACOLOGICAL STUDIES ON STIMULATION-PRODUCED ANALGESIA

W.R. BUCKETT

Centre de Recherche Merrell International, 67084-Strasbourg Cedex, France

ABSTRACT

Peripheral electrical stimulation in mice leads to analgesia of short duration which can be detected in the hot-plate test and which is naloxone-reversible. This effect may represent a functional role of endogenous opioid peptides.

INTRODUCTION

Natural protection against everyday painful stimuli may be afforded by the
rapid release of endogenous substances to provide a situation in which an individual can disregard such stimuli. Although much recent work in the field of
opioid peptides has increased our understanding of the distribution, release,
binding characteristics and degradation of these substances, any functional
relationship to their possible role in antinociception remains to be defined.
This communication presents evidence for analgesia of immediate onset and of
short duration following electrical stimulation in mice. Such analgesia might
be a functional role of opioid peptides.

MATERIALS AND METHODS

Female CD albino mice 20-25 g (Charles River, France) were used. They were
loosely restrained and stimulated electrically by means of a bipolar electrode
placed on the tail surface. Rectangular pulses at threshold voltage for vocalization were delivered for 30 s at 20 Hz and 15 ms pulse width. The voltage and
duration of vocalization were recorded. Control animals were treated identically
but without current. The mice were transferred at various times after stimulation to a hot-plate (52° ; 22.5 x 11 cm surface with 10 cm wall). The times were
measured to (a) first forepaw lick representing an acute pain reaction and (b)
escape from the hot-plate which at this temperature represents reaction to a
more chronic pain.

Drugs studied for their ability to modify the electrically-induced analgesia
were injected i.p. at various times before test. The following were used : naloxone hydrochloride (Endo), D,L-5-hydroxytryptophan (5-HTP ; Sigma) and 4-amino-
hex-5-ynoic acid (RMI 71645) .

RESULTS

Application of peripheral electrical stimulation induces analgesia in the
mouse. This effect is clearly demonstrated in the 52°C hot-plate test where both
presumed acute and chronic pain reactions may be recorded. The data presented
in Fig.1 show an immediate and highly significant increase in reaction times
following a stimulation period of only 30s. The duration of this effect is extremely short, declining rapidly by 60s and totally lost by 5 min. Fig. 1 also
shows that this electrically-induced analgesia is clearly reversed in a dose-
dependent manner by naloxone in a dose-range which is associated with specific
opioid antagonism in mice suggesting that this effect is opioid linked. The time

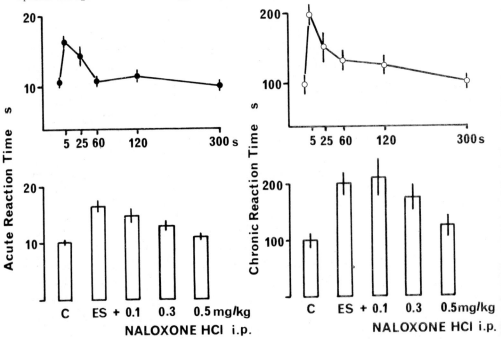

Fig.1.Electrically induced analgesia in mice. Upper panels show duration of effect
(abscissa:time between stimulation and test). Lower panels show reaction times of
control (C) and stimulated (ES) mice and ES after naloxone.Values in s ± s.e. mean.

of vocalization is longer in naloxone treated mice ($P < 0.001$) supporting this hypothesis. Using the chronic reaction times it was found that 5-HTP (120mg/kg i.p.)
and the GABA-transaminase inhibitor RMI 71645 (50 mg/kg i.p.) both potentiated the
analgesia ($P<0.01$).

CONCLUSION

These results indicate that upon stimulation an endogenous substance is released which produces a short protective period of analgesia. Blockade by low doses
of naloxone and enhancement by 5-HTP implicate opioid involvement.

Characteristics and Function of Opioids, editors Van Ree and Terenius
© 1978 Elsevier/North-Holland Biomedical Press

ACUPUNCTURE ANALGESIA IS MEDIATED BY STEREOSPECIFIC OPIATE RECEPTORS.

RICHARD S. S. CHENG and BRUCE POMERANZ
Zoology Department, University of Toronto, Ontario, Canada

ABSTRACT

A newly synthesized stereoisomer, dextronaloxone, having 1/1000 to 1/10000th the affinity of levonaloxone (1), shows no blockade of electro-acupuncture analgesia while levonaloxone inhibits electroacupuncture effects in mice. This result indicates that stereospecific opiate receptors are in-volved in acupuncture analgesia.

INTRODUCTION

It is hypothesized that acupuncture analgesia is mediated by endorphins (2). The endorphins are released from spinal cord, mid-brain or pituitary by acupuncture and will bind to the opiate receptors along the nociceptive pathway in the CNS inducing analgesia (2). The evidence for the acupunc-ture-endorphin hypothesis is mainly based on the observation that naloxone, an opiate antagonist, blocks electroacupuncture analgesia (3)(4)(5). How-ever, it has been criticized (6) that naloxone may have other side effects unrelated to opiate antagonist role; thus the above observation does not necessarily demonstrate that acupuncture is mediated by opiate receptors. To answer this question, we tested the effect of both (-) naloxone and (+) naloxone on acupuncture analgesia in mice. Dextro naloxone, a newly synthesized stereoisomer, has only 1/1000 to 1/10,000[th] the affinity of (-) naloxone in binding to opiate receptors in three systems: (a) rat brain receptor binding assay, (b) electrically stimulated guinea pig ileum assay, (c) neuroblastoma x glioma hybrid cell adenylate cyclase assay (1).

MATERIAL AND METHOD

A similar method as described in the previous study (3) was employed for measuring the behavioural pain threshold in B6AF$_1$/J female mice. Briefly, an audiogram was used to determine the squeak latency in response to noxious heat stimuli applied to the nose. Electroacupuncture (4 Hz, 4-6 volts and 0.1 ms duration) was applied for 20 minutes only to those mice with 4 reproducible responses in the pretreatment tests. The acu-puncture point "Ho-ku (L.I.4)" which is located on the forepaw between the first and second digits are used. Either (+) naloxone (1 mg/kg), (-) naloxone (1 mg/kg) or saline (0.9%) was injected intraperitoneally in a "blind" manner immediately before and after electroacupuncture treatment.

164

RESULT

In 15 saline-treated mice (Fig 1, dotted line), the mean values of
squeak latency were significantly (p <0.05, t-test, two tailed) above
the zero time control value at 30,40,50,60,70,80,90,110 and 120 minutes.
Similarly, this analgesic effect induced by electroacupuncture was seen
in 15 (+) naloxone-treated animals (solid line, Fig 1) at 20,30,40,50,
70 and 110 minutes. However, electroacupuncture analgesia was completely
blocked by (-) naloxone (dashed line, Fig 1). Between group statistical
analyses: the increase in the mean pain thresholds in (+) naloxone-
treated mice was greater than those of (-) naloxone-treated mice at each
time interval, and this analgesia was statistically different between two
groups at 30,40,70 and 110 minutes (p <0.05, t-test, two tailed).

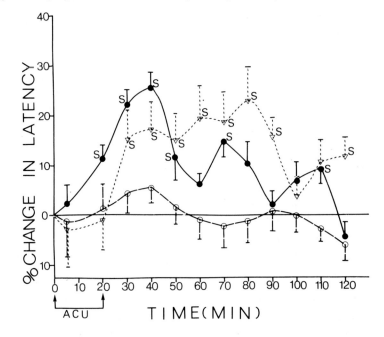

Fig.1. Effect of (+) naloxone, (-) naloxone or saline on electroacupuncture
in mice. Percentage change in latency to squeak as compared to pretreatment
control values. Positive values denote analgesia. Each point is the mean for
15 mice. Bars show S.E. Arrows indicate time of acupuncture treatment.
Injections were given at zero time and again at 20 minutes (booster). "S"
indicates that the mean values were significantly above zero controls at
p <0.05. Dotted line, open triangular show saline plus acupuncture. Solid
line, closed circles show (+) naloxone plus acupuncture. Dashed line, open
circles show (-) naloxone plus acupuncture.

A histogram (Fig. 2) showed that (i) electroacupuncture analgesia was reversed by (-) naloxone in 13 out of 15 mice; (ii) in (+) naloxone-treated animals, only 4 out of 15 animals had no electroacupuncture analgesia, and (iii) in the saline-treated mice, 7 out of 15 animals showed no electroacupuncture effects.

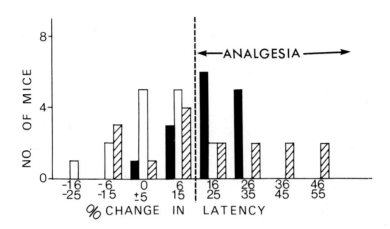

Fig. 2. Abscissa is the average percentage change in squeak threshold (each mouse was averaged for the 30, 40 and 50 minute values, post acupuncture) as compared to the preacupuncture control values. Ordinate is the number of mice with a given percentage change. Solid bars show acupuncture plus (+) naloxone. Open bars show acupuncture plus (-) naloxone. Hatched bars show acupuncture plus saline. (-) naloxone blocks acupuncture analgesia (Analgesia is defined by the % change in squeak latency which is larger than 15%).

DISCUSSION

The results of this study strongly indicate that acupuncture analgesia is mediated by stereospecific receptors. When the opiate receptor sites were occupied by (-) naloxone, electroacupuncture analgesia was blocked. On the other hand, the dextroisomer (+) naloxone, having $1/1000-1/10000^{th}$ the affinity of (-) naloxone for opiate receptors, did not block acupuncture

166

analgesia and this strongly strengthens the previous naloxone results.
Several other lines of evidence (independent of naloxone studies) support
the acupuncture-endorphin hypothesis: (A) poor electroacupuncture analgesia
is shown in mice genetically deficient in opiate receptors (7)(B) endorphin
levels are elevated in human CSF after transcutaneous electroacupuncture (8),
and (C) electroacupuncture analgesia is blocked after removal of the
pituitary (9) or (D) ablation of the raphe system (10). Together, these
add up to 5 lines of evidence for acupuncture-endorphin hypothesis.

ACKNOWLEDGEMENTS

The authors thank John Phelan for his technical assistance and acknowledge
a generous donation of (+) naloxone by Dr. Arthur E. Jacobson. The research
was supported by NRC and MRC of Canada and Ontario Ministry of Health.

REFERENCES

1. Iijima, I. et al. (1978) J. Med. Chem. 21(4), 398-404
2. Pomeranz, B. (1978) Advances in Biochem. Psychopharmacol.Vol.18, Raven
   Press, N.Y. 351-359.
3. Pomeranz, B. and Chiu, D. (1976) Life Sci. 19, 1757-1762.
4. Mayer, D. J. et al. (1977) Brain Res., 121, 368-372.
5. Chapman, C. R. and Benedetti, C. (1977) Life Sci., 21, 1645-1648.
6. Hayes, R. et al. (1977) Science, 196, 600.
7. Peets, J. and Pomeranz, B. Nature (1978) (in press).
8. Sjölund, B. et al. (1977) Acta Physiol. Scand. 100, 382-383
9. Pomeranz, B. et al. (1977) Expt. Neurol., 54, 172-178
10.McLennan H. et al. (1977) Pain 3, 229-238.

Characteristics and Function of Opioids, editors Van Ree and Terenius
© *1978 Elsevier/North-Holland Biomedical Press*

DIFFERENTIAL EFFECTS ON RESPIRATION OF β-ENDORPHIN, D-ALA^2-MET-ENKEPHALINAMIDE AND MET-ENKEPHALIN

JESUS FLOREZ, AFRICA MEDIAVILLA and ANGEL PAZOS

Dept. Pharmacol., Fac. Medicine, Nat. Med. Ctr. 'Valdecilla', Santander (Spain)

ABSTRACT

Respiration is depressed by the three opioid peptides when injected into the lateral ventricles of cats. However, the differences in the time-course of their effects on frequency and amplitude suggest a variability in their access into the brain from the CSF and/or in their interaction with brain structures.

INTRODUCTION

Met-enkephalin (m-E) applied to the ventral surface of the brain stem depresses respiration in an opiate-like way[1]. The purpose of this investigation was twofold: 1) to compare the effects of m-E (900μg) with those of β-endorphin (β-E) (10 μg) and the synthetic derivative D-ala^2-metenkephalinamide (D-alamide) (10 μg), and 2) to analyze the respiratory effects when the drugs are in contact with a more extense area of the central nervous system.

MATERIALS AND METHODS

The peptides, diluted in 100 μl of saline, were administered into a lateral ventricle of 19 lightly anesthetized cats. Respiration, recorded pneumotachographically, blood pressure, and heart rate were continuously monitored. Arterial blood samples were taken to control pCO_2.

RESULTS

M-E induced an immediate drop in frequency and tidal volume. The lowest values were attained at 5 and 1 min and returned to control levels at 60 and 15 min, respectively (fig. 1). D-alamide induced small, inconsistent changes in frequency for the first 15 min whereas tidal volume was markedly decreased, its minimum value being reached at 15 min. Subsequently, frequency was reduced and remained depressed for over 5 hr, but tidal volume slowly returned to control values. β-E elicited stimulation of frequency during the first 30 min, accompanied by a progressive depression of tidal volume. Subsequently frequency steadily declined and remained depressed for over 5 hr, whereas tidal volume returned to control values at about 2 hr. In terms of ventilation, maximal depression was induced by m-E in 1 to 5 min, the recovery being completed in 1 hr. With D-alamide and β-E, peak depressions were attained in 1 and 3 hr, respectively; a

168

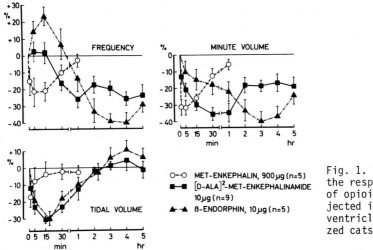

Fig. 1. Time course of the respiratory effects of opioid peptides injected into the lateral ventricle of anesthetized cats (mean±SEM)

substantial depression persisted for over 5 hr.

DISCUSSION

Although the three peptides depress respiration, it is evident that they affect the frequency- and depth-generating respiratory mechanisms differently. Variations in relative affinities of the peptides for the opioid receptor and in the susceptibility to enzymatic degradation may account for the variability in potency[2]. In fact, the prolonged respiratory depression exerted by D-alamide and β-E correlates well with the reported duration of analgesia[2,3]. But there may also exist a dissimilar accessibility for the peptides to penetrate into the brain from the CSF spaces. This would explain the diverse latencies to attain maximal depression for each component of respiration. Furthermore, interaction with opioid receptors located at suprapontine level may elicit stimulatory behavioral effects[4] which will modify the direct action of the peptides upon the respiratory center.

REFERENCES

1. Flórez, J. and Mediavilla, A. (1977) Brain Res., 138, 585-590.
2. Pert, C.B., Pert, A., Chang, J.K. and Fong, B.T.W. (1976) Science, 194, 330-332
3. Meglio, M., Hosobuchi, Y., Loh, H.H., Adams, J.E. and Li, C.H. (1977) Proc. Natl. Acad. Sci., 74, 774-776.
4. Frenk, H., McCarty, B.C. and Liebeskind, J.C. (1978) Science, 335-337.

Characteristics and Function of Opioids, editors Van Ree and Terenius
© *1978 Elsevier/North-Holland Biomedical Press*   169

MOUSE BRAIN ENKEPHALINS: STUDY OF DIURNAL CHANGES CORRELATED WITH CHANGES IN
NOCICEPTIVE SENSITIVITY

R.C.A. Frederickson, D. L. Wesche, and J. A. Richter
Eli Lilly and Company and Indiana University, Indianapolis, IN 46206 and 46202

INTRODUCTION

The endogenous opioid pentapeptides may function as neurotransmitters in
neural systems mediating the reaction to noxious stimuli. We have observed a
diurnal rhythm in responsivity of mice to such stimuli (as measured by jump
latencies of mice on a hot plate) and corresponding diurnal changes in the
degree of naloxone-induced hyperalgesia[1]. A diurnal rhythm in pain tolerance
in human subjects also has been reported[2] and naloxone can decrease the diurnal
variation in pain sensitivity and somatosensory evoked potentials in man[3]. The
present studies were undertaken to examine the role of brain opioid peptides in
mediating these rhythms. The data support the hypothesis that such peptides
modulate nociceptive sensitivity in a diurnally varying fashion but a specific
peptide responsible for this has not yet been unequivocally identified.

METHODS

The hot plate technique for measuring jump latency has been previously
described[1]. For assaying levels of brain opioid peptides mice were sacrificed
by microwave irradiation, the brains homogenized in acid, the homogenate centrifuged and enkephalins extracted from the supernatant over columns of amberlite XAD-2 resin[4,5]. The mouse vas deferens bioassay for opioid activity has
been previously described[6] as has the radioimmunoassay methodology[7]. Mice
weighing 25-27 g were transpharyngeally hypophysectomized under pentobarbital
narcosis[7]. Sham-operated controls were also concurrently prepared.

RESULTS

We perfomed studies on hypophysectomized mice and sham-operated controls to
ascertain whether the pituitary plays a role in mediating the rhythm. The difference in jump latency between the 7:30 AM mean value (minimum) and the 3:30 PM
mean value (maximum) persisted in hypophysectomized mice as did the hyperalgesic
effect of naloxone at the latter time, indicating their origin in brain rather
than pituitary (Table 1). We postulated therefore that the behavioral rhythm
may be mediated by diurnal fluctuations in a brain enkephalinergic system. We
therefore compared whole brain total opioid activity at the times of minimum and

Table 1

| | Jump Latencies (sec) | | | | Enkephalin Levels (pmol/g brain) | |
| | Saline[+] | | Naloxone[+] | | Met[5] | Leu[5] |
	Sham	Hypox	Sham	Hypox		
AM	33.3±7.6	40.1±8.5	31.3±4.9	35.6±5.8	647.0±202.4	185.7±20.7
PM	67.3±8.0*	61.3±8.5*	39.2±9.0	37.0±6.8	995.7±274.3	203.5±23.6

[+]Animals were treated with saline or naloxone (3 mg/kg, sc) 15 minutes before testing on the hot plate; *Significantly different from AM values.

maximum jump latencies using the mouse vas deferens bioassay. The levels were 55.8±3.3 ng/brain for mice sacrificed between 7:30 and 8:00 AM and 93.7±12.1 ng/brain for mice sacrificed between 3:30 and 4:00 PM ($p < 0.01$, df=22, Student's t test). We next utilized RIA methodology to measure specific levels of met[5]-enkephalin and Leu[5]-enkephalin at the two different times. The levels of met[5]-enkephalin were higher in the PM but the increase was not significant due to considerable variability in AM-PM difference between tests (Table 1). When mice were stressed by exposure to a noxious stimulus (left on 52°C hot plate until jump) before sacrifice, however, there was a significant increase compared to unstressed mice in met-enkephalin levels in the PM (1621.8±113.4 vs 750.7±83.8 pmole/g) but not in the AM. This indicated a diurnal variability in response of brain enkephalinergic systems to stress but we cannot yet conclude that the enkephalins are responsible for the behavioral rhythm.

REFERENCES

1. Frederickson, R.C.A., Burgis, V. and Edwards, J. D. (1977). Science 198, 756-758.

2. Procacci, P., Byzelli, G., Passeri, I., Sassi, R., Voegelin, M. R. and Zoppi, M. (1972). Res. Clin. Stud. Headache 3, 260.

3. Davis, G. C., Buchsbaum, M. S. and Bunney, W. E., Jr., Life Sci. (in press).

4. Smith, T. W., Hughes, J., Kosterlitz, H. W. and Sosa, R. P. (1976), pp. 57-62, in Opiates and Endogenous Opioid Peptides, Kosterlitz, H. W., ed., Elsevier, Amsterdam.

5. Frederickson, R.C.A. and Smithwick, E. L. (1978), in Opioid Peptides, Usdin, E., ed., MacMillan Press, London.

6. Frederickson, R.C.A., Schirmer, E. E., Grinnan, E. L., Harrell, C. E. and Hewes, C. R. (1976). Life Sci. 19, 1181-1190.

7. Wesche, D. L., Höllt, V. and Herz, A. (1977). Naun. Schmied. Arch. Pharmacol. 301, 79-82.

Antibodies were kindly provided by Dr. Lars Terenius and Prof. Dr. A. Herz

Characteristics and Function of Opioids, editors Van Ree and Terenius
© 1978 Elsevier/North-Holland Biomedical Press

ENDORPHINS, TRAINING AND BEHAVIOURAL THERMOREGULATION.

JOSEPH JACOB, KRISHNASWAMI RAMABADRAN, JEANNE-MARIE GIRAULT, CHARLES SUAUDEAU
and GERARD MICHAUD.
Laboratory of Pharmacology. Pasteur Institute. F 75724 PARIS CEDEX 15.

ABSTRACT

In the hot plate test, naloxone reduced the latency to jump in moderately but
not in intensively trained mice; further, late (several days) effects were observed, as if enhancement of learning or prolonged peripheral sensitization had occurred. Opiate antagonists injected into the preoptic-anterior hypothalamic region (po.ah) in rats stereospecifically shortened the latency to flight in a
progressively warmed alley.

INTRODUCTION

Earlier studies[1,2] have shown that opiate antagonists stereospecifically shortened the latencies to jump of mice and rats in the hot plate test. The present
work was undertaken to assess a) the interactions between this enhancing effect
of naloxone and training, as training might have been the reason for the failure
of Goldstein et al[3] to observe a similar effect on shock escape threshold in rats
and b) the effects of opiate antagonists on the so-called "behavioural thermoregulation" (technique of Cox et al[4]) a particular thermonociceptive reaction.

RESULTS AND DISCUSSION

Training obtained with several pre-exposures at short intervals diminished or
abolished the enhancing effect of naloxone (TABLE I). It might either diminish
the amount of enkephalin released, as it shortens itself the latency to jump and
(or) switch off enkephalin interneurons through "*Bahnung*" of direct pathways.

TABLE I

INFLUENCE OF TRAINING ON THE PRONOCICEPTIVE EFFECT OF NALOXONE (HOT PLATE TEST)

Test described earlier[1,2]. Groups of 10 or more Swiss OF1 male mice (18-25g).
Saline or naloxone (1 mgkg^{-1} s.c.) was injected 10 min before the test. In naive
mice the average latency was 79 sec for controls and 47 sec for treated.

Preexposures		Jump latency (sec)		Preexposures		Jump latency (sec)	
Number	Interval	Saline	Naloxone	Number	Interval	Saline	Naloxone
1	1 day	44	19[a]	4	30 min	22	14
3	6 h	48	13[a]	6	30 min	23	30
5	2 h	35	21	4[b]	30 min	3	6

a, shortening significant for $p < 0.05$ b, mice selected as fast-responders.

On the other hand when animals had experienced an exposure on the hot plate 10 min after a single injection of naloxone (1 mgkg^{-1} s.c.), they still jumped more readily than the saline controls when re-exposed after 1 to 30 days without further naloxone injection; e.g. one of these experiments gave the following results: days of exposures: 1 - 3 - 5 - 9 - 17 - 33; latencies to jump, controls: 80 ± 18, 44 ± 6, 44 ± 5, 40 ± 5, 41 ± 6, 23 ± 4 sec; mice treated with naloxone only on day 1: 47 ± 4, 19 ± 3, 25 ± 6, 20 ± 4, 21 ± 5, 11 ± 3 sec. Thus by retarding the response, the endogenous ligands might also retard its learning and (or) some peripheral sensitization processes.

TABLE II

STEREOSPECIFIC ENHANCEMENT OF BEHAVIOURAL THERMOREGULATION (PO.AH INJECTION)

Ambient temperature at the time of flight: $\simeq 35°C$. Each animal served as its own control. The antagonist was injected 20 min before the test. Bilateral canulae were stereotaxically implanted at least 10 days before the experiments.

Drug	Dose in μg/animal	Volume (in μl)	n	Latency to flight (in min.) Controls	Treated
Naloxone	20	0.1	7	3.95	2.62[a]
Mr 2266	20[b]	5	10	3.70	2.15[a]
	10[b]	2.5	11	3.80	2.32[a]
	10	1	10	3.81	2.89[a]
	5	2.5	5	4.17	3.47[a]
Mr 2267	10-20	2.5-5	10	3.15	4.05

a, shortening significant for $p < 0.05$ b, behavioural signs (see text).

Opiate antagonists also shortened the latency to flight in rats (Sprague Dawley) put in a progressively warmed alley. This action was stereospecific as it was observed with Mr 2266 but not with its non antagonistic (+) stereoisomer Mr 2267. It was obtained after administration into po.ah (TABLE II), indicating that endogenous ligands might be involved in reactions to thermic stimuli which are not necessarily algesic. Various behavioural signs were also noticed after Mr 2266 but not after Mr 2267 with relatively high doses or volumes: screaming to touch, aggression, circling, tremor, backward locomotion; this suggest some influence of endogenous ligands in the functions of structures adjacent to po.ah.

REFERENCES

1.Jacob, J., Tremblay, E. and Colombel, MC. (1974) Psychopharmacologia, 38, 217.
2.Jacob, J., and Ramabadran, K. (1978) Brit. J. Pharmacol., in press.
3.Goldstein, A., Pryor, G.T., Otis, L.S. and Larsen, F. (1976) Life Sci., 18, 599
4.Cox, B., Green, M.D. and Lomax, P. (1975) Pharmacol. Biochem. Behav., 3, 1051

Supported by grants of the INSERM and the DRET

NALOXONE RELATED ATTENUATION OF MANIC SYMPTOMS IN CERTAIN BIPOLAR DEPRESSIVES

LEWIS L. JUDD, M.D., David S. Janowsky, M.D., David S. Segal, Ph.D., Leighton
Y. Huey, M.D.; Department of Psychiatry, UCSD, La Jolla, CA 92093

ABSTRACT

Eight normal controls and 12 patients with manic or hypomanic signs were
studied in a two day, counterbalanced, double-blind, crossover study of the
effects of naloxone HCl (20 mg) and placebo IV infusions. Increased lethargy
and drowsiness were noted in both samples following naloxone. An attenuation
of manic symptoms was observed in 4 of 12 manic patients. Responders were significantly more manic during baseline ratings. These data suggest a potential
role of opioid peptides in manic symptomotology of some Bipolar depressives.

INTRODUCTION

Reports have suggested directly and indirectly a possible role of opioid
peptides in the regulation of affect.[1,2,3] These together with anecdotal
observations of ours and others suggest that opioid peptides may be involved
in affect disorder with an excess and deficiency of opiate receptor activity
being responsible for mania and depression respectively.

MATERIALS AND METHODS

Subjects were screened with diagnoses derived from the SADS-RDC by two
psychiatrists.[4] Eight normal controls (age 22-31, $\bar{x}$ 27) and 12 patients (age
22-57, $\bar{x}$ 26.7) clinically manifesting mania or hypomania (Bipolar depression
Type I, N=7; Bipolar II, N=4; and Manic Disorder, N=1) were studied. Intravenous naloxone HCl (20 mg) and an inert placebo were administered on two
consecutive days, in a counterbalanced, double-blind crossover. Data were
collected at regular intervals for 45 minutes prior to and for 2 hours following the infusion. Pulse, blood pressure, two self-rated mood scales (Profile
of Mood States,[5] and Subjective High Assessment Scale[6]), and three behavior
ratings (Beigel-Murphy Mania Rating Scale,[7] NIMH Behavioral Rating Scale,[8]
and the Behavioral Rating Scale - Judd[5]) were obtained. An analysis of
variance for repeated measures was used.

RESULTS

Naloxone significantly increased lethargy and drowsiness on the Beigel-
Murphy and decreased the pulse rate in the combined patient and normal sample.
The manic patient group, analyzed separately, showed a significant reduction
in manic symptoms as rated by the Beigel-Murphy Mania Scale. A more detailed

174

examination of the data revealed that 4 of the 8 manics were naloxone responders. These responders were rated as less irritable, angry, restless, tense,
hostile, and sarcastic, with parallel findings in the self-report data. The
time course of the responders was strikingly similar; the response was fully
manifested in 15-30 minutes and returned to baseline levels within one to two
hours. There were no differences between responders and non-responders in
clinical characteristics, familial history, or other demographic variables.
The pre-infusion baseline data showed that the manic responders were rated as
being significantly more grandiose, restless, and panicky, made more unrealis-
tic plans and rated themselves as being higher (100 ml "high" line) than the
non-responder manics.

SUMMARY

The data reported here suggest a sub-population (4 of 12 manics) responded
to naloxone HC1 (20 mg) with an attenuation in manic symptoms. Pre-treatment
analysis indicated that responders were those who were significantly more
extreme in their manic behavior than non-responders. These results suggest
that abnormalities in opioid peptide systems may be responsible for manic
symptoms in a sub-population of patients with Bipolar Depression.

ACKNOWLEDGEMENTS

This research was in part supported by Veterans Administration Hospital, San
Diego, Ca. and by an NIMH Mental Health Clinical Research Center Grant.

REFERENCES

1. Bych, R. (1976) Lancet, 2:72-73.
2. Segal, D.S., et al., (1977) Science, 198:411-414.
3. Holtzman, S.G. (1974) J. Pharmac. exp. Ther., 189, 51-60.
4. Gershon, A., and Deer, R. (eds.) (1975) Prediction in Psychopharmacology,
   N.Y. Raven Press.
5. McNair, D., et al.,(1971) EITS Manual for Profile of Mood States, San
   Diego, CA. Educational and Industrial Testing Service.
6. Judd, L.L., et al., (1977) Arch. Gen. Psych. 34:346-351.
7. Beigel, A., and Murphy, D. (1971) Amer. J. Psychiat. 128:688-694.
8. Wolf, S. and Berle, R.B. (eds.) (1976) The Biology of the Schizophrenic
   Process. pp. 104-133. Plenem Press, N.Y.

Characteristics and Function of Opioids, editors Van Ree and Terenius
© 1978 Elsevier/North-Holland Biomedical Press

A PRESYNAPTIC ACTION OF THE RAPHE ON TOOTH PULP FIBRE TERMINALS: IS THIS MEDIATED BY AN OPIOID PEPTIDE?

T. A. LOVICK, D. C. WEST and J. H. WOLSTENCROFT

Department of Physiology, Medical School, University of Birmingham, U.K.

Analgesia can be produced in man and experimental animals by electrical stimulation of the periaqueductal grey matter (PAG) in the midbrain or the raphe nuclei in the lower brain stem[1,2]. It has been reported that in cats the analgesia produced by raphe stimulation can be blocked by intravenous injection of naloxone[3], suggesting that the effect is mediated by an opioid. This view has been strengthened by the demonstration that enkephalin containing neurones are present in the brain and spinal cord and that there is a close correlation between the distribution of enkephalin-containing terminals and opiate receptors in the regions where afferent nociceptive fibres terminate in the dorsal horn of the spinal cord and spinal trigeminal nucleus. Lamotte et al[4] and Jessel and Iversen[5] have recently put forward the hypothesis that enkephalin is a neurotransmitter with a presynaptic site of action, reducing transmitter release from nociceptive fibres by causing depolarisation of their terminals. In the present study we have investigated this hypothesis with respect to the action of the raphe on the input from the tooth-pulp in the cat.

It has been shown electrophysiologically that there is an excitatory projection from the PAG to cells in the raphe and that many raphe cells project directly to the spinal cord or spinal trigeminal nucleus[6,7]. This pathway appears to be activated during stimulus produced analgesia from the PAG[8]. We have also shown that stimulation of the raphe can inhibit single unit responses to sensory stimuli in the spinal trigeminal nucleus[9]. By using Wall's method for testing the excitability of afferent terminal we have investigated the possibility that the inhibition from the raphe may be mediated presynaptically by an opioid.

The experiments were carried out on paralysed decerebrate cats from which the cerebellum had been removed. Stimulating electrodes were positioned in the midline of the brainstem between 3 and 6mm rostral to the obex and also in the caudal division of the spinal trigeminal nucleus. Recording electrodes were placed either on the ipsilateral inferior dental nerve (crushed peripherally) or the ipsilateral canine tooth pulp. The compound action potential in the nerve, or single units in the pulp, were recorded following antidromic activation of the primary afferent terminals in nucleus caudalis. Averaged records (20 sweeps) of the compound action potential were used. Prior stimulation in nucleus raphe magnus (8–15 pulses, 50–150 µA, 0.5 msec duration, 2–3 msec interval) caused an increase in the amplitude of the peak in the compound action potential which represented conduction in Aβ fibres (conduction velocities 50–56 m/sec) indicating increased excitability of the Aβ terminals. The effect was maximal 0–30 msec following the raphe stimulus train and often lasted for up to 200 msec. The effect of the raphe on the amplitude of the later Aδ peaks in the response was less consistent and usually produced a decrease in their size or no change. To assess the effect of the raphe on individual Aδ fibres the threshold for anti-dromic activation of tooth pulp afferent terminals in the caudal trigeminal nucleus was tested before and after raphe stimulation. In all cases the threshold was lower following stimulation in the raphe indicating increased excitability and primary afferent depolarizat-ion.

Thus at least some of the inhibitory effect of the raphe on trigeminal sensory input appears to be mediated presynaptically. However, naloxone, at doses up to 2–5 mg/Kg i.v., had no effect on either the change in amplitude of the compound action potential or on the change in threshold of tooth pulp fibre terminals following raphe stimulation. We conclude that although raphe stimulation produces presynaptic inhibition of trigeminal primary affer-ent terminals in the decerebrate cat, this is not mediated by an opioid acting on opiate receptors.

It should be stressed that these results do not disprove the hypothesis that there is a pre-synaptic action of enkephalinergic neurones on nociceptive fibres. Our experiments were made in decerebrate cats and it is possible that under other conditions an enkephalinergic mechanism may act to produce presynaptic inhibition. However it is also possible that the effects of naloxone in freely moving cats[3] may be due to blockade of a different type of presynaptic or postsynaptic action by e.g. β endorphin, or another endogenous opioid peptide, being released into the blood stream or the cerebrospinal fluid.

ACKNOWLEDGEMENT

This work was supported by the Medical Research Council.

REFERENCES

1. Richardson, D. E. and Akil, H. (1977) Pain reduction by electrical brain stimulation in man. J. Neurosurg., 47, 178–183.

2. Oliveras, J. L., Redjemi, F., Guilbaud, G. and Besson, J. M. (1975) Analgesia induced by electrical stimulation of the inferior centralis nucleus of the raphe in the cat. Pain, 1, 139-145.

3. Oliveras, J. L., Hosobuchi, Y., Redjemi, F., Guilbaud, G. and Besson, J. M. (1977) Opiate antagonist, naloxone, strongly reduces analgesia induced by stimulation of a raphe nucleus (centralis inferior). Brain Res., 120, 221-229.

4. Lamotte, C., Pert, C. B. and Snyder, S. H. (1976) Opiate receptor binding in primate spinal cord: distribution and changes after dorsal root section. Brain Res., 112, 407-412.

5. Jessell, T. M. and Iversen, L. L. (1977) Opiate analgesics inhibit substance P release from rat trigeminal nucleus. Nature, 268, 549-551.

6. Lovick, T. A., West, D. C. and Wolstencroft, J. H. (1978) Responses of raphespinal and other bulbar raphe neurones to stimulation of the periaqueductal gray in the cat. Neurosci. Lett., 8, 45-49.

7. Lovick, T. A., West, D. C. and Wolstencroft, J. H. (1978) Bulbar raphe neurones with projections to the spinal trigeminal nucleus and the lumbar cord in the cat. J. Physiol., 277, 61-62P.

8. Oleson, T. D., Twombly, D. A. and Liebeskind, J. C. (1978) Effects of pain-attenuating brain stimulation and morphine on electrical activity in the raphe nuclei of the awake rat. Pain, 4, 211-230.

9. Lovick, T. A., West, D. C. and Wolstencroft, J. H. (1977) Interactions between brain stem raphe nuclei and the trigeminal nuclei. pp. 307-317 in "Pain in the Trigeminal Region" eds. Anderson, D. J. and Mathews, B. Elsevier/North Holland.

Characteristics and Function of Opioids, editors Van Ree and Terenius
© *1978 Elsevier/North-Holland Biomedical Press*

EFFECTS OF ENDORPHINS ON DIFFERENT PARTS OF THE GASTRO-INTESTINAL TRACT IN
VITRO

FRANS P. NIJKAMP AND JAN M. VAN REE

Rudolf Magnus Institute for Pharmacology, University of Utrecht, Utrecht
(The Netherlands)

INTRODUCTION

Hughes et al. (1975) demonstrated the existence of opiate-like peptides
(met-enkephalin and leu-enkephalin) in brain tissue which mimic the influence
of morphine on the electrical induced contraction of the guinea pig ileum. We
investigated the spasmogenic and spasmolytic effects of met-enkephalin, leu-
enkephalin, α-endorphin, γ-endorphin, β-LPH 80-91 and (D-Ala^2)met-enkephalin on
different parts of the gastro-intestinal tract of guinea pig and rat in vitro.

METHODS

Male Wistar rats (CPB, TNO, Zeist) weighing between 200-300 g and male guinea
pigs weighing between 250-400 g were used for all experiments. After the animals
were stunned and bled, segments of the gastro-intestinal tract were removed and
superfused in a cascade of 4 tissues^2 with Krebs bicarbonate solution at 37°C
at 5 ml/min. Changes in tone of the intestinal parts were recorded with auxo-
tonic levers. The initial load on the tissues was 2 g.

RESULTS AND DISCUSSION

The endorphins, in a dose of 10 ng and 1 μg, caused changes in muscle tone
in colon and rectum and to a lesser extent in jejunum and ileum of both species.
Intestinal tissue from the rat contracted to the peptides, while relaxations
were induced in the isolated tissues from the guinea pig. In guinea pig colon
and rectum relaxation was preceeded by an initial short lasting contraction.
From the tested endorphins (D-Ala^2)met-enkephalin, met-enkephalin and leu-
enkephalin appeared to be the most potent entities, already showing profound
effect with 10 ng on colon and rectum. For further experiments, the rat rectum
was selected because of the amplitude of the response on enkephalins. On this
tissue (D-Ala^2)met-enkephalin, met-enkephalin, leu-enkephalin, γ-endorphin, α-
endorphin and β-LPH 80-91 caused dose-dependent contractions. ED50 (in mole)
were found resp. 0.96×10^{-12}, 1.05×10^{-11}, 1.22×10^{-11}, 1.08×10^{-10}, 2.65×10^{-10} and
6.5×10^{-9}. Regression lines of the different endorphins appeared to be parallel

180

to that of met-enkephalin. Naloxone (10^{-7}-10^{-5}M) dose-dependently shifted the
dose-response curve of met-enkephalin to the right (fig. 1). Subsequently, we
have tested the effect of several non-opiate inhibitors on the response to met-
enkephalin by adding the inhibitors to the superfusion fluid. Cholinergic
blockade by atropine, ganglionergic blockade by hexamethonium, β-adrenoceptor
blockade by propranolol or prostaglandin synthesis inhibition by indomethacin
in doses ranging from 2-7.7x10^{-6}M did not substantially affect the dose-response curve to met-enkephalin. Blockade of histamine H1 and H2 receptors by
resp. mepyramine and burimamide, although non significantly, increased maximal
contractions to met-enkephalin. Profound effects were observed with the α-
adrenoceptor blocking agent phentolamine. In the presence of phentolamine (2x
10^{-6}M) the maximal response to met-enkephalin was doubled (fig. 2). In contrast,
the serotonin antagonists methysergide and cyproheptadine (2x10^{-6}M) reduced the
contractile response to met-enkephalin in a non-competitive manner (fig. 2).

The present results demonstrate that longitudinal smooth muscle of the
gastro-intestinal tract of guinea pig and rat, in particular rectum and colon,
are sensitive to opioid-like peptides. In contrast to the electrically stimulated guinea pig ileum the effects of the opioid-like peptides in the rat rectum may not be mediated by acetylcholine since atropine does not inhibit the
response to met-enkephalin. Noradrenergic and serotonergic systems however
might be involved in the changes in muscle tone induced by met-enkephalin.

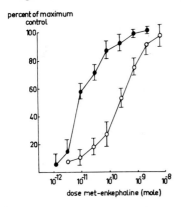

Fig. 1. Effect of naloxone (10^{-6}M) on the contractor response to met-enkephalin of the rat rectum in vitro. ●-● met-enkephalin; 0-0 met-enkephalin + naloxone.

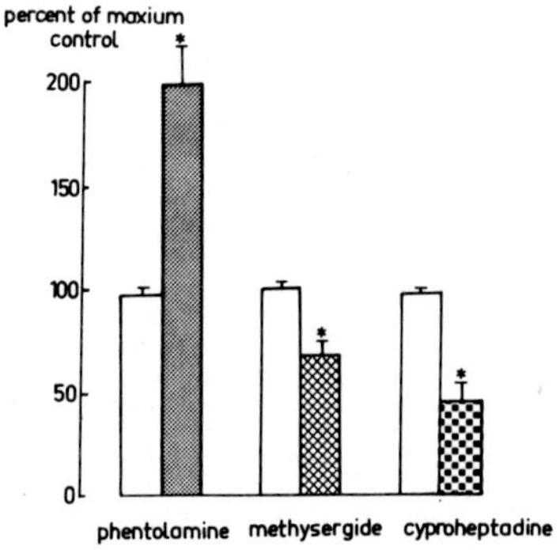

Fig. 2. Effect of 2x10^{-6}M phentolamine, methysergide and cyproheptadine on the maximal contractor response to met-enkephalin of the rat rectum in vitro. □ met-enkephalin control. x $p < 0.05$.

REFERENCES
1. Hughes, J. et al. (1975) Nature (London), 258, 577-579.
2. Vane, J.R. (1964) Brit. J. Pharmacol., 23, 360-373.

Characteristics and Function of Opioids, editors Van Ree and Terenius
© *1978 Elsevier/North-Holland Biomedical Press*

ANTIPSYCHOTIC ACTION OF [DES-TYR¹]-γ-ENDORPHIN (β-LPH$_{62-77}$)

JAN M. VAN REE, WIM M.A. VERHOEVEN[1], HERMAN M. VAN PRAAG[1] & DAVID DE WIED
Rudolf Magnus Institute for Pharmacology and Department of Psychiatry,
State University of Utrecht, The Netherlands.

In animals, [des-Tyr¹]-γ-endorphin (DTγE, β-lipotropin 62-77) produces behavioral effects reminiscent of those caused by neuroleptic drugs. DTγE, a non-opiate-like analogue of γ-endorphin, facilitates the extinction of pole-jumping avoidance behavior, attenuates the retention of a passive avoidance response and is active in various 'grip tests'[1,2]. Similar effects followed the injection of haloperidol, but in contrast to DTγE, haloperidol also caused sedation and suppression of locomotor activity of rats. To demonstrate the purported antipsychotic action of DTγE, two groups of schizophrenic patients were treated with this neuropeptide and their psychotic symptoms were followed carefully.

SUBJECTS AND METHODS

Study 1: This study comprised 6 patients suffering from long-lasting psychosis and at least partly resistant to treatment with various neuroleptic drugs. Most of the subjects showed clear signs of hallucinations and/or delusions. One week after neuroleptic medication had been discontinued, the patients were treated with DTγE (obtained from Organon International B.V.) for 10 days using an open design. In most cases 1 mg DTγE was injected intramuscularly (i.m.) once daily as a zinc-phosphate preparation. During the experimental trial, three-point rating scales were used in order to assess the symptoms of the subjects. The items scored were: hallucinations, delusions, emotional flattening, train of thought, orientation and motor activity.

Study 2: This study dealt with 6 patients with a course of illness generally similar to that described for the subjects of study 1. In this study 2, however, medication with conventional neuroleptics was maintained during experimentation. The patients were given i.m. 1 mg DTγE dissolved in saline or placebo once daily for 16 days using a double-blind, cross-over design. Before and after the experimental trial the subjects were injected with placebo for 4 days (single-blind). Scoring of the symptoms was done the same way as in study 1.

Two patients suffering from a relapsing schizo-affective disorder and admitted because of an acute episode of psychosis and who were free of antipsychotic medication were added to study 2.

RESULTS

The subjects of study 1 could be divided into two groups of 3 patients each on the basis of their response to treatment with DTγE. In the first group the psychotic symptoms were markedly diminished on days 3 and 4 of treatment. The subjects then relapsed and became more or less aggressive and/or agitated. The other three patients improved from day 4 of treatment on and their psychotic symptoms disappeared completely for 2 weeks after treatment had been discontinued. Two of these three subjects were slightly euphoric and DTγE dissolved in saline was injected for 4 days about three weeks after the end of the first experimental trial when symptoms such as a delusional mood and thought disturbances had returned. The symptoms disappeared completely on day 3 of this second treatment and had not recurred up to 4 weeks after experimentation.

In study 2 the psychotic symptoms were not altered by placebo injection for 4 or 12 days. However, from the first day of DTγE treatment on, the patients became progressively less psychotic in that symptoms such as hallucinations and delusions diminished. On the first day of DTγE treatment the scored items hallucinations/delusions decreased slightly as compared to the day before starting DTγE injection ($P < 0.05$). This effect was more pronounced from day 5 of treatment on ($P < 0.005$). In some patients, the psychotic symptoms returned 5 - 7 days after DTγE injections, although at a moderate level. Other patients remained without symptoms for several weeks. The two patients with an acute episode of schizophrenia characterized by profound psychotic symptoms and with no neuroleptic medication at admission showed a distinct improvement on treatment with DTγE. Their psychotic symptoms disappeared with the same time-course as in the patients who had been kept on conventional neuroleptic medication during DTγE treatment.

In summary, 8 of the 13 patients showed clear-cut improvement following treatment with DTγE in that their psychotic symptoms disappeared completely (table 1). DTγE treatment was less effective in the other 5 subjects. In fact, in these patients mild psychotic symptoms were present before experimentation (3 subjects) or the symptoms, although markedly decreased, did not disappear completely (2 subjects).

DISCUSSION

The present data indicate that the neuropeptide DTγE has potential antipsychotic activity as had been predicted from animal experiments. Most, if not all of the patients improved upon treatment, i.e., their psychotic symptoms diminished or even disappeared. In some patients this improvement was only present during and some days after medication, whereas others remained free of psychotic symptoms for a longer period of time. Together, the postulate that DTγE or a closely related neuropeptide is an endogenous neuroleptic and the

TABLE 1

IMPROVEMENT OF PSYCHOTIC SYMPTOMS IN 13 SCHIZOPHRENIC PATIENTS FOLLOWING TREATMENT WITH DTγE [Des-Tyr[1]]-γ-endorphin, β-LPH$_{62-77}$)

improvement[a]	marked		moderate		slight
duration[b]	semi-permanent	transient	semi-permanent	transient	transient
number of patients	5	3	2	2	1

a) marked: profound psychotic symptoms disappeared completely.
   moderate: mild psychotic symptoms disappeared completely or profound psychotic symptoms diminished temporarily.
   slight: mild psychotic symptoms diminished temporarily.
b) psychotic symptoms recurred (transient) or did not recur (semi-permanent) within 14 days after treatment.

finding of a beneficial effect of DTγE in schizophrenic patients suggest that derangements in lipotropin-endorphin homeostasis may be responsible for psychosis of the schizophrenic type. This suggestion must be verified by comparing the activity of endorphin and closely related peptide systems of patients and of control subjects. Such a study may also elucidate the mechanism underlying the differential responses of the patients to DTγE treatment, i.e., the transient versus the semipermanent improvement.

The finding of a beneficial effect of DTγE in patients suffering from psychosis of the schizophrenic type leads to important theoretical and practical considerations:

1. The neuroleptic activity of DTγE is not contingent on the typical morphine-like action of endorphins, since DTγE is practically devoid of morphinomimetic action[1]; 2. To date, animal experiments indicate that the amino acid residue leucine at the C-terminal side of DTγE is particularly important for the purported neuroleptic activity of DTγE.; 3. These observations support the validity of the neuropeptide concept i.e. that peptides involved in behavioral homeostasis may be generated enzymatically from precursor molecules[3].

In fact, the morphinomimetic peptide β-endorphin may be generated from β-lipotropin and have its opiate-like activity dramatically decreased by removal of the N-terminal tyrosine residue. The neuroleptic peptide DTγE may be formed from β-lipotropin and its neuroleptic-like activity may be destroyed when the C-terminal residue leucine is removed; 4. Schizophrenia may have as biochemical background a disturbance in the balance between the activity of DTγE and related peptides and that of β- and α-endorphin and related peptides. Since α- and β-endorphin have behavioral effects opposite to those of DTγE, this balance may

184

be physiologically important for brain functions; 5. A disbalance may lead, at least in some cases, to accumulation of β-endorphin, a peptide which induces a catatonic-like syndrome in experimental animals[4,5] and, which would be responsible for the catatonic symptomatology of schizophrenic patients; 6. Although we assume that decreased availability of DTγE or a closely related peptide is the most important factor in the induction of psychotic symptoms, it might be that increased levels of endorphins of the α- and β-type in the brain contribute to the symptomatology of the psychotic syndrome. These increased levels could also explain the beneficial effect of high, but not of low, doses of naloxone[6-9]. However, other explanations of the temporary relief subsequent to naloxone injection may be possible, particularly since narcotic antagonists seem to affect the extinction of avoidance in the same way as does DTγE[10]; 7. The possibility that such a balance may be physiologically operative in the brain is supported by findings showing that neither pure opiate agonists nor pure antagonists induce typical psychotic symptoms in man, but that, in contrast, partial opiate antagonists, such as cyclazocine, nalorphine and SKF 10.047 produce hallucinations[11,12]; 8. The semi-permanent improvement observed in a number of patients treated with DTγE may be the result of bringing the presumably disbalanced lipotropin-endorphin system into physiological equilibrium, probably by adjusting feedback systems for the generation of the various endorphins. This might be verified by studies on the metabolism of β-endorphin in normal and in psychotic patients. Such studies may contribute to elucidate the disturbances in the brain which are responsible for the psychopathology of schizophrenia; 9. DTγE or a closely related neuropeptide may be an endogenous peptide with neuroleptic activity or a naturally occurring antipsychotic. Entities with such characteristics could be termed endoleptic, naturoleptic, naturopsycholytic or endopsycholytic.

REFERENCES
1. De Wied D. et al. (1978) Europ. J. Pharmacol. 49, 427-436.
2. De Wied, D. (1978) This Volume.
3. De Wied, D. (1977) Life Sci. 20, 195-204.
4. Segal, D.S. et al. (1977) Science 198, 411-414.
5. Jacquet, Y.F. & Marks, N. (1976) Science 194, 632-635.
6. Akil, H. et al. (1978) Adv. Biochem. Psychopharmacol. 18, 125-139.
7. Herz, A. et al. (1978) Adv. Biochem. Psychopharmacol. 18, 333-339.
8. Davis, G.C. et al (1977) Science 197, 74-77.
9. Volavka, J. et al. (1977) Science 196, 1227-1228.
10. De Wied, D. et al. (1978) J. Pharmacol. Exp. Ther. 204, 507-580.
11. Jasinski, D.R. et al. (1967) J. Pharmacol. Exp. Ther. 157, 420-426.
12. Martin, W.R. et al. (1976) J. Pharmacol. Exp. Ther. 197, 517-532.

Characteristics and Function of Opioids, editors Van Ree and Terenius
© *1978 Elsevier/North-Holland Biomedical Press*

A STRUCTURE-ACTIVITY STUDY WITH ENKEPHALIN ANALOGUES: FURTHER EVIDENCE FOR
MULTIPLE OPIATE RECEPTOR TYPES

J.S. SHAW and M.J. TURNBULL
BIOLOGY DEPARTMENT

A.S. DUTTA, J.J. GORMLEY, C.F. HAYWARD and G.J. STACEY
CHEMISTRY DEPARTMENT

ICI Ltd., Pharmaceuticals Division, Alderley Park, Macclesfield, Cheshire,
England.

INTRODUCTION

The in vitro characteristics of both the classical opiate drugs and the
enkephalins differ when results obtained on the guinea pig ileum are compared
with those obtained with the mouse vas deferens preparation[1,2,3,4]. Thus
the enkephalins are considerably more potent on the mouse vas deferens, when
compared with normorphine, than on the guinea pig ileum. In addition, the
activity of the enkephalins on the vas deferens is relatively resistant to
the antagonist action of naloxone whereas normorphine is readily antagonised.
This is not the case with the ileum preparation where both classes of compound
are readily antagonised by naloxone.   Lord et al.[1] suggested that in the
ileum a single type of opiate receptor - the μ receptor - predominates and
this is sensitive to 'classical' agonists and antagonists and also to the
opioid peptides.   In the vas, a second type of receptor - the δ receptor -
predominates and this site is less sensitive to the classical opiates whilst
being fully sensitive to the enkephalins.   Accordingly in the guinea pig
ileum most of the action of the enkephalins is mediated via μ receptors whilst
on the vas the enkephalins act predominantly at δ-receptors, thus accounting
for their insensitivity to the antagonist action of naloxone on the latter
tissue.   The classical opiates on the other hand, are readily antagonised
by naloxone on the vas and this suggests that a proportion of the receptors
in this organ are of the μ type, and that the classical compounds act at
these receptors.

Not all enkephalin analogues however behave like the endogenous peptides[2,3,5].
Whilst the endogenous peptides are considerably less potent on the guinea pig
ileum than on the mouse vas deferens, a few analogues have been reported to
be more potent on the ileum.   Indeed Székely et al.[3] have reported one

analogue with an ileum/vas ratio similar to that of normorphine and β-endorphin In another recent study[5] a number of pentapeptide analogues have been described with ileum/vas ratios spanning a 250-fold range. This clearly supports the hypothesis that the receptors in the two preparations are different. In addition, it demonstrates that not all the enkephalin analogues have the same receptor specificity as the endogenous pentapeptides.

The purpose of the present study was to investigate the effects of some modifications to the enkephalin molecule on the relative potency in the two in vitro assays, and to study the relationship between ileum and vas potencies and analgesic activity. Additional structure-function data obtained with these analogues has been reported elsewhere[5,6,7].

MATERIALS AND METHODS

Drugs. Peptides were synthesised by solution methods in the Peptide Group of ICI Pharmaceuticals Division; the purity of each was established as previously described[6]. Normorphine was a gift from Burroughs Wellcome. All drugs were prepared as solutions in distilled water for the in vitro assays, and in saline for in vivo testing (one equivalent of 0.1 N HCl was added where necessary).

Guinea Pig Ileum Assay. The coaxially-stimulated guinea pig ileum preparation was similar to that described by Kosterlitz and Watt[8]. Segments of ileum approximately 2 cm. in length were mounted under a tension of 1 g. in a 50 cm^3 organ bath containing Krebs solution at 37° and aerated with 95% O_2/5% CO_2. The stimuli (0.5 m.sec square wave, 0.1 HZ at 1.5 x maximal voltage) were generated by a Grass S88 stimulator and were delivered to the bath via platinum electrodes. The contractions were recorded isometrically using an Ether UF1 force transducer and a Devices M X 4 recorder.

Mouse Vas Deferens Assay. This was a modification of the method described by Hughes et al.[9]. The vas was mounted in a 9 cm^3 organ bath containing Mg^{++}-free Krebs solution and aerated with 95% O_2/5% CO_2. Except during the addition of drugs, a flow rate of 3 cm^3. min.$^{-1}$ was maintained through the bath. Contractions were induced by short trains of stimuli (1 m.sec pulses at 50 H_Z for 100 m.sec) at 1.25 x maximal voltage and repeated at 10 sec. intervals. Recordings were made using a Palmer 411/1326 isotonic transducer with 100 mg tension, and a Servoscribe chart recorder.

In both the vas and ileum preparations, agonist activity was calculated as the ratio between the IC_{50} of the test compound and the IC_{50} of met-enkephalin measured immediately before and after the test compound. Met-enkephalin had a mean IC_{50} value of 67.9 ± 6.6 nM on the mouse vas deferens and 190.3 ± 18.9 nM on the guinea pig ileum.

Mouse Hot Plate Test.   Analgesic activity was assessed after intravenous injection of the peptides into female mice of the Alderley Park strain weighing 20-23 g.   Mice were placed on a hot plate maintained at 56° and their reaction time was recorded both before and at 5, 10, 15 and 30 min. after dosing.   The mean pre-dose latency was 3.89 ± 0.125 s.e.m. sec. (n = 70). Saline-treated mice displayed a maximal increase in reaction time of 0.64 ± 0.18 s.e.m. sec. (n = 32).   The ED_{50} was defined as the dose which produced a doubling of the mean reaction time compared to the pre-dose value, and was measured at the time of peak activity.   Groups of at least nine mice were used at each dose level.

RESULTS

Both the natural enkephalins show relatively low ileum/vas ratios and the ratio produced by Leu-enkephalin is significantly lower than that produced by Met-enkephalin (Table 1).   In contrast, β-endorphin has a profile similar to that of the classical opiate agonist normorphine and is almost 70 times more selective for the ileum receptor than is Leu-enkephalin.   These observations indicate that even the endogenous pentapeptides cover a wide range of receptor specificities.   As Leu- and Met-enkephalin differ only at the C-terminal end we decided to investigate the effect of substitutions at position 5 of $[D-Ser^2]-$ and $[D-Ala^2]-$enkephalins.

TABLE 1

COMPARISON BETWEEN GUINEA PIG ILEUM AND MOUSE VAS DEFERENS POTENCIES OF STANDARD OPIOIDS

Drug	Relative Potency*		Ileum/Vas
	Ileum	Vas	
Met-enkephalin	1	1	1
Leu-enkephalin	0.48 ($\pm$ 0.02)	3.63 ($\pm$ 1.02)	0.13
β-endorphin	4.52 ($\pm$ 1.23)	0.50 ($\pm$ 0.02)	9.04
Normorphine	2.17 ($\pm$ 0.27)	0.25 ($\pm$ 0.06)	8.68

* In this and subsequent tables, potencies are expressed as the ratio between the IC_{50} of the test compound and the IC_{50} of Met-enkephalin determined in the same tissue.   The mean IC_{50} values for Met-enkephalin were 67.9 ± 6.6 nM in the mouse vas deferens and 190.3 ± 18.9 nM in the guinea pig ileum.

Analogues with D-amino acids in position 2 were chosen as these have been demonstrated by us, and by others[10,11], to be relatively resistant to enzymic degradation.   As shown in table 2 it is clear that analogues with leucine or methionine in position 5 have low ratios, whilst the analogues with proline ethylamide in this position have greatly increased ratios.   Both the compounds with proline amide in position 5 have the largest ratios, and these compounds show a degree of selectivity for the ileum comparable with that of β-endorphin and normorphine.

TABLE 2

EFFECT OF SUBSTITUTION AT POSITION 5 ON GUINEA PIG ILEUM/MOUSE VAS DEFERENS POTENCY RATIO

Analogue				Potency (met-enkephalin = 1)		Ileum/Vas
				Ileum	Vas	
Tyr-D-Ala-Gly-Phe-Leu-OMe				0.89 ($\pm$ 0.06)	0.89 ($\pm$ 0.17)	1
"	"	"	" Leu-NH$_2$	13.1 ($\pm$ 2.4)	10.1 ($\pm$ 1.75)	1.3
"	"	"	" Met-NH$_2$	7.75 ($\pm$ 0.64)	3.81 ($\pm$ 0.81)	2.04
"	"	"	" Pro-NHEt	2.72 ($\pm$ 0.32)	0.53 ($\pm$ 0.09)	5.2
"	"	"	" Pro-NH$_2$	5.49 ($\pm$ 0.89)	0.49 ($\pm$ 0.07)	11.2
"	D-Ser	"	" Met OMe	14.3 ($\pm$ 2.2)	29.5 ($\pm$ 3.9)	0.48
"	"	"	" Pro-NHEt	2.11 ($\pm$ 0.42)	0.31 ($\pm$ 0.06)	6.8
"	"	"	" Pro-NH$_2$	2.20 ($\pm$ 0.18)	0.19 ($\pm$ 0.09)	11.6

Having demonstrated that specificity for the ileum was increased by the inclusion of a proline in position 5 we proceeded to investigate the effect of modifications at position 2 of [Pro^5]-enkephalinamide.   All of the 5 analogues in this series have relatively high ratios (table 3) indicating that proline does, indeed, produce specificity for μ-receptors.   However, the analogues with D-methionine and D-aspartic acid at position 2 have extremely high ratios indicating that modifications at position 2 may also influence the ileum/vas potency ratio.   To test this possibility we compared 3 peptides with D-alanine in position 2 with their D-methionine analogues (table 4).   In each pair of compounds the [D-Met^2] analogue had the higher ratio indicating that this substitution can contribute to specificity for the μ-receptor.   However, in both the [D-Ala^2] and [D-Met^2] groups of analogues it was the compounds with proline at position 5 which had the largest ratios, indicating that the effects of proline and D-methionine may be, at least partially, additive.

TABLE 3

EFFECT OF SUBSTITUTION AT POSITION 2 ON GUINEA PIG ILEUM/MOUSE VAS DEFERENS POTENCY RATIO

Analogue	Potency (met-enkephalin = 1)		Ileum/vas
	Ileum	Vas	
Tyr-Gly-Gly-Phe-Pro-NH$_2$	0.06 ($\pm$ 0.02)	0.009 ($\pm$ 0.003)	6.9
" D-Ala " " " "	5.49 ($\pm$ 0.89)	0.49 ($\pm$ 0.07)	11.2
" D-Ser " " " "	2.20 ($\pm$ 0.18)	0.19 ($\pm$ 0.09)	11.6
" D-Met " " " "	29.2 ($\pm$ 2.94)	0.97 ($\pm$ 0.10)	30.1
" D-Asp " " " "	8.5 ($\pm$ 1.42)	0.24 ($\pm$ 0.07)	35.4

TABLE 4

COMPARISON BETWEEN D-MET AND D-ALA SUBSTITUTION IN POSITION 2 ON GUINEA PIG ILEUM/MOUSE VAS DEFERENS POTENCY RATIO

Analogue	Potency (met-enkephalin = 1)		Ileum/Vas
	Ileum	Vas	
Tyr-D-Met-Gly-Phe-Leu-NH$_2$	27.5 ($\pm$ 4.7)	3.68 ($\pm$ 0.39)	7.4
" D-Ala " " " "	13.1 ($\pm$ 2.4)	10.1 ($\pm$ 1.75)	1.3
" D-Met " " " OMe	63.1 ($\pm$ 12.3)	2.99 ($\pm$ 0.25)	21.1
" D-Ala " " " "	0.89 ($\pm$ 0.06)	0.89 ($\pm$ 0.17)	1
" D-Met " " Pro-NH$_2$	29.2 ($\pm$ 2.9)	0.97 ($\pm$ 0.1)	30.1
" D-Ala " " " "	5.49 ($\pm$ 0.89)	0.49 ($\pm$ 0.067)	11.2

Another further substitution which we have studied is the N-methylation of tyrosine. In both Leu-enkephalin amide and [D-Ser[2], Pro[5]]-enkephalin ethylamide the inclusion of a methyl on the terminal amino increases the selectivity for the ileum. However in D-Ala[2] leu-enkephalin amide and [D-Met[2], Pro[5]]-enkephalin amide N-methylation of tyrosine has little, if any effect on this ratio.

The analgesic activity of our enkephalin analogues is summarised in table 6. From these results it is clear that analogues with glycine in position 2

and [D-Ala^2]-Met-enkephalin amide are devoid of analgesic activity at doses
up to 50 mg/kg. However, this latter compound was significantly analgesic
at 100 mg/kg. The remaining compounds can conveniently be divided into
three groups. All the compounds tested with proline amide at position 5
have ED_{50} values of <2 mg/kg; the [Pro^5]-ethylamide analogues are analgesic
at approximately 5 mg/kg, and the [Leu^5] and [Met^5] compounds are only active
at doses above 10 mg/kg.

TABLE 5

EFFECT OF N-METHYLATION OF TYROSINE ON GUINEA PIG ILEUM/MOUSE VAS DEFERENS
POTENCY RATIO

Analogue	Potency (met-enkephalin = 1)		Ileum/Vas
	Ileum	Vas	
Tyr-Gly-Gly-Phe-Leu-NH$_2$	1.06 ($\pm$ 0.29)	1.30 ($\pm$ 0.8)	0.82
Me Tyr " " " " "	4.85 ($\pm$ 0.84)	0.85 ($\pm$ 0.16)	5.71
Tyr-D-Ser-Gly-Phe-Pro-NHEt	2.11 ($\pm$ 0.42)	0.31 ($\pm$ 0.06)	6.8
Me Tyr " " " " " "	2.18 ($\pm$ 0.37)	0.07 ($\pm$ 0.01)	31.1
Tyr-D-Ala-Gly-Phe-Leu-NH$_2$	13.1 ($\pm$ 2.4)	10.1 ($\pm$ 1.75)	1.3
Me Tyr " " " " " "	10.8 ($\pm$ 2.7)	6.4 ($\pm$ 0.66)	1.7
Tyr-D-Met-Gly-Phe-Pro-NH$_2$	29.2 ($\pm$ 2.94)	0.97 ($\pm$ 0.1)	30.1
Me Tyr " " " " " "	45.2 ($\pm$ 4.5)	2.16 ($\pm$ 0.31)	20.9

The one exception to these groupings is [D-Met^2]-Leu-enkephalinamide which
has an ED_{50} of 2.2 mg/kg. For comparison the ED_{50} of morphine is 0.82
(0.61 - 1.09) mg/kg. No correlation emerged between analgesic activity
and potency on either the vas or the ileum. However, there is a significant
(p 0.05) correlation between the ileum/vas potency ratio and analgesia.
Table 7 presents the correlation coefficients between these three parameters.
For the purpose of these calculations analogues with glycine in position 2
were omitted in order to reduce the influence of enzymic instability on the
analgesic data.

TABLE 6

ANALGESIC POTENCY OF ENKEPHALIN ANALOGUES DETERMINED IN THE MOUSE HOT PLATE
ASSAY FOLLOWING INTRAVENOUS ADMINISTRATION

| Substituent at | | | ED_{50} (mg/kg i.v.) * |
Tyr[1]	Gly[2]	Leu[5]	(95% confidence limits)
-	-	-	>50
-	-	Met	>50
-	-	Leu-NH$_2$	>50
Me-Tyr	-	Leu-NH$_2$	>50
-	-	Pro-NH$_2$	>50
-	D-Ala	Met-NH$_2$	>50
-	D-Ala	Leu-OMe	34.2 (28.2-41.4)
-	D-Met	Leu-OMe	30.0 (16.1-57.0)
Me-Tyr	D-Ala	Leu-NH$_2$	16.4 (12.0-22.5)
-	D-Ser	Met-OMe	13.6 (10.3-18.0)
Me-Tyr	D-Ser	Pro-NHEt	5.5 (3.2- 9.4)
-	D-Ala	Pro-NHEt	4.4 (2.2- 9.0)
-	D-Ser	Pro-NHEt	4.0 (2.9- 5.6)
-	D-Met	Leu-NH$_2$	2.2 (1.0- 5.2)
-	D-Ser	Pro-NH$_2$	1.7 (1.3- 2.4)
-	D-ASp	Pro-NH$_2$	1.04(0.68- 1.6)
-	D-Ala	Pro-NH$_2$	0.95(0.47- 1.9)
-	D-Met	Pro-NH$_2$	0.93(0.41- 1.9)
Me-Tyr	D-Met	Pro-NH$_2$	0.72(0.46-1.13)

* ED_{50} values were calculated at the time of maximal activity.   See methods
section for further details.

192

TABLE 7

RELATIONSHIP BETWEEN GUINEA PIG ILEUM, MOUSE VAS DEFERENS AND ANALGESIC
ACTIVITIES OF 2-SUBSTITUTED ENKEPHALIN ANALOGUES

Comparison	Correlation Coefficient (r)
Analgesia vs. ileum potency	0.225
Analgesia vs. vas potency	-0.30
Analgesia vs. relative ileum/vas potency	0.56 *
Ileum potency vs. vas potency	0.062

* Significant correlation $p < 0.05$

DISCUSSION

Székely et al.[3] have demonstrated that [D-Met^2,Pro^5]-enkephalin amide has
a greater effect on the ileum than the vas and this potency ratio is of the
same order as that for normorphine and β-endorphin. In addition Bajusz et al.
[12,13] have reported that several enkephalin analogues with proline amide or
ethylamide in position 5 are potent analgesics. We have confirmed these
findings with 4 published and 4 novel analogues, and in addition have
demonstrated that all of the [Pro^5]-enkephalin analogues have high ileum/vas
ratios. Similar ratios have also been reported by Lord et al.[4] for the
N-methyltyrosine analogues of Met-enkephalin and Met-enkephalin amide. We
have found that N-methylation of the tyrosine of Leu-enkephalin amide or
[D-Ser^2, Pro^5]-enkephalin ethylamide increases the selectivity for the ileum.
However, the same substitution applied to [D-Ala^2]-Leu-enkephalin amide and
[D-Met^2,Pro^5]-enkephalin amide has no effect on the ileum/vas ratio.
Therefore this substitution cannot be relied upon to produce this effect in
all circumstances. Thus, in addition to the substitution of proline in
position 5, the only other change to consistently produce an increase in the
selectivity for the ileum was that of replacing the amino acid at position 2
with D-methionine. Thus, all three [D-Met^2] compounds examined had
significantly higher ileum/vas ratios than the [D-Ala^2] analogues. It is
of interest to note that whilst all these [D-Met^2] analogues had high ratios,
the largest effect occured in the compound with proline amide at position 5.
Thus the effects of [D-Met^2] and [Pro^5] substitutions appear to be, at least
in part, additive.

Of the compounds tested only those with leucine or methionine in position 5 had ileum/vas ratios of less than two. Baxter et al.[14] have also reported that [D-Ala^2, D-Leu^5]-enkephalin is considerably less potent on the ileum than on the vas, whilst Beddell et al.[15] have shown that the [D-Ala^2] analogues of [Leu^5]-,[Met^5]- and [D-Met^5]-enkephalins are similarly selective for the vas.

Whilst several authors have explained the variation in relative potency between the opioids in terms of different types of opiate receptor, the possibility remains that the lower ileum/vas ratios observed with some enkephalin analogues could be due to enzymic inactivation in the guinea pig ileum. However, several of our results indicate that the relative potency on the two tissues is unrelated to enzymic stability. Thus [D-Ser^2]-Met-enkephalin methyl ester, which is protected by its D-amino acid from enzymic cleavage of its tyrosine (the major site of enkephalin degradation[11]), is relatively more potent on the vas deferens, indicating that an increase in stability does not necessarily produce a corresponding increase in selectivity for the ileum. Similarly, the analogues [D-Ala^2]-Leu-enkephalin amide and the corresponding [Met^5] compound have ileum/vas potency ratios of 1.3 and 2 respectively although they should be considerably more stable than the endogenous peptides. However, the much less stable analogue [Pro^5]-enkephalin amide is apparently much more selective for the ileum. Such an increase in ileum/vas ratio can only be explained in terms of a change in receptor specificity. A final point concerns the effect of the N-methylation of tyrosine. This substitution, which could be expected to reduce enzymic cleavage of tyrosine, should have had a similar effect in both [D-Ser^2,Pro^5]-enkephalin ethylamide and [D-Ala^2]-Leu-enkephalin amide. However, N-methylation of the former compound produces a large increase in ileum/vas potency ratio whilst in the latter case the effect is minimal. Thus we conclude that the ileum/vas ratio is an index of relative specificity for the two receptor types.

The relationship between in vitro potency and analgesic activity is not immediately clear. In the case of the classical opiate agonists, activity on the vas or the ileum appears to correlate well with in vivo analgesic potency[9,16]. However, since for the enkephalins the ratio between vas and ileum potency is subject to considerably variation it is clear that only one of these assays could be predictive of analgesia. In a recent study, Frederickson[17] compared the activites of several analogues on the vas deferens with their potencies as analgesics after intracerebroventricular injection (thus minimising, although not eliminating, any influence of enzymic stability). No significant correlation was found between the two assay systems thus suggesting that the δ-receptors which predominate in the vas are not responsible for the production of analgesia. Using similar techniques, Morgan et al.[8] demonstrated that activity on the vas was unrelated to either ileum or analgesic potency. However, there appeared to be some correlation between the latter two parameters.

In another study Baxter et al.[14] demonstrated that the analogue [D-Ala^2, D-Leu^5]-enkephalin has approximately 3 times the analgesic potency of morphine by the intracerebroventricular route and is twice as potent as morphine on the guinea pig ileum. However, this compound is 1227 times the potency of morphine on the vas deferens, indicating that the δ-receptors in the vas and the receptors which mediate analgesia are dissimilar. However, Beddell et al.[15] were able to demonstrate a good correlation between mouse vas deferens potency and affinity for opiate receptors in rat brain. Since almost all of the compounds in his study were [Leu^5] or [Met^5] analogues, and none had D-methionine in position 2, the analogues were all likely to possess specificty for the δ-receptor, thus accounting for this correlation. Thus, unless there is a third, as yet uncharacterised, opiate receptor it would appear that the μ-receptor is responsible for the analgesic activity of the opiates.

In the present study we have failed to demonstrate any direct relationship between activity on the guinea pig ileum and analgesia in the mouse. This is undoubtedly due to several factors such as enzymic instability of the peptides, distribution within the body and penetration of the blood/brain barrier. However, we have shown a significant correlation between analgesia and the ileum/vas potency ratio. Thus selectivity for the ileum is, in some way, related to analgesic activity. Nevertheless, this finding is difficult to explain since it implies that analgesic potency is to some extent determined by inactivity on the mouse vas deferens preparation. However, if it is assumed that both preparations contain a mixture of the two receptor types, and that the ileum contains predominatly μ-receptors, it is possible that a potent δ-receptor agonist may possess activity on the ileum by virtue of its affinity for the δ-receptors in this preparation. Thus activity on the ileum may not be an adequate measure of μ-receptor activity without the additional information provided by the ileum/vas ratio. A pure μ-receptor agonist would therefore possess activity on the ileum and a high ileum/vas ratio. This profile is typical of the most potent analgesics amongst the enkephalin analogues and also of the classical opiate agonists, thus supporting the hypothesis that analgesia is mediated via the μ-receptor.

Thus, studies by several authors with analogues of enkephalin have demonstrated that compounds can be synthesised which are selective for either μ or δ-receptors. Evidence from studies of the analgesic activity of these compounds suggests that analgesia is mediated via the μ-receptor. The role of the δ-receptor remains to be elucidated.

REFERENCES

1. J.A.H. Lord, A.A. Waterfield, J. Hughes and H.W. Kosterlitz (1976) in Opiates and Endogenous Opioid Peptides, H.W. Kosterlitz, Ed., pp 275-280, Elsevier/North-Holland Biomedical Press, Amsterdam.

2. A.A. Waterfield, R.J. Smokum, J. Hughes, H.W. Kosterlitz and G. Henderson (1977) European J. Pharmacol. 43, 107-116.

3. J.I. Székely, A.Z. Rónai, Z. Dunai-Kovács, E. Miglécz, I. Berzétri, J. Bajusz and L. Gráf (1977) European J. Pharmacol. 43, 293-294.

4. J.A.H. Lord, A.A. Waterfield, J. Hughes and H.W. Kosterlitz (1977) Nature 267, 495-499.

5. J.S. Shaw and M.J. Turnbull (1978) European J. Pharmacol., 49, 313-317

6. A.S. Dutta, J.J. Gormley, C.F. Hayward, J.S. Morley, J.S. Shaw, G.J. Stacey and M.J. Turnbull (1977) Life Sci. 21, 559-562

7. A.S. Dutta, J.J. Gormley, C.F. Hayward, J.S. Morley, J.S. Shaw, G.J. Stacey and M.J. Turnbull (1978) Acta Pharm. Suecica 14, Suppl., 14-15.

8. H.W. Kosterlitz and A.J. Watt (1968) Brit. J. Pharmacol. 33, 266-276.

9. J. Hughes H.W. Kosterlitz and F.M. Leslie (1975) Brit. J. Pharmacol. 53, 371-381.

10. C.B. Pert, A. Pert, J.K. Chang and B.T.W. Fong (1976) Science 194, 330-332.

11. J.M. Hambrook, B.A. Morgan, M.J. Rance and C.F.C. Smith (1976) Nature 262, 782-783.

12. S. Bajusz, A.Z. Rónai, J.I. Székely, Z. Dunai-Kovács, I. Berzétei and L. Gráf (1976) Acta Biochem. et Biophys. Acad. Sci. Hung. 11, 305-309.

13. S. Bajusz, A.Z. Rónai, J.I. Székely, L. Gráf, Z. Dunai-Kovács and I. Berzétei (1977) FEBS Lett. 76, 91-92

14. M.G. Baxter, D. Goff, A.A. Miller and I.A. Saunders (1977) Br. J. Pharmacol. 59, 455P-456P.

15. C.R. Beddell, R.B. Clark, G.W. Hardy, L.A. Lowe, F.B. Ubatuba, J.R. Vane, S. Wilkinson, K.J. Chang, P. Cuatrecasas and R.J. Miller (1977) Proc. R. Soc. Lond. 198, 249-265.

16. H.W. Kosterlitz and A.A. Waterfield (1975) Ann. Rev. Pharmacol. 29-47.

17. R.C.A. Frederickson (1977) Life Sci. 21, 23-42

18. B.A. Morgan, J.D. Bower, K.P. Guest, B.K. Handa, G. Metcalf and C.F.C. Smith (1977) in Proceedings of the 5th American Peptide Symposium, M. Goodman and J. Meienhefer Eds., pp 111-113, John Wiley and Sons, New York.

Characteristics and Function of Opioids, editors Van Ree and Terenius
© *1978 Elsevier/North-Holland Biomedical Press*

NOVEL DEVELOPMENTS OF N-METHYLBENZOMORPHAN NARCOTIC ANTAGONISTS

W.F. MICHNE, T.R. LEWIS, and S.J. MICHALEC
Department of Medicinal Chemistry

A.K. PIERSON
Department of Pharmacology, Sterling-Winthrop Research Institute, Rensselaer,
N.Y. 12144

M.G.C. GILLAN, S.J. PATERSON, L.E. ROBSON and H.W. KOSTERLITZ
Unit for Research on Addictive Drugs, University of Aberdeen, Aberdeen
AB9 1AS, Scotland

ABSTRACT

Attachment of a 3-alkanone ($-CH_2CH_2COR$) side chain to position 9β of
metazocine results in potent compounds which range from pure agonists to
pure antagonists. The balance of these two activities is a function of the
R group. Among the members of the series are a compound with considerable
κ-antagonist activity and two of the most potent pure antagonists prepared
so far.

INTRODUCTION

It is well known that the change of an N-methyl group in compounds
which are narcotic agonists to an allyl, cyclopropylmethyl or similar group,
in general, results in compounds with narcotic antagonist activity. On the
other hand only a few compounds which retain the N-methyl group are known
to show narcotic antagonism. Figure 1 shows some examples from the benzomorphan literature. The (-)-isomer of 1 is one-tenth as potent as nalorphine in precipitating abstinence symptoms in nonwithdrawn morphine
dependent monkeys[1]. The (-)-isomer of 2 partially antagonizes the
analgesic effect of morphine in the mouse hot plate test[2]. However, based
on single dose and substitution studies in man, 1[3] and 2[4] were found to be
morphine-like agents. The (-)-isomer of 3 appears to have some antagonist
activity[5]. Compound 4 is the first reported N-methylbenzomorphan racemate
with antagonist activity, 4-24 mg/kg precipitating abstinence symptoms of

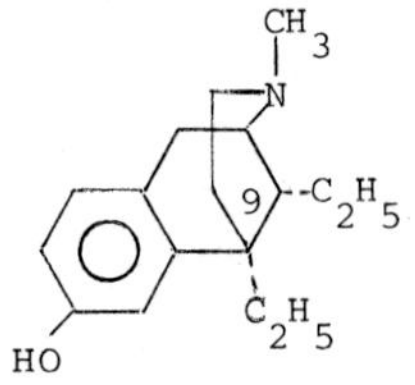

FIGURE 1. N-Methylbenzomorphans which show narcotic antagonist activity and the structure of prostaglandin E$_2$.

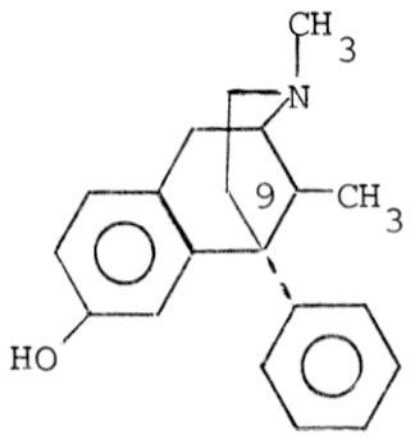

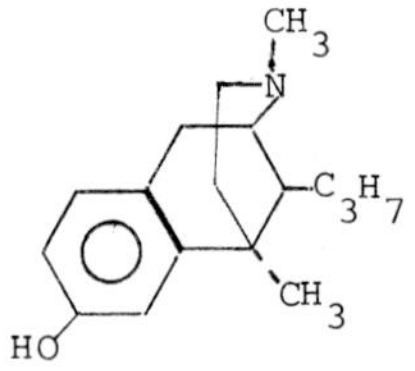

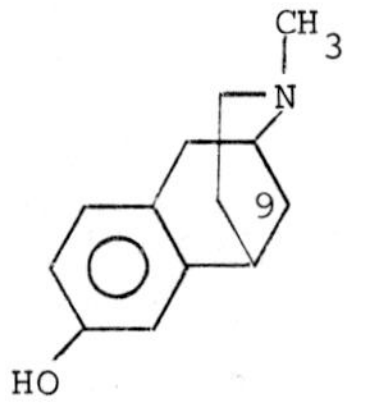

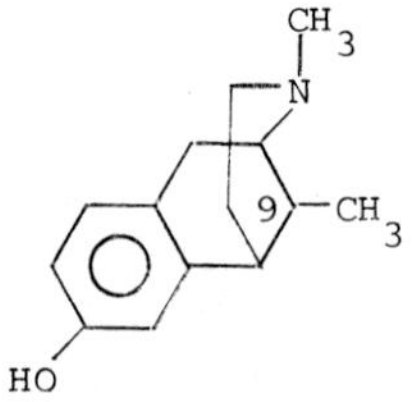

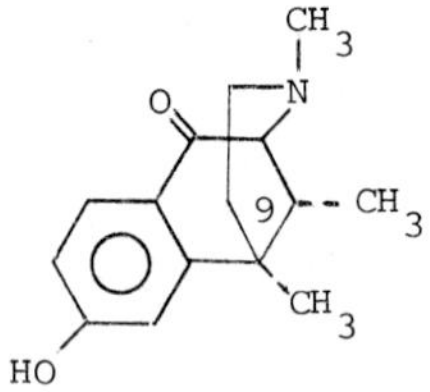

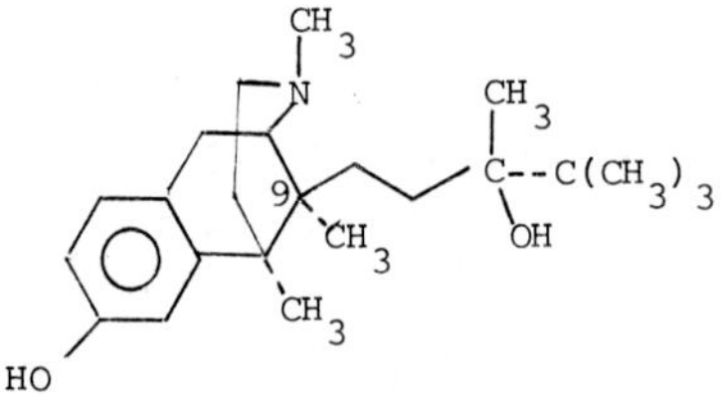

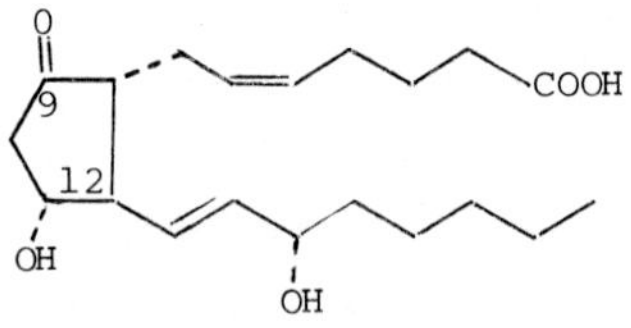

mild to intermediate severity in morphine dependent monkeys[6]. This activity
is enhanced in 5, abstinence symptoms being precipitated at 1 mg/kg[7].
Ketometazocine 6 shows weak antagonism of meperidine in the rat tail flick
test[8]. The rather complex metazocine derivative 7 is about three-tenths as
potent as nalorphine in antagonizing phenazocine in the rat tail flick test[9]
and is the most potent N-methylbenzomorphan antagonist reported so far[10].
The goal of our research was to find N-methylbenzomorphans with greater
antagonist potencies than those just described. This paper highlights the
results of our investigations over the past three years.

In addition to the N-methyl and phenolic hydroxyl groups of structures
1 - 7, substitution at position 9 appears in six of them and, as mentioned
above, antagonist activity is enhanced on going from 4 to 5. Thus, we
focused our attention on this position. With respect to the choice of
substituents which may elicit antagonist activity when attached to this
position we reasoned as follows. Prostaglandins with a ketone at
position 9 (particularly PGE_2 and to lesser extents PGE_1, PGA_1 and PGB_1)
can reverse the morphine block of electrically stimulated contractions of
the guinea pig ileum and evidence has been presented that the mechanism of
this reversal appears to involve displacement of morphine by the prostaglandin from a common receptor[11]. Further, it has been hypothesized that
the binding of an opiate to its receptor uncouples the interaction between
prostaglandin and adenyl cyclase either by occupation of a common binding
site, or allosterically, or in some other way[12]. Assuming a common receptor
we were led to superimpose a model of PGE_2 on a model of 6 aligning the
ketone groups and found that in one of the possible orientations of the two
models position 12 of the prostaglandin corresponded to position 9 of 6.
When the prostaglandin model and one of 7 were compared in the same way we
found that the alcohol side chains of both molecules were identically
oriented on their respective ring carbons and that the configurations of
the alcohol bearing carbons were the same. We therefore decided to attach
to position 9β of metazocine side chains analogous to the eight carbon
alcohol side chains of the prostaglandins choosing initially to work with
saturated ketones rather than unsaturated alcohols for chemical simplicity.

200

MATERIALS AND METHODS

Compounds. A process reported for a simple analog[13] was found to give
the desired compounds in low yield. A more efficient synthesis was developed
to allow wide variation of side chain structures. The full details of this
synthesis will be reported elsewhere.

In Vivo Assays. The agonist and antagonist potencies of the compounds
were determined by the following procedures: acetylcholine writhing test
in mice[14], tail flick test for agonism and phenazocine antagonism in rats[15],
and the intracarotid bradykinin test in rats[16].

In Vitro Assays. The agonist and antagonist potencies of the compounds
were determined at 36° C in the guinea-pig ileum[17] and mouse vas deferens[18]
preparations. Since peptidases degrade $[^3H]$-leucine-enkephalin at body
temperature the assays for inhibition of binding of $[^3H]$-leucine-
enkephalin and $[^3H]$-naltrexone were carried out at $0-4^{\circ}$ C; the incubation
period of homogenates of guinea-pig brain was 150 minutes and Na^+ was
absent[19].

RESULTS AND DISCUSSION

In Vivo Assays. Table 1 shows the results of the in vivo assays for
agonist and antagonist potencies of (±)-Win 42,156. *The singular outstanding
characteristic of this racemic N-methyl compound's pharmacology is its
potent phenazocine antagonist activity, being equal to naloxone in this
regard.* In addition, the compound is twice morphine in the acetylcholine
test and about 50X morphine in the bradykinin test.

Table 2 shows the effect of overall side chain length for an alkyl and
aralkyl series on agonism and phenazocine antagonism in the rat tail flick
test. Note particularly the abrupt reversal of agonist to antagonist
activity in both series when the chain length increases from 7 to 8. This
contrasts with a series of N-cyclopropylmethyl bridged thebaine alkanones
in which a change from antagonism to agonism was observed on going from
propyl to butyl ketone[20], comparable to a change in chain length from 6 to
7.

Table 3 shows the results of in vivo biological testing of some representative metazocinealkanones along with comparative data for morphine,
buprenorphine and naloxone. (-)-Win 42,156 is about twice as potent as
the racemate (Table 1). (-)-Win 42,964 compares favorably with buprenorphine,

TABLE 1

RESULTS OF IN VIVO ASSAYS OF AGONIST AND ANTAGONIST POTENCIES OF (±)-
WIN 42,156

Compound	ED$_{50}$ mg(base)/kg sc [a]			
	ANTAG [b]	TF [c]	ACH [d]	BRDK [e]
(±)-Win 42,156	0.008 (0.004-0.015)	Inactive	0.24 (0.16-0.36)	0.043 (0.031-0.073)
Naloxone	0.008 (0.006-0.012)		60 (50-76)	
Morphine	Inactive	3.9±0.5	0.60 (0.43-0.85)	2.3 (1.1-4.0)

[a] Numbers in parentheses are 95% confidence limits.
[b] Phenazocine antagonism, rat tail flick test.
[c] Rat tail flick test.
[d] Acetylcholine writhing test, mouse.
[e] Intracarotid bradykinin test, rat.

being slightly more potent in the acetylcholine writhing test and slightly
less potent in the bradykinin test. (±)-Wins 43,632 and 44,441 are very
potent antagonists; their lack of activity in the bradykinin test suggests
that the activity observed in the acetylcholine writhing test is non-
specific and the compounds are therefore pure antagonists.

In Vitro Assays. These results are shown in Table 4. (-)-Wins 42,156
and 42,964 have some agonist activity which unexpectedly is more pronounced
in the mouse vas deferens than in the guinea-pig ileum; in the latter model
the dose-response curves were flat and no reliable estimate of the relative
agonist potency could be obtained. Both compounds are potent antagonists
in the guinea-pig ileum but, because of the powerful agonist activity, the
antagonist activity in the mouse vas deferens could not be measured.
(±)-Wins 43,632 and 44,441 were found to be pure antagonists in both pharmacological models. Their potencies lie between those of naloxone and
naltrexone.

TABLE 2

EFFECT OF CHAIN LENGTH(n)[a] OF METAZOCINEALKANONES ON TAIL FLICK AGONISM AND PHENAZOCINE ANTAGONISM

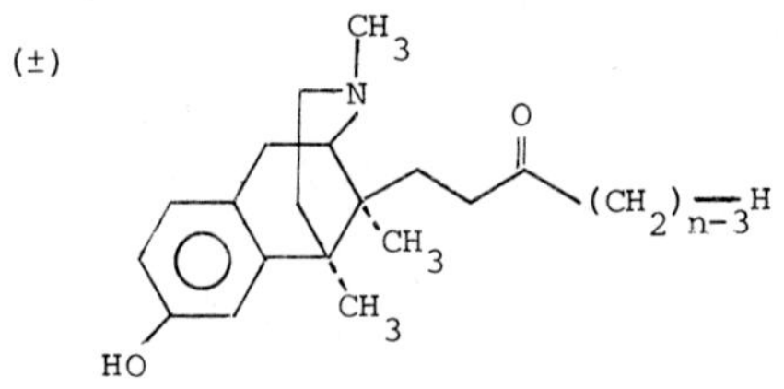

(±)

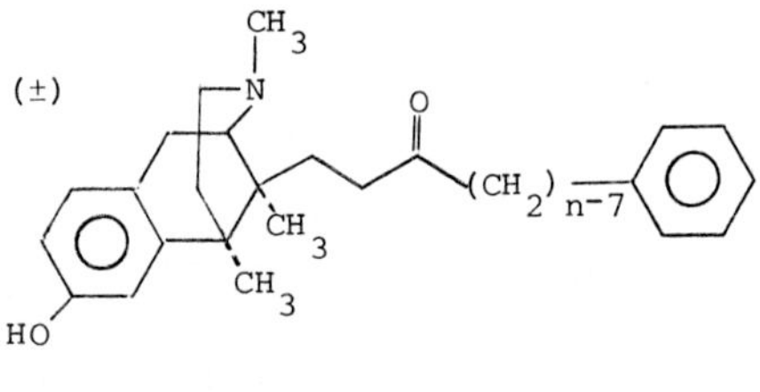

n	Agonism (Morphine = 1)	Antagonism (Naloxone = 1)
4	1.7	0
5	4.3	0
6	43	0
7	110	0
8	0	1
9	0	0.2

(±)

7	3185	0
8	0	2.2
9	0	0.5

[a] A benzene ring contributes four carbon atoms to overall chain length.

TABLE 3

RESULTS OF IN VIVO ASSAYS OF REPRESENTATIVE METAZOCINEALKANONES

Win No. R	ED$_{50}$ mg(base)/kg s.c. (95% confidence limits) or ± S.E.			
	ANT [a]	TF [a]	ACH [a]	BRDK [a]
(-)-42,156 (CH$_2$)$_4$CH$_3$	0.005 (0.003-0.009)	Inactive	0.19 (0.11-0.43)	0.022 (0.012-0.039)
(-)-42,964 (CH$_2$)$_2$CH(CH$_3$)$_2$	0.09 [b]	Minimal [c]	0.016 (0.011-0.021)	0.026 (0.012-0.044)
(±)-43,632 (CH$_2$)$_2$-⬡	0.015 (0.009-0.025)	Inactive	8.1 (5.8-11)	Inactive
(±)-44,441 (CH$_2$)$_2$-◻	0.012 (0.007-0.020)	Inactive	∿25	Inactive
Morphine	Inactive	3.9±0.5	0.60 (0.43-0.85)	2.3 (1.1-4.0)
Buprenorphine	0.11 [b]	Minimal [c]	0.059 (0.031-0.095)	0.0043 (0.0021-0.0082)
Naloxone	0.008 (0.006-0.012)		60 (50-76)	

[a] See Footnotes to Table 1 for a definition of these tests.
[b] Dose response curve too flat for the determination of confidence limits.
[c] At the screening dose of 120 mg/kg sc.

The IC$_{50}$ values for inhibition of [^{3}H]-naltrexone binding are similar to the dissociation equilibrium constants, K$_e$, in the guinea-pig ileum, (±)-Win 44,441 being an exception; the IC$_{50}$ values for inhibition of [^{3}H]-leucine-enkephalin are more similar to the K$_e$ values observed in the mouse vas deferens. (±)-Wins 43,632 and 44,441 are racemates and it will be interesting to obtain the ratios of the antagonist activities of the (-)-isomers to those of the (+)-isomers. These compounds are probably the most potent pure antagonists synthesized so far. It was therefore of

TABLE 4

ASSESSMENT OF THE POTENCIES OF METAZOCINEALKANONES BY THE DEPRESSION OF THE
CONTRACTIONS OF THE GUINEA-PIG ILEUM AND MOUSE VAS DEFERENS AND THE INHIBITION
OF [^{3}H]-LEUCINE-ENKEPHALIN AND [^{3}H]-NALTREXONE BINDING IN BRAIN HOMOGENATES

The values are the means ± S.E.; the number of observations is given in
parentheses. 43,632 and 44,441 did not show any agonist activity in the
guinea-pig ileum or mouse vas deferens. In the guinea-pig ileum, the
agonist potency of (-)-42,156 could not be determined as the dose-response
curve was too flat; (-)-42,964 also had a flat dose-response curve, the
agonist potency at the lowest concentration being 47.9±8.5(5) larger than
that of normorphine. On the mouse vas deferens, the dose-response curves
were parallel to those of normorphine, (-)-42,156 being 52.6±11.5(8) and
(-)-42,964 49.6±13.6(6) times more potent than normorphine. Tested against
ethylketazocine as agonist, the K_e values in the guinea-pig ileum were
3.35±0.84 nM (4) for 43,632 and 0.76±0.11 nM (5) for 44,441, and in the
mouse vas deferens 6.7±0.6(3) and 15.8±1.7(3), respectively. Tested
against methionine-enkephalin in the mouse vas deferens, the K_e value of
43,632 was 22.5±4.1(3) and that of 44,441 was 34.1±11.2 nM (3).

	Antagonist potencies K_e (nM)		Inhibition of binding in brain homogenates (IC_{50}, nM) of	
Win No.	Guinea-pig ileum	Mouse vas deferens	[^{3}H]-Naltrexone	[^{3}H]-Leu-enkephalin
(-)-42,156	0.30±0.05(4)	–	0.45±0.10(4)	1.89±0.37(5)
(-)-42,964	0.42±0.10(5)	–	0.49±0.11(4)	5.66±1.32(4)
(±)-43,632	0.43±0.03(4)	1.67±0.19(3)	0.69±0.34(3)	2.94±0.27(6)
(±)-44,441	0.51±0.12(4)	2.37±0.58(3)	3.62±9.43(3)	4.97±1.53(4)

interest to examine whether their antagonist patterns differ from those of
naloxone and naltrexone[19]. It was somewhat disappointing that neither
compound shows a greater specificity as an antagonist of opioid peptides
than does naloxone. (±)-Win 43,632 has about the same relative potency as
naloxone to antagonize the κ-agonist ethylketazocine[21] whereas (±)-
Win 44,441 has considerable κ-antagonist activity.

SUMMARY

A series of metazocine derivatives in which the 9β position is substituted with a ketonic chain has been described. Narcotic antagonism appears at a chain length of eight carbons. The observation of narcotic antagonism among these N-methyl compounds violates classical structure-activity relationships for opiates[22]. This is particularly true for (±)-Wins 43,632 and 44,441, the most potent pure antagonists so far reported, which also do not support a recent model explaining structure-activity relationships of opiate agonists and antagonists[23]. (±)-Win 44,441 is more potent than naloxone against ethylketazocine and may be of interest as a κ-antagonist. Further study of this series may contribute to our knowledge of the biochemical mechanisms of narcotic antagonism and opiate tolerance and physical dependence.

ACKNOWLEDGEMENTS

The authors wish to thank H. C. Bentley, M. D. Corrigan, H. S. Lawyer and C. A. Luczkowec for their expert technical assistance, and Dr. W. R. Martin for his permission to quote from his paper presented at the meeting of the Committee on Problems of Drug Dependence.

REFERENCES

1. Ager, J.H., Jacobson, A.E. and May, E.L. (1969) J. Med. Chem., 12, 288.

2. Yokoyama, N., Block, F.B. and Clarke, F.H. (1970) J. Med. Chem., 13, 488.

3. Jasinski, D.R., Martin, W.R. and Mansky, P.A. (1971) in Report to the Committee on Problems of Drug Dependence, p. 143.

4. Jasinski, D.R., Martin, W.R. and Hoeldtke, R.D. (1971) Clin. Pharmacol. Ther., 12, 613.

5. Rice, K.C. and Jacobson, A.E. (1976) J. Med. Chem., 19, 430.

6. May, E.L. and Takeda, M. (1970) J. Med. Chem., 13, 805.

7. Inoue, H., Oh-ishi, T. and May, E.L. (1975) J. Med. Chem., 18, 787.

8. Michne, W.F. and Albertson, N.F. (1972) J. Med. Chem., 15, 1278.

9. Michne, W.F., Salsbury, R.L. and Michalec, S.J. (1977) J. Med. Chem., 20, 682.

10. Ziering, A., Malatestinic, N., Williams, T. and Brossi, A. (1970) J. Med. Chem. 13,9 reported that 2'-hydroxy-2,5,8,9-tetramethyl-6,7-benzomorphan was about equipotent to nalorphine in antagonizing morphine in the mouse tail flick test. In our hands neither this compound nor its C-8 isomer were antagonists of phenazocine in the rat tail flick test. In fact both compounds were observed to be typical morphine-like agonists in this test.

11. Ehrenpreis, S. and Greenberg, J. (1973) Nature, New Biology, 245, 280.

12. Collier, H.O.J. and A.C. Roy (1974) Prostaglandins, 7, 361.

13. Michne, W.F. (1976) J. Org. Chem., 41, 894.

14. Collier, H.O.J., Dineen, E., Johnson, C.A. and Schneider, C. (1968) Br. J. Pharmacol. Chemother., 32, 295.

15. Harris, L.S. and Pierson, A.K. (1964) J. Pharmacol. Exp. Ther., 143, 141.

16. Deffenu, G., Pegrassi, L. and Lumachi, B. (1966) J. Pharm. Pharmacol., 18, 135.

17. Kosterlitz, H.W. and Watt, A.J. (1968) Br. J. Pharmacol. 33, 266.

18. Hughes, J., Kosterlitz, H.W. and Leslie, F.M. (1975) Br. J. Pharmacol. 53, 371.

19. Lord, J.A.H., Waterfield, A.A., Hughes, J. and Kosterlitz, H.W. (1977) Nature, London, 267, 495.

20. Lewis, J.W. (1973) in Narcotic Antagonists, Braude, M.C., Harris, L.S., May, E.L., Smith, J.P. and Villareal, J.E. eds., Raven Press, New York, p. 123.

21. Hutchinson, M., Kosterlitz, H.W., Leslie, F.M., Waterfield, A.A. and Terenius, L. (1975) Br. J. Pharmacol., 55, 541.

22. Archer, S. and Harris, L.S. (1965) in Progress in Drug Research, Jucker, E. ed., Birkhäuser Verlag, Basel, pp. 273-285.

23. Feinberg, A.P., Creese, I. and Snyder, S.H. (1976) Proc. Nat. Acad. Sci. USA, 73, 4215.

CHEMICAL AND BIOLOGICAL COMPARISON OF SYNTHETIC AND ISOLATED LEU^5-β_H-ENDORPHIN

J.-K. Chang, B.T.W. Fong, W.J. Peterson, M. Shimizu, F.R. Ervin and R.M. Palmour

Peninsula Laboratories, Inc., San Carlos, CA, Neuropsychiatric Institute,U.C.L.A

CA., and Department of Genetics, Univ. of California, Berkeley, CA., U.S.A.

Palmour et.al.[1] have recently reported the isolation and characterization
of a β_h-endorphin with leucine in position 5. In order to compare the chemical
properties and the biological activities of this molecule with a synthetic
molecule of the proposed structure, we have prepared Leu^5-β_h-endorphin by
solid-phase method.[2] The comparative biochemistry is reported here.

Chromatography of the isolated and synthetic Leu^5-β_h-endorphin on Sephadex
G 75 in 1 M formic acid yielded single symmetrical peaks with a molecular
weight of approximately 3200. Chromatography on Whatman CM cellulose and
elution with an NH_4OAc gradient buffer system likewise revealed similar
elution patterns and single symmetrical peaks for both peptides. Chromatographic behavior of the two peptides is a variety of standard thin layer
solvent systems failed to distinguish any differences. Electrophoresis on
Whatman #1 paper, at pH 2.0 (formate-acetate buffer), 3000V for 45 minutes,
isolated Leu^5-β_h-endorphin has a faster mobility than synthetic Leu^5-β_h-
endorphin. The amino acid content of peptide isolated from one individual
and that of synthetic peptide are displayed in Table 1. Values for each
amino acid are presented as nanomoles present, mole fractions and numbers of
residues, assuming a chain molecular weight of 3500. Within experimental
limits, the values are identical.

Each peptide was hydrolyzed separately with trypsin and chymotrypsin
at an enzyme:substrate ratio of 1:50; digestions were performed for 3 hours
at 37° in a 0.5 M NH_4HCO_3 buffer. Tryptic digests of isolated and synthetic
Leu^5-β_h-endorphin are shown in figure 1, while chymotryptic digests may be
seen in figure 2. Although the isolated peptide maps exhibit somewhat more
streaking, the maps of the isolated and the synthetic compounds are very
similar. The amino acid sequence of isolated and synthetic Leu^5-β_h-endorphin
is presented in Table 2. Samples containing 120 uM of each peptide were
sequenced; yields for each residue are denoted below the residue. Average
repetitive yield for the sequencing of the isolated peptide was 91.1%, and
for the synthetic peptide was 95.5%.

Biological activity was tested following intraventricular administration
of 10-30 nM peptide to 2 Kg cats implanted with recording electrodes in the

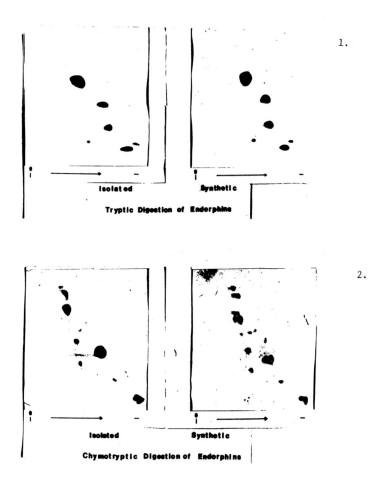

1.

2.

Figure 1 and 2. Tryptic and chymotryptic digests
of isolated and synthetic Leu^5-β_h-endorphin. Micro-
peptide maps were prepared on cellulose thin layer
plates (EM Reagents). Approximately 20μg digested
endorphin was applied to each plate. Electrophoresis
at pH 2.0 formate-acetate buffer was performed in the
horizontal direction and chromatography in pyridine:
n-BuOH:HOAc:H$_2$O (5:5:1:4) in the vertical direction.

frontal cortex, the reticular formation, the left amygdala and the right
entorhinneal cortex. Baseline recordings for each cat were obtained before
drug administration and after injection of similar volumes of saline and of
peritoneal dialysis fluid. No behavioral or electrophysiological changes
were observed following these administrations. Electroencephalograms and
behavioral recordings were obtained for each cat several times each day until
electrophysiological and behavioral effects of endorphins subsided. Administration of both isolated and synthetic Leu^5-β_h-endorphin elicited paroxysmal
hypersynchronous firing in the amygdala, reticular formation and entorhinneal
cortex, and occasional interictal spiking in the frontal cortex. Bursts of
electrical activity were accompanied by frozen stares, which clinically
resemble epileptiform "absences". Alternately, cats displayed frequent,
obsessive grooming activity, increased motility and motor stereotypies;
during such times, the electrical recordings are essentially normal. The
duration of electrophysiological behavioral changes varies from 10 to 30
hours with the isolated Leu^5-β_h-endorphin, while with the synthetic Leu^5-
β_h-endorphin it ranges from 6 to 12 hours.

Thus we report that, in general, the chemical and biological properties
of isolated and synthetic Leu^5-β_h-endorphin are quite similar. The possibility of the differences in electrophoretic moblilty is due to a difference
in amidination of a Glu or Asp residue remains to be disproved, but at least
two lines of evidence suggest that this is not the case. First, when tryptic
and chymotryptic peptides from isolated and synthetic Leu^5-β_h-endorphin are
compared following high voltage electrophoresis, there are no apparent differences; were there an amide difference, this should be apparent electrophoretic-
ally. Secondly, when isolated Leu^5-β_h-endorphin is subjected to extensive
solvent extraction, the electrophoretic mobility is increased to one more
nearly that of the synthetic molecule. Inasmuch as the original Leu^5-β_h-
endorphin was isolated from a solution containing high concentrations of salt,
it is not unreasonable to postulate that it was isolated in salt complex.
Studies now in progress with chelating agents tentatively support this hypothesis. The prolonged electrophysiological activity of the isolated Leu^5-
β_h-endorphin will of course have to be re-evaluated in light ot this
observation.

TABLE 1. Amino acid analysis of isolated and synthetic Leu^5-β_h-endorphin. Amino acids were determined on a Beckman Model 121M Automatic Amino Acid Analyzer. Samples were hydrolyzed by 6N HCl in a sealed tube at 110°C for 18 hours. Each value is the mean of three separate determinations from each of two hydrolyses.

Amino Acid	Isolated Leu^5-Endorphin			Synthetic Leu^5-Endorphin		
	nmole	mole frac	residues	nmole	mole frac	residues
Asp	.3215	.0744	2.35	.9359	.0740	2.33
Thr	.5256	.1147	3.17	1.3057	.1024	3.23
Ser	.2719	.0633	1.99	.8866	.0679	2.14
Glu	.4019	.0947	2.97	1.2265	.0962	3.03
Pro	.1456	.0340	1.07	.4288	.0346	1.09
Gly	.4290	.0992	3.10	1.2767	.1008	3.18
Ala	.2860	.0661	2.09	.8198	.0646	2.04
Val	.1251	.0296	0.93	.3727	.0297	0.94
Ile	.2051	.0445	1.41	.6017	.0477	1.50
Leu	.2493	.0997	3.14	1.2334	.0970	3.06
Tyr	.2736	.0631	1.99	.7756	.0605	2.11
Phe	.2783	.0637	2.01	.7914	.0615	1.94
Lys	.6584	.1505	4.74	2.0693	.1619	5.11
	4.324	.9975	30.98	12.7242	.9988	31.70

TABLE 2. Automated sequence analysis of isolated and synthetic Leu^5-β_h-endorphin on Beckman Model 890C Sequencer.

SEQUENCE ANALYSIS OF HUMAN LEU^5-ENDORPHIN

	Tyr.	Gly.	Gly.	Phe.	Leu.	Thr.	Ser.	Glx.	Lys.	Ser.
ISOLATED	96	83	100	100	104	90	75	81	72	53
SYNTHETIC	101	94	108	102	113	92	86	75	48	61

	Glx.	Thr.	Pro.	Leu.	Val.	Thr.	Leu.	Phe.	Lys.	Asx.
ISOLATED	64	70	48	50	48	37	48	50	41	38
SYNTHETIC	53	68	63	59	56	48	48	43	30	39

	Ala.	Ile.	Ile.	Lys.	Asx.	Ala.	Tyr.	Lys.	Lys.	Gly.	Glx.
ISOLATED	33	25	33	22	28	33	20	18	18	9	12
SYNTHETIC	30	32	33	30	29	28	28	22	19	10	14

REFERENCES

1. Palmour, R.M., et. al., Submitted for publication.

2. Coy, D. H., et. al., Peptides, Proceedings of the Fifth American Peptide Symposium, Edited by M. Goodman and J. Meinhofer, John Wiley and Sons, p. 107.

Characteristics and Function of Opioids, editors Van Ree and Terenius
© *1978 Elsevier/North-Holland Biomedical Press*

FLUORESCENT ENKEPHALIN DERIVATIVES WITH OPIATE-LIKE PROPERTIES AND THEIR USE IN CONFORMATIONAL ANALYSIS AND STUDY OF BRAIN PEPTIDASES.

M.C. FOURNIE-ZALUSKI, G. GACEL, A. GUYON and B.P. ROQUES *Université René Descartes, 4 avenue de l'Observatoire, 75006 Paris, France.*
B. SENAULT, J.M. LECOMTE *Centre de Recherche LEBRUN, 5 rue de Lübeck, 75016 Paris.*
B. MALFROY, J.P. SWERTS and J.C. SCHWARTZ *Unité 109 de l'INSERM, 2ter rue d'Alésia, 75014 Paris, France.*

ABSTRACT

The synthesis, spectroscopic and opiate-like properties of fluorescent enkephalin derivatives and their use as probes for conformational studies and as subtrates to evaluate the activity of enkephalins degradation enzymes are reported. The dansyl group has been introduced at the C-terminal moiety of methionine-enkephalin (Met-E) or of the peptidase-resistant analogue, D-Ala$_2$-Met-E. These derivatives exhibit opiate-like activity on two different biological systems, *i.e.* inhibition of electrically-induced contractions of guinea-pig *ileum* and inhibition of ^{3}H-Leu-E binding to striatal membranes. Met-E-(CH$_2$)$_2$-dansyl and D-Ala$_2$-Met-E-(CH$_2$)$_2$-dansyl show on both tests an activity similar to that of Leu-E. The D.Ala$_2$ derivative present significant analgesic activity in rat after *i.v.* administration (about 35% that of morphine). The conformational analysis of these peptides from quantitative measurements of energy transfer is presented. Furthermore, the energy transfer between the Tyr and the dansyl groups provides an indirect index of the integrity of the molecule and so Met-E-(CH$_2$)$_2$-dansyl has been used as a substrate for the cleaving enzymes and monitoring the *in vitro* changes in fluorescence, has proved to be a convenient mean to evaluate the activity of these enzymes.

INTRODUCTION

Fluorescent derivatives of enkephalins potentially represent useful experimental tools for the visualization of opiate receptors[1] and the exploration of ligand-receptor interactions[2]. The dansyl, 1-(5-dimethylaminonaphtalene) sulfonyl group, D, has been selected as fluorescent probe in view i) the marked changes in spectral properties induced by the modifications of its environment, particularly as a consequence of ligand-receptor interaction[1,2] ii) the good energy transfer with tyrosine (or tryptophane) residues it allows iii) its relatively easy covalent attachment to peptides. Met-E-C$_2$-D, I, Met-E-C$_5$-D, II, the peptidase-resistant D.Ala$_2$-Met-E-C$_2$-D[3], III, and the enzyme degradation product Gly-

Gly-Phe-Met-C$_2$-D, <u>IV</u> were synthesized[4]. In a first time, the conformational beha-viour of <u>I</u> was studied quantitatively by energy transfer experiments and the large increase of the Tyr fluorescence of <u>I</u> after breakdown of the Tyr-Gly bond was used to study brain peptidases.

MATERIALS AND METHODS

<u>Synthesis</u>. Met-E and D-Ala$_2$-Met-E were prepared by liquid phase method as previously described[5]. The synthesis of Met-E-(CH$_2$)$_2$-dansyl, <u>I</u>, D-Ala$_2$-Met-E-(CH$_2$)$_2$-dansyl, <u>II</u>, Met-E-(CH$_2$)$_5$-dansyl, <u>III</u>, and Gly-Gly-Phe-Met-(CH$_2$)$_2$-dansyl, <u>IV</u>, were performed by coupling the t.boc protected peptides with the corresponding N-aminoalkyl dansylamides in the presence of DCC, and purified by chromatography on silicagel column using CHCl$_3$:MeOH (9:1) as eluent. Deprotection was performed using trifluoroacetic acid. The structure of the compounds used as trifluoroacetates, was confirmed by NMR spectroscopy and their purity was checked by TLC[4].

<u>Fluorescence experiments</u>. The fluorescence spectra were recorded on a Perkin Elmer MPF 44A equiped with a differential corrected spectra unit. Degradation studies were performed at 37°C with tris-HCl buffer (pH:7.4) in a sample volume of 3 ml. 100 µl of S$_2$ (~30 µg of proteins) were added at t$_o$ and the fluorescence intensity (λem = 305 nm) recorded in a continous mode.

<u>Biological activities</u>. *Opioid peptide activity* was measured on the guinea-pig *ileum* as described[6]. 5 different conc of each compound (3-6 assays for each) were tested and inhibition specificity established by reversal with naloxone. Relative potencies represent the ratio expressed in percent of IC$_{50}$ of the peptide/IC$_{50}$ of Leu-E measured on the same preparation. *Binding studies* were made on mice striatum as described[14]. In all experiments, 20 µM bacitracin was added in the incubation medium. The IC$_{50}$ of each compound was estimated from the effects of 6 conc with triplicate assays and Ki's calculated assuming a competitive inhibition.

RESULTS

<u>Biological properties</u>. The opiate-like activity of the fluorescent derivatives is reported in table I. Both test gave similar results as regard the potency of the various compounds relatively to that of Leu-E(or Met-E which was of the same magnitude).

Compound	Guinea-pig *ileum*		^{3}H-Leu-E binding
	IC$_{50}$ (nM)	Relative Potency	Ki (nM)
Leu-E	67 $\pm$ 12	100	5 $\pm$ 1
Met-E-(CH$_2$)$_2$ dansyl, <u>I</u>.	50 $\pm$ 11	86	10 $\pm$ 3
D-Ala$_2$-Met-E-(CH$_2$)$_2$ dansyl, <u>II</u>.	27 $\pm$ 4	147	5 $\pm$ 2
Met-E-(CH$_2$)$_5$ dansyl, <u>III</u>.	288 $\pm$ 15	13	21 $\pm$ 5

The D-Ala$_2$-Met-E-(CH$_2$)$_2$-dansyl, III, is able to cross the blood-brain barrier as shown by its significant analgesic properties after $i.v.$ administration. So, III at 10 mg/kg elicits the same potency as morphine at 1mg/kg (35% of the activity of morphine on a molar basis) in the mouse hot-plate test, the duration of action being equivalent.

Fluorescent properties. Spectral properties of Met-E-(CH$_2$)$_2$-dansyl, I, are shown in Fig.1. The energy transfer from the Tyr to the dansyl group is evidenced: i) by an increase (~26%) in the fluorescence emission of dansyl by excitation in the Tyr absorption (λexc:277nm) as compared to the Gly-Gly-Phe-Met-C$_2$-dansyl, IV. ii) by a dramatic decrease (~90%) in the fluorescence emission of Tyr at 305 nm for λexc:277nm as compared to Met-E alone, Fig.2. The difference in the transfer efficiencies measured on Tyr$_1$ or dansyl is related to an additional quenching.

Conformational study by energy transfer experiments. Energy-transfer from donor to acceptor chromophores is distance-dependent and can be used for calculation of intramolecular distances in biomolecules[7]. The distance calculated here for I is r=13.7Å and is to be compared with those evaluated from molecular models i) in folded conformation, G-P β-turn[5], 3.4Å<r<17.6Å, ii) in full-extended conformation, 3.4Å<r<24Å. Due to the mobility of the chain linking the dansyl group to the backbone a large variation of r is expected and the energy transfer must be interpreted using energy calculations from potential functions[11]. However, NMR studies and semiquantitative estimations are in favor of a folded conformation for I.

Use of fluorescent enkephalin for study of brain peptidases. Many studies have shown that natural enkephalins are degradated by an initial breakdown between Tyr$_1$ and Gly$_2$[8-10]. Such a process was essentialy studied using tritiated enkephalins. With Met-E-C$_2$-D the hydrolysis of Tyr$_1$-Gly$_2$ bond leads to a disappearance of the energy transfer wich can be followed very nicely from the increase of the Tyr$_1$ emission fluorescence (λem=305nm). In the same conditions, no change occurs with the D.Ala^2 derivative III. The Tyr$_1$ fluorescence quantum yields varies from 0.0038 in I to 0.14 in free tyrosine. Fig.3 show the kinetic of enzyme degradation of I by striatum homogenates (S$_2$). Some remarks can be made on these preliminary studies of brain peptidases using fluorescent-E, i) at the end of the reaction (~3h) only Gly-Gly-Phe-Met-C$_2$-dansyl, IV, is detected by TLC, ii) the sensibility of the method permits to use substrate-concentration as low as 10^{-7}M when using S$_2$ fraction and 2.10^{-6}M with P$_2$ fraction. iii) such a method allows a continuous recording and appears very usefull to study the effects of pH, temperature, inhibitors... iii) preliminary results on S$_2$ leads to the following constants : V$_M$ 3.5mM/mn/mg Prot, K$_M$ 6.10^{-6}M. The values are closed to those eva-

214

luated on Met-E. iiii) this method prevents the use of titriated material and can be extended to many neuropeptides containing one Tyr or Trp residue by sim-

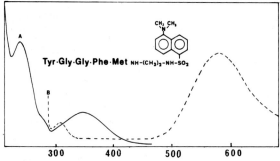

Fig.1. Spectral properties of Met-E-(CH₂)₂ dansyl at 2.10⁻⁵M in tris buffer (5.10⁻²M, pH:7.4) A. Absorption spectrum. B. Fluorescence spectrum (λexc:277nm).

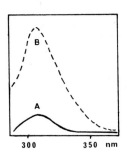

Fig.2. Emission intensity of Tyr upon excitation at 277nm for Met-E-(CH₂)₂-dansyl (A) and Met-E (B) at the same concentration (4.10⁻⁵M) in 0.05M tris-HCl buffer.

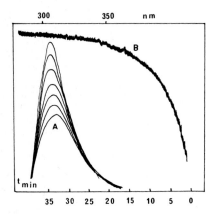

Fig.3. Kinetic of the degration of I by striatal peptidases using increase of the Tyr fluorescence-emission (λem=305nm). A. recorded from 280 to 380nm (λexc=277nm). B. in continuous mode at fixed λem=305nm. (λexc=277nm).

REFERENCES
1. Atlas, D. and Levitzki,A., (1977) Proc. Natl. Acad. Sci.(USA) 74, 5290-5294.
2. Waksman, G., Fournié-Zaluski, M.C., Roques, B.P., Heidmann, T., Grunhagen, H. H. and Changeux, J.P., (1976) FEBS Letters, 67, 335-342.
3. Pert, C.B., Pert, A., Chang, J.K. and Fong, V.T.W.,(1976) Science, 194, 330.
4. Fournié-Zaluski, M.C., Gacel, G., Roques, B.P., Senault, B., Lecomte, J.M., Malfroy, B., Swerts, J.P. and Schwartz, J.C. (1978) Biochem. Biophys. Res. Comm., in press.
5. Garbay-Jaureguiberry, C., Roques, B.P., Oberlin, R., Anteunis, M. and Lala, A.K. (1976) Biochem. Biophys. Res. Comm. 71, 558-565.
6. Paton, W.D.M., Brit. J. Pharmac. Chemother. 12, 119-127 (1957).
7. Schiller, T.W. and Yam, C.F. (1977) in Peptides, Eds Goodman, M. and Meienhofer, J., John Wiley and Sons, p.92-95 and ref cited herein.
8. Hambrook, J.M., Morgan, B.A., Rance, M.J. and Smith, C.F.C., (1976) Nature, 262, 782-783.
9. Vogel, Z. and Altstein, M.,(1977) FEBS Letters, 80, 332-336.
10.Meek, J.L., Yang, H.Y.T. and Costa, E. (1977) Neuropharmacology, 16, 151-154.
11.Work in progress in coll with Englert,A. and Maigret, B.

OPIOID PEPTIDES: STRUCTURE ACTIVITY STUDIES AND DEVELOPMENT OF ANALOGUES WITH CLINICAL POTENTIAL

R.C.A. FREDERICKSON, E. L. SMITHWICK AND R. SHUMAN

Eli Lilly and Company, Indianapolis, IN 46206

INTRODUCTION

There is evidence that the endogenous brain opioid peptides[1,2] are neuro-transmitters[3] and thus may provide the substrate for development of unique therapeutic entities. The natural peptides are too labile to study effectively but if they do have physiological role(s) in brain then analogues modified to reach receptors in brain should have appropriate pharmacology. Since there is a danger with such modifications of altering receptor interaction in a qualitative manner, we first examined a large series of peptides in vitro to determine the structure activity requirements then introduced modifications to provide enzy-matic protection. pA_2 values for naloxone were determined to facilitate judg-ment whether particular compounds were interacting with similar receptors as were the natural peptides. Peptides were prepared that were >100,000 x more potent as analgesics by the intracerebroventricular (ICV) route as were the natural materials. Many compounds were potent analgesics after systemic injection. One compound, D-ala^2-5[N-Me] enkephalin amide, was of similar potency to analgesics such as morphine, meperidine, codeine or pentazocine and had lesser tendency to produce respiratory depression or tolerance and physical dependence.

METHODS

The methods utilized for the synthesis and testing of the peptides discussed have been described previously[4,5].

RESULTS

A portion of the data is shown in the table. Some of the SAR data has been already published[3-5]. Replacement with D-amino acids in position 1, 3 or 4 results in complete loss of activity, in position 5 this results in some loss of activity. Substitution in position 2, however, with D-ala or several other D-amino acids protects this critical bond from cleavage and provides a substantial increase in receptor activation. Similarly, N-methylation at position 5 of enkephalin provides protection from enzymatic cleavage at the C-terminal without interference with receptor activity. Determination of pA_2 values for naloxone (7.3-7.8) indicated that the D-ala^2 and 5[N-Me] substituted analogues utilize the same receptor as does unmodified Met^5-enkephalin. This analysis, further-more, indicated a second receptor in the vas deferens (pA_2 = 8.1-8.4) used by

| | Mouse vas deferens | Mouse Hot Plate | | | | Mouse writing test |
| | | Hind Paw Lick | | Jump | | |
		ICV	SC	ICV	SC	
1.Morphine (M)	NT	1	1	1	1	1
2.Normorphine (NM, $IC_{50}=3.6\times10^{-7}$M)	1 (8.24)	NT	NT	NT	NT	NT
3.Pentazocine	0.02	NT	0.2	NT	0.4	0.4
4.Met^5-E*	21 (7.55)	0.003	NA	0.001	NA	NT
5.Met^5-EA*	11	0.004	<0.02	0.002	<0.02	NT
6.D-Ala^2-Met^5-EA	60 (7.47)	2.0	<0.04	0.3	0.03	NT
7.D-Ala^2-D-met^5-EA	8	21	<0.1	4	0.4	NT
8.D-Ala^2-5(N-ME)Met^5-EA	54 (7.60)	238	0.3	144	4	1.5
9.(OAC)Tyr'-(8)	6 (7.32)	NT	0.2	NT	0.9	NT
10.(N-Allyl)Tyr'-(8)	0.3	NT	<<0.1	NT	<<0.1	NT
11.des-met^5-EA	0.1	NT	NA	NT	NA	NT
12.D-Ala^2-des-Met^5-EA	2.4(8.35)	50	0.4	15	0.7	NT

Data are expressed as molar potency ratios cf. M or NM as unity. ED_{50}'s for M were 2, 1.5 and 1.0 mg/kg, sc and 0.25, 0.030 and NT µg/mouse ICV for the mouse hot plate hind paw lick, jump and mouse writhing tests, resp. M was tested 30 min and the peptides at 15 min (3 min for the starred materials). E = enkephalin, A = amide, NA = not active, NT = not tested. Brackets in first data column contain pA_2 values.

normorphine and various modified tetra- and pentapeptides. Many of the protected peptides were potent analgesics administered either ICV or systemically. The [N-allyl]Tyr' compound was inactive and demonstrated no antagonist properties. The modified pentapeptide, D-ala^2-5[N-Me]-enkephalin amide was a potent parenteral analgesic with relatively little respiratory depressant properties or tendency to development of tolerance or physical dependence.

REFERENCES

1. Hughes, J. (1975) Brain Res. 88, 295-308.
2. Terenius, L. and Wahlstrom, A. (1975) Acta Physiol. Scand. 94, 74-81.
3. Frederickson, R.C.A. (1977) Life Sci 21, 23-42.
4. Frederickson, R.C.A., Nickander, R., Smithwick, E.L., Shuman, R. and Norris, F.H. (1976) in Opiates and Endogenous Opioid Peptides, Kosterlitz, H., ed., Elsevier/North-Holland Biomedical Press, Amsterdam, pp. 239-246.
5. Frederickson, R.C.A. and Smithwick, E.L. (1978) in Opioid Peptides, Usdin, E., ed., MacMillan Press, London.

Characteristics and Function of Opioids, editors Van Ree and Terenius
© *1978 Elsevier/North-Holland Biomedical Press*

RESPECTIVE ROLES OF THE AMMONIUM AND HYDROXYL GROUPS OF TYROSINE IN THE CONFORMATION AND ACTIVITY OF ENKEPHALINS

G. GACEL, M.C. FOURNIE-ZALUSKI, E. FEILLON and B.P. ROQUES, *Université René Descartes, 4 avenue de l'Observatoire, 75006 Paris, France.*
B. SENAULT, J.M. LECOMTE, *Centre de Recherche LEBRUN, 5 rue de Lübeck, 75016 Paris, France.*
B. MALFROY, J.P. SWERTS and J.C. SCHWARTZ, *Unité 109 de l'INSERM, 2ter rue d'Alésia, 75014 Paris, France.*

ABSTRACT

In order to explore the induced role of the additional Arg or Tyr residue in the activity of Arg-Met-E and Tyr-Met-E, a series of analogs were prepared and their binding properties to striatal membranes and biological activities on guinea-pig *ileum* and mouse *vas deferens* were analyzed. From these studies the following general conclusions can be drawn i) the presence of an ammonium group located on the CH_α of the N-terminal aminoacid is absolutely required for activity whereas its position relative to the backbone can be somewhat modified, ii) the presence of an OH group strictly on Tyr_1 of E is an absolute requirement. RMN studies indicate that the characteristic conformation of E backbone is retained in the analogs (β-bend between CO of Gly_3 and NH of Met_6) ruling out that the observed changes in activity are related to modified conformation of this part of the molecule. A model for the variation of the activity of E and analogs impliyng a stepwise conformational process for the receptor-recognition with a possible modulation of the electrostatic potential but a precise location of the Tyr residue in its subsite can be proposed.

INTRODUCTION

Various structure-activity studies have previously demonstrated that only the aminoacids in positions 2 and 5 can be safely manipulated to yield compounds retaining potent activity. Particularly the terminal amino group of enkephalins (E) seems essential for receptor recognition [1]. However anomalies to this last rule are observed since N-substitution of E by a Tyr or Arg residue leads to hexapeptides retaining significant activity [2,3]. This property could be due i) for Arg-E to a bent conformation of the Arg side chain allowing interaction of the guanidino group with a postulated negatively charged site in the receptor ii) for Tyr-E to an interaction of the additional Tyr with the receptor instead of Tyr_1 of E. In order to explore these hypothesis, a series of analogs were prepared and their binding properties to striatal membranes and biological activities on guinea-pig *ileum* and mouse *vas deferens* were analyzed. The following peptides were studied : X-Y-Gly-Gly-Phe-Met with (X=Tyr, Y=Tyr) I ; (X=Desamino-Tyr, Y=Tyr) II ; (X=Phe, Y=Tyr) III ; (X=Tyr, Y=Phe) IV ; (X=Arg, Y=Tyr) V ; (X=Lys, Y=Tyr) VI ; (X=Gly, Y=Tyr) VIII. In addition the ammonium group was separated from the E backbone in the following compounds : $H_3N^+-(CH_2)_n-CO-NH-Tyr-Gly-Gly-Phe-Met$ with n=2,3,5 (<u>IX</u>, <u>VII</u>, <u>X</u>). In the other hand, the apparent anomalies reported above are related to the addition of an aminoacid on the N-terminal moiety of Met-E or Leu-E which exhibit in solution folded conformations with a large degree of freedom for the tyrosine residue [4,5]. Such conformational behaviour might be modified in the hexapeptides and it was necessary to determine by PMR spectroscopy their preferential conformations in solution.

MATERIALS AND METHODS

<u>Synthesis</u>. The hexapeptides I to IV were prepared by liquid phase method as described [5,6]. The different derivatives $NH_2-(CH_2)_n-CO-NH-Met-E$ with n=1,2,3 and 5 (VIII, IX, VII, X) were synthetized by coupling the corresponding t.boc $NH-(CH_2)_n-COOH$ with TFA, Met-E in the presence of DCC. Arg-Met-E, V and Lys-Met, VI, have been prepared by solid phase synthesis as described [2,3]. The structure of the different compounds was confirmed by NMR spectroscopy and their purity was checked by thin layer chromatography. [12]

<u>PMR studies</u>. ^1H NMR spectra were recorded on a Brüker WH 270 spectrometer operating at 270 MHz in FT mode and equiped with decoupler unit and variable temperature accessories. NMR spectra were obtained on the zwitterionic forms in DMSO-d_6 (100%) solutions ($10^{-2}M$) using convolution-differences techniques.

<u>Biological activities</u>. *Opioid peptide activity* was measured on the guinea-pig *ileum* as described [7] and evaluated on the mouse stimulated *vas deferens* by the method of Hughes et al [8]. 5 different conc of each compound (3-6 assays for each) were tested and inhibition specificity established by reversal with naloxone for the G.P.I. test. Relative potencies represent the ratio expressed in percent of IC_{50} of the peptide/IC_{50} of morphine for G.P.I. test and IC_{50} of the peptide/IC_{50} of Met-E for MVD. These ratio were measured on the *same* preparation.

Binding studies were made on mice striatum as described [9]. In all experiments, 20 µM bacitracin was added in the incubation medium. The IC_{50} of each compound was estimated from the effects of 6 conc with triplicate assays and Ki's calculated assuming a competitive inhibition.

RESULTS

<u>Biological properties</u>. The affinity constants and the activity on guinea-pig *ileum* and mouse *vas deferens* are reported in table I for all studied compounds.

<u>Conformational states of compounds I, III, VI, VIII in DMSO-d_6 solution</u>. Backbone conformational informations were obtained from ^3J coupling constants as described[4,5]. For the studied compounds, the couple of ϕ, ψ angles for the Gly_3 and Phe_4 residues are in agreement with a G-P β-bend. These results are strongly corroborated by the very low Met_6-NH's temperature dependencies ($< 2.10^{-3}$ ppm/°C).

TABLE I

INHIBITORY POTENCIES OF MET-ENKEPHALIN DERIVATIVES ON THE CONTRACTION OF GUINEA-PIG
ILEUM AND MOUSE *VAS DEFERENS* AND ON THE BINDING OF ^{3}H-LEU-ENKEPHALIN BY MEMBRANES
FROM MOUSE STRIATUM.

Assays			^{3}H Leu-E binding	Guinea-pig ileum		mouse vas deferens	
Compounds			K_i	IC50 (nM)	relative potency	IC50 (nM)	relative potency
	morphine				100		
	Met-E =	Tyr-Gly-Gly-Phe-Met	3	19	210	8.2	100
(I)		Tyr-Tyr-Gly-Gly-Phe-Met	30	120	32.4	380	28
(II)	D.amino	Tyr-Tyr-Gly-Gly-Phe-Met	1600	>1500	0	>3000	0
(III)		Phe-Tyr-Gly-Gly-Phe-Met	30	125	44	144	25
(IV)		Tyr-Phe-Gly-Gly-Phe-Met	200	>1500	0	2100	0
(V)		Arg-Tyr-Gly-Gly-Phe-Met	40	155	40	165	22
(VI)		Lys-Tyr-Gly-Gly-Phe-Met	40	225	41	145	25
(VII)	D.amino	Lys-Tyr-Gly-Gly-Phe-Met	1400	>1500	0	>3000	0
(VIII)		Gly-Tyr-Gly-Gly-Phe-Met	20	175	40	135	30
(IX)		β Ala-Tyr-Gly-Gly-Phe-Met	280	>1500	0	>3000	0
(X)		(pip)-Tyr-Gly-Gly-Phe-Met	900	>1500	0	>3000	0

DISCUSSION

From the results reported in table I, some conclusions about the structure activity
relationships of hexapeptides can be proposed ; i) the addition of an aminoacid on the
N-terminal residue of Met-E leads to either a decrease of about 60% or a whole inhibition of activity ; ii) the complete loss of activity of desamino Tyr-Met-E, II and desamino Lys-Met-E, VII while Tyr-Met-E, I and Lys-Met-E, VI, retain high biological potencies prove that the N-terminal ammonium group of the peptide backbone is necessary and
that it cannot be replaced by the NH_3^+ group located at the end of the side chain. So,
it can be ascertained that the guanidinium or ammonium groups in V or VI, does not
interact with the postulated negatively charged receptor site by a favourable folded
conformation of their side-chains ; iii) the activity of the hexapeptides Gly-Met-E,
VIII, Tyr-Met-E, I, Lys-Met-E, VI, Arg-Met-E, V and Phet-Met-E, III, demonstrate that
the terminal NH_3^+ is not necessarily borne by the Tyr residue of the endogenous pentapeptide but can be located on the preceeding aminoacid. However, the space between
the phenyl ring of the Tyr and the NH_3^+ is relatively critical while in the series
$NH_3^+(CH_2)_n-CO-Met-E$ with n=1,2,3 or 5 corresponding to the derivatives VIII, IX, X,
VII only the first compound Gly-Met-E (n=1) present some opiate-like activity. iiii)
the difference in the activity of the two peptides Tyr-Phe-Gly-Gly-Met-E, IV and
Phe-Tyr-Gly-Gly-Phe-Met-E, III, indicates that in order to retain some opiate-like
properties, the phenol can be placed on the second aminoacid of the hexapeptide and
so in the same position as in the pentapeptides Met-E or Leu-E.

At the receptor, it was assumed that the tyrosine side chain of enkephalin adopts
the conformation observed for the tyramine moiety in rigid opiates molecules with the
same precise distance between the ammonium group and the phenol ring found in these
later[10]. Due to the addition of one aminoacid, such precise distance cannot be so stric-
kly fitted in any conformation of the active hexapeptides. However it must be also
stressed that such acute structural requirement cannot be brought about in many flexible opiates like fentanyl, etonitazene, diampromide[11]. Due to the simple inverse
relation (1/r) of the electrostatic potential of an opiate for its anionic site, the
interaction energy must not be greatly modified from penta- to hexapeptides. On the
contrary it can be assumed that the role of the Tyr moiety appears to be one of the
key topological anchor for the proper orientation of the entire molecule at the receptor. Such Tyr residue would interact strongly by its phenyl ring to a flat and hydrophobic portion of the receptor through van der Waals forces exhibiting an acute
variation $(1/r^6)$ in function of the distance. In order to allow the binding of Tyr
to its site, the additional preceeding aminoacid must not interfere by steric hindran-
ce to this attachment. In accordance with this notion, the conformational study of
the hexapeptides by ^{1}H NMR show a highly preferential folded conformation with a
G-P β-bend involving the CO of Gly_3 and the NH of Met_6 as in Met-E and Leu-E[4,5].
So, as in these later the X-Tyr moiety exhibits a large defree of freedom allowing
the binding of the essential groups by a stepwise process with sucessive conformational reorientations.

REFERENCES

1. Beddell, C.R., Clark, R.B., Hardy, G.W., Lowe, L.A., Ubatuba, F.B., Vane, J.R., Wilkinson, S., Chang, K.J., Watrelasas, P. and Miller, R.J. (1977) Proc. R. Soc. London B. 198, 249-265.
2. Terenius, L., Wahlstrom, A., Lindeberg, G., Karlsson, S. and Ragnarsson, U. (1976) Biochem. Biophys. Res. Comm. 71, 173-179.
3. Chang, J.K., Cong, B.T.W., Pert, A. and Pert, C.B. (1976) Life Sciences 18, 1473.
4. Roques, B.P., Garbay-Jaureguiberry, C., Oberlin, R., Anteunis, M. and Lala, A.K., (1976) Nature ,(London) 262, 778-779.
5. Garbay-Jaureguiberry, C., Roques, B.P., Oberlin, R., Anteunis, M., Combrisson, S. Lallemand, J.Y. (1977) F.E.B.S. Letters, 76, 93-98.
6. Gacel, G., Fournié-Zaluski, M.C., Feillon, E., Roques, B.P., Senault, B., Lecomte, J.M., Malfroy, B., Swerts, J.P. and Schwartz, J.C. (1978) Life Sciences, submitted.
7. Paton, W.D.M., (1957) Brit. J. Pharm. Chemiother. 12, 119-127.
8. Hughes, J., Kosterlitz, H.W. and Leslie, F., (1975) Brit. J. Pharm. 53, 371-381.
9. Schwartz, J.C., Pollard, H., Llorens, C., Malfroy, B., Gros, C., Pradelles, P. and Dray, F. (1978) in The endorphins, eds. Costa and Trabucchi, Raven Press, N-Y, p.245-264.
10.Bradbury, A.F., Smyth, D.G. and Snell, C.R. (1976) Nature, 260, 165-166.
11.Horn, A.S. and Rodgers, J.R., (1977) J. Pharm. Pharmac. 29, 257-265.
12.We acknowledge Dr Rivaille, P., for help in solid phase synthesis.

Characteristics and Function of Opioids, editors Van Ree and Terenius
© *1978 Elsevier/North-Holland Biomedical Press*

NARCOTIC LEVELS IN CEREBROSPINAL FLUID AND PLASMA IN MAN

R. F. KAIKO, K. M. FOLEY, R. W. HOUDE AND C. E. INTURRISI
Memorial Sloan-Kettering Cancer Center, New York, New York (USA)

ABSTRACT

The time course of morphine levels in cerebrospinal fluid (CSF) and plasma following therapeutic doses are subjected to pharmacokinetic analysis and compared to the time action of drug effects. We propose that the peak intensity of drug effects such as miosis, decreased respiratory rate, analgesia and improved mood be assigned to a peripheral pharmacokinetic compartment.

INTRODUCTION

CSF is contiguous with extracellular fluid of cells of the central nervous system, some of which possess opiate receptors. There is no information available concerning CSF levels of narcotic analgesic drugs following therapeutic doses. The purpose of this study is to determine the relationships of CSF and plasma morphine levels to the time action of drug effects in patients with pain.

MATERIALS AND METHODS

CSF is collected serially via an indwelling intraventricular catheter after intravenous injection of morphine sulfate. Morphine is quantitated by radio-immunoassay[1]. Estimates of analgesia[2], mood[3], miosis[4] and vital signs are obtained prior to and following intravenous injection.

RESULTS

Figure 1 shows the mean plasma morphine time course (adjusted to a dose of 10 mg per 70 kg) following intravenous injection in 9 cancer patients. The levels decline rapidly during the first 15 to 30 minutes and then more slowly through 8 hours. Morphine persists in plasma for at least 48 to 72 hours. In 6 of these patients CSF morphine levels were determined. The mean level rises rapidly during the first 15 minutes to a peak at 1 hour and then declines. At 8 hours the CSF morphine level approximates the calculated free plasma morphine concentration (assuming 65% free drug). Using the two-compartment model the time course of CSF morphine most closely approximates the time course of morphine in the peripheral compartment (P). Alternately, using a three-compartment model reveals that the time course of CSF morphine most closely

Fig. 1. The time course of morphine in plasma and cerebrospinal fluid (CSF). P is the theoretical time course of morphine in the peripheral compartment of a two-compartment open pharmacokinetic model. P_1 and P_2 are the theoretical time course of morphine in the shallow and deep peripheral compartments, respectively, of a three-compartment open mammillary model.

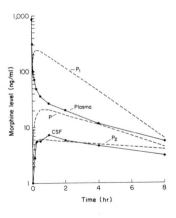

approximates drug levels in the deep peripheral compartment (P_2). Table 1 shows the median time of peak intensity of effects following intravenous morphine.

TABLE 1

TIME OF PEAK INTENSITY OF EFFECT AFTER INTRAVENOUS MORPHINE

		Time (minutes) (median; N = 6)			
↑ Pulse	↓ Blood Pressure	Miosis	↓ Respiratory Rate	Analgesia	Improved Mood
6	15	30	75	75	100

SUMMARY

We find that the peak intensity of morphine's effects occur from 6 to 100 minutes after drug injection. Assuming that peak intensity is a function of peak drug level in a compartment then our data suggest that different effects may be associated with different compartments. It would appear that effects such as miosis and changes in respiration, analgesia and mood correspond most closely to the time course of morphine in a peripheral compartment.

ACKNOWLEDGEMENT

This work was supported by NIDA Grant #DA-01707.

REFERENCES

1. Spector, S. (1971) J. Pharmacol. Exp. Ther., 178, 253-258.

2. Houde, R. W., Wallenstein, S. L. and Rogers, A. (1960) Clin. Pharmacol. Ther., 1, 163-174.

3. Wallenstein, S. L., Heidrich III, G., Rogers, A. and Houde, R.W. (1978) in Proc. 7th Intern'l Congr. Pharmacol., Paris, France, abst. (in press).

4. Marquardt, W. G., Martin, W. R. and Jasinski, D. R. (1967) Intern'l J. Addict., 2, 301-304.

EFFECT OF C_7 SUBSTITUTION ON AGONIST/ANTAGONIST ACTIVITY IN ORIPAVINES

GILDA H. LOEW & DONALD S. BERKOWITZ

Molecular Theory Laboratory, Dept. of Genetics, Stanford Univ.,Stanford,CA94305

ABSTRACT

Quantum mechanical energy-conformation studies of tertiary carbinol C_7-substituents are used to explain modulation of agonist/antagonist potency in oripavines.

INTRODUCTION & METHODS

In the potent oripavine and thebaine series of synthetic opiates shown (A):

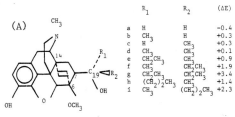

	R_1	R_2	(ΔE)
a	H	H	-0.4
b	CH_3	H	+0.3
c	H	CH_3	+0.3
d	CH_3	CH_3	+0.1
e	CH_2CH_3	CH_3	+0.9
f	CH_3	CH_2CH_3	+1.9
g	CH_2CH_3	CH_2CH_3	+3.4
h	$(CH_2)_2CH_3$	CH_3	+1.4
i	CH_3	$(CH_2)_2CH_3$	+2.3

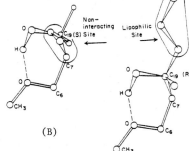

(B)

Energy difference (kcal/mole) between optimized H-bonded and non H-bonded conformers

Lowest energy conformers of C_7R- and S-substituents diastereoisomers for etorphine showing by complementarity the lipophilic site for accommodation of the most potent isomer.

tertiary carbinol substituents on C_7 confer unexpectedly high agonist[>1000 x morphine(M)]and antagonist[>100 x nalorphine(N)] potencies[1]. As the allyl groups increase in length from methyl(d) to n propyl(i);an increasing disparity occurs in activities of R and S isomers; activities of N-allyl and N-methyl cyclopropyl compounds change from potent antagonist[50;2xN]to potent agonist[100;60xM].

Sensitivity of agonist/antagonist potency ratio to C_7-substituent is probably related to binding and interaction of C_7-substituent at receptor site. Lipophilic character[1]and more recently aromatic groups[2],e.g., phenethyl substituent on C_{19} were proposed as essential to enhanced agonist potency. To provide additional insight into how substituents modulate agonist/antagonist activity, conformational studies of the C_7 substituents a-i were made, using quantum mechanical techniques to determine the most energetically feasible conformations. In the studies attention was given to possible hydrogen bonding interactions between C_6-OCH_3 & C_7-OH.

Energy conformation calculations were performed, using an all valence electron semiemperical quantum mechanical method called Perturbative Configuration Interaction using Localized Orbitals (PCILO) described in detail elsewhere[3] and developed specifically for such studies of large molecules.

Torsion angles for all but the C_6 and C_7 substituents were determined by independent variation. Coupled rotation of the C_6 and C_7 substituents, together with geometry relaxation were performed to obtain energy optimized hydrogen bonded and nonhydrogen bonded conformers.

RESULTS AND DISCUSSION

The results of conformation studies shown above indicate that intramolecular hydrogen bonding to the C_6-OCH_3 in oripavines does not appear to play a dominant role in determining the conformation of C_{19} carbinol substituents on C_7 if R_1 and R_2 are hydrogen or methyl groups (a-d). This result of substantial conformational freedom is in keeping with the observation of several conformers of these C_7 substituents in the NMR spectra,[4] with their similar apparent potencies, increasing somewhat with lipophilicity of the alcohol group (17,15,37 and 63 x M for a-d, respectively) and with the fact that relative agonist/antagonist activities conferred by different N-substituents are consistent with structure activity relationships found in other fused-ring opiates.

In compounds with tertiary carbinol substituents of the type $C_{19}CH_3(CH_2)_nCH_3OH$ with $n \geq 1$ hydrogen bonding is favored in both diastereoisomers (A-ΔE). This constraint fixes the C_7 substituent in one of two distinct spatial regions which are different for the (R)- and (S)-diastereoisomers (B). It is suggested that the difference in orientation determines the extent to which the long allyl group of C_{19}-carbinol can be accommodated at the postulated lipophilic receptor and could account for the enhanced agonist potencies of the (R) over (S) isomers of N-CH_3 compounds, (e>f;h>i) and over compounds (a-d) with smaller allyl groups. It is further suggested that interaction of these conformationally restricted groups with this site   directs the overall orientation of these compounds at the receptor and imposes a change in N-substituent binding relative to morphine-like compounds, interfering with the antagonist "type" of N-substituent binding mode while enhancing the agonist "type". If this hypothesis is correct, replacement of the C_6OCH_3 or the C_{19}-OH group by an H or CH_3 substituent should enhance or restore antagonist potency to N-allyl and N-cyclopropylmethyl derivatives of oripavines and thebaines with long chain, C_7-carbinol substituents.

We gratefully acknowledge support of this work from NIDA #DA-00770

REFERENCES

1. Lewis, J.W.,Bentley, K.W., & Cowan, A. (1971) Annu.Rev.Pharmacol.,11,241-70.

2. Feinberg, A.P., Creese, I., & Snyder, S.H. (1976) Proc.Nat.Acad.Sci. USA 73 (11), 4215-19.

3. Fulmore, W., Lancaster, J.E., Morton, G.O., Brown, J.J., Howell, C.F., Nora, C.T., Hardy, Jr., R.A. J. Am.Chem.Soc. 89(13), 322-30.

4. Diner,S., Malrieu,J.P.,Jordan,F. & Gilbert,M. Theoret.Chim. Acta (Berl), 15, 100-10.

Characteristics and Function of Opioids, editors Van Ree and Terenius
© *1978 Elsevier/North-Holland Biomedical Press*

RAT BRAIN LEVELS AND SUBCELLULAR DISTRIBUTION OF IN VIVO ADMINISTERED BUPRENOR-PHINE: EFFECT OF NALOXONE.

L. Manara, C. Cerletti, A. Luini and A. Tavani
Mario Negri Pharmacological Research Inst., Via Eritrea, 62 - 20157 Milan, Italy

ABSTRACT

Buprenorphine levels in rat cerebrum (brain without cerebellum), but not in cerebellum and plasma, remain the same from 5 to 75 min, but decrease after naloxone pretreatment which has more effect than naloxone given after the opiate both in this respect and in altering buprenorphine brain subcellular distribution.

INTRODUCTION

We have shown that after systemic administration brain levels and subcellular distribution of tritium labelled etorphine reflect drug effectiveness and in vivo stereospecific binding, tentatively located in the microsomal (P_3) fraction[1,2]. We report here similar studies on the newer compound buprenorphine, with special reference to the reversibility of its pharmacological action[3].

MATERIALS AND METHODS

Buprenorphine, tritiated in 15 and 16 positions — donated by Dr. M.J. Rance, Reckitt and Colman, Hull, U.K. — 5 μg, 20-40 μCi/kg, was given to control male Sprague Dawley rats or to rats receiving naloxone; the drugs were administered i.v. dissolved in 2 ml/kg saline. Buprenorphine was assayed, as reported for etorphine[1,2] by individual TLC chromatography of all specimens followed by LSC radioassay. Brain subcellular primary fractions were obtained as described earlier[1].

RESULTS AND DISCUSSION

The table shows the time course of i.v. administered buprenorphine in CNS and plasma from 5 to 75 min; in cerebrum (brain without cerebellum) the drug concentration remained unchaged. Conversely cerebellum, which at 5 min had drug levels similar to the rest of the brain, lost 75% of buprenorphine within 75 min; plasma had the lowest levels and fastest drug disappearance rate. Naloxone pretreatment (N-pre), 500 μg/kg 5 min before, had no effect at any interval on plasma and cerebellum levels of buprenorphine but rendered the time course in cerebrum similar to that in cerebellum; naloxone given 15 min after buprenorphine (N-post) was less effective. Assay of in vivo administered buprenorphine (5 μg/kg) in primary fractions from whole brain (see figure) showed that the subcellular

TABLE. Buprenorphine levels (ng/g or ml $\pm$ S.D. n = 4) after 5 μg/kg i.v.

Time (min)		5	15	20	30	45	75*
Cere-brum	Control	2.32+0.57	3.40+1.03	3.53+0.91	2.94+0.77	2.81+0.91	2.91+0.50
	N-pre	2.76+0.43	1.94+0.21	1.55+0.49	1.40+0.23	1.06+0.09	0.55+0.09
	N-post	-	-	2.72+0.54	2.53+0.88	2.06+0.52	1.31+0.30
Cere-bellum	Control	2.12+0.60	2.07+0.72	1.85+0.46	1.25+0.23	0.83+0.17	0.53+0.14
	N-pre	2.93+0.44	1.89+0.10	1.46+0.36	1.13+0.16	0.73+0.09	0.40+0.10
	N-post	-	-	1.48+0.33	1.31+0.24	0.88+0.27	0.47+0.09
Plasma	Control	0.97+0.19	0.56+0.07	0.50+0.13	0.33+0.05	0.20+0.03	0.14+0.04
	N-pre	0.99+0.21	0.55+0.06	0.41+0.10	0.35+0.03	0.22+0.06	0.11+0.01
	N-post	-	-	0.46+0.07	0.29+0.04	0.25+0.12	0.14+0.04

distribution profile was altered more markedly by naloxone (500 μg/kg) given before the opiate than after it. The overall results reflect in vivo binding of buprenorphine presumably to functionally relevant sites and appear consistent with reports on the long duration and limited reversibility of this drug's pharmacological action[3].

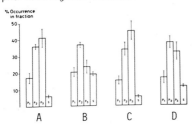

FIGURE. Brain subcellular distribution of in vivo administered buprenorphine. A and C: controls at 30 and 45 min; B: naloxone 35 min prior to A; D: naloxone 30 min prior to C; results are means and S.D., n = 4 for each experimental group.

ACKNOWLEDGEMENT

Supported by Italian CNR Contract No. 77.01661.04

REFERENCES

1. Cerletti, C., Coccia, P., Manara, L., Mennini, T. and Recchia, M. (1978) Br.J.Pharmacol., 62, 31-38.

2. Manara, L., Aldinio, C., Cerletti, C., Coccia, P., Luini, A. and Serra, G. (1978) in Factors affecting the Action of Narcotics, Adler, M.W., Manara, L. and Samanin, R. eds., Raven Press, New York, pp. 271-296.

3. Cowan, A., Lewis, J.W. and MacFarlane, I.R. (1977) Br.J.Pharmacol., 60, 537-545.

* N-pre and N-post received an additional injection of naloxone s.c. at 30 min.

Characteristics and Function of Opioids, editors Van Ree and Terenius
© *1978 Elsevier/North-Holland Biomedical Press*

STRUCTURE-ACTIVITY RELATIONSHIPS IN OPIOIDS OF THE (-)-(1R,5R,9R)-2-ALKOXY-ALKYL-5,9-DIMETHYL-2'-HYDROXY-6,7-BENZOMORPHAN SERIES

HERBERT MERZ and KLAUS STOCKHAUS
Department of Medicinal Chemistry and Department of Pharmacology,
C.H. Boehringer Sohn, D-6507 Ingelheim, Federal Republic of Germany

ABSTRACT

Depending on the nature of the N-alkoxyalkyl substituent the (-)-nor-metazocine derivatives 1 are morphine-like agonists, non-morphine-like agonists, or opioid agonist-antagonists. Their action profiles are closely related to position and size of the alkoxy residue, degree and type of branching at the carbon bearing the alkoxy residue, and configuration of the branched carbon if chiral. These SAR suggest interactions of high stereospecificity between the ether oxygen of the N-substituent and supplementary binding sites of opioid receptors.

INTRODUCTION

The unique action profiles of stereoisomeric N-tetrahydrofurfuryl substituted 5,9-dimethyl-2'-hydroxy-6,7-benzomorphans[1] and noroxymorphones[2] prompted us to modify the obviously crucial N-tetrahydro-furfuryl group by preparation of (-)-N-alkoxyalkyl-normetazocines 1 and to study their opioid properties.

METHODS

The new compounds were synthesized from (-)-normetazocine according to well established procedures[3]. Aqueous solutions of their hydrochlorides and those of appropriate standards were tested sc for analgesia (tail-clip[4], hot-plate[5], and writhing[6] methods), morphine antagonism (tail-clip[7]), and Straub tail activity[8] in mice (NMRI mice, both sexes, 19-24 g). ED_{50} and AD_{50} values were calculated with 95 % confidence limits according to approved statistical methods.

RESULTS

The structures of the compounds 1, their opioid properties and those of the reference substances are summarized in Table 1 (confidence limits omitted for want of space). "Inactive" means that the effect in question was not observed up to doses causing side-effects. Straub tail activity was rated to be presend (+) or absent (-) according as observed or not in the range of the hot plate ED_{50}.

DISCUSSION

The compounds 1 may be divided into three groups with differentiated action profiles: (a) Typical morphine-like agonists which show analgesic activity in all three assays and pronounced Straub tail activity. (b) Nonmorphine-like agonists which exert analgesic activity at least in the writing test and generally also in the two other (more rigorous) assays but fail to induce the typical Straub tail phenomenon. 1a-1[1] which has been suggested[9] to be a κ-receptor agonist may tentatively be regarded as a reference compound for this group. (c) Opioid agonist-antagonists (like nalorphine or pentazocine) which reveal their analgesic action only in the sensitive writhing test, suppress morphine analgesia in the tail-clip test, and do not elicit the Straub phenomenon.

Structure-Activity Relationships (SAR). The following SAR are observed: (1) Maximum analgesic activity (either morphine-like or not) is obtained if nitrogen and oxygen are linked by a two-carbon alkylene chain (n = 1) and the alkoxy is small. With growing length of the alkylene chain (n = 1, 2, 3) and/or size of the alkoxy $O-R^3$ (R^3 = Me, Et, Pr) potency markedly decreases and the Straub tail phenomenon becomes less pronounced. (2) The action profiles of those compounds with maximum analgesic potency due to a two-carbon chain (n = 1) between nitrogen and oxygen are not morphine-like if carbon C-2" bearing the alkoxy is branched, either by one or two methyl groups or by its incorporation into a tetrahydrofuran ring. Compounds with homologous alkylene chains (n = 2, 3), however, are morphine-like even if the corresponding carbon is incorporated into a tetrahydrofuran ring. (3) If such branching of the two-carbon chain (n = 1) renders C-2" chiral and thus gives rise to the existence of diastereoisomeric pairs, the 2"S forms are by far more potent analgesics than their 2"R counterparts which may even be inactive[10]. This close configuration-activity relationship is not observed with compounds with homologous alkylene chains (n = 2, 3). (4) Antagonist activity is induced only by the N-tetrahydrofurfuryl substituent, in particular if fitted out with a 2-methyl group.

TABLE 1

CHEMICAL STRUCTURES AND OPIOID
PROPERTIES OF THE (-)-(1R,5R,9R)-
2-ALKOXYALKYL-5,9-DIMETHYL-2'-
HYDROXY-6,7-BENZOMORPHANS

1a: -R = -(CH$_2$)$_n$

1b: -R = -(CH$_2$)$_n$-O-R^3

Compd.	R^1	R^2	R^3	n	C-2"	Analgesia (ED$_{50}$, mg/kg, sc) Tail clip	Hot plate	Writhing	M. antagonism AD$_{50}$, mg/kg sc	Straub tail	Action profile
1a-1	H	-	-	1	S	0.22	0.11	0.015	inactive	-	(b)
1a-2	H	-	-	1	R	inactive	inactive	3.9	4.7	-	(c)
1a-3	Me	-	-	1	S	inactive	inactive	0.051	1.5	-	(c)
1a-4	Me	-	-	1	R	inactive	inactive	9.3	7.1	-	(c)
1a-5	H	-	-	2	S	16.9	6.8	0.4	inactive	+	(a)
1a-6	H	-	-	2	R	17.0	13.6	1.3	inactive	+	(a)
1a-7	H	-	-	3	S	21.3	15.5	4.5	inactive	-	(b)
1a-8	H	-	-	3	R	118.6	65.6	7.5	inactive	-	(b)
1b-1	H	H	Me	1	-	0.19	0.11	0.003	inactive	+	(a)
1b-2	H	H	Et	1	-	2.1	1.3	0.066	inactive	+	(b)
1b-3	H	H	n-Pr	1	-	7.5	3.5	0.65	inactive	-	(b)
1b-4	H	H	i-Pr	1	-	3.9	2.1	0.25	inactive	-	(b)
1b-5	H	H	Me	2	-	5.6	3.6	0.29	inactive	+	(a)
1b-6	H	H	Me	3	-	17.7	15.5	1.0	inactive	+	(a)
1b-7	H	H	Me	1	S	0.04	0.02	0.004	inactive	-	(b)
1b-8	H	H	Me	1	R	inactive	inactive	inactive	inactive	-	(b)
1b-9	Me	Me	Me	1	-	10.9	2.3	0.15	inactive	+	(a)
Morphine						inactive	inactive	0.47	inactive	-	(a)
Nalorphine						inactive	inactive	0.35	0.8	-	(c)
Pentazocine						inactive	inactive	1.3	7.4	-	(c)

CONCLUSIONS

These SAR demonstrate that potencies as well as action profiles of the compounds 1 are closely related to the nature of the N-alkoxyalkyl substitution, in particular to the position of the ether oxygen and steric demands of its environment, thus suggesting interactions of high sterespecificty between the ether oxygen and supplementary binding sites of opioid receptors. It should be noted that N-alkoxy-alkyl-norpethidine analogues of 1 have already been known for twenty years[11, 12] and that hydrogen bonding of the ether oxygen (to a receptor) has been proposed to account for their enhanced analgesic activity[12]. The SAR described, however, are quite different from those we have found with the (-)-normetazocine congeners 1 and, moreover, all the norpethidine derivatives in question seem to have the same morphine-like action profile. The considerable differences in molecular flexibility in the two series of opioids may be responsible for the different SAR following from parallel modifications of the N-alkoxyalkyl substituent.

REFENCES AND NOTES

1. Merz, H., Stockhaus, K., and Wick, H., J. Med. Chem., 18, 996 (1975).

2. Merz, H., Stockhaus, K., and Wick, H., J. Med. Chem., 20, 844 (1977).

3. Merz, H., and Stockaus, K., to be published in detail elsewhere.

4. Haffner, F., Dtsch. Med. Wochenschr., 55, 731 (1929).

5. Eddy, N.B., and Leimbach, D.G., J. Pharmacol. Exp. Ther., 107, 385 (1953).

6. Blumberg, H., Wolf, P.S., and Dayton, H.B., Proc. Soc. Exp. Biol. Med. 118, 763 (1965).

7. Merz, H., Langbein, A., Stockhaus, K., Walther, G., and Wick, H., Adv. Biochem. Psychopharmacol., 8, 91 (1974).

8. Straub, W., Dtsch. Med. Wochenstr., 37, 1462 (1911).

9. Lord, J.A.H., Waterfield, A.A., Hughes, J., and Kosterlitz, H.W., in "Opiates and Endogenous Opioid Peptides", H.W. Kosterlitz, Ed., Elsevier/ North-Holland Biomedical Press, Amsterdam, 1976, pp 275-280.

10. In the publications cited in the references 1 and 2 erroneous configurational assignments have been occurred and have to be corrected. (+)-L-te-trahydrofurfuryl alcohol has been shown by Defaye et al. (ref. 1, loc. cit.) to have S configuration (and not R configuration as erroneously cited). Consequently, all benzomorphans (ref. 1) and noroxymorphones (ref. 2) described to have 2"R configuration truely are 2"S compounds and vice versa.

11. Frearson, P.M., and Stern, E.S., J. Chem. Soc., 1958, 3062.

12. Frearson, P.M., Hardy, D.G., and Stern, E.S., J. Chem. Soc., 1960, 2103.

Characteristics and Function of Opioids, editors Van Ree and Terenius
© *1978 Elsevier/North-Holland Biomedical Press*

CORRELATION BETWEEN BRAIN SUBCORTEX LEVELS OF FENTANYL AND ITS ANTINOCICEPTION

GERDA J.J. PLOMP, ROBERT A.A. MAES, BERT KWAKERNAAK AND JAN M. VAN REE

Centre for Human Toxicology and Rudolf Magnus Institute for Pharmacology, Pharmaceutical and Medical Faculty, University of Utrecht (The Netherlands)

ABSTRACT

Fentanyl levels in rat brain subcortex and plasma were determined by a radio-immunoassay procedure and were correlated with the analgesic activity of this drug. The data indicated a very rapid penetration of fentanyl into brain tissue and a correlation (r=0.96) appeared to exist between the brain subcortex level of fentanyl and its antinociceptive activity.

INTRODUCTION

Studies concerning self-administration of morphinomimetics (morphine, heroin, fentanyl) in rats suggest that the penetration of these drugs into brain tissue and the amount of drug presented per injection (unit dose) are important factors in initiating and maintaining self-injecting behavior and probably in narcotic dependence[1]. There was a linear relationship between the amount of the narcotic drug self-administered and the unit dose presented.

The purpose of the present study was to determine whether brain subcortex levels of fentanyl in rats were related to the amount of drug injected and possibly to the potency of the drug to exhibit biological activity.

MATERIALS AND METHODS

Fentanyl levels in brain subcortex and plasma were determined by a radio-immunoassay procedure (Janssen Pharmaceutica) after a single intravenous injection of fentanyl citrate. Four groups of 30 male Wistar rats were treated with 22.6, 11.3, 5.63 and 2.5 µg/kg fentanyl as base, respectively. Rats were decapitated at 5, 10, 15, 30 or 60 min after drug administration. The brains were quickly removed and dissected. Part of the brainstem, including medulla spinalis, medulla oblongata, thalamus, hypothalamus and mesencephalon, was homogenized in 0.01 N HCl, centrifuged and the supernatant was decanted. These samples, as well as plasma were used for measuring fentanyl concentrations.

Four groups of 10 rats each were injected i.v. with 22.6, 11.3, 5.63 and 2.5 µg/kg fentanyl as base, respectively and one group of 10 rats received placebo (saline 0.3 ml). The degree of analgesia was assessed by the hot plate technique at 5, 10, 15, 30 and 60 min after drug administration. The response latency of the animals to heat was measured on a hot plate (54.2°+0.1°C) according to Eddy and Leimbach[2], before and 5, 10, 15, 30 and 60 min after the treatment with fentanyl or saline. The citerion of the response was the licking of one paw or intensive jerking with lifting off or jumping on the hind legs. The trial was terminated if the latency exceeded 60 sec.

RESULTS

Fentanyl levels in brain subcortex and plasma were related to the amount of drug administered. The highest concentration in brain, as well as in plasma, was found 5 min after i.v. injection of the various doses. Thereafter, the fentanyl levels declined rapidly over the next 10 min. Between 15 min and 60 min after injection, both brain and plasma levels decreased more slowly, but fentanyl was still detectable 60 min after treatment. The ratio of brain and plasma fentanyl levels peaked 15 min after the administration of 22.6 and 11.3 µg/kg fentanyl and reached a maximum value of approximately 3, whereas after 5.63 and 2.5 µg/kg this ratio reached its highest value (approximately 3) 5 min after drug administration.

The analgesic response to fentanyl appeared to be related to the amount of drug injected. A maximum analgesic effect was obtained 5 min after the injection of the various doses. Thereafter, the analgesic response declined progressively.

There was an extremely good correlation ($r = 0.96$, $P < 0.001$) between the brain subcortex level of fentanyl and its antinociceptive activity, as determined 5, 10 and 15 min after treatment. Detailed analysis of the data revealed that although a certain analgesic response corresponded with a given brain level of fentanyl, this correlation was influenced by the dose of fentanyl administered. The correlation was apparently superimposed on a set-point level determined by the unit dose injected.

DISCUSSION

The data indicate that there is a very rapid penetration of fentanyl into brain tissue and a highly significant correlation between the brain level of fentanyl and its antinociceptive activity. The doses of fentanyl given to rats in this study have been shown to induce self-administering behavior. This behavior was related to the unit dose of the drug. A relation has been shown between the analgesic activity of narcotics and the drug-seeking behavior they induce[1]. Thus, the present data may also indicate the presence of a relation between fentanyl levels and the effectiveness of fentanyl in inducing self-injecting behavior. The relationship between unit dose and biological activity of fentanyl with respect to antinociception and self-administration may be the result of a common mechanism. This phenomenon is reminiscent of a biological set-point induced and determined by the unit dose.

REFERENCES
1. Van Ree, J.M., Slangen,J.L. & De Wied,D. (1978)J.Pharm.exp.Ther. 204,547-557.
2. Eddy, N.B. and Leimbach, D. (1953) J. Pharmacol. exp. Ther. 107, 385-393.

ANALGESIC ACTIVITY OF L-5-OH TRYPTOPHAN L-GLUTAMATE: INTERACTION
WITH OTHER ANALGESICS

RABADAN PEINADO F., GALAN CANO J., GARRIDO GARCIA J. M.ROLDAN, C.
Departamento de Farmacología. Laboratorios Made, S.A. Madrid,SPAIN

Brain serotonine precursors have been suggested in the
treatment of endogen depressions[3,1,4]. L-5-hydroxytryptophan
L-glutamate is a synthetic drug precursor of brain serotonine[2]. Its
main pharmacological effects are: increase of excitability in mice
(Irwin scheme), inhibition of the responses of isolated uterus of
rat to serotonine, and potentiation of the effect of catecholamines
in guinea pig deferens duct. This study aims to study the effect
of the drug on the pain, and the modifications of this effect when
the drug is associated to various narcotic and non-narcotic
analgesics. We also study the reflection of this effect on the
acute toxicity and other side effects of narcotic analgesics, e.g.
on the intestinal passage. The narcotic analgesics assayed were:
morphine, pentazocine, fentanyl and dextropropoxyphene, and the
non-narcotic analgesic were salycilamide, acetylsalicylic acid,
aminopyrine, antipyrine and phenacetin.

The experimental technics used were:

1. Acute toxicity.- Litchfield and Wilcoxon, 1949[5]
2. Analgesic.- Writing test induced by acetic acid[6]
3. Intestinal passage with activated charcoal.

The period elapsed from the administration of the analgesic drug
until the evaluation of its effect (administration of acetic acid),
was 30 minutes in the case of narcotic analgesics (with the
exception of fentanyl which was evaluated after 5 minutes), and 60
minutes in the case of non-narcotic analgesics.

RESULTS

1. Acute toxicity

Made-1932 increases significantly the toxicity of morphine (*),
dextropropoxyphene and fentanyl (*); the drug decreases the toxicity of pentazocine and does not modify the toxicity of non-narcotic
analgesics.

2. Analgesia

Made-1932 potentiates significantly the analgesic activity of all the hypnotic analgesics assayed, and of the non-narcotic analgesics derivatives of pyrazol.

3. Intestinal Passage

The depressive effect of the narcotic analgesics is not modified by Made-1932.

CONCLUSSIONS

L-5-hydroxytryptophan L-glutamate produces:

1. An increase of toxicity of morphine, dextropropoxyphene and fentanyl and a decrease of pentazocine, which could be due to a partial agonist effect of the analgesia. The drug does not modify the non-narcotic analgesics.

2. A potentiation of the analgesic activity of all the hypnotic analgesics derivative from pyrazol. This effect backs the theory of participation of serotonine in this mechanism of action. This potentiation does not occur with the non-hypnotic analgesics which are not pyrazol derivatives.

3. The product does not modify the depressive effect of the narcotic analgesics on the intestinal passage.

REFERENCES

1. Coppen A. Serotonine in the affective disorder in "Factors in Depression" edit by N.S. Kline, Raven Press, New York (1974).

2. García de Jalón, P.D. y col. Deuxieme Rencontre Franco-Espagnole de Pharmacologia. Madrid. (1977).

3. Goodwin F.K., Murphy D.L. "Biological factors in the affective disorders and schizophrenia", Psychopharmacological Agents col. 3., edit by M. Gordon, Academic Press, N.Y. (1974).

4. Kline N.S. Shah B.K., Blanda J. An application of Bayés theorem: tryptophan is as good as imipramine, in "Factors in depression" edit by N.S. Kline, Raveu Press, New York (1974).

5. Litchfield J.R. and Wilcoxon F.J. Pharmacol Exptl. Therapeut. 96, 99 (1949).

6. Siegmund E.A., Cadmus A. and Lu G. J. Pharmacol. Exptl. Therapeutic 119, 453 (1957).

Characteristics and Function of Opioids, editors Van Ree and Terenius
© *1978 Elsevier/North-Holland Biomedical Press*   235

PHARMACODINAMIC STUDY OF A NEW ANALGESIC: GR-119

RABADAN F.P., GARRIDO J., MARTINEZ ROLDAN C.
Dept. Farmacología. Laboratorios Made,S.A. Madrid. SPAIN

INTRODUCTION

After the studies on the analgesig drug 2-(2-phenyl)-4 methyl-pyridine[3], we have followed a line of investigation and, because of its analgesic activity, we have selected the product 1,4,4a-trimethyl-1,2,4a,4b,9a,10a-hexahydro-1-OH-benzo b thieno 2',3':4,3 cyclopenta 1,2-b pyridine or GR-119, also synthetized by Granados and col. We state in this study the major results obtained in our experiment with GR-119.

EXPERIMENT

Acute toxicity

The LD_{50} in male and female white mice of Swiss ICR strain is 232.9 mg/kg and 465 mg/kg, by intraperitoneal and oral route respectively[2].

Analgesic activity

White mice of Swiss ICR strain were used. We used dextropropoxy phene as comparative drug.

Analgesic activity against thermic stimulus. Hot plate test at 55ºC was used[1]. The activity of GR-119 was similar to the activity of dextropropoxyphene.

Analgesic activity against a chemical stimulus. The Wrighting test was used administering 0.25 ml of a 1% solution of acetic acid[4].

The drug GR-119 was active both by oral and intraperitoneal route. The ED_{50} by oral route was 51.29 mg/kg.

Interaction with L-5-hydroxytryptophan L-glutamate (Made 1932). The L-5-hydroxytryptophan L-glutamate potentiates the analgesic activity of GR-119.

Intestinal passage

Doses of 25 mg/kg of GR-119 did not modify the intestinal passage of 0.25 ml of 1% activated charcoal in mices.

236

Blood pressure

a) The drug did not modify the blood pressure in anaesthetized rats.

b) The drug did not modify the hypertension produced by 5-HT in pithed rats.

Action in isolated organs

The product GR-119 inhibits the responses to histamine, acetylcholine, barium chloride, adrenaline and serotonine.

Stimulation of ileum in guinea pig

Bath of Krebs solution at 37ºC, flow of carbogen (95% O_2 and 5% CO_2) at 37ºC.

Platinum electrodes, battery of impulses 0.2 Hertzs, duration 2 mseg., voltage 50% higher than threshold.

GR-119 inhibits the responses of guinea pig ileum to electric stimulations. The effect is antagonized in 84,2% when 1 mcg/ml of naloxone is previously added to the incubation bath.

Other studies

GR-119 does not modify the Irwin scheme; it has no anti-convulsivant or anti-inflammatory activity.

DISCUSSION AND SUMMARY

We feel that GR-119 can be included among the group of analgesic narcotic drugs, due to the following facts:

a) it has shown to be active in both the tests tried (Hot plate method and Writing test),

b) its effect is potentiated by L-5-hydroxy-tryptophan L-glutamate,

c) it inhibits the responses of guinea pig ileum to electric stimulation,

d) Naloxone is a reversible antagonist of GR-119.

REFERENCES

1. Janssen P.A.J.and Jageneau A.J.Pharm,Pharmacol.9,381 (1957).
2. Litchfield J.J.and Wilcoxon T.J.Pharm.Exptl.Therap. 96,99 (1949)
3. Martínez Roldán y col. XVI Congreso Nacional SECF.Barcelona 1977
4. Siegmund A. Cadmus A. and Lu G.J.Pharm.Exptl. Therap.119, 453 (1957).

ACTIONS OF FURYL BENZOMORPHAN DERIVATIVES UPON THE ISOLATED MOUSE VAS DEFERENS [1]

CHARLES B. SMITH

Department of Pharmacology, The Univ. of Michigan, Ann Arbor, Mich. 48109 U.S.A.

When administered to the rhesus monkey, certain furyl benzomorphan derivatives cause a behavioral depression which is reversed to varying degrees by different narcotic antagonists. These drugs do not suppress the abstinence syndrome in the morphine-dependent rhesus monkey. In these two respects they resemble the ketazocines pharmacologically. The isolated mouse vas deferens possesses at least two types of narcotic receptors, one of which has a high affinity for ketazocine[1]. In the present studies, a series of furyl benzomorphan derivatives were evaluated for their effects upon the isolated, electrically stimulated mouse vas deferens and were compared to ethylketazocine and morphine. The purpose of this study was to determine whether actions of these drugs upon the two types of receptors could be differentiated by the use of the antagonists, naltrexone and UM 979 [(-)-5,9 α-dimethyl-2(3-furylmethyl)-2'-hydroxy-6,7-benzomorphan], a furyl benzomorphan antagonist which precipitates abstinence in the morphine-dependent rhesus monkey. The drugs studied were UM 909 [2-(2-methyl-3-furyl)-2'-hydroxy-α -5,9-dimethyl-6,7-benzomorphan], UM 911 [2-(3-methylfurfuryl)-2'-hydroxy- α-5,9-dimethyl-6,7-benzomorphan], UM 1070 [(±)-5-9 α-dimethyl-2'-hydroxy-2-tetrahydrofurfuryl-6,7-benzomorphan], and UM 1072 [(±)-5,9 β-dimethyl-2'-hydroxy-2-tetrahydrofurfuryl-6,7-benzomorphan], as well as morphine and ethylketazocine.

MATERIALS AND METHODS

Male, albino Swiss-Webster mice, weighing between 25 and 30 g, were sacrificed by decapitation. The vasa deferentia were removed, and 1.5 cm segments were suspended in organ baths which contained a modified Krebs' physiological buffer. The buffer contained the following: NaCl, 118 mM; KCl, 4.75 mM; $CaCl_2$, 2.54 mM; $MgSO_4$, 1.19 mM; KH_2PO_4, 1.19 mM; glucose, 11 mM; $NaHCO_3$, 25 mM, hexamethonium bromide, 0.07 mM; pargyline, 0.3 mM; tyrosine, 0.2 mM; ascorbic acid, 0.1 mM and disodium edetate, 0.03 mM. The buffer was saturated with 95% O_2-5% CO_2 and kept at 37°C. The segments were attached to a strain gauge transducer and suspended between two platinum electrodes. After a 15-minute equilibration period, the segments were stimulated once every ten seconds with pairs of pulses of 1 msec duration, 1 msec apart and at supramaximal voltage. The segments were stimulated for 30 min or until a stable twitch height was achieved. Cumulated concentration-response curves were determined for the various drugs. EC 50's were calculated by probit analysis.

RESULTS

Ethylketazocine was approximately ten times more potent than morphine upon the isolated vas deferens. Similarly, all of the furyl benzomorphans except 909 were more

[1] This study was supported by USPHS grants DA 00254 and DA 10474. Valuable technical assistance was provided by John Evaldson

238

potent than morphine. The least potent of these compounds was UM 909, and the most potent was UM 1070 (Table1).

TABLE I

EC 50's FOR THE EFFECT OF NARCOTIC AGONISTS UPON THE ISOLATED MOUSE VAS DEFERENS. DIFFERENTIAL ANTAGONISM BY NALTREXONE AND UM 979.

Drug	EC 50	EC 50 after naltrexone, 10^{-8}M.	EC 50 after UM 979, 10^{-7}M.
UM 1070	5.88×10^{-10} M ± 0.85	1.62×10^{-9} M ± 1.40	2.18×10^{-9} M ± 0.60
Ethylketazocine	1.56×10^{-9} M ± 0.81	1.12×10^{-8} M ± 0.66	7.32×10^{-9} M ± 3.00
UM 1072	2.58×10^{-9} M ± 0.42	2.56×10^{-9} M ± 0.43	4.04×10^{-8} M ± 0.06
UM 911	1.21×10^{-8} M ± 0.23	8.68×10^{-9} M ± 0.77	2.49×10^{-8} M ± 0.63
Morphine	1.83×10^{-8} M ± 0.42	7.52×10^{-8} M ± 0.24	1.62×10^{-7} M ± 0.11
UM 909	6.17×10^{-8} M ± 0.85	2.89×10^{-7} M ± 0.45	1.28×10^{-7} M ± 0.36

[a]Each value represents the mean of at least six determinations $\pm$ the standard error

Naltrexone, 10^{-8} M, antagonized the effects of ethylketazocine, morphine, UM 1070 and UM 909, but it did not antagonize the effects of UM 1072 or UM 911. In contrast, UM 979, 10^{-7} M, antagonized all of the agonists which were studied. It was most effective against UM 1072 and morphine, and least effective against UM 1070 and UM 909.

SUMMARY
1. Like ethylketazocine and morphine, the furyl benzomorphans suppressed the twitch elicited by electrical stimulation of the isolated mouse vas deferens.
2. All of these compounds were more potent than morphine except for UM 909 which was only slightly less potent.
3. UM 979 antagonized the effects of all of the agonists studied. However, naltrexone only antagonized the effects of ethylketazocine, morphine, UM 1070 and UM 909.
4. These results suggest that by the use of appropriate antagonists it is possible to differentiate between the two types of narcotic receptors which are present in the mouse vas deferens.

REFERENCES
1. Lord, J.A.H., Waterfield, A.A., Hughes, J. and Kosterlitz, H.W. (1977) Nature (Lond), 267, 495-499.

ARTERIO-VENOUS DIFFERENCE OF MEPERIDINE ACROSS THE FETAL BRAIN

H. Szeto, R. Kaiko, J. Clapp, R. Abrams, L. Mann and C. Inturrisi
Dept. Obstet-Gynecol., U. of Vermont Coll. of Med., Burlington, VT (H.S., J.C.,
L.M.), Dept. Pharmacology, Cornell U. Med. Coll., New York, NY (R.K., C.I.) and
Dept. Obstet-Gynecol., U. of Florida Med. Coll., Gainesville, FL (R.A.), USA

ABSTRACT

The time course of the arterio-venous(A-V) difference of meperidine(M) across
the fetal lamb brain is compared following intravenous(i.v.) and intramuscular
(i.m.) administration of M to the mother. A-V equilibration occurs at 10-15 min
following an i.v. dose, and at 20-25 min following an i.m. dose.

INTRODUCTION

M rapidly crosses the placenta and is distributed to the fetus following i.v.
administration to the mother[1]. Both the rate and extent of drug distribution to
the fetus are decreased when M is administered i.m. to the mother[1]. The influence of the route of administration of M on the distribution of M to the fetal
brain was assessed by measuring the time course of M across the fetal brain (A-V
difference) following i.v. or i.m. administration to the mother.

MATERIALS & METHODS

Using the technique of Mann et al.[2], 5 pregnant ewes at 116-137 days gestation
were surgically prepared with chronic indwelling catheters in the maternal aorta
(MA) and vena cava (MV), and the fetal brachiocephalic artery (FA) and sagittal
vein (SV). 24 hrs or more after surgery, M (2.5 mg/kg) was administered i.v.
into MV, or i.m. into the maternal gluteal region. Plasma M concentration was
determined using the gas-liquid chromatographic method of Szeto & Inturrisi[3].

RESULTS

An example of plasma M levels in MA(●—●), FA(✗—✗) and SV(○—○) after
i.v. and i.m. administration of M to the mother are given in Fig. 1(i.v.) and
Fig. 2(i.m.). M in SV rises until a point in time when SV achieves its maximum
concentration, and FA and SV are in equilibrium (M in SV = M in FA)(see Table I).
At equilibrium, the concentration of free drug in FA, SV and brain are equal[4] i.e:

$$C_{FA,eq} = C_{brain, eq} = C_{SV,eq}$$

$C_{brain,eq}$ can therefore be estimated from Fig. 1 and Fig. 2 (see Table I).

240

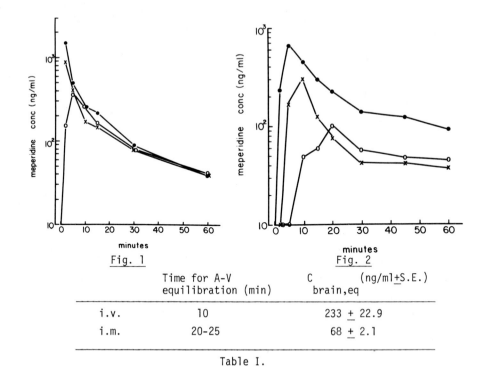

Fig. 1   Fig. 2

	Time for A-V equilibration (min)	$C_{brain,eq}$ (ng/ml$\pm$S.E.)
i.v.	10	233 ± 22.9
i.m.	20-25	68 ± 2.1

Table I.

SUMMARY

We have previously shown that the pharmacokinetics of M in the fetus can be described by a 2-compartment open model, consisting of central and peripheral compartments[1]. The lag time required for plasma-brain equilibration of M suggests that the fetal brain behaves as if it is part of the peripheral compartment. The rate of plasma-brain equibration and $C_{brain,eq}$ of M are a function of the route of administration of M to the mother. These data suggest that during labor the route of administration of M will determine the time course of M in the fetal brain, and the time action of effects seen in the neonate.

REFERENCES

1. Szeto, H.H., Mann, L.I., Bhakthavathsalan, A., Liu, M. and Inturrisi, C.E. (in press) J. Pharmacol. Exp. Ther.
2. Mann, L.I., Carmichael, A. and Duchin, S. (1972) Am. J. Ob-Gyn. 114, 546.
3. Szeto, H.H. and Inturrisi, C.E. (1976) J. Chromatogr. 125, 503.
4. Riggs, D.S. (1963) The Mathematical Approach to Physiological Problems, pp. 216-229. The Williams & Wilkins Co., Baltimore, Maryland.
Supported in part by NIDA Grants DA-01825 and DA-01707.

Characteristics and Function of Opioids, editors Van Ree and Terenius
© 1978 Elsevier/North-Holland Biomedical Press

SOME STRUCTURE ACTIVITY RELATIONSHIPS IN THE DIAZADITWISTANE SERIES

J. TEN BROEKE, R. L. HUDGIN,[*] A. A. PATCHETT, A. RACKHAM,[*] F. M. ROBINSON, AND
M. WILLIAMS[†]

Merck Sharp & Dohme Research Laboratories, Rahway, New Jersey 07065, and West
Point, Pennsylvania 19486[†] USA. Merck-Frosst Research Laboratories, Montreal,
Quebec, Canada[*]

ABSTRACT

Testing of a new series of diazaditwistanes has confirmed the unusual structure activity relationships in this series of analgesics. They appear structurally to be more similar to the enkephalins than to known opiates.

INTRODUCTION

The synthesis of a series of analogs of 5,11-diazaditwistane (Ia) and the
finding that one isomer of one of them (Ib) was an analgesic more potent than
morphine has been reported.[1] It appeared to be a typical morphine-like compound,
but analogs did not show typical opiate structure activity relationships. The

$$\text{Ia} \quad R_1, R_2, R_3, R_4 = H$$
$$\text{b} \quad R_1 = R_2 = C_6H_5CH_2CO$$
$$R_3 = R_4 = CH_3$$

activities of some additional analogs based on the structure of enkephalin[2] are
reported here.

MATERIALS AND METHODS

Synthesis. The compounds in Table I were prepared using the basic synthetic
procedures previously reported.[1]

Receptor Binding. The ^3H naloxone binding assay was carried out by a variation of a published method.[3] Five concentrations were used in triplicate and
ED_{50}'s calculated from log probit analysis.

Analgesic Testing. Analgesia was measured by the increase in the pain reaction threshold to pressure applied to the normal hind paw of rats.[4] Thresholds were determined 30 minutes after administration of vehicle or test compounds i.p. The ED_{50} was the dose at which 50% of the animals showed a reaction pressure 150% of the vehicle control.

RESULTS AND DISCUSSION

TABLE I

	R_1	R_2	R_3	R_4	Receptor Binding ED_{50} nM $(-Na^+)$	Analgesia ED_{50} mg/kg
Ib	$C_6H_5CH_2CO$ (-) isomer	$C_6H_5CH_2CO$	CH_3	CH_3	122	1.2 (0.9-1.6)[b]
II	"	"	$-CH_2CH=CH_2$	"	4350	>80[a]
III	"	"	"	$-CH_2CH=CH_2$	inactive	>80[a]
IV	$o(OH)C_6H_4CH_2CO$	"	CH_3	CH_3	135	7.8 (7.0-8.7)
V	$m(OH)C_6H_4CH_2CO$	"	"	"	833	15.9 (9.9-26.3)
VI	$p(OH)C_6H_4CH_2CO$	"	"	"	245	>32
VII	$C_6H_5CH_2CH_2-$	$C_6H_5CH_2CO-$	"	"	435	17.9 (12.8-25)
VIII	$C_6H_5CH_2-$	$C_6H_5CH_2-$			70	8-16
Morphine					11.2	2.2 (1.7-2.9)

[a]Data from Ref. 2.

[b]95% Confidence limits.

As shown in Table I, N-allyl groups (II & III) severely interfere with receptor binding--unlike known opiate antagonists. In only one case (IV) did the introduction of a phenolic hydroxyl increase binding (assuming one enantiomer is inactive). (Symmetrical bisphenolic analogs showed reduced activity.)

Structural comparisons of Ib with probable conformations of enkephalins, and of their crystal structures[5,6] suggest that the primary binding sites for Ib may correspond to the basic nitrogen and the Phe of enkephalin rather than the Tyr as is thought to be the case with morphine.

REFERENCES

1. Fisher, M. H., Grabowski, E. J. J., Patchett, A. A., ten Broeke, J., Flataker, L. M., Lotti, V. J. and Robinson, F. M. (1977) J. Med. Chem., 20, 63-66.

2. Hughes, J., Smith, T. W., Kosterlitz, H. W., Fothergill, L. A., Morgan, B. A., Morris, H. R. (1975) Nature (London), 258, 577-579.

3. Pasternak, G., Wilson, H. and Snyder, S. (1975) Mol. Pharmacol., 11, 340-351.

4. Winter, C. A. and Flataker, L. M. (1965) J. Pharmacol., 150, 165-168.

5. Hirschfield, J., Hoogsteen, K., Springer, J. and van der Veen, J., in press.

6. Smith, G. D. and Griffin, J. F. (1978) Science, 199, 1214-1216.

Characteristics and Function of Opioids, editors Van Ree and Terenius
© *1978 Elsevier/North-Holland Biomedical Press*   243

EXORPHINS - PEPTIDES WITH OPIOID ACTIVITY DERIVED FROM

α - CASEIN AND WHEAT GLUTEN

CHRISTINE ZIOUDROU* AND WERNER A. KLEE

Laboratory of General and Comparative Biochemstry NIMH Bethesda, Md 20014

We have isolated peptides with opioid activities from pepsin hydrolysates
of food proteins, such as wheat gluten and α-casein. Like the endogenous
opiates these peptides, the exorphins, inhibit the adenylate cyclase activity
of neuroblastoma x gloma hybrid cells as well as the electrically stimulated
contractions of the mouse vas deferens. (Fig 1) These inhibitions are blocked
or reversed by (-) - naloxone but not by its enantiomer. In addition, the
exorphins compete with dihydromorphine and D-ala^2 - Met-enkephalin amide for
binding to rat brain opiate receptors. The peptide nature of the exorphins is
demonstrated by their loss of activity after pronase treatment (Table I).

TABLE 1. EFFECT OF PRONASE ON THE ACTIVITIES OF GLUTEN EXORPHIN$^\alpha$
CASEIN EXORPHIN$^\alpha$ AND THE GLUTEN STIMULATORY FRACTION$^\alpha$

Adenylate cyclase activity (pmol cyclic AMP/min/mg)

	Untreated	Naloxone	Pronase-treated	Naloxone
Gluten Exorphin	12.4	16.5	15.2	16.4
Casein Exorphin	14.5	18.2	17.8	17.7
Control	16.5	16.9	17.0	18.1
Gluten Stimulatory Fraction	48.5	50.3	45.2	48.5
Control	32.5	32.3	29.0	33.5

$^\alpha$Pepsin hydrolysis, peptide purification and opiate assays are all described in detail elsewhere (1).

Also present in pepsin hydrolysates of gluten is a substance which stimulates adenylate cyclase (Table 1) and the vas deferens (Fig 1 B). These stimulatory actions. are not affected by naloxone. Furthermore the activity of the
stimulatory material is not affected by pronase (Table 1), but is destroyed by
periodate oxidation and by treatment with glycosidases. Thus, the stimulatory
activity is associated with a carbohydrate moiety. Analysis of this, partially
purfied, material showed the presence of hexoses as well as amino acids.

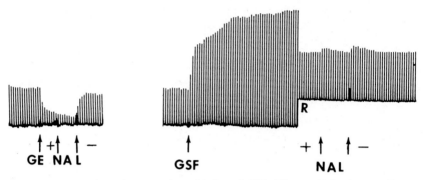

Fig 1. The effects of GE (Gluten Exorphin) and GSF (Gluten Stimulatory Fraction) on the electrically stimulated mouse vas deferens. (+) or (–) refer to the two enantiomers of Naloxone.

A comparison of the potencies of two purified exorphins in three different opiate assays is shown in Table II. Gluten exorphin is comparable to met-enkephalin in its potencies in these assays, whereas casein exorphin is less active.

Table II. CONCENTRATIONS$^{\alpha}$ OF EXORPHINS FOR HALF MAXIMAL
INHIBITIONS IN SEVERAL OPIATE ASSAYS

	Brain receptor Binding	Adenylate cyclase	Vas deferens
Gluten Exorphin	2	30	2
Casein Exorphin	3500	320	8000
Met-Enkephalin	20	7	7
Morphine Sulfate	1	570	190

$^{\alpha}$Concentration in nanograms per ml.

Opiate activity has also been found in pepsin hydrolysates of maize zein, barley hordein and bovine serum albumin but not in hydrolysates of many other proteins. All grain proteins examined proved to have stimulatory activity. The physiological roles of these exogenously derived peptides remain to be determined but may, in some respects at least resemble those of endorphins.

REFERENCE.

W. A. Klee, C. Zioudrou and R. A. Streaty, in Endorphins in Mental Health Research, (eds) E. Usdin, W. E. Bunney, N. S. Kline; Macmillan, N. Y. p. 209–218 (1978).

*Visiting Scientist NRC "Democritos, Aghia Paraskeri, Attikis, Greece.

Characteristics and Function of Opioids, editors Van Ree and Terenius
© *1978 Elsevier/North-Holland Biomedical Press*

BIOSYNTHESIS OF BETA-ENDORPHIN FROM BETA-LIPOTROPIN AND A LARGER PRECURSOR MOLECULE.

M. CHRETIEN, P. CRINE, M. LIS, C. GIANOULAKIS, F. GOSSARD, S. BEN-JANNET AND N.G. SEIDAH.
Protein and Pituitary Hormone Laboratory, Clinical Research Institute of Montreal, 110 Pine Avenue West, Montreal H2W 1R7 (Canada).

ABSTRACT

The pars intermedia is known to be made almost exclusively of cells containing ACTH and LPH peptides. It was thus used to study their biosynthesis. Results show that rat pituitary pars intermedia cells synthetize in large amount a large protein (M.W. 28,500 ± 1,500 daltons) which bears antigenic determinant for both beta-MSH and ACTH. Pulse chase experiments revealed that this molecule is matured into several products including beta-endorphin and beta-LPH. These studies show for the first time in pulse-chase experiments, the release of beta-endorphin from a larger precursor molecule. In conclusion, the pituitary gland and most importantly the pars intermedia might be the primary source of beta-endorphin.

INTRODUCTION

Beta-lipotropin, a 91 amino acid peptide, had been considered to be a precursor molecule instead of a biologically active hormone. The subject has been recently reviewed[1]. This assumption was based on the fact that it contains beta-MSH within it and that the proposed sites of cleavage are similar to those of proinsulin and finally, that it has only minimal biological activities (Table 1). Until 1975, its C-terminus portion had not attracted too much attention until the astonishing discovery of enkephalins by Hughes et al.[2]. They described the isolation of two peptides, called enkephalins, from hog brains that are agonists of morphine. The first one, Tyr-Gly-Gly-Phe-Met, has a methionine residue in the fifth position and was therefore named Met-enkephalin. In the second one, a leucine residue replaces the methionine in the fifth position. The sequence of Met-enkephalin is identical to the fragment containing residues 61-65 of beta-lipotropin, a lipolytic hormone pro-

246

TABLE 1

BIOLOGICAL ACTIVITIES OF BETA-LPH AND RELATED PEPTIDES

	Beta-LPH	Gamma-LPH	Beta-MSH	Beta-endorphin
MSH (units/g)	2×10^{-7}	1.6×10^{-7}	1.2×10^{-9}	nil
Lipolytic (MED) ug	0.01 to 0.1	0.01 to 0.1	0.006	-
Morphinomimetic (MED) 1 Molar	$< 1 \times 10^{-5}$	-	nil	1×10^{-7}

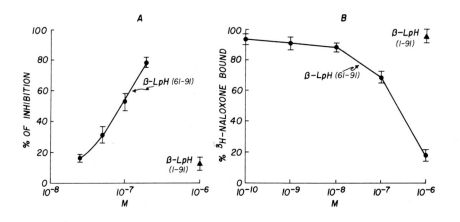

Fig. 1. Morphine-like activity assay of beta-LPH (1-91) and beta$_h$-LPH (61-91). (A) Vas deferans. (B) Receptor.

duced by the pituitary gland. This discovery prompted several groups to look in pituitary glands for endogenous morphine-like substances structurally related to beta-lipotropin. Several investigators[2-6] were able to show the presence of such morphine-like substances in human as well as in camel, sheep, and hog pituitaries. Most of them have sequences corresponding to the segment 61-91 of their respective beta-lipotropin and were named beta-endorphin. The segments 61-76 and 61-77 of beta-lipotropin were also extracted from fragments of pig hypothalamus-neurohypophysis[7,8]. It was moreover observed that while beta-lipotropin had no morphine-like activity, even at high doses[9], the portion 61-91 had considerable activity in the morphine bioassay and opiate-receptor-binding assays[3,5,9] (Fig. 1). These findings also clearly indicate that the relationship between beta-lipotropins and the opioid peptides is more than accidental.

The pituitary gland is also known to contain another lipotropic hormone, gamma-lipotropin, which is made of the first 58 residues of the beta-lipotropin molecule[10]. Gamma-lipotropin contains as its COOH-terminus the complete structure of beta-melanotropin, a 18-amino-acid peptide that is 100 times more potent than either beta or gamma-lipotropin in lipolysis and melanophore stimulation[1] (Table 1).

The discovery of gamma-LPH in 1967[10] and the demonstration, in 1970[11], that beta-LPH was unlikely to be a degradation product led us to consider beta-LPH as a prohormone for beta-MSH. With the discovery of the endorphins, beta-lipotropin now appears to be a unique molecule containing the structure of two biologically active peptides.

The prohormone hypothesis proposed for beta-lipotropin is further supported by the analogy between its sequence and the sequence of proinsulin at their respective cleavage sites (Fig. 2), which in both cases contain two basic amino acids, a feature likely to be recognized by a trypsin-like enzyme[12], which, in association with a carboxypeptidase B-like enzyme will release beta-endorphin and beta-MSH (Fig. 3).

Recently, it was shown that cells of whole bovine pituitaries[13-16] and of bovine pars intermedia[17] actively incorporate radiolabeled amino acids into beta-lipotropin, gamma-lipotropin and beta-

248

AMINO ACID SEQUENCES OF β-LPH AND PROINSULIN AT THEIR SITE OF ENZYMATIC CLEAVAGE

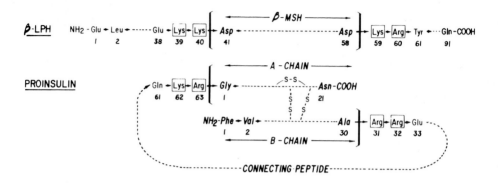

Fig. 2

ALL POSSIBLE STAGES OF BIOSYNTHESIS OF β-ENDORPHIN, γ-LPH AND β-MSH FROM β-LPH

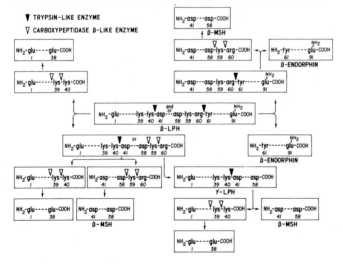

Fig. 3

endorphin. The pars intermedia of pituitary glands synthesized relatively large amounts of lipotropin (LPH) and adrenocorticotropin
(ACTH) and their related fragments[18-19]. Such a rich source of
these peptides was thus chosen as a model to study their in vitro
biosynthesis in the rat. The anterior and whole rat pituitaries
were recently shown, by an elegant micropurification technique, to
contain both beta-LPH[20] and beta-endorphin[21]. The beta-endorphin
segment was found to be homologous to the corresponding peptide
from sheep, bovine and camel, by amino acid analysis and peptide
mapping[21].

Immunocytochemical studies have shown that ACTH and beta-LPH immunoreactive peptides occur in all of the parenchymal cells of the
pars intermedia[22-24]. Furthermore, when these cells were observed
under the electron microscope, staining for ACTH and beta-LPH was
seen in all the granules and in the structures of the rough endo-
plasmic reticulum[19,23]. These results agree with the hypothesis
of a common precursor for ACTH and beta-LPH, which has recently
found two good experimental confirmations[25-27].

In both studies, the experimental model was the ACTH-secreting
mouse pituitary cell line AtT-20. Mains et al.[25] used a double
immunoprecipitation technique to isolate labeled proteins from
cells incubated with radioactive amino acids. Roberts and Herbert[26,27] prepared a cell free translation product from a polyA
containing mRNA fraction obtained from AtT-20 cells. In both cases, the ACTH - beta-LPH precursor seems to be a 28,000 to 31,000
dalton protein which would be cleaved into beta-LPH, beta-endorphin
and several high molecular weight forms of ACTH[25,28,29].

The primary purpose of this study was to investigate the ACTH -
beta-endorphin biosynthetic pattern in the intermediate lobe of rat
pituitaries. We report that during short incubations with labeled
amino acids, rat pituitary intermediate lobe cells synthesize predominantly one 28,500 ± 1,500 dalton protein which bears antigenic
determinants for both beta-MSH and ACTH. Pulse-chase labeling experiments show that this peptide is matured into several products
including beta-LPH and beta-endorphin.

MATERIALS AND METHODS
Preparation of rat pars intermedia cells. Pituitary glands from

Sprague-Dawley male rats were removed immediately after decapitation. The posterior lobe (pars nervosa plus pars intermedia) was
carefully separated from the anterior lobe with fine needles. They
were washed several times with fresh buffer (Krebs Ringer buffer
containing bicarbonate, 0.2% glucose and 0.1% bovine serum albumin
- Fraction V, Sigma) (KRBGA). The cells were dispersed by mechanical agitation and were harvested by low speed centrifugation, resuspended in 1 to 5 ml of gassed KRBGA and preincubated for 1 hr
at $37^{O}C$ in an atmosphere of O_2/CO_2 (95:5 vol/vol).

Incorporation of labeled amino acids in vitro and pulse-chase
experiments. At the end of the preincubation, the cells were
resuspended either in 1 ml of prewarmed KRBGA containing 2 mCi/ml
of ^{35}S-methionine (New England Nuclear, 596 Ci/mmol) or 5 ml of the
same medium containing 0.5 mCi/ml of ^{3}H-phenylalanine (115 Ci/mmol)
(NEN). Pulse-chase labeling experiments were performed with ^{35}S-
methionine. At the end of the labeling period (10 min), unlabeled
methionine was added to the incubation medium at a final concentration of 2 mM. This reduced 300 fold the incorporation of ^{35}S-
methionine into TCA insoluble proteins within the next 10 minutes.
This result agrees with previous reports[28,31].

Protein extraction. After the incubation, the cell was centrifuged at low speed. The cell pellet was washed once with cold
saline and directly extracted in 5 N acetic acid containing 0.3 mg/
ml phenylmethyl sulfonyl fluoride, 0.3 mg/ml iodoacetate, 0.5 mg/
ml BSA and 5 uMol/ml of the corresponding unlabeled amino acid[31].
The cell extract was desalted on a 9.1 ml Sephadex G-25.

Disc electrophoresis. Samples from various chromatographic
fractions during the purification of labeled products or total cell
extracts were analyzed by disc electrophoresis in acidic polyacrylamide gels according to Reisfield et al.[32]. For the identification of beta-LPH and beta-endorphin, purified labeled rat beta-LPH
and beta-endorphin obtained from a separate incubation and characterized as described recently[33] were run on separate gels. Sodium
dodecyl sulfate (SDS) polyacrylamide gels were prepared and used
according to Weber and Osborn[34]. The molecular weight determination was made by comparing the relative mobility of the unknown
molecular species with a set of standard proteins (Pharmacia).
SDS-urea polyacrylamide gel electrophoresis according to Swank and

Munkres[35] was performed as described elsewhere[33]. Gels containing radioactive proteins were cut into 2-mm slices immediately after the electrophoresis and counted.

Immunoprecipitation. Labeled peptides obtained after a 10 min incubation with ^{3}H-phenylalanine were used for immunoprecipitation studies. An aliquot of the ^{3}H-labeled cell extract which had been previously desalted on Sephadex G-25 was mixed with an excess of either beta-MSH antiserum[36] or ACTH antiserum[37]. The mixture was incubated for 16 hours at 4°C in a phosphate saline buffer (0.01 M sodium phosphate, 0.15 M NaCl, 0.025 M EDTA) (SPB, EDTA) and 2% Triton X-100 after which an immunoprecipitate was formed by addition of goat antiserum to rabbit immunoglobulins (Calbiochem). The immunoprecipitate was collected and dissolved in a solution containing 12 mg Tris, 15 mg DTT and 10 mg SDS per ml and analyzed by SDS gel electrophoresis.

Sequencing of labeled peptides. Automatic Edman degradations on the purified peptides were done as described elsewhere[33].

RESULTS

Identification of a large precursor for ACTH and beta-LPH. Intermediate lobe cells were incubated with ^{3}H-phenylalanine (115 Ci/ mmol, 0.5 mCi/ml) for 10 min and the proteins extracted from the cells were desalted on Sephadex G-25 and directly analyzed by SDS-gel electrophoresis. One major peptide with an apparent molecular weight of 28,500 ± 1,500 was found. This major radioactive cell product was immunoprecipitated with either anti beta-MSH serum or anti-ACTH serum as shown by SDS-gel electrophoresis (data not shown). In each case, immunoprecipitation of labeled material was shown to be specific since the radioactive peaks on the gels were abolished by the addition of an excess of cold beta-MSH or ACTH to the sample before adding the corresponding immunoserum. Moreover, a non immune rabbit serum failed to precipitate any radioactivity.

Pulse-chase studies. In another experiment, intermediate lobe cells were incubated with ^{35}S-methionine (596 Ci/mmol, 2 mCi/ml) in 1 ml of KRBGA at 37° for 10 min, after which excess unlabeled methionine (final concentration 2 mM) was added and the incubation continued. Aliquots of the cell suspension were withdrawn at the

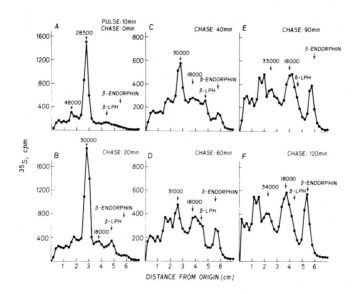

Fig. 4. SDS gel electrophoresis of desalted extracts obtained during a pulse-chase labeling experiment.

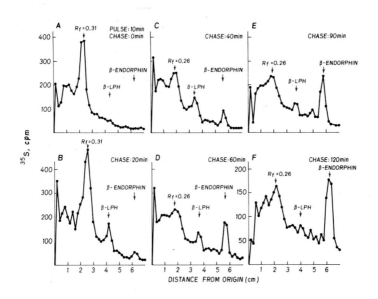

Fig. 5. Polyacrylamide gel electrophoresis (pH 4.5) of the same extracts as in Fig. 4.

end of the 10 min labeling period and then 20, 40, 60, 90 and 120
min later. Fig. 4 shows that during the chase period with unlabeled methionine, the 28,500 dalton peptide progressively disappeared,
giving rise to smaller fragments. After 20 min of chase, two fragments were observed: a 18,000 dalton fragment and another smaller
peptide comigrating with beta-LPH. After 40 min of incubation in
the presence of unlabeled methionine, a new peptide comigrating
with standard beta-endorphin appeared. As the incubation with unlabeled methionine proceeded, two fragments increased in importance, the 18,000 dalton peptide and the beta-endorphin. Meanwhile,
the 28,500 daltons protein slowly disappeared as its apparent molecular weight slightly increased. The fragment corresponding to
beta-LPH seemed to have a transient existence. The 40,000 to
50,000 dalton protein remained constant and represented about 10
to 20% of the total cpm recovered from the gel throughout the
chase-incubation.

When cell extract from the same pulse-chase experiment were also
analyzed by acidic gel electrophoresis (Fig. 5), the major molecular species present after 10 min of ^{35}S-methionine incorporation
has an Rf of 0.31. During the chase, it diminished and gave rise
to three peptides: a first one comigrating with standard labeled
rat beta-LPH, a second one with beta-endorphin, and a third peptide which had an Rf of 0.26. At 20 and 40 min of chase, the peptide
comigrating with standard rat beta-LPH was clearly apparent as a
well characterized peak on the acidic gels; however, it diminished
in importance as the chase proceeded and was barely detectable, but
still present after 2 hrs. The beta-endorphin remained as a major
peak and did not seem to be further transformed.

DISCUSSION

Previous studies involving labeled amino acid incorporation in
whole pituitary slices had proved that beta-endorphin was biosynthesized in the pituitary gland[16]. However, the elucidation of the
detailed biosynthetic pathway requires the use of a more specific
system where beta-endorphin biosynthesis would represent a high
percentage of the total protein synthesis. Immunohistochemical
studies have shown that beta-lipotropin and beta-endorphin are most
concentrated in cells of the pars intermedia[23]. These observations

led us to reinvestigate the study of the biosynthesis of beta-endorphin in isolated pars intermedia cells from beef[17] or rats[33]. We have recently shown that, in both species, this tissue can indeed synthesize beta-LPH together with its two fragments gamma-LPH and beta-endorphin[17,33]. This beta-endorphin[33] has been chemically characterized at its residues 5, 9, 14 and 17. A computer data search showed that these key amino acids allowed the unambiguous identification of this peptide as beta-endorphin (see this volume Seidah et al.)

The results presented in this report prove that in 10 min pulse experiments, one major labeled protein has a molecular weight of 28,500 ± 1,500 and contains antigenic determinants for both ACTH and beta-MSH.

When the radioactivity incorporated in the cells within the first 10 min of the incubation is chased for 2 hrs by an excess of unlabeled amino acid, several fragments are formed from the initial 28,500 dalton peptide and can be separated on SDS gel as well as on acid gel electrophoresis. In both systems, one of them, which is produced in high yield, comigrates with standard rat beta-endorphin isolated from a 3 hrs continuous incubation experiment which has been characterized by electrophoresis and by microsequencing[33]. Considering the extremely high resolution of the acidic gels for intermediate lobe peptides[33], we can unambiguously identify this fragment coming from the precursor as beta-endorphin (see this volume, Seidah et al.).

If the chase incubation is performed for shorter time (20 min), only two major fragments are formed from the initial 28,500 dalton protein and can be separated by electrophoresis on SDS gels. One fragment comigrates with standard rat beta-LPH, purified and characterized as described in reference 33, and the other has an apparent molecular weight of 18,000. This peptide is believed to be a high molecular weight form of ACTH. This is in agreement with the results of Mains and Eipper[29] who have studied the biosynthesis of ACTH and beta-endorphin in AtT-20 tumor cells. As soon as beta-LPH is cleaved from the precursor, its maturation into beta-endorphin is very fast. Even after a 20 min chase when beta-LPH is the predominant form, a small peak is probably formed by the same enzymatic cleavage step.

Even after a 2 hrs chase, a fraction of the initial precursor still remained in the cells but its apparent molecular weight has increased from 30,000 to 36,000. This result has also been observed in AtT-20 tumor cell and could be explained by an increased glycosylation of the peptide backbone[27]. The extensively glycosylated precursor could represent a stable form which could have its own biological role.

Beta-endorphin biosynthesis in the rat intermediate lobe is very similar to the mechanism of ACTH and beta-LPH biosynthesis proposed by Mains and Eipper[29] for AtT-20 cells, a tumor cell line derived from the adenohypophysis. However, the control of hormone secretion in the intermediate lobe seems to be different from the anterior lobe[38,39]. The experiments described in this report conclusively show that the pars intermedia of the pituitary is a highly specialized tissue for the synthesis of the large molecular weight precursor which is transformed into beta-endorphin with beta-LPH as an intermediate. There seems to be no further maturation of beta-endorphin into enkephalin. This constitutes an excellent model, if not the best so far, to study the biosynthesis of beta-endorphin in normal tissue. Moreover, in view of the recent demonstration that pituitary hormones can be directly transferred into the brain[40,41], the pituitary gland might be the main source, if not the only one, of brain beta-endorphin.

SUMMARY

Rat pars intermedia cells incubated for 10 min with radioactive amino acids produced one major labeled protein with a m.w. of 28,500 ± 1,500. It contains in its sequence the antigenic determinants for ACTH and beta-MSH by immunoprecipitation. This large molecular weight protein was chased by a further incubation in presence of an excess of unlabeled amino acid and the initial protein was degraded mainly into beta-endorphin and beta-LPH. Another 18,000 daltons peptide was also observed which could be a large molecular form of ACTH. From the kinetics of the maturation of the initial precursor, it is concluded that the initial cleavage of the 28,500 dalton peptide gives rise to beta-LPH and the 18,000 dalton form of ACTH and beta-LPH is subsequently cleaved to form beta-endorphin.

ACKNOWLEDGMENTS

This work was supported by a MRC Program Grant, and the CRSQ.

REFERENCES

1. Chrétien, M., Seidah, N.G., Benjannet, S., Dragon, M., Routhier, R., Motomatsu, T., Crine, P., & Lis, M. (1977) Ann. N.Y. Acad. Sci. 297, 84-107

2. Hughes, J., Smith, T.W., Kosterlitz, H.W., Fothergill, L.A., Morgan, B.A. & Morris, H.R. (1975) Nature 258, 577-579.

3. Chrétien, M., Benjannet, S., Dragon, N., Seidah, N.G. & Lis, M. (1976) Biochem. Biophys. Res. Commun. 72, 472-478.

4. Li, C.H., Chung, D. & Doneen, B.A. (1976) Biochem. Biophys. Res. Commun. 72, 1542-1547.

5. Li, C.H. & Chung, D. (1976) Proc. Natl. Acad. Sci. USA 73, 1145-1148.

6. Bradbury, A.F., Smyth, D.G., Snell, G.R., Birdsell, N.J.M. & Hulme, E.C. (1976) Nature 260, 793-795.

7. Lazarus, L.H., Ling, N. & Guillemin, R. (1976) Proc. Natl. Acad. Sci. USA 73, 2156-2159.

8. Guillemin, R., Ling, N. & Burgus, R. (1976) C.R. Hebd. Seances Acad. Sci. Ser. D 282, 783-785.

9. Cox, B.M., Goldstein, A. & Li, C.H. (1976) Proc. Natl. Acad. Sci. USA 73, 1821-1823.

10. Chrétien, M. & Li, C.H. (1967) Can. J. Biochem. 45, 1163-1174.

11. Chrétien, M. & Gilardeau, C. (1970) Can. J. Biochem. 48, 511-516.

12. Steiner, D.F., Kemmley, W., Tager, H.S. & Peterson, J.D. (1974) Fed. Proc. 33, 2105-2115.

13. Bertagna, X., Lis, M., Gilardeau, C. and Chrétien, M. (1974) Can. J. Biochem. 52, 349-358.

14. Chrétien, M., Benjannet, S., Bertagna, X., Lis, M. & Chrétien, M. (1974) Clin. Res. 22, 730.

15. Chrétien, M., Lis, M., Gilardeau, C. & Benjannet, S. (1976) Can. J. Biochem. 54, 566-570.

16. Crine, P., Benjannet, S., Seidah, N.G., Lis, M. & Chrétien, M. (1977) Proc. Natl. Acad. Sci. USA 74, 1403-1406.

17. Crine, P., Benjannet, S., Seidah, N.G., Lis, M. & Chrétien, M. (1977) Proc. Natl. Acad. Sci. USA 74, 4276-4280.

18. LaBella, F., Queen, G., Senyshyn, J., Lis, M. & Chrétien, M. (1977) Biochem. Biophys. Res. Commun. 75, 350-357.

19. Moriarty, G.C. (1973) J. Histochem. Cytochem. 21, 855-894.

20. Rubinstein, M., Stein, S., Gerber, L.D. & Udenfriend, S. (1977) Proc. Natl. Acad. Sci. USA 74, 3052-3055.

21. Rubinstein, M., Stein, S. & Udenfriend, S. (1977) Proc. Natl. Acad. Sci. USA 74, 4969-4972.

22. Moon, H.D., Li, C.H. & Jennings, B.M. (1973) Anat. Res. 175, 529-538.

23. Pelletier, G., Leclerc, R., Labrie, F., Côté, J., Chrétien, M. & Lis, M. (1977) Endocrinology 100, 770-776.

24. Bloom, F., Battenberg, E.O., Rossier, J., Ling, N., Leppeluoto, J., Vargo, T.M. & Guillemin, R. (1977) Life Sci. 20, 43-48.

25. Mains, R.E., Eipper, B.A. & Ling, N. (1977) Proc. Natl. Acad. Sci. USA 74, 3014-3018.

26. Roberts, J.L. & Herbert (1977) Proc. Natl. Acad. Sci. USA 74, 4826-4830.

27. Roberts, J.L. & Herbert, E. (1977) Proc. Natl. Acad. Sci. USA 74, 5300-5304.

28. Mains, R.E. & Eipper, B.A. (1976) J. Biol. Chem. 251, 4115-4120.

29. Mains, R.E. & Eipper, B.A. (1978) J. Biol. Chem. 253, 651-655.

30. Kraicer, J. & Morris, A.R. (1976) Neuroendocrinology 20, 79-96.

31. Richelson, E. & Thompson, E.F. (1973) Nature New Biol. 241, 201-204.

32. Reisfield, R.A., Lewis, U.J. & Williams, E.D. (1962) Nature 195, 281-283.

33. Seidah, N.G., Gianoulakis, C., Crine, P., Lis, M., Benjannet, S., Routhier, R. & Chrétien, M. Proc. Natl. Acad. Sci. USA (In Press).

34. Weber, K. & Osborn, M. (1969) J. Biol. Chem. 244, 4406-4412.

35. Swank, R.T. & Munkres, K.D. (1971) Anal. Biochem. 39, 462-477.

36. Pezalla, P.D., Clarke, W.C., Lis, M., Seidah, N.G. & Chrétien, M. (1978) Gen. Comp. Endocrinol. 39, 163-168.

37. Lis, M. & Chrétien, M. (Unpublished results).

38. Kraicer, J., Gosbee, J.L. & Bencosme, S.A. (1973) Neuroendocrinology 11, 156-176.

39. Moriarty, C.M. and Moriarty, G.C. (1975) Endocrinology 96, 1419-1425.

40. Oliver, D., Mical, R.S. & Porter, J.C. (1977) Endocrinology 101, 598-604.

41. Bergland, R.M. & Page, R.B. (1978) Endocrinology 78, 1325-1337.

Characteristics and Function of Opioids, editors Van Ree and Terenius
© 1978 Elsevier/North-Holland Biomedical Press

BIOSYNTHESIS AND RELEASE OF ENKEPHALINS

A.T. McKNIGHT, R.P. SOSA, J. HUGHES* and H.W. KOSTERLITZ
Unit for Research on Addictive Drugs, University of Aberdeen, Aberdeen AB9 1AS,
Scotland and *Imperial College of Science and Technology, Department of
Biochemistry, South Kensington, London, SW7, England

ABSTRACT

The evidence for synthesis and release of enkephalins is reviewed.   Methods
for studying enkephalin synthesis in guinea-pig striatum and ileum and release
from guinea-pig ileum in vitro are described.

INTRODUCTION

Two important criteria which must be fulfilled before any substance can be
established as a neurotransmitter are that the substance itself and the means
for its synthesis must be present in neurones and the substance must be released following activation of these neurones.   There is much good evidence
from immunohistochemical studies that enkephalins are contained in neurones in
the central and peripheral nervous systems[1,2].   The purpose of this paper is
to review the existing evidence, and in particular to present our own recent
evidence that the remaining criteria are fulfilled for the enkephalins.

ENKEPHALIN BIOSYNTHESIS

When the enkephalins were originally isolated and their structures elucidated it was proposed, since the methionine enkephalin (ME) pentapeptide sequence
occurred between residues 61 and 65 of the β-lipotropin (β-LPH) structure, that
ME synthesis might proceed through β-LPH as precursor[3] and by analogy that a
similar precursor might exist for leucine enkephalin (LE)[4].   Attractive as
this hypothesis may be, there is no experimental evidence in its favour.
Since long term hypophysectomy does not alter the distribution or levels of
enkephalins in rat brain[5,6,7,8], circulating β-LPH of pituitary origin is
clearly not the source of the ME which is widely distributed in the central and
peripheral nervous system as has been proposed[9].   There is also some doubt
whether ME can be derived from β-LPH of local origin since there is no clear
correlation between the distributions of ME and β-LPH-like immunoreactive
material in rat brain[10,11].   For similar reasons β-endorphin is an unlikely
source of ME[12,13].

Several groups have attacked the problem of enkephalin biosynthesis by attempting to study the incorporation of radio-isotopically labelled amino acids into the enkephalins.   The short term goals of these experiments must first be to determine whether the synthetic pathway involves ribosomal or non-ribosomal assembly and whether enkephalins are in fact derived from larger precursor peptides.   One approach has been to study the incorporation of labelled amino acid after in vivo administration.   Such experiments, by providing data for the time courses of appearance and subsequent disappearance of labelled enkephalins, may yield information about the rate of turnover of enkephalins in vivo.   From the first study of this type Clouet and Ratner[14] concluded that there was a rapid incorporation into the enkephalins of rat brain 15-30 min after intracisternal administration of {^{3}H}-glycine and that the turnover time was less than 3 h.   In contrast, Sosa et al.[15] reported that maximum incorporation of {^{3}H}-tyrosine into enkephalins of rat brain occurred in less than one hour but remained constant for 16 hours after intracisternal administration. More recently, Yang et al.[16] reported that the maximum incorporation of {^{3}H}-glycine into rat striatal enkephalins after intracerebroventricular administration was reached after 15 min while the incorporation of {^{3}H}-tyrosine into whole brain minus striatum and cerebellum was reached within 30 min and remained constant for at least 2 h.   Valuable as these results are and those from future studies - comparing, say, turnover rates in different brain areas or comparing the effects of different drug treatments undoubtedly will be - these methods are somewhat limited in their usefulness.   The degree of labelling of enkephalins is usually small and variable and these methods can give no information about the synthesis of enkephalins in peripheral sites such as the gut. To overcome these problems, we have recently turned our attention to the use of two in vitro systems for the study of enkephalin biosynthesis: the myenteric plexus-longitudinal muscle from the guinea-pig ileum and striatal slices from guinea-pig brain [15,17].   Although these preparations are undeniably less physiological than the in vivo models, they are more versatile and the former provides the only obvious means of studying enkephalin synthesis at a peripheral site.   Our methods for obtaining incorporation of labelled amino acids into the enkephalins of these tissues and for isolating the labelled enkephalins are outlined below and some preliminary results from our use of these preparations are also described.

Synthesis of enkephalins by guinea-pig ileum and striatum in vitro.   As in the in vivo studies, the incorporation of labelled amino acids into the enkephalin stores of isolated guinea-pig myenteric plexus or striatum was taken as an

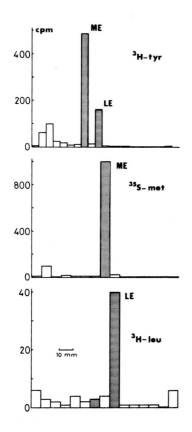

Fig. 1. Thin layer chromatographic separation of labelled enkephalins from myenteric plexus extracts. The labelling period with $\{^3H\}$-Tyr (80 µCi), $\{^{35}S\}$-Met (175 µCi) or $\{^3H\}$-Leu (80 µCi) was 4 h followed by incubation for 3 h with cold amino acids.

index of enkephalin synthesis in these tissues in vitro. After an initial "labelling period" in Krebs-bicarbonate solution at $36^{\circ}C$, saturated with 5% CO_2 in oxygen and containing 11 mM glucose for preparations of myenteric plexus or 22 mM glucose for the striatum plus the appropriate labelled amino acid (L-$\{2,3,5,6-^3H\}$-Tyr, 80 Ci/mmol, L-$\{4,5-^3H\}$-Leu, 20 Ci/mmol or L-$\{^{35}S\}$-Met, 800-1200 Ci/mmol; Radiochemical Centre, Amersham), incubation was continued in fresh medium lacking the labelled amino acid but containing a high concentration (1 µg/ml) of a mixture of cold amino acids (Ala, Arg, Asp, Cys, Glu, Gly, His, Ileu, Leu, Lys, Met, Phe, Pro, Ser, Thr, Trp, Tyr and Val). Preparations of myenteric plexus-longitudinal muscle (300-500 mg) from guinea-pig ileum were suspended under an initial resting tension of 0.5 g in 3 ml organ baths while 0.5 mm thick slices from individual guinea-pig striata were incubated in 10 ml

Krebs solution in 25 ml measuring cylinders. With the preparation of guinea-pig striatum the flow of the O_2/CO_2 gas mixture through the medium was just sufficient to prevent settling and clumping of the slices. In preliminary experiments with this preparation, the incorporation of {^{3}H}-Tyr into the enkephalins of sagittally sectioned slices was greater than that into coronally sectioned slices, and the former were used thereafter. At the end of the appropriate post-labelling incubation time, tissues were homogenised in 15-20 ml of ice-cold 0.1 M HCl containing synthetic carrier enkephalins (20-40 μg of each of ME and LE). The homogenates were centrifuged at 50,000 g for 20 min and the enkephalins were isolated from the supernatants by progressive chromatographic purification by adsorption onto Amberlite XAD-2, eluting with methanol, cation exchange on HC-Pellionex-SCX, desalting the enkephalin-containing fraction from the cation exchange column by a second XAD-2 adsorption step (striatum only) and anion exchange on AE-Pellionex-SAX[15]. Finally, resolution of ME and LE was achieved by thin layer chromatography on silica gel plates (Fig. 1) developed with ethyl acetate/pyridine/water/acetic acid (100:43:25:11) containing either ethane-1,2-dithiol 0.01% (v/v) or dithiothreitol 0.01% (w/v) to minimize oxidation of the sulphur of ME. The spots corresponding to the enkephalins were located for elution with 1 ml of 80% (v/v) methanol and subsequent scintillation counting by spraying the plates with ninhydrin-cadmium

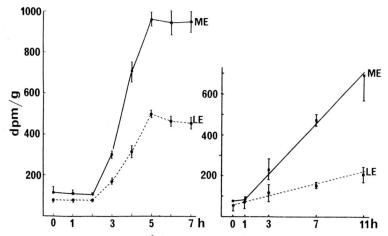

Fig. 2.   Time courses of {^{3}H}-Tyr incorporation into ME and LE of striatal slices (left) and myenteric plexus (right).   The times are for incubation after a labelling period of 30 min (striatum, 50 μCi) or 1 h (myenteric plexus, 10 μCi).

acetate reagent.

Using these methods we have obtained reproducible values for incorporation of labelled amino acids into enkephalins in both tissues (Figs. 1 & 2). In preliminary experiments with the myenteric plexus we observed that {^{3}H}-Tyr was incorporated into both ME and LE while {^{35}S}-Met was incorporated only into ME and {^{3}H}-Leu only into LE (Fig. 1). More recently we have concentrated in particular on the use of {^{3}H}-Tyr since both ME and LE incorporate this amino acid, and we have found that the time courses of incorporation into both enkephalins are similar (Fig. 2). The incorporation of {^{3}H}-Tyr into ME is always at least twice that into LE which probably only reflects the higher content of ME in both sites[18]. Comparing the time courses of incorporation of {^{3}H}-Tyr into the myenteric plexus and striatum, we have shown that the rate of incorporation increases linearly in both tissues after an apparent lag phase (Fig. 2). This is more obvious with the striatum, which may be a result of the shorter labelling time in this tissue, or may be due to an impaired condition of the slices, compared to the more robust myenteric plexus preparation. This explanation may also account for the fact that the incorporation levels off after 5 h in the striatum while it is still increasing even after 11 h in the myenteric plexus (Fig. 2). It is probable that the incorporation of {^{3}H}-Tyr into enkephalin involves ribosomal synthesis since both puromycin and cycloheximide (both 0.1 mM) will inhibit incorporation by more than 90% in the myenteric plexus if they are present throughout the incubations, but hardly affect incorporation at all if they are present only during the post-labelling

TABLE 1

EFFECT OF PUROMYCIN OR CYCLOHEXIMIDE ON INCORPORATION OF {^{3}H}-TYROSINE INTO THE ENKEPHALINS OF THE MYENTERIC PLEXUS

Paired experiments (n = 3). In (A) and (B) puromycin or cycloheximide (0.1 mM) were present throughout the labelling (4 h, 80 µCi) and incubation (2 h) periods. In (C) puromycin was present only during the post-labelling (2 h, 40 µCi) incubation period (4 h).

		ME (dpm g^{-1})	LE (dpm g^{-1})
(A)	Control	3752 ± 240	1424 ± 64
	Puromycin	312 ± 56	200 ± 128
(B)	Control	2888 ± 312	1436 ± 192
	Cycloheximide	544 ± 160	197 ± 72
(C)	Control	1360 ± 188	740 ± 132
	Puromycin	1312 ± 160	560 ± 48

incubation period (Table 1). Similar experiments with the striatal slices have shown that incorporation of {^{3}H}-Tyr can be blocked if cycloheximide is present during the labelling period of 30 min and also the first 2 h of a 5 h-incubation (the "lag phase"), but not at all if the protein synthesis inhibitor is present only during the latter 3 h of the 5-h incubation. We have concluded from these results that the enkephalins of guinea-pig ileum and striatum can be synthesized locally from a precursor or precursors also produced locally and that the synthetic pathway involves ribosomal assembly of the precursor peptide and conversion to enkephalin from this precursor. Since the rate of incorporation of {^{3}H}-Tyr into enkephalins remains constant for a long time, particularly in the myenteric plexus, it may be that there is a large pool of rapidly synthesized precursor which is only comparatively slowly converted to enkephalin and these methods may therefore prove useful in future attempts to identify the precursors of the enkephalins.

RELEASE OF ENKEPHALINS

The evidence for release of enkephalins, or more correctly of opiate-like substances, in the whole animal is circumstantial since it comes largely from the results of experiments where the effects of opiate antagonists in avoidance-behaviour tests are observed. It is implied that where naloxone, for example, by itself produces an effect in a particular test, then that effect is due to antagonism of the action of released opioid peptides (for examples, see ref. 19). In addition, analgesia following periaqueductal grey stimulation in animals[20] and in man[21], and also during acupuncture[22,23], may involve the release of opiate-like substances since the analgesia is at least partially blocked by naloxone. For a number of reasons, beyond the scope of this review, it is more likely that if these effects do involve the release of an opioid peptide, this will be β-endorphin rather than enkephalin. All the direct evidence for neurally-evoked release of enkephalins has come from experiments using isolated tissues, either from brain or from gut.

Release of enkephalins from isolated preparations of brain has been demonstrated by several groups after depolarization either by excess K$^+$ (50 mM) or by veratridine (50 μM). In support of the claim that the enkephalins are neurotransmitters, it was shown that the K$^+$-induced release from rat brain synaptosomes[24], rabbit striatal synaptosomes[25], rat globus pallidus slices[26] and rat striatal slices[27], was calcium-dependent and that veratridine-induced release from guinea-pig striatal slices was blocked by tetrodotoxin[25]. In these experiments, the preparations were exposed to the depolarizing agent for varying times and the amount of enkephalin released during these exposures, estimated either by bioassay on the mouse vas deferens or by radioimmunoassay, ranged from 2-30% of the total tissue contents. The use of the myenteric plexus-longitudinal muscle preparation of guinea-pig ileum was expected to yield data for release of enkephalins by more physiological means, i.e. after field stimulation of intramural nerves at various frequencies. Although there is good indirect evidence for release of opiate-like material from the myenteric plexus after stimulation at 10 Hz[28], a number of attempts in various laboratories to demonstrate any such release directly have been notably unsuccessful, with a single reported exception. Schulz et al.[29] have been able to detect variable, but in some instances unexpectedly large amounts of enkephalins in the bath fluid after stimulating preparations of myenteric plexus for one hour at 0.1 Hz. In view of our own lack of success in detecting release of enkephalins from the myenteric plexus directly, we have resorted to the following indirect method for estimating stimulation evoked release[30]. The rationale for this method is that in the presence of a protein synthesis inhibitor, any enkephalin mobilized from the tissue stores by nerve stimulation will not be replaced by de nouveau synthesis and a measure of the tissue content at the end of the stimulation period compared to an unstimulated control, will provide an indication of the amount of enkephalin released.

Enkephalin release from the myenteric plexus of the guinea-pig ileum in the presence of cycloheximide. Preparations of myenteric plexus-longitudinal muscle were set up as described above in Krebs-bicarbonate solution containing 1 μg/ml of each of the amino acids already listed and also 20 μg/ml ascorbic acid. After 30 min preincubation, cycloheximide (0.1 mM) was added and the incubation was continued for a further 30 min when field stimulation (0.5 ms, supramaximal voltage) was started. Stimulation at all frequencies was continuous for periods of 0.5 to 4 h and during this time the bathing fluid was replaced by overflow every 20 min. At the end of the stimulation period, tissues were homogenised in 0.1 M HCl and centrifuged and enkephalins were extracted from the supernatants by adsorption onto XAD-2 and elution with methanol. The total tissue contents of enkephalins were measured by bracket assay against ME standards on the mouse vas deferens; the reversal by the opiate antagonist naloxone (900 nM) was used to test for the specificity of ME-like activity in the tissue extracts[18]. The results are shown in Table 2. Stimulation at 10 Hz reduced the content by 18% in 30 min and by 46% in 1 h; but continuing stimulation at this frequency for up to 2 h produced no further decrease. Stimulation at 1 Hz for 2 and 4 h reduced the content by 5 and 14%, respectively,

TABLE 2

ENKEPHALIN CONTENT OF THE MYENTERIC PLEXUS AFTER ELECTRICAL FIELD STIMULATION IN THE PRESENCE OF CYCLOHEXIMIDE (0.1 mM)

	Duration (min)	Enkephalin content as ME (pmol g^{-1})	Differences
Unstimulated 0.1 Hz	240	428 ± 38 436 ± 19	8.7 ± 24.3(5)
Unstimulated 1 Hz	120	539 ± 41 511 ± 37	28.8 ± 5.2(3)[a]
Unstimulated 1 Hz	240	510 ± 49.1 440 ± 50	70 ± 12.5(5)[a]
Unstimulated 10 Hz	30	506 ± 77 416 ± 74	90 ± 10.1(3)[b]
Unstimulated 10 Hz	60	434 ± 36 237 ± 37	197 ± 14.7(4)[b]
Unstimulated 10 Hz	120	446 ± 59 247 ± 22	199 ± 43.3(5)[b]

[a] $p < 0.05$

[b] $p < 0.01$

while with 0.1 Hz no reduction was observed even after 4 h. We confirmed that these reductions in enkephalin content were due to loss from the tissue stores after stimulation-evoked release by the finding that tetrodotoxin (0.3 μM) blocked the decrease caused by stimulation at 10 Hz for 1 h (Table 3). From

TABLE 3

INHIBITION BY TETRODOTOXIN OF THE DECREASE IN ENKEPHALIN CONTENT DUE TO ELECTRICAL STIMULATION IN THE PRESENCE OF CYCLOHEXIMIDE (0.1 mM)

	Enkephalin content as ME (pmol g^{-1})	Differences
Unstimulated	381 ± 39	
		174 ± 29(4)[a]
10 Hz	207 ± 22	
		182 ± 39(4)[a]
10 Hz, TTX (0.3 μM	389 ± 53	

[a] $p < 0.01$

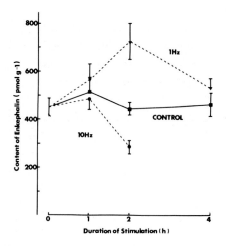

Fig. 3. Enkephalin content of the myenteric plexus longitudinal muscle after electrical stimulation in the absence of cycloheximide. The differences between the contents of the stimulated and non-stimulated (control) preparations were significant for 1 Hz after 2 h ($P < 0.005$) and 4 h ($P < 0.05$), and for 10 Hz after 2 h ($P < 0.0005$) ($n = 4$).

these results we have estimated that the amount of enkephalin released per pulse during stimulation at 1 and 10 Hz is about 4-5 fmol/g (fractional release of the order of 10^5). This estimate may be too low since it has not been established that 0.1 mM cycloheximide blocks synthesis completely and also the possible existence of a large store of precursor may mean that the tissue's demands for releaseable enkephalin may be met for a considerable time. By repeating these experiments in the absence of cycloheximide we were able to assess whether de nouveau synthesis of enkephalin could offset the loss due to release and by how much. The difference between corresponding values for enkephalin contents obtained in the presence (Table 2) and in the absence of cycloheximide (Fig. 3) would give an indication of the turnover of enkephalins during stimulation at that frequency for that time. Thus the maximum turnover occurs after stimulation at 1 Hz for 2 h. Since there is an increase in content after stimulation in the absence of cycloheximide of about 340 pmol/g (Fig. 3) and in the corresponding experiment with cycloheximide present the content was decreased by 28.8 pmol/g (Table 2), it follows that the turnover during 2 h was about 370 pmol enkephalin/g tissue. Since the enkephalin content is increased after stimulation at 1 Hz for 2 h in the absence of cycloheximide (Fig. 3) it appears that enkephalin synthesis is stimulated and actually overcompensates for the loss due to release, while stimulation at 10 Hz for the same duration still produces a reduction (36%) only 6% less than that observed in the presence of cycloheximide, implying that enkephalin synthesis may be inhibited under these conditions.

SUMMARY

A method for obtaining incorporation of labelled amino acids into the enkephalin stores of guinea-pig striatum and ileum in vitro is described. Results obtained using this method are consistent with the view that enkephalins are synthesized locally from precursors also synthesized locally by ribosomal assembly.

An indirect method for measuring stimulation-evoked enkephalin release and turnover in preparations of the myenteric plexus from guinea-pig ileum is described. At stimulation frequencies of 1 and 10 Hz the release of enkephalin per pulse is about 4-5 fmol/g and the turnover during stimulation at 1 Hz for 2 h is 300-400 pmol/g.

ACKNOWLEDGEMENTS

Supported by grants from the Medical Research Council, the U.S. National Institute on Drug Abuse and the U.S. Committee on Problems of Drug Dependence.

REFERENCES

1. Elde, R., Hökfelt, T., Johansson, O. and Terenius, L. (1976) Neuroscience, 1, 349-351.

2. Simantov, R., Kuhar, M.J., Uhl, G.R. and Snyder, S.H. (1977) Proc. natn. Acad. Sci. U.S.A., 74, 2167-2171.

3. Hughes, J., Smith, T.W., Kosterlitz, H.W., Fothergill, L.A., Morgan, B.A. and Morris, H.R. (1975) Nature, Lond., 258, 577-579.

4. Hughes, J., Kosterlitz, H.W., McKnight, A.T., Sosa, R.P., Lord, J.A.H., Waterfield, A.A. (1978) in Centrally Acting Peptides, Hughes, J. ed., Macmillan Press Ltd., London, pp. 179-194.

5. Cheung, A.L. and Goldstein, A. (1976) Life Sci., 19, 1005-1008.

6. Hong, J.S., Yang, H.-Y.T., Fratta, W. and Costa, E. (1977) Brain Res., 134, 383-386.

7. Wesche, D., Höllt, V. and Herz, A. (1977) Naunyn-Schmiedeberg's Arch. Pharmac., 301, 79-82.

8. Kobayashi, R.M., Palkovits, M., Miller, R.J., Chang, K.-J. and Cuatrecasas, P. (1978) Life Sci., 22, 527-530.

9. Lazarus, L.H., Ling, N. and Guillemin, R. (1976) Proc. natn. Acad. Sci. U.S.A., 73, 2156-2159.

10. Watson, S.J., Barchas, J.D. and Li, C.H. (1977) Proc. natn. Acad. Sci. U.S.A., 74, 5155-5158.

11. Watson, S.J., Akil, H., Sullivan, S. and Barchas, J.D. (1977) Life Sci., 21, 733-738.

12. Rossier, J., Vargo, T.M., Minick, S., Ling, N., Bloom, F.E. and Guillemin, R. (1977) Proc. natn. Acad. Sci. U.S.A., 74, 5162-5165.

13. Bloom, F., Battenberg, E., Rossier, J., Ling, N. and Guillemin, R. (1978) Proc. natn. Acad. Sci., 75, 1591-1595.

14. Clouet, D.H. and Ratner, M. (1976) in Opiates and Endogenous Opioid Peptides, Kosterlitz, H.W. ed., Elsevier/North Holland Press, Amsterdam, pp. 71-78.

15. Sosa, R.P., McKnight, A.T., Hughes, J. and Kosterlitz, H.W. (1977) FEBS Lett., 84, 195-198.

16. Yang, H.-Y.T., Hong, J.S., Fratta, W. and Costa, E. (1978) in Endorphins, Costa, E. and Trabucchi, M. eds., Raven Press, New York, pp. 149-160.

17. Hughes, J., Kosterlitz, H.W. and McKnight, A.T. (1978) Br. J. Pharmac., 63, 396P.

18. Hughes, J., Kosterlitz, H.W. and Smith, T.W. (1977) Br. J. Pharmac., 61, 639-647.

19. Frederickson, R.C.A. (1977) Life Sci., 21, 23-42.

20. Akil, H., Mayer, D.J. and Liebeskind, J.C. (1976) Science N.Y., 191, 961-962.

21. Adams, J.E. (1976) Pain, 2, 161-166.

22. Sjölund, B. and Eriksson, M. (1976) Lancet, ii, 1085.

23. Pomeranz, B. and Chiu, D. (1976) Life Sci., 19, 1757-1762.

24. Smith, T.W., Hughes, J., Kosterlitz, H.W. and Sosa, R.P. (1976) in Opiates and Endogenous Opioid Peptides, Kosterlitz, H.W. ed., Elsevier/North Holland Press, Amsterdam, pp. 57-62.

25. Henderson, G., Hughes, J. and Kosterlitz, H.W. (1978) Nature, Lond., 271, 677-679.

26. Iversen, L.L., Iversen, S.D., Bloom, F.E., Vargo, T. and Guillemin, R. (1978) Nature, Lond., 271, 679-681.

27. Osborne, H., Höllt, V. and Herz, A. (1978) Eur. J. Pharmac., 48, 219-221.

28. Puig, M.M., Gascón, P., Craviso, G.L. and Musacchio, J.M. (1977) Science N.Y., 195, 419-420.

29. Schulz, R., Wüster, M., Simantov, R., Snyder, S. and Herz, A. (1977) Eur. J. Pharmac., 41, 347-348.

30. Hughes, J., Kosterlitz, H.W. and Sosa, R.P. (1978) Br. J. Pharmac., 63, 397P.

Characteristics and Function of Opioids, editors Van Ree and Terenius
© *1978 Elsevier/North-Holland Biomedical Press*

CHARACTERIZATION OF THE OPIOID EFFECTS OF CEREBROSPINAL FLUID FROM MORPHINE TREATED RABBITS ON RODENTS.

WILLIAM L. DEWEY, TSU-CHING FU, CONSUELO IZAZOLA-CONDE and STEPHEN HALENDA
Department of Pharmacology, Medical College of Virginia, MCV Station 726,
Richmond, Virginia   23298

Introduction

Previous experiments have demonstrated that humoral mechanisms are involved in morphine's antinociceptive activity as quantitated by the mouse tail-flick test. Antinociceptive doses of morphine were inactive in mice spinalized by ligation or cauterization but were as potent as when given to intact mice when the neural component of the spinal cord was destroyed and the humoral component kept intact, i.e., spinalization with dura mater intact. A partial interruption of the humoral component without damage to the neural component significantly reduced the antinociceptive activity of morphine in mice, i.e., removal of a portion of the dura mater at T11-13 or making an opening in the cisterna magnum allowed the CSF to leak out rather than be transported to more caudal regions of the spinal cord. The purpose of the experiments reported here was to quantitate the opioid activity of cerebrospinal fluid taken prior to and 60 minutes after the subcutaneous injection of 10 mg/kg morphine to rabbits.

Methods

The opioid activity of the CSF was quantitated in the phenylquinone (ppq) induced writhing and coaxially stimulated guinea pig ileum assays. Mice were injected intracerebroventricularly with 5 µl of CSF which was followed 10 minutes later by the i.p. injection of 3 mg/kg ppq. The number of writhes during the 10th and 15th minute after the injections were counted. Other samples of CSF (0.1 - 0.4 ml) were added to a 10 ml tissue bath which contained the coaxially stimulated guinea pig ileum.

Results

The data presented in table 1 show that the CSF taken prior to the injection of morphine significantly reduced the number of writhes induced by ppq indicating that control rabbit CSF contains a substance with antinociceptive activity. CSF taken after morphine had a much greater inhibitory effect.

TABLE 1

EFFECTS OF CSF FROM MORPHINE TREATED RABBITS ON PHENYLQUINONE INDUCED WRITHING
IN MICE

Treatment	# of groups of 6 mice	# of Writhes $\bar{x} \pm$ S.E.M.	Percent Inhibition
1. Control	6	37 ± 1.30	0
2. CSF before MSO$_4$	10	32 ± 1.07	13%
3. CSF after MSO$_4$	10	21 ± 1.29	42%
4. Naloxone pretreated (mice)			
1. CSF before MSO$_4$	3	37 ± 1.20	0
2. CSF after MSO$_4$	8	37 ± 0.78	0

The inhibitory effect of both samples of CSF were antagonized by 2 mg/kg
naloxone given i.p. to the mice 10 minutes prior to the injection of the CSF.
These data support the hypothesis that an endogenous substance with opioid
activity is released into the CSF by morphine.

CSF taken from rabbits prior to the injection of morphine caused an inhibition of the coaxially stimulated induced contractions of guinea pig ileum
and CSF taken after morphine had a greater inhibitory effect. Naloxone added
to the bath prior to the addition of either sample of CSF blocked their
inhibitory activity. Preliminary experiments in rats confirmed the results
described above in rabbits.

The increased opioid activity of CSF after the injection of morphine could
be due to the presence of morphine in the CSF. Rabbits were injected with
radiolabelled dihydromorphine (40 CimM) and the quantity found in the CSF of
three rabbits ranged from 3×10^{-9} M to 10^{-11} M. These concentrations are
inactive in the phenylquinone assay and at least 10-fold less than the mini-
mally effective dose in the guinea pig ileum assay.

Therefore, we conclude from these studies that an endogenous substance
which exists·in CSF has opiate activity and the injection of morphine
increases the activity of this material probably due to an increase in its
release from the brain.

Characteristics and Function of Opioids, editors Van Ree and Terenius
© 1978 Elsevier/North-Holland Biomedical Press

RADIOIMMUNOASSAY FOR β-ENDORPHIN IN HUMAN PLASMA

VARTAN GHAZAROSSIAN, R.R.DENT, M.ROSS, B.M.COX, AVRAM GOLDSTEIN

Addiction Research Foundation, Palo Alto, California 94304 U.S.A.

In our view there are seven minimum necessary criteria for asserting that one has a valid assay for β-endorphin (in contrast to "β-endorphin immunoreactivity") in plasma. The procedure we describe here does not yet fully meet these criteria, but a progress report seems in order.

Method: Heparinized human plasma (5 ml) is adjusted to pH 4, and silicic acid (300 mg) is added in a glass tube. After centrifuging and washing twice with water then with 1N HCl, the gel is eluted in 50% acetone. Evaporation under N_2 at 45° yields a barely visible glassy residue, which is taken up in 0.5 ml of neutral phosphate buffer saline with 0.1% BSA and assayed in triplicate using an antiserum to α-endorphin and ^{125}I-α-endorphin trace, as described elsewhere.

Criteria: (1) The material in plasma should react with the antiserum in the same manner as authentic β-endorphin and should yield a parallel dilution curve. This criterion is met. Our antiserum recognizes β_h-endorphin with IC_{50}=180 pM. Opiate alkaloid agonists and antagonists do not react. Direct assays in plasma or cerebrospinal fluid were abandoned; we found trace displacement (or degradation) equivalent to β-endorphin in the nanomolar range, resistant to pronase, and yielding nonparallel dilution curves. A parallel dilution curve is obtained with plasma extracts.

(2) Blanks not containing plasma should give no reactivity. This criterion is met, except that trace displacement of a few percent is not unusual, especially in the presence of salt. As with other immunoassays, results are only reliable in the steep central part of the standard curve (e.g., 25-75%). This requirement accounts for the need to extract a full 5 ml of human plasma.

(3) Immunoreactivity of the material in plasma should be destroyed by proteases. This criterion remains to be tested.

(4) β-endorphin added to plasma in different amounts, down to endogenous levels, should be recovered adequately. This criterion is met. With ^{125}I-β_h-endorphin, overall recovery was about 60%. Addition of nonradioactive β_h-endorphin followed by radioimmunoassay yields a good linear relationship between fmoles added and fmoles recovered, with a y-axis intercept corresponding to 30 pM β_h-endorphin equivalent per ml original plasma.

(5) The material in plasma should closely resemble β_h-endorphin in its chemical and physical properties. This criterion is thus far partially met. On Bio-Gel P-10 columns, material from 40 ml of pooled human plasma yielded

two major peaks of immunoreactivity corresponding to elution positions of β_h-LPH and β_h-endorphin. Variable amounts of a third, as yet unidentified, component are also found.

(6) <u>Plasma from hypophysectomized humans should yield much less (or none) of the immunoreactive material</u>. This criterion is not yet fully met. A 24-hr postoperative sample contained much less immunoreactivity, but not zero. Further studies will assay other pituitary hormones to validate the completeness of hypophysectomy.

(7) <u>The assay should have acceptably low variance between replicates.</u> In the immunoassay itself, agreement among triplicates is within a few percent. However, agreement between assays of independent parallel extractions of the same plasma is not yet satisfactory.

<u>Conclusions</u>: We are able to measure by radioimmunoassay a substance in human plasma, which appears to be β-endorphin. In some ambulatory normal males and females during the daytime we have found a concentration around 10-20 pM β-endorphin, exclusive of other immunoreactive substances. β-LPH appears to be present also, in about the same concentration range.

This low basal concentration is nearly 1000 times less than required for significant occupancy of known opiate receptors or for producing a small degree of analgesia in man.[2] Thus, β-endorphin in plasma may only be a by-product of ACTH secretion. Alternatively, β-endorphin might be secreted from pituitary back into the cerebroventricular system, eventually entering blood at great dilution. Although β-endorphin in peripheral plasma may not be enroute to physiologic targets, its level there could nonetheless be indicative of the functional status of the endorphin system.

This work was supported by HEW grant DA-1199.

References:

1. M.Ross, V.Ghazarossian, B.M.Cox, A.Goldstein; Life Sci. 22:1123, 1978.

2. D.H.Catlin, K.K.Hui, H.H.Loh, C.H.Li; Comm. Psychopharm 1:493, 1977.

Characteristics and Function of Opioids, editors Van Ree and Terenius
© 1978 Elsevier/North-Holland Biomedical Press

ADRENALECTOMY CHANGES ENDOGENOUS OPIOID CONTENT IN RAT HYPOTHALAMUS

A. Gibson, M. Ginsburg, M. Hall, S.L. Hart and I. Kitchen.
Department of Pharmacology, Chelsea College, London, SW3 6LX, U.K.

INTRODUCTION

Naloxone inhibits, and normorphine enhances the ether induced rise in plasma corticosteroids in mice suggesting the involvement of endogenous opioids in the hypothalamus-pituitary-adrenal (HPA) axis[1]. This has been investigated further by measurement of rat hypothalamic enkephalin levels in altered functional states of the HPA axis.

MATERIALS AND METHODS

Male Wistar albino rats (200-250g) were housed in a controlled light cycle room. Sham operations and bilateral adrenalectomies (ADX) were performed under ether anaesthesia. All animals were maintained on 0.9% NaCl. Extraction of enkephalin, assay procedures, and apparent M.W. determinations by gel filtration, were essentially as described by Hughes et al[2]. The estimated recovery was 96.1% ± 5.5, n = 9.

RESULTS AND DISCUSSION

TABLE 1

Enkephalin content of hypothalamus in sham operated and ADX rats

Ng met-enkephalin equivalents g^{-1} wet weight ± S.E.M. Number of animals in parentheses. t-test, sham vs ADX, *$P<0.05$; control vs operated, †$P<0.05$.

		24h	3 day	6 day	11 day	18 day
Series I	Sham		397± 32 (9)†*	1297±130 (6)†*	576±132 (6)	717± 55 (6)
Control 671±30 (10)	ADX		510± 32 (8)†*	570± 73 (6)*	905± 83 (8)†	1160±308 (5)
Series II	Sham	613±75 (6)†	1114± 79 (8)	1180±136 (8)*	779± 84 (9)	1003± 89 (8)
Control 940±63 (21)	ADX	511±41 (6)†	976±109 (9)	765±103 (7)*	922± 81 (10)	927± 76 (8)

Control levels of enkephalin differed significantly between two series of experiments (P<0.001) and although the overall pattern of post-operative changes was similar there were differences in the time course. Enkephalin levels fell initially after both operations but the repletion of enkephalin was more rapid in intact rats. Addition of dexamethasone to drinking water (20μg ml^{-1}) of unoperated rats for 24h increased hypothalamic enkephalin significantly (P<0.002).

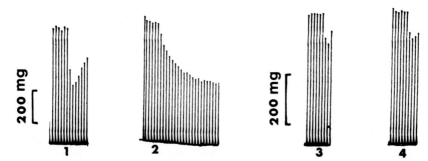

FIG.1: Isometric contractions of mouse vas deferens to field stimulation (0.1Hz, 1ms, 530mA:200mg tension). Effect of 1)40nM met-enkephalin 2)50μl atypical extract 3)16nM met-enkephalin 4)50μl enkephalin-like extract. All inhibitions were reversed by naloxone (900nM).

Experiments in which the most striking changes seen after ADX are excluded from Table 1; in 9 out of the 69 hypothalamic extracts from ADX rats the vas deferens response was atypically prolonged (Fig.1). This was not seen in any of the 97 extracts from intact rats. The apparent M.W. estimated by gel filtration was c.600. The amounts of atypical opioid were variable and in terms of met-enkephalin equivalent, often very large - as much as 60 times that of enkephalin in control hypothalamus.

These results suggest that hypothalamic enkephalin is involved in laparotomy stress; that glucocorticosteroids may participate in short-term regulation of enkephalin in some hypothalamic neurones; and that an atypical opioid may be involved in this regulation.

ACKNOWLEDGEMENTS: This work was supported by the Medical Research Council. I.K. is an MRC student.

REFERENCES

1. Gibson, A., Ginsburg, M., Hall, M. and Hart, S.L. (1977) J.Physiol., 270, 28P.

2. Hughes, J., Kosterlitz, H.W. and Smith, T.W. (1977) Brit.J.Pharm., 61, 639-647.

Characteristics and Function of Opioids, editors Van Ree and Terenius
© *1978 Elsevier/North-Holland Biomedical Press*   277

REGIONAL DISTRIBUTION OF ENDORPHINS IN HUMAN BRAIN AND PITUITARY

CH. GRAMSCH, V. HÖLLT, P. MEHRAEIN, A. PASI* AND A. HERZ
Department of Neuropharmacology, Max-Planck-Institut für Psychia-
trie, Kraepelinstrasse 2, D-8000 München 40 (F.R.G.)
Gerichtlich Medizinisches Institut der Universität Zürich,
Zürichbergstrasse 8, CH-8028 Zürich 7

ABSTRACT
    Concentrations of methionine-enkephalin- (met-enkephalin) and ß-
endorphin immunoreactivity were determined in 33 areas of human
brain and in pituitary and found to have quite different distribution patterns, suggesting their existence in independent systems in
the central nervous system.

INTRODUCTION
    Met-enkephalin and ß-endorphin are biologically active peptide
fragments of ß-lipotropin (LPH). It is, therefore, possible that
met-enkephalin arises as a breakdown product of ß-endorphin in the
brain. To investigate this question and in general interest in obtaining data from humans we measured the concentrations of both
peptides in brain and pituitary.

MATERIAL AND METHODS
    RIA for met-enkephalin (0.3% cross-reactivity to leu-enkephalin)
and ß-endorphin (50% cross-reactivity to LPH) were performed according to (1) and (2), resptl. In order to increase the sensitivity of
the RIA for ß-endorphin we developed an affinity chromatographic
procedure for the purification of tissue extracts from human brain,
which were frozen at -70°C between 2 1/2 and 3 h after death.

RESULTS
    Table 1 compares the concentrations of ß-endorphin- and enkepha-
lin-immunoreactivity in various regions of brain and pituitary.
Several other structures not listed, such as the mid brain, pons,
medulla, area postrema, inferior olivary nucleus, geniculate nucleus and red nucleus were also found to contain detectable amounts of
ß-endorphin. Concentrations in various parts of the cerebral cortices (frontal lobe, occipital lobe), cerebellum (vermis, quadrangul-
ar lobe, dentate nucleus) hippocampus, cerebral white matter,

TABLE 1

MET-ENKEPHALIN- AND ß-ENDORPHIN-IMMUNOREACTIVITIES IN HUMAN BRAIN
AND PITUITARY

Values represent the mean ± S.E.M.; number of determination in
parenthesis.

	met-enkephalin pmoles/g	ß-endorphin pmoles/g
Caudate nucleus	1721 ± 530(4)	O (6)
Pallidum	1930 ± 400(5)	O (6)
Putamen	462 ± 70(4)	O (6)
Substantia nigra	1138 ± 340(4)	7 ± 3(3)
Olfactory bulb	170 ± 80(4)	31 ± 9(3)
Periaqueductal gray	168 ± 42(4)	8 ± 4(6)
Superior colliculus	180 ± 80(4)	6 ± 3(4)
Anterior hypothalamus	240 ± 63(5)	82 ± 12(4)
Posterior hypothalamus	195 ± 48(5)	47 ± 11(5)
Mammillary bodies	137 ± 40(4)	19 ± 6(5)
Medial amygdaloid nuclei	70 ± 18(5)	5 ± 2(6)
Septum	O	6 ± 2(2)
Pulvinar of thalamus	70 ± 20(5)	8 ± 3(4)
Pineal gland	50 ± 25(2)	13 ± 8(2)
Pituitary		
Pars distalis	5200 ± 1700(8)	26000 ± 4700(8)
Pars nervosa	642 ± 75(3)	5200 ± 2050(4)
Stalk	2830 ± 890(3)	2680 ± 820(3)

medial and lateral nuclei of thalamus were below the limits of detection of the RIA (0.5 pmole/g). Certain parallels can be seen
between the distribution of the two endorphins measured in the present study and the distribution of opiate receptor binding in human
brain. The periaqueductal gray, containing high concentrations of
met-enkephalin, ß-endorphin and opiate receptors, is particularly
interesting, especially in view of the supposed role of this structure in both drug- and stimulation-produced analgesia[3].

1. Wesche, D. et al. (1977) Naunyn-Schmiedeberg's Arch.Pharmacol., 301, 79-82.
2. Höllt, V. et al. (1978) Naunyn-Schmiedeberg's Arch. Pharmacol., 303,171-174.
3. Herz, A., in A. Herz (Ed.) (1978) Developments in Opiate Research, Dekker, New York, pp. 153-191.

ß-ENDORPHIN-LIKE IMMUNOREACTIVITY (ß-ELI) IN HUMAN PLASMA AND
CEREBROSPINAL FLUID (CSF)

V. HÖLLT*, H.M. EMRICH*, O.A. MÜLLER** AND R. FAHLBUSCH***
*Max-Planck-Institut für Psychiatrie, Kraepelinstrasse 2,
D-8000 München 40; **Med. Klinik Innenstadt, ***Neurochir. Klinik,
Universität München (F.R.G.)

INTRODUCTION

In rats, ACTH and ß-endorphin concentrations in plasma are altered concomitantly in response to stress and after adrenalectomy[1].
We now studied whether or not such a correlation between immunoreactive ACTH and ß-endorphin also exists in the plasma of humans
with pathologically elevated ACTH levels. In addition, since endorphin levels have been found to be altered in the CSF of schizophrenics[2] and since considerable amounts of leucine-ß-endorphin
have been detected in plasma and haemodialysates of schizophrenics
(R. Palmour, personal communication), we have studied the levels of
ß-ELI in plasma and CSF of schizophrenic patients.

MATERIALS AND METHODS

ACTH and ß-endorphin were measured by radioimmunoassay (RIA)
following the extraction of plasma and CSF with silicic acid[3,4].
The RIA for ß-endorphin had a sensitivity of 40 pg/ml plasma or 20
pg/ml CSF. Cross-reactivities: human leucine-ß-endorphin 100%,
human ß-lipotropin 50%, α-, γ-endorphin < 1%, methionine-enkephalin
< 0.1%, human ACTH 1-39 < 0.1%. The RIA for ACTH had a sensitivity
of 2-10 pg ACTH/ml extracted plasma. Cross-reactivities: human
ß-endorphin < 0.1%, human ß-lipotropin < 1%.

RESULTS

Figure 1 shows a close correlation between the ACTH- and ß-endorphin-like immunoreactivity in plasma of patients with Nelson's
syndrome, Cushing's disease and Addison's disease. Gel-filtration
of the immunoreactive components in plasma of a patient with Nelson's syndrome, however, revealed that ß-ELI was to a high percentage (60%) due to substances not distinguishable from ß-lipotropin
and only to a minor extent (15%) due to substances which elute with
ß-endorphin from the column.

280

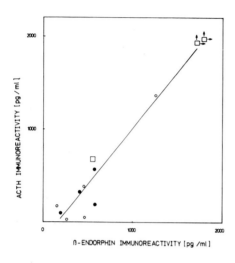

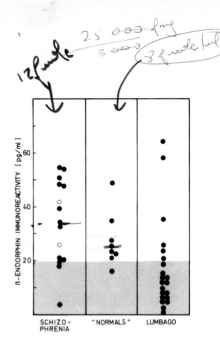

Fig. 1. Correlation between ACTH- and ß-ELI in plasma of patients with Addison's disease (●), Cushing's disease (○) and Nelson's syndrome (□). R = 0.91.

Fig. 2. ß-ELI in CSF of schizophrenics (closed circles: treated with neuroleptics; open circles: without treatment), patients with lumbago and "normals". Sensitivity limit shaded.

Figure 2 shows no significant difference between ß-ELI in the CSF of schizophrenic patients and "normals" (patients suspected to have meningitis which was not confirmed upon subsequent examination). A tendency to lower ß-ELI levels is observed in patients with lumbago (treated with 10 mg diazepam). Similarly, no significant difference was found between ß-ELI in the plasma of schizophrenic (< 40-160 pg/ml) and neurotic patients (< 40-100 pg/ml). Although small differences of ß-ELI in plasma and CSF between these groups cannot be excluded, since some of the ß-ELI levels were below the detection limit of the RIA, our results provide no evidence for markedly elevated ß-ELI levels (comprising ß-endorphin, ß-lipotropin and leucine-ß-endorphin) in plasma and CSF of schizophrenics.

1. Guillemin, R., Vargo, T., Rossier, J., Minick, S., Ling, N., Rivier, C., Vale, W. and Bloom, F.E. (1977) Science, 197, 1367-1369.
2. Lindström, L.H., Widerlöv, E., Gunne, L.M., Wahlström, A. and Terenius, L. (1978) Acta psychiatr. scand., 57, 153-164.
3. Höllt, V., Przewłocki, R. and Herz, A. (1978) Naunyn-Schmiedeberg's Arch. Pharmacol., 303, 171-174.
4. Müller, O.A., Fink, R., Baur, X., Ehbauer, M., Madler, M. and Scriba, P.C. (1978) GIT Labor-Medizin, 2, 117-124.

Characteristics and Function of Opioids, editors Van Ree and Terenius
© 1978 Elsevier/North-Holland Biomedical Press

INDICATION FOR A POSSIBLE ROLE OF ENDORPHINS IN PREGNANCY.

W.Kromer[+], H.Teschemacher[++], C.Fischer[++], V.Höllt[++], R.Schulz[++]
and K.H.Voigt[+++]
[+]) Pharmakol.Inst., Univ. 8000 München 2, Nußbaumstr. 26,
[++]) Max Planck-Inst. f. Psychiatrie, Department of Neuropharmacology
8000 München 40, Kraepelinstr. 2, [+++]) SFB 87-Endokrinologie,
Universität, 7900 Ulm, Parkstr. 11 (FRG)

INTRODUCTION

There is to date, little information concerning the physiological role of endorphins. To us a role of endorphins in pregnancy and
childbirth seemed to be a possibility. We therefore looked for a
material in the uterus that was able to stimulate endorphin release
from the pituitary and searched for evidence for a dependent state
of maternal and fetal small intestine, as might occur as a result
of enhanced endorphin release during pregnancy.

MATERIALS AND METHODS

a) Demonstration of releasing activity. Guinea pigs, non-pregnant, pregnant or up to one day after parturition were decapitated.
Both uterus horns and pieces of skeletal muscle were dissected out,
homogenized in 0.1 M HCl at $0°C$ and lyophilized. The residues were
tested for releasing activity with porcine ant.pituitary lobes.
The latter were teased into small pieces, washed and subsequently
superfused with a modified Krebs-Ringer-Bicarbonate (KRB) solution
at $37°C$. After collection of superfusate for determination of the
basal endorphin and ACTH release, superfusion was continued with
residues from lyophilization taken up into KRB and, subsequently,
with KRB only. See Kromer et al.[1] for details. Opioid activity in
the superfusates was determined by radioreceptor assay. Scatchard
analysis provided evidence for the competitive inhibition of ^{3}H-
naloxone binding. The concentrations of ß-endorphin-like immunoreactivity (ß-ELI) and ACTH were determined by radioimmuno assay.

b) Demonstration of opioid dependence. Male, female non-pregnant
or pregnant and fetal guinea pigs were decapitated and segments of
their ileum placed in an organ bath. After 15 min. the electrical

Correspondence to W.Kromer at the above address.

stimulation was switched off, and (+)naloxone (2.8×10^{-7}M) was added, followed after 1-4 min. by (-)naloxone (final concentration 1.4×10^{-7}M). A contracture evoked by the opiate antagonist (-)naloxone[2] was used as an indicator for opioid dependence. See Kromer and Teschemacher[3] for details.

RESULTS AND DISCUSSION

a) Upon superfusion of ant.pituitary tissue with uterine extracts from animals just prior or up to one day after parturition the release of ACTH and opioid activity increased up to tenfold. Uterine extracts from animals post partum, however, failed to enhance the release of ß-ELI significantly. On the other hand, uterine extracts from non-pregnant animals caused a slight stimulation of the release of ß-ELI and ACTH, but not of opioid activity as determined by radioreceptor assay. Skeletal muscle extract did not cause any enhancement of release.

b) Upon challenge with (+)naloxone, no effect could be elicited in any of the ileum preparations. Upon challenge with (-)naloxone however, 11 of 14 ileum preparations from fetuses and 4 of 9 preparations from pregnant guinea pigs 1-3 days prior to parturition displayed contractures, which were prevented by atropine and diminished by extensive washing; only 1 of 16 or 3 of 16 preparations from non-pregnant or male animals, respectively, showed this withdrawal sign.

Our results point to a role of endorphins in pregnancy and childbirth, possibly controlled by a uterine releasing factor. Preliminary experiments[1] seemed to favour a peptide nature of this releasing material, but our subsequent experiments have not yet confirmed this possibility. Gut experiments indicate an increased concentration of endorphins in the fetal guinea pig small intestine and may demonstrate a natural state of opioid dependence.

REFERENCES
1. Kromer, W., Fischer, C. and Teschemacher, H. (1978) Neuroscience Letters, in press.
2. Schulz, R. and Herz, A. (1976) Life Sci., 19, 1117-1128
3. Kromer, W. and Teschemacher, H. (1978) Europ.J.Pharmacol., 49, 445-446

We thank Dr.A.E. Jacobson, N.I.H. Bethesda, Md. USA for his generous donation of (+)naloxone.
Supported by Deutsche Forschungsgemeinschaft,SP Neuroendokrinologie

Characteristics and Function of Opioids, editors Van Ree and Terenius
© *1978 Elsevier/North-Holland Biomedical Press*

IN VITRO DEGRADATION OF SYTHETIC MET^{5}ENDORPHIN AND LEU^{5}ENDORPHIN

R. M. PALMOUR, F. R. ERVIN, J.-K. CHANG AND B. FONG

Genetics, U. California, Berkeley (USA); NPI, UCLA, Los Angeles (USA); Peninsula Laboratories, San Carlos, California (USA).

The primary biological effects of a drug or hormone are presumed to be directly related to its half-life in the pertinent tissue. We have recently identified, in human hemodialysate, an endorphin with leu rather than met in position 5;[1] its increased (100-1000 x normal) concentration and long duration of electrophysiological action (>30 hr IVT in the cat) might be parsimoniously explained by a decreased rate of degradation. We present here preliminary experiments assessing the differential rates of degradation of met^5- and leu^5-β-endorphin (ME, LE) in rat brain homogenate and membranes, and identification of the ^{125}I-tyr^1-containing fragments generated.

MATERIALS AND METHODS

ME and LE were iodinated by the chloramine T method to a SA of 8 and 13 Cu/mmol, respectively. Degradations contained 0.5 µg ^{125}I-endorphin and 0-50 µg cold endorphin. Tissues were washed in saline, cooled to 0°, minced and homogenized. The supernatant from a 20,000 x g preparation was dialyzed before use, while membrane fractions were washed 3x with incubation buffer. Incubations were at 25° and 37°, at pH 7.4 and 5.0, for 0.1, 0.5, 1, 2, 3 and 6 hr. Products were identified by thin-layer electrophoresis in the presence of a standard mix of known degradation products, followed by visualization and autoradiography. Degradation was quantitated by counting dpm in eluted peptides.

RESULTS

Degradation of ME and LE occurs very rapidly at pH 7.4 in supernatants from brain, liver and kidney, with the major products being ^{125}I-tyr and 61-64 (+61-65, for LE). The $T_{\frac{1}{2}}$ for the intact molecule in the absence of bacitracin is 9 ±1.8 min for ME and 12 ±2.1 min for LE in dialyzed brain supernatant; $T_{\frac{1}{2}}$'s are slightly longer in dialyzed kidney supernatant. Washed membrane preparations yield a variety of peptides with opiate receptor activity; $T_{\frac{1}{2}}$ estimates for ME and LE are 1.8 and 2.3 hr, respectively, with brain membranes in the absence of bacitracin, but 20-30% of the ^{125}I-containing fragments display receptor activity. At pH 5 in the presence of bacitracin (10 µg/ml), 61-65^{met} is generated in a yield of about 30%, as previously reported;[2] $61\text{-}65^{leu}$ is produced from LE in somewhat lower yield. The $T_{\frac{1}{2}}$ ranges from 2.8 to 4.5 hr, depending on the specific preparation. Washed membranes from kidney (a tissue with specific opiate receptors[3,4]) yield predominantly ^{125}I-tyr and undegraded LE or ME at pH 7.4. Quantitative data for various degradations is summarized in Table 1.

TABLE I. DEGRADATION OF ENDORPHIN PEPTIDES

Tissue	Substrate	Conditions	61-91	61-77	61-68	61-65	61-64	Tyr
Brain	ME	1 hr, pH7.4	---	1.4	0.3	---	12.1	86.2
supernatant	LE	- bacitracin	---	2.2	0.8	14.0	8.3	74.7
Brain	ME	2 hr, pH7.4	45.0	20.3	1.4	3.6	2.3	28.4
membranes	LE	- bacitracin	54.4	18.9	7.6	1.8	1.9	17.3
Brain	ME	6 hr, pH 5	20.7	26.1	7.2	29.0	1.4	15.6
membranes	LE	+ bacitracin	32.3	28.3	9.1	13.7	2.6	14.0
Kidney	ME	1 hr, pH7.4	6.3	2.1	0.2	---	9.2	82.2
supernatant	LE	- bacitracin	5.1	12.6	2.1	11.7	6.9	61.6
Kidney	ME	2 hr, pH7.4	55.3	3.8	0.9	---	6.6	33.4
membrane	LE	- bacitracin	71.2	---	6.8	3.1	0.7	18.2

Preliminary results of degradations of ME and LE by tissue supernatants and membrane preparations are in general agreement with those obtained by Austen et al.[2] $T_{\frac{1}{2}}$ values obtained in the present experiments for ME and LE in brain membranes are in general agreement with those suggested by earlier pharmacological studies;[5] they do not support the hypothesis that LE is degraded more slowly than ME. Definitive evaluations of this possibility will require similar experiments in intact animals. These studies, and other unpublished data, do suggest that endorphins are bound by kidney membrane fractions, and are degraded very slowly at these sites.

REFERENCES

1. Palmour, R. et al. (1978) in Endorphins in Mental Health Research, Usdin, E., ed., Macmillan Press, in press.
2. Austen, B. M. et al. (1977) Nature 269, 619-621.
3. Simantov, R. et al. (1977) Mol. Pharmacol., in press.
4. Landau, C. et al. (1978) Unpublished observations.
5. Cox, B. M. et al. (1978) Life Sci., in press.

SUBSTANCES MODULATING THE RELEASE OF ß-ENDORPHIN-LIKE IMMUNOREACTI-
VITY (ß-ELI) FROM RAT PITUITARY IN VITRO

R. PRZEWŁOCKI, V. HÖLLT AND A. HERZ
Department of Neuropharmacology, Max-Planck-Institut für Psychiatrie, Kraepelinstrasse 2, D-8000 München 40 (F.R.G.)

INTRODUCTION

The opiate-like peptide ß-endorphin is found at a high concentration in the pituitary gland of rats from which it has been shown
to be released in response to stress[1,2]. We have previously reported that high potassium containing media augmented the release of
ß-ELI from anterior lobes of rat pituitaries in a calcium dependent
manner in vitro[3]. The aim of the present study was to explore the
influence of different neurohumoral substances on the release of
ß-ELI from anterior and intermediate lobes of rat pituitaries in
vitro.

MATERIAL AND METHODS

Anterior and intermediate/posterior lobes of rat pituitaries
were incubated in Krebs-Ringer medium as previously described[3].
Media from the following incubation periods: pretest base line
(1 h) and test period (1 h) were collected and subsequently assayed
for ß-endorphin content by means of a RIA[2]. The antiserum used exhibited a negligible avidity for α- and γ-endorphin and methionine-
enkephalin. Human ß-lipotropin, however, showed a 50% molar cross-
reactivity.

RESULTS AND DISCUSSION

Standardized rat hypothalamic extract (NIAMDD-Rat HE-RP-1,
kindly supplied by The National Pituitary Agency) induced secretion
of ß-ELI from the anterior lobe in a dose-dependent manner (Fig.1).
We suggest that at least a part of this ß-endorphin releasing activity reflects the presence of a putative endorphinergic releasing
factor (ERF).Lys-vasopressin was a very potent releasor of ß-ELI
(Fig.1), suggesting that this peptide is a putative ERF. Norepinephrine also causes a slight stimulation of secretion of ß-ELI
from the anterior lobe (Fig.1). ACTH, substance P, D-ala-met-enkephalin and substances such as GABA, dopamine, carbachol, morphine,

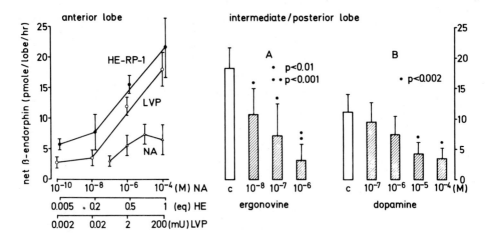

Fig.1. Release of ß-ELI from anterior lobe by: hypothalamic extract (HE); lys-vasopressin (LVP); noradrenaline (NA). Each point represents the mean value ± S.D. of 4-5 experiments.
Fig.2. Inhibition of ß-ELI release from intermediate/posterior lobe by ergonovine (A) and dopamine (B). Each bar represents the mean value ± S.D. of 4-5 experiments.

etorphine and naloxone were found to have no effect on the secretion of ß-ELI from anterior lobe $\underline{in}$ $\underline{vitro}$ when tested over a concentration range (10^{-5}-10^{-6} M).

Substances which release ß-ELI from anterior lobe were without effect on the secretion from intermediate/posterior lobe. Release from intermediate lobe was inhibited by dopamine and the ergot alkaloid, ergonovine (Fig.2), indicating that this release might be controlled by a dopaminergic innervation.

Similarities between the findings presented here and those reported the release of ACTH $\underline{in}$ $\underline{vitro}$, together with the evidence for a concomitant release of ß-endorphin and ACTH $\underline{in}$ $\underline{vivo}$[1], suggest a common mechanism for the secretion of these peptides. This hypothesis is supported by the recent observation that corticosterone at physiological concentrations ($5 \cdot 10^{-7}$ M) suppresses the stimulating effect of hypothalamic extracts on ß-ELI release from the anterior lobe of the pituitary.

1. Rossier, J., French, E.O., Rivier, C., Ling, N., Guillemin, R. and Bloom, F.E. (1977) Science, 197, 1367-1369.
2. Höllt, V., Przewłocki, R. and Herz, A. (1978) Naunyn-Schmiedeberg's Arch. Pharmacol., 303, 171-174.
3. Przewłocki, R., Höllt, V. and Herz, A. (1978) Europ. J. Pharmacol., in press.

PARALLEL RELEASE OF β-ENDORPHIN + β-LPH AND ACTH IN RAT ANTERIOR PITUITARY
CELLS IN CULTURE.

VINCENT RAYMOND, LOUISE FERLAND, JEROME LEPINE, JEAN-CLAUDE LISSITZKY and
FERNAND LABRIE,
Medical Research Council Group in Molecular Endocrinology, Le Centre Hospitalier
de l'Université Laval, Québec G1V 4G2, Canada.

It has been found that β-LPH (β-lipotropin), β-endorphin, ACTH (adrenocorticotropin) and their fragments originate from the same common precursor molecule
(31K) (1) and are present in the same anterior pituitary cells and secretory
granules (2). In order to characterize the factors controlling the processing
and release of these peptides, we have studied control of the secretion of
β-LPH, β-endorphin, β-MSH (β-melanotropin), ACTH and α-MSH using rat anterior
pituitary cells in primary culture and specific radioimmunoassays (RIAs) for
the mentioned peptides (3) after Sephadex G-75 gel filtration.

Chromatography of pituitary cellular extracts and secretion products showed
almost identical elution profiles. Using the β-endorphin RIA, 2 peaks of immunoreactivity were resolved: the fastest component comigrated with the β-LPH
marker, while the other ran at the position of β-endorphin. Using the β-MSH
RIA, a major peak eluting at the position of γ-LPH was found and a small shoul-
der corresponding to β-LPH could also be resolved.

In order to study control of the secretion of the above-mentioned peptides,
rat anterior pituitary cells were then incubated during a 4-h period in the
presence or absence of the substances to be tested. A purified porcine hypothalamic CRF fraction (provided by A.V. Schally) led to a parallel stimulation
(~ 3-fold) of β-endorphin + β-LPH and ACTH release. Increasing concentrations
of N^6, $O^{2'}$ -dibutyryl cyclic AMP (dbcAMP) or theophylline, a cyclic nucleotide
phosphodiesterase inhibitor, led to a maximal 8-fold stimulation of β-endorphin
+ β-LPH and ACTH release. When cells were preincubated for 12 or 24 h in the
presence of 10 nM dexamethasone, spontaneous and stimulated release of β-endorphin + β-LPH and ACTH induced by the purified CRF fraction, dbcAMP or theophylline were decreased to approximately 60% of controls. When the α- and β-MSH
RIAs were used, changes of release similar to those measured with the β-endorphin and ACTH RIAs were observed.

Increasing concentrations of L-norepinephrine (NE) led to a parallel stimulation of β-endorphin + β-LPH and ACTH release. The decreasing order of poten-

cy of a series of compounds, as measured by their ED_{50} values on ACTH release,
was typically α-adrenergic: L-epinephrine (L-E) ≥ L-NE > phenylephrine >> D-Ne =
isoproterenol = dopamine. Increasing concentrations of phentolamine, an α-adrenergic antagonist, in the presence of 0.3 μM L-E, completely reversed the stimulatory effect of L-E on ACTH release. Propranolol, a β-adrenergic antagonist,
had no effect up to 10 μM. Similar results were obtained when the incubation
with the 2 antagonists was performed in the presence of 3 μM phenylephrine instead of L-E. Parallel effects were observed when β-endorphin + β-LPH release
was measured.

The present data clearly demonstrate that almost very identical elution patterns were found in adenohypophyseal cellular extracts and released products.
The pattern of peptides released upon stimulation or inhibition of corticotrophs
is similar to that of the cellular pool. Thus, acute changes of release do not
affect the processing of precursor peptides. In species where the intermediate
lobe is absent, it is to be expected that the secretion of ACTH parallels that
of β-LPH and/or its fragments. In fact, human plasma ACTH and β-MSH immunoreactive levels have shown parallel changes under a variety of stimuli in
both normal and pathological states (4-6). The present findings extend previous observations of the effect of NE on ACTH release (7) and show that the
release of β-endorphin + β-LPH is also stimulated by an α-adrenergic mechanism
as well as by purified CRF.

REFERENCES

1. Mains, R.E., Eipper, B.A. and Ling, N.(1977) Proc. Natl. Acad. Sci. USA
   74, 3014-3018.

2. Pelletier, G., Leclerc, R., Labrie, F., Côté, J., Chrétien, M. and Lis, M.
   (1977) Endocrinology 100, 770-776.

3. Lissitzky, J.C., Morin, O., Dupont, A., Labrie, F., Seidah, N.C., Chrétien,
   M., Lis, M. and Coy, D.H. (1978) Life Sci. 22, 1715-1722.

4. Abe, K., Nicholson, W.E., Liddle, G.W., Orth,D.N.and Island, D.P. (1969)
   J. Clin. Invest. 48, 1580-1585.

5. Gilkes, J.J.H., Bloomfield, G.A., Scott, A.P., Lowry, P.J., Ratcliffe, J.G.,
   Landon, J. and Rees, L.H. (1975) J. Clin. Endocrinol. Metab. 40, 450-457.

6. Tanaka, K., Nicholson, W.E. and Orth, D.N. (1977) Proc. 59th Meeting of the
   Endocrine Soc., Chicago, Abstract 73.

7. Vale, W. and Rivier, C. (1977) Federation Proc. 36, 2094-2099.

Characteristics and Function of Opioids, editors Van Ree and Terenius
© 1978 Elsevier/North-Holland Biomedical Press

K^+-STIMULATED RELEASE OF LEU- AND MET-ENKEPHALIN FROM RAT STRIATAL SLICES IN VITRO

J.A. Richter, D.L. Wesche, and R.C.A. Frederickson
Indiana Univ. Med. Sch. and Eli Lilly & Co., Indianapolis, IN, USA

INTRODUCTION

Since the discovery of the endogenous opiate peptides it has been suggested they they may serve as neurotransmitters in the central nervous system[1,2]. The present experiments were undertaken to determine if the stimulated release of leu- and met-enkephalin could be demonstrated in vitro. The results show that this does occur during stimulation with high potassium and add further support to the possible transmitter role of these peptides.

METHODS

Male Wistar rats (200-300 g) were decapitated and the striata from two rats were sliced in two directions with a McIlwain chopper at 0.4 mm and loaded into a perfusion chamber[3]. Up to 6 chambers were superfused at one time at 2 ml/min at 37° with medium bubbled with 95% O_2-5% CO_2. The normal low K medium contained (mM): 120 NaCl, 25 $NaHCO_3$, 10 glucose, 5 KCl, 1.2 KH_2PO_4, 1.2 $MgCl_2$, 2 CaCl. The effluents from the chambers were run directly over columns of Amberlite XAD2 from which the pentapeptides were eluted with methanol and measured by radioimmunoassay[4]. Some of the antibodies were kind gifts from Dr. Lars Terenius (Uppsala) and also Dr. Albert Herz (Max-Planck Inst.); further supplies were puchased from Immunonuclear Corp. (MN.) or produced at Eli Lilly and Co. (IN.). Reported values have been corrected for cross reactivity.

RESULTS

After 30 min of preperfusion with normal low K medium release of leu- and met-enkephalin during a second 30 min period of perfusion with high K medium (50 mM KCl) was significantly greater than that during a similar period of perfusion with low K medium (Table 1).

TABLE 1. RESTING AND K^+-STIMULATED RELEASE OF MET- AND LEU-ENKEPHALIN FROM SUPERFUSED RAT STRIATAL SLICES[+]

	Resting Release	K^+-Stimulated Release
Met-enkephalin	4.78 ± 0.94 (6)	12.2 ± 2.38* (6)
Leu-enkephalin	0.650 ± 0.070 (5)	1.34 ± 0.23* (6)

[+]Values are ng/g/30 min, given as the mean ± S.E.M. (N).
*Significantly different from corresponding resting release rate.

When Ca^{++} was removed from the medium after the initial 30 min perfusion period (and 2 mM EGTA added), the K^+-stimulated portion of met-enkephalin release was reduced 51% and that of leu-enkephalin was decreased by 43%. Increasing the Mg^{++} concentration to 20 mM completely inhibited the K^+-stimulated release of both met- and leu-enkephalin. These ionic changes did not alter the resting release of either peptide (Table 2).

TABLE 2. EFFECT OF CA^{++} AND MG^{++} ON RESTING AND K^+-STIMULATED RELEASE OF MET- AND LEU-ENKEPHALIN[+]

	Hi K^+,0 Ca^{++}	Hi K^+,Hi Mg^{++}	Low K^+	Low K^+,0 Ca^{++}	Low K^+,Hi Mg^{++}
Met-enk	65.0 ± 13.2*	30.8 ± 8.8	29.1 ± 10.2	28.4 ± 12.1	18.5 ± 7.8
Leu-enk	85.4 ± 6.0*	59.9 ± 7.8	65.1 ± 2.4	65.0 ± 7.0	68.1 ± 7.2

[+]Values are expressed as a percent of the release found in high K medium and are given as the mean ± S.E.M. (n=5). All values are significantly different from 100%.
*Significantly different from the value for low K.

The stimulated release of the peptides was not sustained over successive 30 min periods; therefore a new paradigm was used for the following experiments. After a preliminary 30 min superfusion with low K medium separate collections were made for 30 min with low K medium followed by 5 min with high K medium. The increase in met-enkephalin release caused by high K (ng/g/min) was 30-50 fold compared to 3-8 fold as measured before. The effects of naloxone and morphine were tested using the 30 min-5 min schedule with Bacitracin (30 µg/ml) included in all the media. Neither naloxone (1 x 10^{-5}M) nor morphine (1 x 10^{-5} or 3 x 10^{-7}M) altered the resting or stimulated release of leu- or met-enkephalin significantly.

SUMMARY

Our results demonstrate a Ca^{++}-dependent K^+-stimulated release of met- and leu-enkephalin from rat striata in vitro. This confirms the findings of others[5,6] published while this work was in progress. In addition we have found that the release is not altered by naloxone or morphine.

ACKNOWLEDGMENTS

Supported in parts by USPHS Grant DA 00796 and a Grant-in-Aid from Eli Lilly and Co. The technical assistance of Ms. Linda Werling is gratefully acknowledged.

REFERENCES

1. Kosterlitz, H.W. and Hughes, J. (1975) Life Sci. 17: 91-96.
2. Frederickson, R.C.A. (1977) Life Sci. 21: 23-42.
3. Richter, J.A. (1976) J. Neurochem. 26: 791-797.
4. Wesche, D., Hollt, V. and Herz, A. (1977) Arch. Pharmacol. 301: 79-82.
5. Henderson, G., Hughes, J. and Kosterlitz, H.W. (1978) Nature 271: 677-679.
6. Iversen, L.L., Iversen, S.D., Bloom, F.E., Vargo, T., and Guillemin, R. (1978) Nature 271: 677-681.

BIOSYNTHESIS AND CHEMICAL CHARACTERIZATION OF β-LPH, β-ENDORPHIN, γ-LPH AND ACTH
IN RAT PITUITARY PARS INTERMEDIA.

N.G. SEIDAH, C. GIANOULAKIS, P. CRINE, S. BENJANNET, R. ROUTHIER, M. LIS AND
M. CHRETIEN. Protein and Pituitary Hormone Laboratory, Clinical Research Institute of Montreal, 110 Pine Avenue West, Montreal H2W 1R7, P.Q., Canada.

ABSTRACT

Four incubations of cells of pars intermedia obtained from 40 pituitaries
with ^{35}S-Met, ^{3}H-Lys, ^{3}H-Leu and ^{35}S-Met + ^{3}H-Phe sufficed for the purification
on CMC columns and characterization of newly biosynthesized β-LPH, γ-LPH, β-endorphin and ACTH. The purified radiolabeled β-endorphin was shown to have a
sequence Phe 4, Met 5, Lys 9 and Leu 14, 17 and was identical to its sheep homologue. Both β-LPH and γ-LPH were different from the corresponding sheep peptides and showed Leu 2, 10, 14, Lys 20 and Phe 6 at their N-terminus. Rat ACTH
was purified in minor amounts and showed Met 4, Phe 7.

INTRODUCTION

Rat pars intermedia, known to be a rich source of ACTH-LPH peptides[1] was chosen as a model tissue to study the mode of their in vitro biosynthesis. In this
study the biosynthesis and chemical characterization of rat β-LPH, γ-LPH and
β-endorphin is undertaken, in a similar fashion as their recent biosynthesis
in bovine pars intermedia[2], in addition to the biosynthesis of rat ACTH.

MATERIALS AND METHODS

The isolation of rat (Sprague Dawley) pars intermedia cells and incubation
conditions with various labeled amino acids has been presented elsewhere[2,3,4].
Four 3 hrs incubations of isolated cells of rat pars intermedia obtained from
40 rat pituitaries with ^{35}S-Met, ^{3}H-Lys, ^{3}H-Leu and ^{35}S-Met + ^{3}H-Phe were performed. The desalted 5 N acetic acid extract of the cells following each incubation was purified on CMC column (1 x 25 cm). The peptides analyzed were
each repurified under the same conditions on a shorter CMC column (1 x 10 cm).
Purity was judged by migration on polyacrylamide gels (PAGE) at pH 4.5 and molecular weights were obtained on PAGE/SDS/urea gels. Comparisons with standard
ovine peptides were done in each case. Microsequencing of these purified peptides was done as reported elsewhere[2,3,4].

292

RESULTS

Four main fractions were repurified from each protein extract, corresponding to labeled peptides eluting with or slightly before ovine β-LPH, γ-LPH, β-endorphin and ACTH on the CMC chromatogram:

(1) the rat γ-LPH peptide showed an amino terminal sequence of Leu 2, 10, 14, Lys 20 and Phe 6. It eluted slightly before its sheep homologue on the CMC and was slightly more acidic on PAGE, but had the same molecular weight on PAGE/SDS/urea. However, no Met-labeled γ-LPH could be seen indicating a β-MSH (β-LPH 41-58) sequence lacking methionine.

(2) The rat β-LPH showed the same amino terminal sequence as γ-LPH but eluted slightly before ovine β-LPH on CMC. However, its molecular weight and migration on PAGE was identical. The final proof of its identity was obtained after blocking the ε-NH$_2$ group of lysines via citraconylation, followed by selective tryptic cleavage at arginine residues whereby its C-terminal segment β-endorphin (β-LPH 61-91) was released[5], a property not observed with rat γ-LPH. Both rat β-LPH and γ-LPH possess different N-terminal sequences from ovine, bovine, porcine and human peptides.

(3) The β-endorphin peptide behaved in all respects identically to its sheep homologue, showing a sequence of Phe 4, Met 5, Lys 9, Leu 14, 17. A computer data bank search showed that the probability of finding other molecules with identically positioned key amino acids is less than one in a hundred million. However, no indication of the presence of Leu 5-β-endorphin was seen on sequencing of the ^{3}H-Leu labeled peptide.

(4) Rat ACTH was partially purified on CMC and was found to be present in minor amounts and eluted slightly before its sheep homologue. Its sequence showed Met 4, Phe 7 identical to what we would expect from the N-terminal 1-24 segment of ACTH of which sequence is conserved between species.

(5) These peptides were then used as markers for pulse-chase experiments on the 31,000 dalton precursor of ACTH-LPH (in this volume, M. Chrétien et al.).

ACKNOWLEDGMENTS

This work was supported by a Program Grant from Canada M.R.C.

REFERENCES

1. Pelletier, G. et al. (1977), Endocrinology 100, 770-776.
2. Crine, P. et al. (1977) Proc. Natl. Acad. Sci. USA 74, 4276-4280.
3. Seidah, N.G. et al. (1978) Proc. Natl. Acad. Sci. USA (In Press).
4. Crine, P. et al. (1978) Proc. Natl. Acad. Sci. USA (Submitted).
5. Seidah, N.G. et al. (1977) Can. J. Biochem. 55, 35-40.

Characteristics and Function of Opioids, editors Van Ree and Terenius
© *1978 Elsevier/North-Holland Biomedical Press*

N-ACYL DERIVATIVES OF ENDORPHINS; BIOLOGICAL PROPERTIES AND
DISTRIBUTION

D.G. SMYTH and S. ZAKARIAN
National Institute for Medical Research, Mill Hill, London, NW7 1AA

α,N-Acyl derivatives of the C-Fragment of lipotropin
(β-endorphin, residues 61-91) and of the C'-Fragment (61-87) have
recently been shown to occur in porcine pituitary.[1] Unlike the
parent peptides, the acyl forms do not exhibit analgesic activity
in the rat tail flick assay and do not show the cardiovascular
actions of morphine in the cat. The acylation reaction appears to
take place intracellularly since no conversion of $|^{125}I|$C-Fragment
to the acyl derivative could be detected after ICV injection and
similarly no deacylation of the acyl form was observed in the
C.S.F. Although the acyl peptides are inert as opiates they

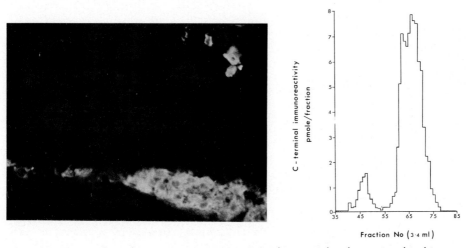

Fig. 1. Localization of fragments of lipotropin in rat pituitary
by immunofluorescence. All cells stain in the pars intermedia;
individual cells stain in the anterior lobe.

Fig. 2. Resolution of peptides present in rat anterior pituitary
which have lipotropin C-terminal immunoreactivity. Gel filtration was on a column (70 x 2·4cm) in 50% acetic acid and fractions
were analysed by immunoassay.

retain the full immunoreactivity of the respective NH$_2$-peptides.

Our immunofluorescent study of rat pituitary, which employed an antibody to natural porcine C-Fragment, shows that the pars intermedia stains densely and that the anterior pituitary stains in individual cells (Fig 1). Other fluorescence studies employing antisera to lipotropin[2] or synthetic C-Fragment[3] have given similar results. In order to identify the nature of the immuno-active peptides, we have performed immunoassay of regions of rat pituitary, and also of brain, after separation of the endogenous peptides by chromatography. The procedure involved acid acetone homogenization of 60 anterior and 60 posterior pituitary lobes and the peptides were resolved by gel filtration on Sephadex G75 in a dissociating solvent. Subsequent fractionation was on Sephadex G100 in 4M guanidine or by chromatography on SP Sephadex C-25. The peptides were detected with the aid of the C-Fragment antiserum which has a C-terminal specificity; its affinity for C'-Fragment was one quarter that for C-Fragment and its affinity for lipotropin one sixth.

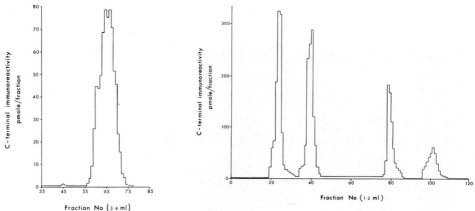

Fig. 3 Resolution of immunoreactive peptides present in rat pars intermedia + posterior pituitary. Gel filtration was as in Fig.2.

Fig. 4. Chromatography of β-endorphin' peptides present in pars intermedia on SP-Sephadex C-25. The column (70 x 0·6 cm) was in 0.01M sodium phosphate at pH7 with a zero to 0.5M sodium chloride gradient. Fractions were analysed by immunoassay. The molar amounts of the first two peaks (N-acyl C'-Fragment and C'-Fragment). are 4 times greater than is indicated by their immunoreactivity.

The anterior pituitary was shown to contain two groups of immunoactive peptides (Fig. 2). The first fraction contained lipotropin together with a larger polypeptide, presumably the 31K molecule,[4] and they were resolved on Sephadex G-100. The second fraction contained peptides of the size of β-endorphin; on SP Sephadex C-25 these resolved into four components with elution positions corresponding to N-acyl C'-Fragment, C'-Fragment, N-acyl C-Fragment and C-Fragment. Parallel experiments on the pars intermedia plus posterior pituitary showed that they contain essentially no lipotropin or 31K molecule (Fig. 3) but these regions were found to have 10 times as much immunoactive peptide the size of β-endorphin as the anterior pituitary. Ion exchange chromatography showed again the four components (Fig. 4) and it was notable that C-Fragment was present in the least amount, accounting for less than 4% of the four peptides. Thus the heavy staining of the pars intermedia seen by immunofluorescence should not be attributed to the presence of lipotropin or β-endorphin (C-Fragment); it appears to be due principally to the C'-Fragment and the acyl derivatives.

Immunofluorescent studies of rat brain[5,6,7] shows that the react-material is concentrated mainly in the hypothalamus (Fig. 5). Gel

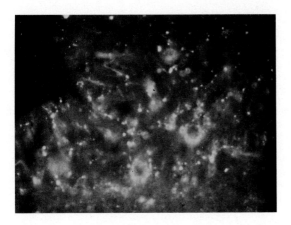

Fig. 5. Localization of lipotropin C-Fragment in rat hypothalamus by immunofluorescence; the peptide is present in cell bodies, axons and terminals.

filtration of the immunoactive peptides in 30 hypothalami revealed a small amount of lipotropin but the 'β-endorphin' fraction, which included the four peptides, contained principally the C-Fragment. This result stands in contrast to the much larger proportions of C'-Fragment and acyl derivatives which we have demonstrated in pituitary.

The results suggest that in the pituitary the 31K precursor molecule may be processed to produce corticotropin in preference to the opiate peptide C-Fragment. In the brain, on the other hand, it appears that the 31K molecule may be activated for the production of lipotropin C-Fragment, to function there as a neurotransmitter.

REFERENCES

1. Smyth, D.G. and Zakarian, Siraik (1978) in Endorphins in Mental Health, Usdin, E. ed., MacMillan, in the press.

2. Pelletier, F., Lecterc, R., Labri, F., Cote, J.,Chretien, M. and Lis, M. (1977) Endocrinology, 100, 770-776

3. Bloom, F.E., Rossier, J., Battenberg, L.F., Bayou, A., French, E., Henriksen, S.J., Siggins, G.R., Segal, D., Browne, R., Ling, N and Guillemin, R. (1978) Advances in Biochemical Psychopharmacology, Costa, E. and Trabucchi, M. eds., 18, 89-109

4. Mains, R.E., Eipper, B.A. and Ling, N. (1977) Proc. Natl. Acad. Sci. U.S.A. 74, 3014-3018

5. Watson, S.J., Barchas, J.D. and Li, C.H. (1977) Proc. Natl. Acad. Sci. U.S.A. 74, 5155-5158

6. Zimmerman, E.A., Liotta, A. and Krieger, D.T. (1978) Cell Tiss. Res. 186, 393-398

7. Bloom, F., Battenberg, E., Rossier, J., Ling, N. and Guillemin, R. (1977) Proc. Natl. Acad. Sci. U.S.A., 75, 1591-1595

8. Akil, H., Watson, S.J., Berger, P.A. and Barchas, J.D. (1978) Advances in Biochemical Psychopharmacology, Costa, E. and Trabucchi, M., eds. 18, 125-139

THE EFFECTS OF NARCOTIC AGENTS ON ENKEPHALIN LEVELS IN THE RAT BRAIN

BEN AVI WEISSMAN*, FELIX BERGMANN and RAYA ALTSTETER

Dept. of Pharmacology, Israel Inst. for Bio. Res., P.O.B. 19, Ness-Ziona*, and

Dept. of Pharmacology, The Hebrew University-Hadassah Medical School, Jerusalem,

Israel

INTRODUCTION

It was suggested that following morphine administration enkephalin levels in the CNS decrease and the deficiency brought about might be caused by or related to physical dependence and the withdrawal syndrome[1]. Lower enkephalin concentrations following morphine pellet implantation were recently reported[2]. Some authors failed to detect any changes in enkephalin levels as a result of various regimens of morphine administration[3,4]. It seems likely that enkephalins released from distinct sites in the CNS may be found in the CSF. Moreover, the presence of endogenous opioid peptides in the CSF has been demonstrated[5,6]. Thus, enkephalin concentrations in the CSF may serve as indicators for the interactions between exogenous opiates and endogenous opioid peptides.

MATERIALS AND METHODS

"Sabra" male rats weighing 400-500 g were operated under light ether anesthesia. A 20 gauge, 10 mm long cannula was inserted into the right lateral ventricle and a 21 gauge needle pierced the atlanto-occipital membrane to create a direct outlet from the fourth ventricle. Artificial CSF was infused into the lateral ventricle at a rate of 0.09 ml/min. Samples (1.5-1.7 ml) were collected over the period of 20 min and assayed for enkephalins as previously described[6].

RESULTS

Enkephalin content in the CSF remains constant during perfusion of the ventricular system with artificial CSF (up to 5 hrs). An i.v. injection of morphine (6 mg/kg) elicits an immediate elevation of the opioid level in the perfusate (60 to 125% above basal levels); this marked change is followed by a fall below basal value. A second rise (60 to 190%) is observed 80-120 min after the opiate is applied. Naloxone (1 mg/kg) given i.p. fails to produce the initial rise described above but causes a delayed response similar but not identical to the second peak appearing after morphine administration. A naloxone injection followed by morphine (same doses and routes of administration) exhibits a pattern of enkephalin content which differs from that expected after either drug, namely, a single peak appearing 40 min after the morphine application and its height is about 50% above basal value.

DISCUSSION

The separate peaks of enkephalin levels appearing after morphine administration may indicate two distinct sites of action of this drug. It seems likely that there are two pools of enkephalins, one which is readily accessible and another one responding in a much slower fashion. These data can be interpreted by relating the immediate rise to the release of enkephalins present in the synaptic cleft while the later may be due to an intracellular pool. Indeed, naloxone fails to cause the first peak, probably because of its inability to activate the opiate receptors, still it may displace enkephalins from intracellular pools. Naloxone, the opiate antagonist, also postpones the appearance of the immediate peak expected following morphine injections. The fact that the second peak observed after both drugs is completely suppressed when the combination is administered remains unexplained.

REFERENCES

1. Kosterlitz, H.W. and Hughes, J. (1975) Life Sci., 17, 91-96.
2. Weissman, B.A., Azov, R. and Shani, J. (1977) Proc. Int. Soc. Neurochem. Vol. 6, p. 302.
3. Frata, W., Yang, H.-Y.T., Hong, J. and Costa, E. (1977) Nature, 268, 452-453.
4. Childers, S.R., Simantov, R. and Snyder, S.H. (1977) Europ. J. Pharmacol., 46, 289-293.
5. Terenius, L. and Wahlstrom, A. (1975) Life Sci., 16, 1759-1764.
6. Sarne, Y., Azov, R. and Weissman, B.A. (1978) Brain Res. (in press).

Characteristics and Function of Opioids, editors Van Ree and Terenius
© *1978 Elsevier/North-Holland Biomedical Press*

NEUROBLASTOMA X GLIOMA HYBRID CELLS AS A MODEL SYSTEM FOR STUDYING
OPIOID ACTION

Michael Brandt, Claudia Buchen and Bernd Hamprecht
Max-Planck-Institut für Biochemie, 8033 Martinsried (Federal Republic
of Germany)

ABSTRACT

Neuroblastoma x glioma hybrid cells have been shown to display
many neuronal properties. Among these is their susceptibility to
opioids. These compounds prevent the increase in the cellular level
of cyclic AMP that is elicited by prostaglandin E_1 (PGE_1). Besides
these short-term effects, opioids cause long-term effects, i.e., an
increased maximal response to PGE_1. The acute and chronic effects
on the hybrids may be considered as biochemical correlates of opiate
analgesia and tolerance, respectively. The review of this work is
followed by some more recent results that show the importance of
calcium and sodium ions for the short- and of Ca^{2+} for the long-term
regulation of the cyclic AMP-level in the hybrid cells.

INTRODUCTION

The complex construction of the brain is a serious obstacle to
studies of the molecular events underlying the activity of this organ.
A biochemist engaged in such efforts would like to investigate the
different cell types of the brain first separately and then in stepwise recombinations. This would most likely provide insight into the
factors and events which are required to organize the constituing cell
types into such an effective instrument of information storage, retrieval and processing. In recent years progress is gaining momentum in
the field of cell separation. Till the time various cell types will be
at hand in quantities sufficient for biochemical studies, model systems will have to be employed for studying basic mechanisms of nervous
activity in a paradigmatic way. Permanent cell lines derived from
tumors of the nervous system are such models. One of these model
systems is the neuroblastoma x glioma hybrid line 108CC15 [1,3]. It has
been employed for studying the mechanisms of opioid action and in
the quest for answers to other problems. The research carried out
with these hybrid cells has been reviewed from time to time [1-3].
Therefore, the work compiled within these reviews will only be
summarized here, in order to lay the basis for the more recent work on

opioids dealt with in this article.

The neuroblastoma x glioma hybrid cells are considered as model systems for neurons because they express many properties characteristic of neurons [1-3] (Table 1). To neurohormones they respond by changing their membrane potential [1,3] and/or their intracellular concentration of cyclic AMP [1-3]. It would be important to know if, e.g., the α-adrenergic receptor depressing the level of cyclic AMP [5] is identical with that lowering the membrane potential of these cells [5]. Generally speaking, the question has to be answered if a receptor is constructed to directly regulate only one effector system (e.g., adenylate cyclase or a certain ion channel) or several (e.g., adenylate cyclase and a certain ion channel). This fundamental problem has many implications. The properties of the hybrid cells permit to seek for an answer by using this model system. The principal advantages of working with this hybrid cell system have been summarized elsewhere [6]. Their sensitivity to opioids makes the hybrid cells a useful system for studying actions of opioids (example of an in vivo correlate: tolerance, dependence and withdrawal syndromes). In table 2 the neurohormones are listed that regulate, most likely via specific receptors, the level of cyclic AMP in the hybrid cells.

TABLE 1

NEURONAL PROPERTIES OF NEUROBLASTOMA X GLIOMA HYBRID CELLS

The references for those properties that are not provided with a reference are given in ref. 3.

Property
Extension of neurite-like processes
Excitable membranes
Cholineacetyltransferase
Dopamine-ß-hydroxylase
Clear vesicles
Dense-core vesicles
Uptake systems for neurotransmitters (4)
Formation of functional synapses
Receptors for neurohormones

SHORT-TERM EFFECTS OF OPIOIDS

Characteristic representatives (table 2) of the hormones that respectively elevate the level of cyclic AMP or prevent this elevation (incubation time 10 min) are prostaglandin E_1 (PGE_1) and the opioids,

TABLE 2

HORMONES REGULATING CYCLIC AMP LEVELS IN NEUROBLASTOMA X GLIOMA
HYBRID CELLS 108CC15
The literature references for those hormones that are not provided
with a reference are given in ref. 3.

Level is increased by	Level is decreased by
PGE_1	Opioids
Adenosine	Somatostatin
Secretin (7)	Acetylcholine (muscarinic receptors)
Glucagon (7)	Noradrenaline (α-receptors)

respectively. Thus the interference of an opioid with the action of
PGE_1 can be used as an assay system for effects of opioids. The relationship between opioid and cyclic AMP, including that in the hybrid
cells, has been reviewed recently [9,10].

The inhibition by morphine and its congeners of the action of PGE_1
is stereospecific and it can be blocked by the specific opiate antagonist naloxone. A positive correlation was found between the potency
of an opiate in exerting this biochemical effect and the affinity for
the opiate receptor [11]. Several orders of magnitude more potent than
opiates in the hybrid cell system are the opioid peptides enkephalins
[12,13] and endorphins [14,15]. This sequence of potencies is the reverse
of that found in binding studies on brain cell membranes [16]. This
indicates that different kinds of opioid receptors [17] may be involved.
Curtailing of the pentapeptide chain of the enkephalins at either end
or substitution of the terminal amino group by a hydrogen renders
completely inactive material. Unexpectedly, however, on substitution of
the terminal amino group by an arginyl residue the activity drops only
by a factor of 10. Replacement by hydrogen of the phenolic hydroxyl
group lowers the activity by 3 orders of magnitude. Elongation of the
peptide chain at the carboxyl terminal is well tolerated [16]. In agreement with this is the still high activity of Leu-enkephalinamide or
-methylester [18]. These data demonstrate that the negative charge of
the carboxylate ion is not required for activity.

Somatostatin has been considered as a partial agonist/antagonist at
the opioid receptor. In the hybrid cells this tetradecapeptide with
no resemblance to opioids affects the influence of PGE_1 like the
opioids do. However, opioid receptors were shown not to be involved
in this activity [8]. Thus, at least in these cells opioid and somatostatin receptors must be different species.

Also acetylcholine [19] and noradrenaline [5] exert, via muscarinic and
α-adrenergic receptors, respectively, effects analogous to those of
the opioids and somatostatin (see table 2). This could suggest that
all these hormones act by the same mechanism. There are several ways
in which they could prevent the increase in the level of cyclic AMP
elicited by PGE_1 [6]. The use of one of them, the inhibition of adenylate
cyclase, has been demonstrated [11,20]. Preliminary evidence for a
concurrent activation of cyclic AMP phosphodiesterase has been presented [6]. The possibility has been considered that the hormones listed
in Table 2, after combination with their corresponding receptor, produce a structural change in the plasma membrane, which, in turn,
causes a change in the permeability for a certain ion and thus a

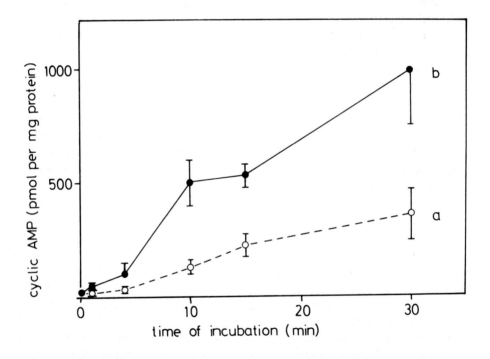

Fig. 1. Time course of the increase in the level of cyclic AMP evoked
by the phosphodiesterase inhibitor RO20-1724 (0.3 mM) in the absence
(curve a) and presence (curve b) of 1.8 mM Ca^{2+}. $1.1x10^6$ viable hybrid
cells 108CC15 per plate 85 mm in diameter, viability 95 %, passage
number 15. After seeding, the cells were grown [3] in 20 ml of growth
medium for 4 days. Thereafter, the growth medium was removed, the cells
were washed 3 times with 3 ml of incubation medium [6] containing or
lacking Ca^{2+}. Then they were incubated (x min, 37° C) with 5 ml of
incubation medium (± Ca^{2+}) containing 0.3 mM RO20-1724. After termination of the incubation the intracellular concentration of cyclic AMP
was determined [6].

possible change in membrane potential and intracellular concentration of the ion. This then might influence the activity of the cyclic AMP enzyme system and thus alter the level of the nucleotide [3,6]. Ca^{2+} ions have been known to functionally antagonize morphine in the generation of analgesia [21] and tolerance [22]. Therefore, the effect of Ca^{2+} on the regulation of the cyclic AMP level has been studied in the hybrid cells.

TABLE 3

EFFECT OF La^{3+} AND Co^{2+} ON THE INCREASE IN THE LEVEL OF CYCLIC AMP EVOKED BY PGE_1.

Experiment 1 (2): 1.7 (4.0)x10^6 viable cells per plate, viability 83 % (80 %), passage number 19 (22). After removal of the growth medium the cells were washed 3 times with 5 ml of a medium[4] containing 6 mM KCl, 25 mM HEPES, 0.8 mM $MgCl_2$, 1.8 mM $CaCl_2$, 20 mM glucose and 145 mM NaCl (pH 7.4 at room temperature). Thereafter, the cells were incubated (10 min, 37° C) with 5 ml of the same medium supplemented with the compounds indicated in the table. Other details as in fig. 1.

Expt. no.	Addition (μM) preincubation	main incubation	Cyclic AMP (pmol per mg protein)	
1	no preincubation	-	17 ± 10	
	no preincubation	$LaCl_3$ (3000)	10 ± 3	
	no preincubation	PGE_1 (3)	1010 ± 230	
	no preincubation	$LaCl_3 + PGE_1$	530 ± 160	
	-	-	36 ± 11	1)
	$LaCl_3$ (3000)	$LaCl_3$	18 ± 4	1)
	-	PGE_1	1340 ± 360	1)
	$LaCl_3$	$LaCl_3 + PGE_1$	180 ± 30	1)
2	no preincubation	Leu-enkephalin (0.1)	7 ± 1	
	no preincubation	$LaCl_3$ (3000)	11 ± 2	
	no preincubation	$CoCl_2$ (3000)	7 ± 1	
	no preincubation	PGE_1 (3)	740 ± 30	
	no preincubation	Leu-enkephalin+PGE_1	290 ± 20	
	no preincubation	$LaCl_3 + PGE_1$	220 ± 60	
	no preincubation	$LaCl_3$+Leu-enkephalin+PGE_1	75 ± 7	
	no preincubation	$CoCl_2 + PGE_1$	85 ± 40	
	no preincubation	$CoCl_2$+Leu-enkephalin+PGE_1	48 ± 30	

1) After a preincubation in the above medium (30 min, 37° C, $\pm$ $LaCl_3$) the main incubation (10 min, 37° C, $\pm$ PGE_1, $\pm$ $LaCl_3$) was carried out without prior change of media.

It turns out that the response of the cells to the stimulating hormones (table 2) is strongly dependent on the presence of external Ca^{2+} ions [6,23]. Even the basal activity of cyclic AMP generation relies on the presence of Ca^{2+}. If cellular phosphodiesterase activity is blocked by the inhibitor RO20-1724 [24], the cyclic AMP level rises more quickly in the presence than in the absence of external Ca^{2+} (Fig. 1). The influence of Ca^{2+} is counteracted by a chelator of Ca^{2+} ions [6], by the Ca^{2+}-antagonists La^{3+} and Co^{2+} (Table 3), and by prenylamine (Segontin), an inhibitor of Ca^{2+}-influx into hybrid cells [4] (Table 4). A comparable situation is the increase in the level of cyclic AMP evoked in adrenal cells by ACTH, since it depends on external Ca^{2+} ions [25].

A change of the extracellular concentrations means a change also of the total intracellular concentration of Ca^{2+} ions [4] and is likely to alter the extremely low cytosolic activity of Ca^{2+} as well. This in

TABLE 4

EFFECT OF THE "Ca^{2+}-BLOCKER" SEGONTIN AND OF LEU-ENKEPHALIN ON THE INCREASE IN THE LEVEL OF CYCLIC AMP EVOKED BY PGE_1

PGE_1 (as always) and Segontin were added as solutions in 95 % and 30 % ethanol, respectively, both giving rise to a final alcohol concentration of 0.3 % (v/v). Therefore, the data for the ethanol controls were included in the table. The details of experiments 1 and 2 are identical to those of experiment 1 and 2, respectively, of table 3.

expt. no.	PGE_1 3μM	Segontin 100μM	Ethanol %(v/v)	Leu-enke-phalin 0.1μM	Cyclic AMP pmol per mg protein
1	-	-	-	-	19 ± 3
	+	-	0.3	-	1080 ± 290
	+	-	0.6	-	2110 ± 130
	+	+	0.6	-	560 ± 90
2	-	-	-	-	10 ± 3
	-	-	0.3	-	14 ± 2
	-	+	0.3	-	4 ± 4
	-	-	-	+	12 ± 3
	+	-	0.3	-	1680 ± 90
	+	-	0.6	-	2020 ± 270
	+	+	0.6	-	940 ± 280
	+	-	0.6	+	970 ± 260
	+	+	0.6	+	300 ± 90

turn, could change the activity, e.g., of adenylate cyclase [26]. The dependence on Ca^{2+} of the basal activity of cyclic AMP formation (Fig. 1) and, less compellingly, the effect of Segontin, point to an intracellular action of Ca^{2+}. A simplified picture of adenylate cyclase activity in the hybrid cells has to deal with at least 4 regulatory factors: Two act via their receptors from outside: the activating (e.g., PGE_1) and the inhibitory (e.g., opioid) hormones. GTP [27] and probably also Ca^{2+} ions [28,29] activate the enzyme from inside the cell. Our results are compatible with the view [6] that a hormone cannot activate adenylate cyclase unless the internal factors are present. In this model no change, by the activating hormone-receptor complex, of Ca^{2+} permeability is required for switching on adenylate cyclase [6].

The activating hormones (Table 2) raise the level of cyclic AMP

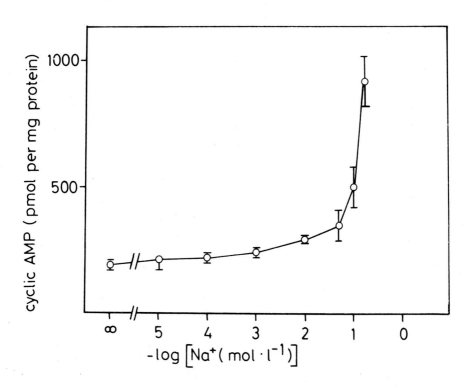

Fig.2. Maximal response to PGE_1 (3µM) of neuroblastoma x glioma hybrid cells 108CC15 at varying concentrations of Na^+, $3.2x10^6$ viable cells per plate, viability 98 %, passage number 17. After removal of the growth medium the cells were washed 3 times with the medium described in table 3 containing (instead of 145 mM NaCl) x mM NaCl + (145-x) mM choline chloride, before they were incubated (10 min, 37° C) with 5 ml of the same medium. Other details as in fig. 1.

markedly even if no Ca^{2+} has been added to the external medium and opioids are still capable of attenuating this raise [6]. Thus, extra-cellular Ca^{2+} ions are not required for the action of opioids on the level of cyclic AMP. Nevertheless, the functional antagonism between morphine and Ca^{2+} ions [21,22] can still be understood, if all that matters for the cell is the resulting level of cyclic AMP. Morphine lowers it, Ca^{2+} raises it [6].

To our surprise also Na^+ ions are required for the stimulatory effect of the hormones (Table 2), as can be seen from Fig. 2. Our pre-liminary evidence points to an extracellular site of action.

LONG-TERM EFFECTS OF OPIOIDS

Once short-term effects of opioids were found in the hybrids, it was not too surprising to encounter long-term effects as well. During

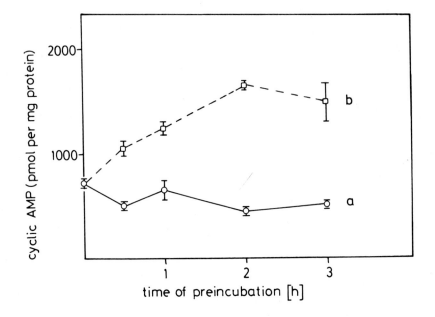

Fig. 3. Maximal response to PGE_1 (3μM) as a function of the time the neuroblastoma x glioma hybrid cells 108CC15 were preincubated in the presence (curve a) or absence (curve b) of 1.8 mM Ca^{2+}. 2.0×10^6 viable cells per plate, viability 76 %, passage number 12. After the removal of the growth medium the cells were washed as in fig. 1. Thereafter, they were preincubated for varying length of time in incubation medium[6] ($- Ca^{2+}$). Subsequently, the medium was removed, the cells were washed 3 times with 3 ml incubation medium[6] containing 1.8mM Ca^{2+} (37° C) and the main incubation (10 min, 37° C) in 5 ml of this medium was started by the addition of PGE_1. Other details as in fig. 1.

chronic (range of hours) exposure to morphine [30,31] or enkephalins [32,33] tolerance to the inhibitory action of opioids develops in
the cells. If one withdraws the opioid, an increased maximal response
to PGE_1 is observed. The development of the tolerance effect can be
inhibited by cycloheximide [30,34]. The long durations of the experiments and the high inhibitor concentrations used let the conclusion
appear premature that protein snythesis is required for the development of tolerance in the hybrid cells.

The analogy in the mode of action of the inhibitory hormones [3]
(Table 2) also holds for the long-term effects, since adrenergic and
cholinergic agents cause the same tolerance effects as opioids [30].
This report has been confirmed [35]. From the analogues between the actions of opioids and that of other neurohormones (Table 2) it has been
concluded [3] that opioids do probably not principally differ from other
neurohormones in their mechanism of action. Thus they assume a special
position only due to the striking effects on the physiology of animals
and man after oral or systemic application.

In short-term experiments (minutes range) opioids and lack of external Ca^{2+} had the same effects on the hybrid cells. This is the case
also in long-term experiments. Chronic exposure of hybrid cells to low
concentrations of Ca^{2+} gradually evokes the same increase in the maximal response to PGE_1 as treatment with opioids. The time course of the
development of this effect is shown in fig. 3, the dependence on the
concentration of Ca^{2+} in fig. 4. For the cell it is obviously unimpor-
tant which way the level of cyclic AMP is lowered, by opioid or by
deficiency of Ca^{2+}. Its reaction is the same in both cases: The specific activity of adenylate cyclase is increased [30] (has the activity of
phosphodiesterase been decreased concomitantly?) to make up for the
loss of activity. The level of cyclic AMP is homeostatically controlled [20]. This points to a presumptively highly important but unfortunately still widely unknown function of cyclic AMP in the regulation of
nerve cell activity.

ACKNOWLEDGEMENTS

The expert technical assistence of Ms. Claudia Buchen is gratefully
acknowledged. We are indebted to Dr. J. Pike, Upjohn Co., Kalamazoo,
for PGE_1, to Hoffmann-La Roche, Grenzach, for RO20-1724 and to the
Sonderforschungsbereich 51 of the Deutsche Forschungsgemeinschaft for
support.

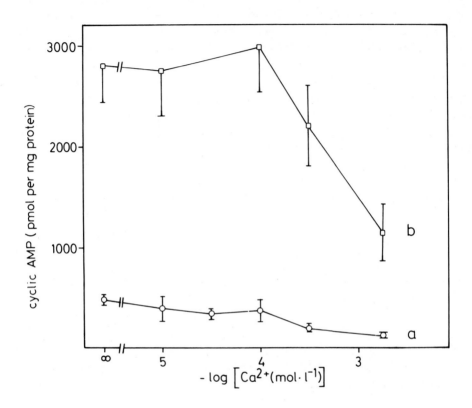

Fig. 4. Effect of the Ca^{2+}-concentration during the preincubation on the maximal response to PGE_1 (3μM) in the subsequent main incubation (10 min, 37° C, ± 1.8 mM calcium ions). 3.2×10^6 viable cells per plate, viability 96 %, passage number 15. The preincubation (2.75 h) was as in fig. 3, except that the concentration of Ca^{2+} in the medium was varied as indicated on the abscissa. After the preincubation the media were replaced by incubation media containing (curve b) or lacking (curve a) 1.8 mM Ca^{2+} and the main incubation (10 min, 37° C) was started by the addition of PGE_1. Other details as in fig. 1.

REFERENCES

1. Hamprecht, B. (1974) in Biochemistry of Sensory Functions, 25th Mosbacher Kolloquium, Jaenicke, L. ed., Springer, Berlin, pp. 391-423.

2. Hamprecht, B. (1976) Angew. Chem. Int. Ed. Engl., 15, 194-206.

3. Hamprecht, B. (1977) Int. Rev. Cytol., 49, 99-170.

4. Kürzinger, K. (1978) Dissertation, Univ. of Munich.

5. Traber, J., Reiser, G., Fischer, K. and Hamprecht, B. (1975) FEBS Lett., 52, 327-332.

6. Brandt, M., Traber, J., Glaser, T. and Hamprecht, B. (1978) Proc. 7th Int. Cong. Pharmacology (Paris) Pergamon Press, Oxford, in press.

7. Propst, F., Moroder, L., Wünsch, E. and Hamprecht, B., in prepn.

8. Traber, J., Glaser, T., Brandt, M., Klebensberger, W. and Hamprecht, B. (1977) FEBS Lett., 81, 351-354.

9. Klee, W. (1977) in Alcohol and Opiates, Blum, K. (ed.) Academic Press, New York, pp. 299-308.

10. Hamprecht, B. (1978) in Developments in Opiate Research, Herz. A. (ed.), M. Dekker, New York.

11. Sharma, S.K., Nirenberg, M. and Klee, W.A. (1975) Proc. Natl. Acad. Sci. U.S.A., 72, 590-594.

12. Brandt, M., Gullis, R.J., Fischer, K., Buchen, C., Hamprecht, B., Moroder, L. and Wünsch, E. (1976) Nature, 262, 311-313.

13. Klee, W.A. and Nirenberg, M. (1976) Nature, 263, 609-612.

14. Brandt, M., Buchen, C. and Hamprecht, B. (1977) FEBS Lett., 80, 251-254.

15. Goldstein, A., Cox, B.M., Klee, W.A. and Nirenberg, M. (1977) Nature, 265, 362-363.

16. Wahlström, A., Brandt, M., Moroder, L., Wünsch, E., Lindeberg, G., Ragnarsson, U., Terenius, L. and Hamprecht, B. (1977) FEBS Lett., 77, 28-32.

17. Lord, J.A.H., Waterfield, A.A., Hughes, J. and Kosterlitz, H.W. (1977) Nature, 267, 495-499.

18. Agarwal, N.S., Hruby, V.S., Katz, R., Klee, W. and Nirenberg, M. (1977) Biochem. Biophys. Res. Comm., 76, 129-135.

19. Traber, J., Fischer, K., Buchen, C. and Hamprecht, B. (1975) Nature, 255, 558-560.

20. Traber, J. (1976) Dissertation, University of Munich.

21. Kaneto, H. (1971) in Narcotic Drugs, Clouet, D. (ed.),Plenum Press New York, pp. 300-309.

22. Weger, P. and Amsler, C. (1936) Arch. Exp. Pathol. Pharmacol., 181, 489-493.

23. Brandt, M. (1976) Diploma thesis, University of Munich.

24. Sheppard, H. and Wiggan, G. (1971) Mol. Pharmacol. 7, 111-115.

25. Sayers, G., Beall, R.J. and Seelig, S. (1972) Science, 175, 1131-1133.

26. Lefkowitz, R.J., Roth, J. and Pastan, I. (1970) Nature, 228, 864-866.

27. Rodbell, M., Birnbaumer, S.L. and Krans, H.M.J. (1971) J. biol. Chem.,246, 1877-1882.

28. Brostrom, C.O., Huang, Y.-C., Breckenridge, B.M.L. and Wolff, D.J. (1975) Proc. Natl. Acad. Sci. U.S.A., 73, 352-355.

29. Cheung, W.Y., Bradham, L.S., Lynch, T.J., Lim, Y.M. and Tallant, E.A. (1975) Biochem. biophys. Res. Comm., 66, 1055-1062.

30. Traber, J., Gullis, R. and Hamprecht, B. (1975) Life Sci., 12, 1863-1868.

31. Klee, W.A., Sharma, S.K. and Nirenberg, M. (1975) Life Sci., 16, 1869-1874.

32. Brandt, M., Fischer, K., Moroder, L., Wünsch, E. and Hamprecht, B. (1976) FEBS Lett., 68, 38-40.

33. Lampert, A., Nirenberg, M. and Klee, W.A. (1976) Proc. Natl. Acad. Sci. U.S.A., 73, 3165-3167.

34. Sharma, S.K., Klee, W.A. and Nirenberg, M. (1977) Proc. Natl. Acad. Sci. U.S.A., 74, 3365-3369.

35. Nathanson, N.M., Klein, W.L. and Nirenberg, M. (1978) Proc. Natl. Acad. Sci. U.S.A., 75, 1788-1791.

Characteristics and Function of Opioids, editors Van Ree and Terenius
© *1978 Elsevier/North-Holland Biomedical Press*

THE EFFECT OF ACUTE AND CHRONIC MORPHINE ADMINISTRATION IN SYNAPTOSOMAL

CALCIUM UPTAKE

F. Guerrero-Munoz, M.L. Guerrero and E.L. Way

Department of Pharmacology, School of Medicine, University of California

San Francisco, San Francisco, California 94143 (U.S.A.)

INTRODUCTION

Several investigations have indicated a role for Ca^{++} in the production of
analgesia by opiate narcotics and in tolerance and physical dependence development. Takemori[1] and Elliott *et al.*[2] reported that Ca^{++} antagonizes the reduction of respiration produced by morphine or rat brain slices. Heimans[3]
determined that Ca^{++} reduced the effects of morphine on the electrically
stimulated guinea pig ileum. Increases in brain Ca^{++}, Mg^{++} and Mn^{++} were
observed to decrease the analgesic effect of morphine *in vivo*[4,5,6]. On the
other hand administration of Ca^{++} chelator EGTA (ethylenebis oxyethylenenitrilo
tetra-acetic acid) potentiated the action of morphine, while the Ca^{++}-Mg^{++}
chelator EDTA (ethylenediamine tetraacetic acid) had little effect on morphine
analgesia[6,7] indicating the importance of Ca^{++} brain levels rather than Mg^{++} in
opiate action. Moreover, increasing the membrane permeability of calcium with
the ionophore X537A greatly antagonized the analgesia produced by morphine[6].
These studies suggest that the brain concentration of Ca^{++} may be involved in
opioid action. In support of such a hypothesis it has been recently found
that the acute administration of morphine or levorphanol in mice and rats decreases Ca^{++} levels in nerve ending fractions (synaptosomes)[8] and in synaptic
vesicles[9,10] and the effects are reversed by naloxone. In contrast to these
acute effects of morphine, chronic morphine treatment by pellet implantation
produced an elevation of Ca^{++} level in synaptic vesicles and lysed

synaptosomes of both rats and mice but not in other subcellular fractions[9].
Changes have also been reported on synaptic plasma membrane (SPM) calcium binding after acute or chronic morphine pellet implantation[10]. Previous studies
in rat brain slices demonstrated that both Ca^{++} influx and efflux could be inhibited by morphine and this inhibition could be partially reversed by
nalorphine[11].

In light of the evidence implicating Ca^{++} in morphine action it appeared of
interest, to investigate calcium fluxes in synaptosomes during acute and
chronic morphine treatment

METHODS

Male ICR mice weighing 20-25 g were sacrified by decapitation and their
brains were rapidly removed. Using a teflon-glass homogenizer, synaptosomes
were prepared from whole brain homogenates (10 vol. 0.32 M sucrose, 5 mM Hepes
buffer, pH 7.5). All procedures were carried out at 4 to 5°C. The crude
homogenate was centrifuged at 1,100 g for 10 min and the supernatant was decanted and recentrifuged at 18,000 g for 15 min. The resulting pellet (P_2)
was washed three times and resuspended in 10 ml sucrose buffer. This
suspension was layered over a gradient of 7.5% and 12% ficoll (w/v) in 0.32 mM
sucrose, 5 mM Hepes, pH 7.5) according to a modification of the procedure of
Cotman and Matthews[12] and Gurd *et al.*[13]. After centrifugation at 65,000 g for
50 minutes, the material between the 7.5% and 12% ficoll interface
(synaptosomes) was removed and recentrifuged at 110,000 g for 30 minutes. The
pellet thus obtained was resuspended in buffer and used immediately for Ca^{++}
uptake studies.

Synaptosomal calcium uptake

(a) Centrifugation technique

Aliquots of synaptosomal suspensions were used for determination of Ca^{++} uptake. After allowing the sample to incubate at 30°C for two minutes in a
Dubnoff shaker the preparation was incubated for fixed intervals between 0.5 to

10 minutes with 1 ml $^{45}Ca^{++}$ (specific activity 0.05 mCi/mg) in a solution containing 0.1 mM $CaCl_2$ (final concentration) 3 mM $MgCl_2$, 3 mM ATP, disodium salt, 50 mM tris pH 7.5 was added at fixed intervals. Ca^{++} uptake was terminated by the addition of 6 ml of ice cold stopping solution (100 mM NaCl 3 mM $MgCl_2$, 0.1 mM $CaCl_2$ 50 mM tris, pH 7.5) and the suspensions were centrifugated at 110,000 g for 30 minutes[14,15]. The supernate was removed as completely as possible by aspiration and each tube carefully dried with cotton swabs. The pellet was dissolved in 0.5 ml of tissue solubilizer (NCS), transferred to glass counting vials containing 10 ml of counting solution (omnifluor 16 g/gallon of toluene), and the $^{45}Ca^{++}$ present determined by liquid scintillation spectrometry. The amount of protein from synaptosomes was determined by the method of Lowry et al.[16] using bovine serum albumin as standard.

The Ca^{++} uptake for the 10 minute period was calculated from the Ca^{++} radioactivity within the synaptosomal pellet and expressed as umoles synaptosomal Ca^{++}/g protein. The initial rate of Ca^{++} uptake along the linear portion of the uptake curve is reported as umole Ca/g protein/min and the plateau level of the uptake curve was taken as maximal Ca^{++} uptake (umole/g). Drug additions to the incubation media and any modification of the method are noted in the legends for each figure.

Animal treatment

Mice were maintained at room temperature, water and food were given ad libitum. The concentration of the drugs added in vitro are expressed as the molar base. For assessing the effects of morphine acutely, mice were given 10 mg/kg morphine sulfate intraperitoneally 30 minutes before sacrifice. Tolerance-dependence was induced by the subcutaneous implantation of a single morphine pellet[17] and three days later mice were sacrificed for preparation of synaptosomes.

RESULTS

Calcium uptake into mouse brain synaptosomes

There is an initial phase of rapid Ca^{++} uptake for about 2-3 minutes and this rapid phase is followed by a slower phase which reaches a plateau in about 6 min.   Calculation of the slope of the linear portion of the curve using the method of linear regression gives a value of 2.35 ± 0.08 umole Ca^{++}/g synaptosomal protein/min for the initial rate of Ca^{++} uptake.   The plateau (steady state) value for control uptake is 5.32 ± 0.40 umole Ca^{++}/g synaptosomal protein.   These data are in good agreement with those reported by Lust and Robinson[14,15] and Blaustein et al.[18] using similar methods to determine Ca^{++} uptake into synaptosomes and are summarized in Table 1.

Effect of morphine on synaptosomal calcium uptake

Morphine significantly reduced the calcium uptake into the synaptosomes. The decrease was observed in both the initial rate and maximal level which was reduced to 60% of control.   As can be seen in Table 1, both the initial and maximal rate of Ca^{++} uptake was decreased in a dose-dependent manner.   A similar effect was produced after acute injection of morphine (10 mg/kg/ip). The inhibition was rapid and near maximal by 6 minutes.   The in vitro and acute morphine effect on synaptosomal Ca^{++} uptake both appear to be a specific opiate action since naloxone pretreatment (1.9 x 10^{-8} M in vitro and 2 mg/kg/sc in vivo) reversed the reduction in Ca^{++} uptake produced by morphine (Table 2).

Effect of levorphanol and dextrorphan on synaptosomal calcium uptake

Preincubation of synaptosomes with the potent opiate agonist, levorphanol, also significantly reduced Ca^{++} uptake.   As can be noted in Table 1, at equivalent concentrations levorphanol decreased both the initial Ca^{++} uptake velocity and the maximum Ca^{++} uptake level to a greater degree than morphine. On the other hand, dextrorphan, the inactive isomer of levorphanol had no effect on the initial or maximal Ca^{++} uptake.

TABLE 1

EFFECT OF OPIATES *IN VITRO* ON THE INITIAL AND MAXIMAL CA^{++} UPTAKE INTO
SYNAPTOSOMES BY THE CENTRIFUGATION TECHNIQUE[a]

Treatment	Calcium uptake[b] (umol/g/min) initial	%I	(umol/g/10 min) maximal	%I
Experiment I				
Control	2.6 ± 0.12	%I	5.10 ± 0.55	
Morphine Sulfate				
0.17 uM	2.2 ± 0.10	15	3.10 ± 0.20^d	39
0.34 uM	1.66 ± 0.08^c	36	1.93 ± 0.30^d	62
Dextrorphan				
0.17 uM	2.60 ± 0.08	-	4.90 ± 0.35	4.0
Levorphanol				
0.17 uM	1.60 ± 0.10^c	38	1.70 ± 0.20^d	69
Experiment II				
Control	2.75 ± 0.10		4.75 ± 0.25	
Morphine Sulfate				
0.17 uM	2.05 ± 0.12	22	2.85 ± 0.30^d	40
Morphine Sulfate 0.17 uM + Naloxone 0.019 uM	2.65 ± 0.10	3.6	4.55 ± 0.20	4.2

[a]See Materials and Methods
[b]Mean S.E.M. for 4 preparations run in triplicate
Values significantly different from Control values
^{c}(P < .01)
^{d}(P < .ool) as determined by Student's t test.

Effect of Ca^{++} concentration on the morphine blockade of calcium uptake

Since the previous data established that morphine could inhibit Ca^{++} uptake
into the synaptosomes, it was of interest to test this effect at several
different external calcium concentrations (Ca^{++})$_o$ to determine whether morphine was acting as a competitive or non-competitive inhibitor of calcium uptake.   A double reciprocal plot of the data obtained from incubating the

316

TABLE 2

EFFECT OF MORPHINE SULFATE *IN VIVO* ON THE UPTAKE OF CA^{++} IN SYNAPTOSOMES[a]

Treatment	Calcium uptake[b] (umol/g/min) initial		(umol/g/10 min) maximal	
Saline	1.94 ± 0.26	%I	4.28 ± 0.18	%I
Morphine Sulfate				
10 mg/kg/ip	1.12 ± 0.18	42	2.49 ± 0.25[c]	41.83
Morphine Sulfate 10 mg/kg/ip + Naloxone 2 mg/kg/sc	2.04 ± 0.11	-	3.77 ± 0.28	12.0

[a]See Materials and Methods
[b]Mean S.E.M. for 4 preparations run in triplicate
[c]$P < .002$

synaptosomes with various calcium concentrations in the presence and absence of morphine indicated a non-competitive inhibition of calcium uptake by morphine.

Additional experiments were performed to corroborate our previous findings in the filtration technique. The data obtained supported those obtained with a centrifugation procedure. However, although the absolute values for $^{45}Ca^{++}$ during initial rate and plateau are greater with filtration techniques than with centrifugation techniques the per cent of inhibition on Ca^{++} uptake produced by addition of morphine *in vitro* using filtration technique was 25%, whereas, with centrifugation morphine decreased the synaptosomal Ca^{++} uptake by 40-45%. On the other hand the inhibition of Ca^{++} uptake produced after single morphine administration (10 mg/kg/ip) was similar with both methods.

Time course of synaptosomal Ca^{++} uptake after chronic morphine

A progressive increase in Ca^{++} uptake was observed after pellet implantation for 1, 2, and 3 days. The time course of synaptosomal Ca^{++} uptake after development of tolerance and dependence was also consistent with earlier observations and with the extent of tolerance and dependence developed after pellet implantation. The maximal Ca^{++} uptake after 3 days of morphine pellet implantation occurred within 1 minute whereas in the non-tolerant control maximal uptake of Ca^{++} did not occur until after 6 minutes of incubation. As shown in Table 3, an inverse relationship was found to exist between the time for maximal calcium uptake and the duration of morphine pellet implantation. The time for maximal Ca^{++} uptake decreased from 6 minutes on day 1 to 3 minutes after 2 days and to 1 minute after 3 days. However, the maximal calcium uptake (5 umole/g) was the same for the morphine treated and control groups. The progressive faster plateau of Ca^{++} reached after morphine pellet implantation for 1, 2, and 3 days suggest the possibility that calcium fluxes are affected during development of tolerance and dependence. To explore this possibility the synaptosomal Ca^{++} efflux is being studied after chronic morphine treatment (manuscript in preparation).

TABLE 3

RELATIONSHIP OF THE TIME AFTER MORPHINE PELLET IMPLANTATION AND SYNAPTOSOMAL $^{45}CA^{++}$ UPTAKE

Duration of pellet implantation[a] (hours)	Maximal $^{45}Ca^{++}$ uptake[b] (umol/g)	Time to reach maximum (min)
0	5.75 ± 0.25 (4)	10
24	4.70 ± 0.20 (4)	6
48	4.90 ± 0.43 (4)	3
72	5.15 ± 0.25 (4)	1

[a] Morphine pellet contains 75 mg of morphine base and was placed subcutaneously (See Methods).
[b] Number of determinations/group and the mean ± S.E.M.

DISCUSSION

The data clearly indicate that synaptosomes have a viable Ca^{++} uptake mechanism and that can be blocked in a dose-dependent manner by *in vitro* or acute morphine treatment and that after tolerant and dependent development synaptosomal Ca^{++} uptake becomes enhanced. These findings support previously reported *in vitro* data from this laboratory[10] and are consistent with our other findings indicating that synaptosomal Ca^{++} content is decreased after acute morphine administration and increased after tolerance development[9,10]. Moreover, the decrease in Ca^{++} after acute morphine administration is accompanied by decreased binding of Ca^{++} by synaptic vesicles and is reversed after chronic morphine administration.   It appears from the present data the decrease in synaptosomal Ca^{++} content after acute morphine treatment could at least be due in part to decreased Ca^{++} uptake.   This is further supported by preliminary data indicating that Ca^{++} efflux is not affected by morphine *in vitro* and only slightly increased after acute morphine injection.

As was mentioned above, increasing Ca^{++} produces a diminution of morphine antinociceptive action[4,5] whereas decreasing neuronal Ca^{++} either with EGTA or lanthanum potentiates morphine analgesia[6,7].   It appears reasonable, therefore, to consider a possible relationship between the decrease of synaptosomal Ca^{++} uptake and the antinociceptive action.   Such a possibility appears plausible since both effects are selective opiate actions.   Thus, dextrorphan, the inactive isomer of levorphanol neither affects Ca^{++} uptake nor possesses anti-nociceptive action.   Furthermore, both the analgesic effects and the inhibi-tion of Ca^{++} uptake produced by opiates are antagonized by naloxone.   Moreover, rank order of potency of levorphanol is higher than that of morphine with respect to both analgesia and inhibition of synaptosomal Ca^{++} uptake and the latter decrease may be due to a reduction in Ca^{++} uptake.   Finally, after chronic morphine treamtment and the development of tolerance to anti-nociceptive action   there is an enhancement of a synaptosomal Ca^{++} uptake after chronic morphine treatment and this increase is proportional to the degree of tolerance developed.   The enhancement of Ca^{++} uptake observed is also consistent with previous reports showing an increase of synaptosomal Ca^{++} content and synaptic vesicular calcium binding after tolerance and dependence development.   Since Ca^{++} antagonizes morphine analgesia, this accumulation of of Ca^{++} after chronic morphine treatment provides a mechanism to explain tolerance.

Although the number of Ca^{++} pools in the synaptosomes that control the internal Ca^{++} levels has not been delineated, it would appear that the changes affected by morphine on Ca^{++} disposition may be due to alteration of specific internal Ca^{++} pools.   Since the mitochondria is the largest Ca-pool localized in the subcellular component it would be only logical to look for changes in this fraction after morphine treatment.   However, Harris *et al.* have reported that mitochondrial content is not affected by morphine acutely or chronically and mitochondrial Ca^{++} uptake is also not affected (unpublished data).   Although small changes in mitochondrial content would be difficult to detect, we believe it significant that no changes were noted after morphine when synaptosomal and synaptic vesicles Ca^{++} content were altered.   Recently it has been reported that there is an ATP-dependent Ca^{++} storage site in synaptosomes which has a much higher affinity for Ca^{++} than mitochondria and it appears to be involved in controlling the internal calcium levels[20].   Our preliminary studies show that the ATP-dependent Ca^{++} storage site in synaptosomes is also affected by morphine.

The functional Ca^{++} which is altered by morphine has not been established but a reasonable inference would be the Ca^{++} pool which is concerned with neurotransmitter release.   It has been demonstrated that morphine inhibits the release of acetylcholine[21,22] and norepinephrine[23] and since it is well-known that Ca^{++} entry is coupled with neurotransmitter release[24,25] a close relationship between these two parameters needs to be considered.   Such an approach is especially appealing since it has also been found that synaptic vesicular Mg^{++} dependent ATPase activity increases with development of tolerance to morphine[26] and it has been reported that this enzyme is associated with neurotransmitter release[27].   Also Blaustein *et al.* suggest that an increase in the intraneuronal Ca^{++} concentration may be involved in in triggering neurotransmitter release[27,28] and if this be the case, morphine could well inhibit neurotransmitter release by decreasing intraneuronal Ca^{++}.

ACKNOWLEDGEMENTS

We are grateful to Mr. Dennis Duncan for able technical assistance and the patient and skilled efforts of Ms. Jacky Carnes were responsible for the preparation of the manuscript.

REFERENCES

1. Takemori, A.E. (1962) J. Pharmacol. Exp. Ther. 135, 89-93.

2. Elliott, H.W., Kokka, N., and Way, E.L. (1963) Proc. Soc. Exp. Biol. Med. 113, 1049-1052.

3. Heimans, R.L.H. (1975) Archiv. int. Pharmacodyn. 215, 13-19.

4. Kakunaga, T., Kaneto, H., and Hano, K. (1966) J. Pharmacol. Exp. Ther. 153, 134-141.

5. Kaneto, H. (1971) in Narcotic Drugs: Biochemical Pharmacology Clouet, D.H., ed., Plenum Publ. Corp., New York, pp. 300-309.

6. Harris, R.A., Loh, H.H. and Way, E.L. (1975) J. Pharmacol. Exp. Ther., 195, 488-498.

7. Cerreta, K.V., Loh, H.H., and Way, E.L. (1977) Fed. Proc. 36(3), 943.

8. Ross, D.H., Medina, M.A., and Cardenas, H.L. (1964) Science 186, 63-65.

9. Harris, R.A., Yamamoto, H., Loh, H.H., and Way, E.L. (1977) Life Sciences 20, 501-506.

10. Yamamoto, H., Harris, R.A., Loh, H.H., and Way, E.L. (1978) J. Pharmacol. Exp. Ther. 205, 255-264.

11. Kakunaga, T., Kaneto, H., and Hano, H. (1966) Folia Pharmacol. Jap. 62, 31-39

12. Cotman, C.W., and Mathews, D.A. (1971) Biochem. Biophys. Acta 249, 380-394.

13. Gurd, J.W., Jones, A.R., Mahler, H.R., and Moore, W.J. (1974) J. Neurochem. 22, 281-290.

14. Lust, W.D., and Robinson, J.D. (1970) J. Neurobiol. 1(3), 303-316.

15. Lust, W.D., and Robinson, J.D. (1970) J. Neurobiol. 1(3), 317-328, 1970.

16. Lowry, O.H., Rorebrough, N.L., Farr, A.J., and Randall, R.J. (1951) J. Biol. Chem. 193, 265-275.

17. Way, E.L., Loh, H.H., and Shen, F.J. (1969) J. Pharmacol. Exp. Ther. 167, 1-8

18. Blaustein, M.P. and Oborn, C.J. (1975) J. Physiol. 247, 657-686.

19. Blaustein, M.P. and Roussell, J.M. (1975) J. Memb. Biol. 22, 285-312.

20. Kendrick, N.C., Blaustein, M.P., Fried, R.C. and Ratzlaff, R.W. (1977) Nature (Lond.) 265, 246-248.

21. Paton, W.D.M. (1957) Brit. J. Pharmacol. 12, 119-127.

22. Schauman, W. (1957) Brit. J. Pharmacol. 12, 115-118.

23. Henderson, G., Hughes, J., and H.W. Kosterlitz, (1976) Brit. J. Pharmacol. 46, 764-766.

24. Douglas, W.W. (1968) Br. J. Pharmacol. 34, 451-474.

25. Rubin, R.P. (1970) Pharmacol. Rev. 22, 389-428.

26. Yamamoto, H., Harris, R.A., Loh, H.H. and Way, E.L. (1977) Life Sciences 20, 1533-1540.

27. Poisner, A.M. and Trifaro, J.M. (1967) Mol. Pharmacol. 3, 561-571.

28. Blaustein, M.P., Johnson, E.M.J., Needleman, P. (1972) Proc. Natl. Acad. Sci. U.S.A. 69, 2237-2240.

Characteristics and Function of Opioids, editors Van Ree and Terenius
© *1978 Elsevier/North-Holland Biomedical Press*

INTERACTION OF ENDORPHINS WITH BRAIN CATECHOLAMINE SYSTEMS

DIRK H.G. VERSTEEG, E. RONALD DE KLOET and DAVID DE WIED
Rudolf Magnus Institute for Pharmacology, Medical Faculty, University of
Utrecht, Vondellaan 6, Utrecht (The Netherlands)

ABSTRACT

Following the intracerebroventricular administration of methionine-enkephalin in a dose of 200 pmoles per rat the α-MPT-induced catecholamine disappearance was found to be altered in distinct brain regions. A significantly
enhanced noradrenaline disappearance was observed in the medial preoptic
nucleus and the central amygdaloid nucleus, whereas noradrenaline disappearance was attenuated in the ventral central gray and the A2-region; dopamine
disappearance following synthesis inhibition was increased in the arcuate
nucleus and decreased in the dorsal central gray. The data obtained support
the suggestion that the endorphins act as modulators of neurotransmission
in specific brain regions. Since the pattern of effects of methionine-enkephalin in forebrain regions is different from that observed for α-endorphin,
β-endorphin and (des-Tyr[1])-γ-endorphin in a previous study, another provisional
conclusion may be that a regional differentiation exists in the interaction
of the various endorphins with catecholamine neurotransmission in the brain.

INTRODUCTION

Using immunocytochemical techniques it has been shown that the rat brain
contains circumscribed neuronal networks containing enkephalin-like[1-3] and
β-LPH-like[4] immunoreactivity. Probably the system containing β-LPH and that
containing enkephalin constitute two separate systems[1-6]. Fibers of both
networks appear to occur in close association with various parts of the catecholamine systems in the brain[1-4]. These neuroanatomical data fit well with the
hypothesis that endorphins may act as modulators of specific transmitter
systems in the brain. Relatively few and sometimes conflicting data are presently available concerning effects of endorphins on the activity of transmitter systems; however, the pattern that emerges from these data is that
effects are not widespread in the brain but occur in distinct brain regions
[7-15]. In this communication the results are presented of a study concerning
the effects of methionine-enkephalin (met-enk), administered i.c.v. in a
relatively low dose, on α-MPT-induced catecholamine disappearance in discrete

brain regions. The results are discussed in relation to those obtained in a similar study with various longer β-LPH fragments[15].

MATERIALS AND METHODS

Male rats weighing 130-150 g were used. They were kept under controlled lighting conditions, with lights on from 7 a.m. to 6 p.m., and had access to water and chow ad lib. Three to four days before the day of the experiment polyethylene canulas were implanted in the lateral ventricle as previously described[16]. On the day of the experiment all rats received α-methy-para-tyrosine methylester HCl (α-MPT; Labkemi AB, Göteborg; 300 mg/kg, i.p.); 30 min after the α-MPT administration half of the rats received 200 pmoles met-enk (Dr. H.M. Greven, Organon International B.V., Oss) in 1 μl saline through the intraventricular canula; the other half received 1 μl saline. Three h later, i.e. 3.5 h following α-MPT, the rats were killed by decapitation.

The brains were taken out rapidly and frozen on dry ice. Discrete brain regions were dissected from 300 μm sections according to Palkovits[17] as pre-viously described[18,19]. Tissue of two rats was pooled. Protein was measured in 10 μl samples of the homogenate of the tissue pellets in 50 μl 0.1 N HClO4 according to Lowry et al.[20]. After centrifugation of the residual homogenates noradrenaline and dopamine were assayed in 20 μl samples of the supernatants according to Van der Gugten et al.[21]. Data are expressed as pg catecholamine per μg protein $\pm$ S.E.M. Tests of significance were performed using Student's t-test. Values of P less than 0.05 were considered as indicating significant differences.

RESULTS

The results show that, following the i.c.v. administration of met-enk in as low a dose as 200 pmoles, α-MPT-induced catecholamine disappearance is altered in distinct brain regions. A significantly enhanced noradrenaline disappearance was observed in the medial preoptic nucleus and the central amygdaloid nucleus, whereas noradrenaline disappearance was attenuated in the ventral central gray and in the A2-region (Table 1). The changes in the nucleus accumbens and the dorsal central gray were close to significance (P < 0.1). Dopamine disappearance following synthesis inhibition with α-MPT was increased in the arcuate nucleus and decreased in the dorsal central gray of rats that had been treated with met-enk (Table 2).

TABLE 1

NORADRENALINE AND DOPAMINE CONTENT OF FOREBRAIN REGIONS OF RATS THAT HAD RE-
CEIVED α-MPT (i.p.) 3.5 h, AND MET-ENK OR SALINE (i.c.v.) 3 h PRIOR TO DE-
CAPITATION

	NORADRENALINE (pg/μg protein)		% change	DOPAMINE (pg/μg protein)		% change
	saline	met-enk		saline	met-enk	
Nucl. accumbens	4.04+0.32[a)	3.01+0.37	-25	20.04+1.09	23.27+1.56	-16
Caudat nucl.	n.d.[b)	n.d.		24.20+2.34	26.76+0.53	+11
Globus pallidus	4.31+0.49	4.81+0.62	+12	2.40+0.56	2.50+0.52	+ 4
Dors. septal nucl.	3.22+0.36	2.46+0.34	-24	1.94+0.28	1.83+0.42	- 6
Lat. septal nucl.	6.92+0.62	7.34+1.04	+ 6	3.41+0.24	3.53+0.33	- 4
Med. septal nucl.	4.69+0.34	5.31+0.47	+13	1.55+0.18	1.78+0.25	+15
Nucl. int. str. term.	20.32+2.47	17.86+3.49	-12	4.60+1.05	4.30+0.86	- 7
Med. preoptic nucl.	18.86+1.18	14.63+1.23*	-22	1.27+0.29	1.10+0.32	-13
Supraoptic nucl.	8.97+0.89	9.72+1.08	+ 8	n.d.	n.d.	
Periventricular nucl.	22.99+3.52	25.55+2.49	+11	1.21+0.17	1.12+0.20	- 7
Paraventricular nucl.	30.41+4.42	22.14+3.21	-27	1.91+0.22	1.90+0.26	- 1
Anterior hypoth. nucl.	7.38+0.37	7.40+0.43	0	n.d.	n.d.	
Med. forebr. bundle	12.17+1.46	12.01+1.30	- 1	n.d.	n.d.	
Arcuate nucl.	8.54+1.69	6.75+1.92	-21	3.59+0.57	1.45+0.28[φ]	-60
Median eminence	13.61+1.82	15.52+1.14	+14	6.50+0.64	8.19+0.72	+26
Ventromedial nucl.	8.95+1.30	10.24+0.89	+14	0.75+0.18	0.82+0.30	+ 9
Dorsomedial nucl.	29.07+1.85	31.27+4.36	+ 8	0.67+0.11	0.75+0.14	+12
Centr. amygd. nucl.	4.44+0.22	3.38+0.23[φ]	-24	n.d.	n.d.	
Parafascicular nucl.	3.33+0.55[a)	3.63+0.32	+ 9	n.d.[b)	n.d.	
Ventr. thal. nucl.	2.39+0.34	2.01+0.20	-16	n.d.	n.d.	
Lat. post. thal. nucl.	1.47+0.20	1.46+0.32	- 1	n.d.	n.d.	
Subiculum	2.35+0.46	2.04+0.49	-13	n.d.	n.d.	
Gyrus dentatus	3.32+0.40	3.51+0.73	+ 6	n.d.	n.d.	
CA2 region	3.35+0.22	3.25+0.23	- 3	n.d.	n.d.	

a) mean $\pm$ S.E.M. (n = 6-7); b) n.d. = not detectable; $*$ P < 0.05;
φ P < 0.01 for differences with saline treated controls (Student's t-test)

TABLE 2

NORADRENALINE AND DOPAMINE CONTENT OF HINDBRAIN REGIONS OF RATS THAT HAD
RECEIVED α-MPT (i.p) 3.5 h, AND MET-ENK OR SALINE (i.c.v.) 3 h PRIOR TO
DECAPITATION

	NORADRENALINE (pg/μg protein)		% change	DOPAMINE (pg/μg protein)		% change
	saline	met-enk		saline	met-enk	
Dors. raphe nucl.	4.68+0.68[a]	5.12+0.86	+ 9	1.98+0.39	1.59+0.52	-20
Dors. central gray	4.90+0.41	3.77+0.33	-23	0.97+0.07	0.62+0.10$^{\emptyset}$	-36
Ventr. central gray	3.71+0.37	6.09+0.45$^{\pm}$	+64	0.57+0.11	0.92+0.21	+61
Nucl. ruber	3.79+0.28	4.40+0.46	+16	n.d.[b]	n.d.	
A8-region	4.72+0.63	4.83+0.71	+ 2	2.05+0.66	1.26+0.34	-39
A9-region	3.12+0.29	2.78+0.32	-11	4.96+1.04	4.15+0.65	-16
A10-region	4.25+0.25	4.02+0.22	- 5	3.98+0.89	2.96+0.71	-26
Subst. nigra (retic.)	3.82+0.43	3.97+0.21	+ 4	1.32+0.38	0.92+0.13	-30
A5-region	5.72+0.77	6.33+0.90	+11	n.d.	n.d.	
Locus coeruleus	16.39+1.67	12.95+2.77	-21	n.d.	n.d.	
Nucl. raphe magnus	4.95+0.66	5.61+0.42	+13	n.d.	n.d.	
Nucl. tract.solitarii	7.63+1.60	6.32+0.66	-17	n.d.	n.d.	
A1-region	4.65+0.71	4.42+0.30	- 5	n.d.	n.d.	
A2-region	16.25+1.74	23.35+2.17*	+44	1.18+0.28	1.27+0.29	+ 7

a) mean $\pm$ S.E.M. (n = 6-7); b) n.d. = not detectable; $*$ P < 0.05;
$\emptyset$ P < 0.02; $\pm$ P < 0.005 for differences with saline treated controls (Student's
t-test).

DISCUSSION

Analgesia can be induced by met-enk, but the doses needed are very high (up
to hundreds of μgs, i.c.v.) and the effects are short lasting[22-27]. This has
been explained as being due to the very rapid enzymatic degradation of met-enk
in the brain[28-31]. Effects of met-enk on avoidance behavior, however, can be
obtained with much lower doses[32]. This and other data have been interpreted
as indicating that interaction with the perception of pain is not the primary
effect of the endorphins[32-34]. The dose employed in the present study was based
on these considerations and is approximately 1000 times lower than those
previously used in studies on effects of met-enk on catecholamine metabolism
in the brain by Ferland et al.[7], Algeri et al.[12], Calderini et al[13],

Biggio et al.[14] and Laska and Fennessy[35]. Nevertheless pronounced effects were observed on α-MPT-induced catecholamine disappearance in discrete brain regions. As far as the regions are concerned where effects were found, it appears that these in general coincide with brain areas rich in enkephalin-like immuno-reactivity[1-3]. This certainly holds for the amygdaloid nucleus and the dorsal and ventral central gray. However, in other areas with enkephalin containing projections[1-3] no significant effects were observed. Although there were tendencies towards a decrease, no significant changes were found in dopamine disappearance in the median eminence in which region Ferland et al.[7] found a significant decrease in α-MPT-induced dopamine disappearance following i.c.v. met-enk administration, or in the caudate nucleus. It is difficult to compare the present results for the caudate nucleus with literature data, since studies on effects of met-enk on dopamine metabolism in this region thus far have led to rather conflicting results: using high doses in the range of 100-200 μg i.c.v. no effects[12] and both a decreased[13] and an increased[14] dopamine synthesis have been reported.

In a similar study we recently measured the effects of i.c.v. administered α-endorphin, β-endorphin and (des-tyrosine[1])-γ-endorphin on α-MPT-induced catecholamine disappearance in forebrain regions in a similar dose range as was used for met-enk in the present study[15]. It appears that in the forebrain the pattern of effects of met-enk clearly differs from that observed for the above mentioned endorphins[15]. The effect of met-enk on noradrenaline disappearance in the central amygdaloid nucleus is opposite to that of α-endorphin and, whereas α-endorphin was found to decrease α-MPT-induced dopamine disappearance in a variety of forebrain regions, among which were the caudate nucleus, globus pallidus, medial septal nucleus, paraventricular nucleus, zona incerta and central amygdaloid nucleus[15], met-enk was without effect in either of these structures.

Clearly, comparisons like the above should be regarded with caution. Differences in dose are likely to contribute to this, but it should be realized that the occurrence and magnitude of effects of endorphins is not only dependent on the dose and the metabolic stability of these compounds in the brain. Factors as the receptor types present in a given region, the affinity and intrinsic activity of the administered compound for these various receptors, the activity of products resulting from the enzymatic degradation of the compound and, finally, the fractional amount of the catecholamine neurons in a region affected by the peptide should also be taken into account. Evidence for the possible involvement of all these factors is available. It is

likely that the enkephalin containing network in the brain and that
containing β-LPH represent two indepent systems with distinct differences
in their projections to various brain regions[1-6]. Differences in affinity
have been observed for representatives of the class of the endorphins
for opiate receptors in brain and peripheral tissues[36-40]. Recently it
was found that γ-endorphin and, even more markedly, its des-tyrosine[1]
analog, (des-Tyr[1])-γ-endorphin, have effects on avoidance behavior
opposite to those of α-endorphin[34,41]. Interestingly, (des-Tyr[1])-γ-
endorphin also has an effect on dopamine disappearance in the paraventricular
nucleus and zona incerta opposite to that of α-endorphin[15]. It might be possible
that in the caudate nucleus, and also in other structures, met-enk at low doses
has no effects or only slight effects resembling those of α-endorphin[15], whereas the effects at analgesic doses are similar to those of morphine[42,43] and the
more stable enkephalin analog D-ala[2]-met-enk[13,14]. Alternatively, it could be
that degradation products of met-enk, e.g. the des-tyrosine analog, have
effects different from those of met-enk itself (cf.[13]).

In addition to analgesic effects[22-27] and effects on avoidance behavior[32,34],
the endorphins have been shown to exert a variety of behavioral, neuroendocrine
and autonomic effects. Endorphin-induced alterations in specific catecholamine
systems have been related to some of these effects. Thus, it was suggested by
Ferland et al.[7] that the decrease in α-MPT-induced dopamine disappearance in
the medial and lateral palisade zones of the median eminence following infusion of met-enk in the lateral ventricle is related to the increase in prolactin release elicited by this compound. Likewise, it is tempting to speculate
that the change induced by met-enk in the disappearance of noradrenaline in
the A2-region has some bearing on the respiratory and cardiovascular effects
of the peptide[44-47]. However, in most cases insufficient evidence is available
to enable to relate specific changes in catecholamine neurotransmission with
the effects of endorphins.Some of the endorphins, but also vasopressin, delay
extinction of pole-jumping avoidance behavior; the influence of vasopressin
has been interpreted as being on memory processes, those of the endorphins
seem to be on adaptive processes[32,34,48,49]. Particularly noradrenaline
neurotransmission in limbic structures as the dorsal septal nucleus and the
parafascicular nucleus of the thalamus seem to be involved in the effects of
vasopressin on avoidance behavior[19,48,49]. Based on the present data and those
concerning the longer endorphins which were presented elsewhere[15] it can
tentatively be concluded that the effects of the endorphins in this respect
are mediated by other neuronal systems than those involved in the effects
of vasopressin.

ACKNOWLEDGEMENT

The skilful technical assistance of Mr. Henk Spierenburg and Mr. Cees C. Creutzburg is gratefully acknowledged. Methionine-enkephalin was kindly supplied by Dr. Henk M. Greven, Organon International B.V., Oss, the Netherlands.

REFERENCES

1. Elde, R., Hökfelt, T., Johansson, O. and Terenius, L. (1976) Neuroscience 1, 349-351.

2. Simantov, R., Kuhar, M.J., Uhl, G.R. and Snyder, S.H. (1977) Proc. Natl. Acad. Sci. USA, 74, 2167-2171.

3. Watson, S.J., Akil, H., Sullivan, S. and Barchas, J.D. (1977) Life Sci. 21, 733-738.

4. Watson, S.J., Barchas, J.D. and Li, C.H. (1977) Proc. Natl. Acad. Sci. USA, 74, 5162-5165.

5. Rossier, J., Vargo, T.M., Minick, S., Ling, N., Bloom, F.E. and Guillemin, R. (1977) Proc. Natl. Acad. Sci. USA 74, 5162-5165.

6. Barchas, J.D., Akil, H., Elliott, G.R., Holman, R.B. and Watson, S.J. (1978) Science 200, 964-973.

7. Ferland, L., Fuxe, K., Eneroth, P., Gustafsson, J.A. and Skett, P. (1976) Europ. J. Pharmacol. 43, 89-90.

8. Izumi, K., Motomatsu, T., Chrétien, M., Butterworth, R.F., Lis, M., Seidah, N. and Barbeau, A. (1977) LIfe Sci. 20, 1149-1156.

9. Moroni, F., Cheney, D.L. and Costa, E. (1977) Nature 267, 267-268.

10. Moroni, F., Cheney, D.L. and Costa, E. (1978) Neuropharmacology 17, 191-196.

11. Arbilla, S. and Langer, S.Z. (1978) Nature, 271, 559-561.

12. Algeri, S., Calderini, G., Consolazione, A. and Garattini, S. (1977) Europ. J. Pharmacol. 45, 207-209.

13. Calderini, G., Consolazione, A., Garattini, S. and Algeri, S. (1978) Brain Res. 146, 392-399.

14. Biggio, G., Casu, M., Corda, M.G., Di Bello, C. and Gessa, G.L. (1978) Science 200, 552-554.

15. Versteeg, D.H.G., De Kloet, E.R. and De Wied, D., Brain Research, Submitted.

16. De Wied, D. (1976) Life Sci. 19, 685-690.

17. Palkovits, M. (1973) Brain Res. 59, 449-450.

18. Versteeg, D.H.G., Van der Gugten, J., De Jong, W. and Palkovits M. (1976) Brain Res. 113, 563-574.

19. Tanaka, M., De Kloet, E.R., De Wied, D. and Versteeg, D.H.G. (1977) Life Sci. 20, 1799-1808.

20. Lowry, O.H., Rosebrough, N.J., Farr, A.L. and Randall, R.J. (1951) J. Biol. Chem. 193, 265-275.

21. Van der Gugten, J., Palkovits, M., Wijnen, H.J.L.M. and Versteeg, D.H.G. (1976) Brain Res. 107, 171-175.

22. Bloom, F., Segal, D., Ling, N. and Guillemin, R. (1976) Science 194, 630-632.

23. Büscher, H.H., Hill, R.C., Römer, D., Cardinaux, F., Closse, A., Hauser, D. and Pless, J. (1976) Nature 261, 423-425.

24. Leybin, L., Pinsky, C., LaBella, F.S., Havlicek, V. and Rezek, M. (1976) Nature 264, 458-459.

25. Van Ree, J.M., De Wied, D., Bradbury, A.F., Hulme, E.C., Smyth, D.G. and Snell, C.R. (1976) Nature, 264, 792-794.

26. Jacquet, Y.F. and Marks, N. (1976) Science 194, 632-635.

27. Bradbury, A.F., Smyth, D.G., Snell, C.R., Deakin, J.F.W. and Wendlandt, S. (1977) Biochem. Biophys. Res. Comm. 74, 748-754.

28. Hambrook, J.M., Morgan, B.A., Rance, M.J. and Smith, C.F.C. (1976) Nature 262, 782-783.

29. Miller, R.J., Chang, K.J. and Cuatrecasas, P. (1977) Biochem. Biophys. Res. Comm. 74, 1311-1317.

30. Marks, N., Greynbaum, A. and Neidle, A. (1977) Biochem. Biophys. Res. Comm. 74, 1552-1559.

31. Meek, J.L. Yang, H.Y.T. and Costa, E. (1977) Neuropharmacology 16, 151-154.

32. De Wied, D., Bohus, B., Van Ree, J.M. and Urban, I. (1978) J. Pharmacol. Exp. Ther. 204, 570-580.

33. Van Ree, J.M. and De Wied, D. (1976) in Opiates and Endogenous Opioid Peptides, Kosterlitz, H.W., ed. North Holland, Amsterdam, pp. 443-445.

34. De Wied, D., Kovacs, G.L., Bohus, B., Van Ree, J.M. and Greven, H.M. (1978) Europ. J. Pharmacol. 49, 427-436.

35. Laska, F.J. and Fennessy, M.R. (1978) Clin. Exp. Pharmacol. Physiol. 5, 95-98.

36. Birdsall, N.J., Bradbury, A.F., Burgen, A.S., Hulme, E.C., Smyth, D.G. and Snell, C.R. (1976) Brit. J. Pharmacol. 58, 460P-461P.

37. Birdsall, N.J. and Hulme E.C. (1976) Nature 260, 793-795.

38. Vall'ee, E., Chambon, J.P. and Delahayes, J. (1977) Cont. Rend. Acad. Sci. 285, 257-260.

39. Lord, J.A., Waterfield, A.A., Hughes, J. and Kosterlitz, H.W. (1977) Nature, 267, 495-499.

40. Waterfield, A.A., Smokcum, R.W., Hughes, J., Kosterlitz, H.W. and Henderson, G. (1977) Europ. J. Pharmacol. 43, 107-116.

41. De Wied, D., Bohus, B., Van Ree, J.M., Kovács, G.L. and Greven, H.M. (1978) The Lancet, May 13, 1046.

42. Sasame, H.A., Perez-Cruet, J., Di Chiara, G., Tagliamonte, A., Tagliamonte, P. and Gessa, G.J. (1972) J. Neurochem. 19, 1953-1957.

43. Kuschinsky, K. and Hornykiewicz, O. (1974) Europ. J. Pharmacol. 26, 41-50.

44. Teschemacher, H., Blässig, J. and Kromer, W. (1976) Naunyn Schmiedeberg's Arch. exp. Path. Pharmak. 294, 293-295.

45. Florêz, J. and Mediaville, A. (1977) Brain Res. 138, 585-590.

46. Bolme, P., Fuxe, K., Agnati, L.F., Bradley, R. and Smythies, J. (1978) Europ. J. Pharmacol. 48, 319-324.

47. Versteeg, D.H.G., Palkovits, M., Van der Gugten, J., Wijnen, H.J.L.M., Smeets, G.W.M. and De Jong, W. (1976) Brain Research 112, 429-434.

48. De Wied, D. (1977) Life Sci. 20, 195-204.

49. Van Ree, J.M., Bohus, B., Versteeg, D.H.G., and De Wied, D. (1978) Biochem. Pharmacol. in press.

Characteristics and Function of Opioids, editors Van Ree and Terenius
© *1978 Elsevier/North-Holland Biomedical Press*

OPIOIDS AND ANTERIOR PITUITARY HORMONE SECRETION

FERNAND LABRIE, LIONEL CUSAN, ANDRE DUPONT, LOUISE FERLAND and
ANDRE LEMAY,
Medical Research Council Group in Molecular Endocrinology, Le
Centre Hospitalier de l'Université Laval, Quebec G1V 4G2, Canada;
Laboratory of Endocrinology of Reproduction, Saint-François
d'Assise Hospital, Quebec G1L 3L5, Canada.

ABSTRACT
   Both methionine-enkephalin and β-endorphin stimulate growth
hormone and prolactin secretion after intraventricular injection
in the rat. Some analogues of methionine-enkephalin substituted
at position 2 were found to be 2000 to 5000 times more potent
than the natural peptide. β-endorphin and the highly active
(more resistant to proteolytic degradation) analogues of methionine-enkephalin can also stimulate growth hormone and prolactin
secretion after parenteral administration. While the stimulatory
effect of endorphins on growth hormone release appears to be
secondary to the stimulated release of growth hormone releasing
activity from the hypothalamus, an inhibition of dopaminergic
activity by endorphins seems to play a major role in mediating
the stimulation of prolactin release. The opiate antagonist
naloxone could completely prevent the stress-induced release of
prolactin and markedly inhibit the rise induced by suckling in
the rat, thus suggesting a physiological role of endorphins in
the stress- and suckling-induced stimulation of prolactin release
in the rat. A role of endorphins in the nocturnal rise of serum
prolactin in the human is suggested by the finding of a marked
reduction of serum prolactin levels during sleep in post-menopausal
women.

INTRODUCTION
   Morphine is well known to be a potent stimulus of growth
hormone (GH)[1,2] and prolactin[3] release in the rat. The opiate
has also been shown to stimulate prolactin secretion in the
human[4]. Since met-enkephalin and β-endorphin bind to the opiate

receptor[5,6] and have potent morphine-like activity in various
biological assays[5,7], the possibility was raised that the endogenous opioid peptides, beside their well-known analgesic potency[8,9]
and activity as behavior modulators[10], could be involved in the
neuroendocrine control of GH and prolactin secretion.

The present paper summarizes data describing the stimulatory
effect of met-enkephalin, β-endorphin and their analogues on GH
and prolactin secretion after intraventricular and parenteral
(met-enkephalin analogues and β-endorphin) administration in the
rat. Moreover, using the opiate antagonist naloxone, the present
data indicate a physiological role of endorphins in the stimulation of prolactin release induced by stress and suckling in the
rat as well as in the nocturnal rise of prolactin secretion in
the human. Recent evidence indicates that dopamine may be the
main or even the only inhibitory substance of hypothalamic origin
controlling prolactin secretion, and we present data suggesting a
role of dopamine in the potent stimulatory action of opiates on
prolactin secretion.

RESULTS AND DISCUSSION

A. Stimulatory effects of β-endorphin, met-enkephalin and
their analogues on GH and prolactin secretion. As illustrated in Fig. 1A, the intraventricular injection of 0.5 to 25 μg
of β-endorphin (β-LPH$_{61-91}$) led to a rapid and marked stimulation
of prolactin release in unanesthetized freely-moving rats. With
the 0.5 μg dose, a significant rise was already measured 5 min
after injection of the peptide and a maximal stimulation (approximately 7-fold) was measured after 10 min with a slow return
toward basal plasma hormone levels at later time intervals. The
higher doses of β-endorphin (2, 5 and 25 μg) led to a progressive
increase of prolactin release, a 30- to 60-fold increase being
measured between 20 and 60 min after injection of 25 μg of the
peptide.

Although inactive at 0.5 μg, doses of 2 μg or higher of β-
endorphin led to a significant stimulation of plasma GH release.
With the 2 μg dose, a 6- to 10-fold stimulation of the plasma GH
concentration was measured 10 and 20 min after injection of β-
endorphin, with a progressive decrease to basal levels at 45 min.

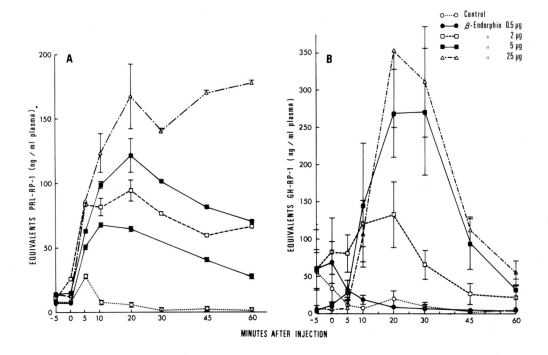

Fig. 1. Effect of increasing doses of β-endorphin on plasma prolactin (A) and GH (B) levels in the rat. Male rats bearing intraventricular and intrajugular cannulae were injected intravenously
with 0.2 ml of sheep somatostatin antiserum 5 min before the
intraventricular injection of the indicated amounts of synthetic
β-endorphin. PRL and GH concentrations were measured at the indicated time intervals after administration of β-endorphin to
8-10 animals per group. Data are presented as mean ± S.E.M.[11,12]

The two highest doses (5 and 25 µg) of β-endorphin led to a maximal 20- to 30-fold stimulation of plasma GH levels measured 20
and 30 min after injection of the peptide[11].

Methionine-enkephalin, the NH_2-terminal pentapeptide of β-
endorphin, was much less potent than β-endorphin to stimulate
prolactin and GH release. In fact, at the 500 to 1000 µg doses,
methionine-enkephalin led to approximately 4- and 6-fold increases
of plasma prolactin levels, respectively. Stimulation of GH release was observed only at the 1000 µg dose, thus indicating again
a greater sensitivity of the prolactin response to the opioid
peptide.

Specificity of the stimulatory effect of β-endorphin on prolactin and GH release is illustrated in Fig. 2 where naloxone, a specific opiate antagonist, completely blocked the stimulation of GH release (B) at a dose of 0.5 mg/kg while the highest dose of naloxone (12.5 mg) was required to completely abolish the rise of prolactin secretion. This higher resistance of the prolactin than GH responses to naloxone might be due to the greater sensitivity of prolactin than GH release to the stimulatory action of opiate peptides. This possibility is supported by the data of Figs 1 and 2 where changes of prolactin release were observed earlier and at lower doses compared to GH after β-endorphin or met-enkephalin injection. A similar preferential release of prolactin has been

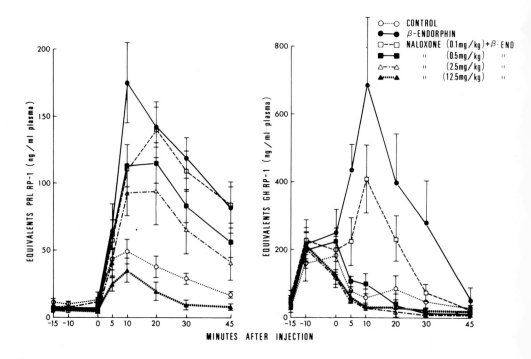

Fig. 2. Effect of increasing doses of naloxone on plasma prolactin and growth hormone release induced by intraventricular injection of 5 μg of β-endorphin in the rat. The experiment was performed as described in Fig. 1 except that naloxone was injected in the indicated groups 10 min before β-endorphin administration.

observed after injection of β-endorphin into the cisterna magna of steroid-primed rats[13]. It is also possible that these effects are secondary to different rates of access of β-endorphin and/or naloxone to their sites of action on prolactin and GH release.

The potency of met-enkephalin as stimulator of prolactin and GH release is however much lower than that of β-endorphin. In fact, the present data demonstrate that β-endorphin is 2000 times more potent than met-enkephalin to stimulate prolactin and GH secretion. This difference of biological activity is in marked contrast with the relative affinities of the two peptides for the opiate receptor; met-enkephalin shows a binding affinity for the opiate receptor approximately three times higher than β-endorphin[14]. These data indicate that the higher potency of β-endorphin is probably due to its higher resistance to degradation. It is of interest, in this connection, to mention that met-enkephalin is rapidly inactivated by plasma and brain tissue. Indeed, 15 sec after i.v. injection of [^{3}H] met-enkephalin, only 5% of total radioactivity comigrated with intact met-enkephalin, while 74% of the radioactivity was eluted in the area corresponding to tyrosine[15]. The highly potent and long-lasting activity of [D-Ala^2]met-enkephalin reported previously[16] indicates the importance of the Tyr-Gly amide bond for action of the degrading enzymes in plasma and various tissues. β-endorphin and its [D-Ala^2] analogue displayed similar potency as stimulators of GH and prolactin release when injected intraventricularly but [D-Ala^2]β-endorphin injected intravenously led to an increased duration of action of the peptide relative to the native molecule[17]. [D-Ala^2]met-enkephalin and [D-Ala^2]met-enkephalin amide were also active on GH and prolactin release after intravenous administration.

The stimulatory effect of morphine[2], β-endorphin[11,12], methionine-enkephalin[11,12] and the endorphin analogues[16] on GH release has been observed in animals where circulating somatostatin was neutralized by excess somatostatin antiserum, thus suggesting that the endogenous tetradecapeptide is not involved in the release of GH induced by opiates. Since opiate peptides cannot stimulate GH release in anterior pituitary cells in _vitro_, it is likely that the observed stimulation of GH release is due to increased release of GH-releasing activity (GH-RH) from the hypothalamus (Fig. 3).

338

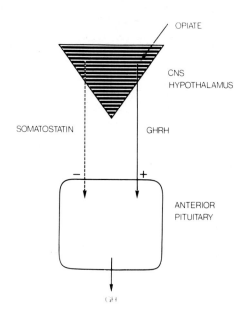

OPIATE

CNS
HYPOTHALAMUS

SOMATOSTATIN

GHRH

ANTERIOR
PITUITARY

GH

Fig. 3. Schematic representation of the stimulatory effect of
endorphins on growth hormone secretion. This effect appears to
be exerted, at least in part, through stimulation of the release
of growth hormone-releasing activity from the hypothalamus.

B. <u>Role of endorphins in stress- and suckling-induced release</u>
<u>of prolactin in the rat</u>. Acute release of prolactin in the rat is
well known to be induced by suckling[18] and a variety of stressful
stimuli such as ether, surgery, restraint, nicotine injection,
exposure to cold, heat or simple venous puncture[19-21]. Stress
also stimulates serum prolactin levels in the human, the response
being higher in women than men[22]. Moreover, suckling increases
prolactin release in women[23]. It was thus of interest to study
the possible role of endorphins in the acute release of prolactin
induced by stress and suckling. Using the specific opiate antagonist naloxone, the present data provide evidence for such a role
of endorphins.

In agreement with previous data[19], it can be seen in Fig. 4
that exposure to ether vapor led to a rapid stimulation of plasma
prolactin release. A maximal effect was already seen at 5 min

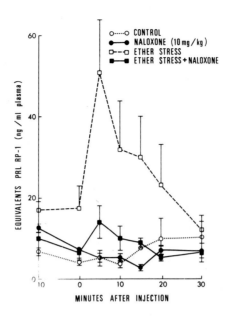

Fig. 4. Effect of naloxone (10 mg/kg) on ether-induced stimulation of plasma prolactin levels in the rat. Animals bearing an intra-jugular cannula were injected with naloxone 10 min before being exposed to ether vapor for 1-2 min. Blood sampling was performed at the indicated time intervals.

with a progressive decrease toward control levels at 30 min. When the opiate antagonist naloxone (10 mg/kg) was injected 10 min before exposure to ether, the stimulation of prolactin release was completely abolished ($p < 0.01$).

As illustrated in a representative experiment shown in Fig. 5, single injection of naloxone (5 mg/kg) 5 min before return of the pups led to a 50 to 95% inhibition of the marked rise of plasma prolactin induced by suckling up to the last time interval studied (90 min). In complementary experiments where naloxone was injected at -10, 45 and 90 min, plasma prolactin levels were still reduced from 600 ± 95 to 115 ± 40 ng/ml two hours after the start of suckl-ing (data not shown).

The present data clearly indicate that endogenous opiate peptides could be involved as mediators of the stimulatory effect of stress and suckling on prolactin release in the rat. Although TRH could

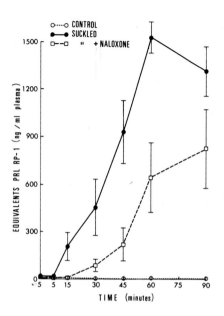

Fig. 5. Effect of naloxone (5 mg/kg) on suckling-induced prolactin release in the rat. Naloxone was injected 5 min before return
of the pups and blood samples taken at the indicated time intervals.

possibly be implicated in the effect of stress and suckling on
prolactin release, indirect evidence suggests that DA is the main
factor involved. The observation that stress elevates plasma
prolactin levels in both male and female rats except in the afternoon of proestrus or other conditions of high prolactin levels[19]
suggests that inhibition of dopaminergic activity is involved in
the response of prolactin to stress. It should be mentioned that a
role of serotonin has also been suggested in the suckling[24]- and
stress[25]-induced release of prolactin.

   C. Role of endorphins in the nocturnal rise of prolactin in the
human. Twenty-four hour studies of plasma prolactin levels in the
human show that this hormone is released episodically and that
plasma concentrations of the hormone increase after the onset of
sleep. The sleep-related increase in prolactin secretion is
dependent upon sleep itself and not related to clock time[26,27].

In an attempt to gain a better understanding of the mechanisms involved in the increased release of this hormone during sleep, we have studied the effect of naloxone infusion on serum prolactin levels.

Six healthy postmenopausal women took part in this study after giving informed consent. Three-ml blood samples were obtained at 20-min intervals through a long brachial intravenous catheter permitting sampling without disturbing the patient. A 24h- basal study showed typical nycthemeral secretory profiles. In a subsequent 24-h study, naloxone was infused continuously between 2300 and 0700h. The marked rise of serum prolactin levels occuring between 2400 and 0700 in six women was 45 to 95% inhibited by naloxone infusion (data not shown). As confirmed in other subjects, the inhibition by naloxone of serum prolactin levels is dose-dependent. No apparent change of sleeping pattern could be noticed during or after naloxone administration.

These data strongly suggest that endorphins are involved as mediators of the nocturnal rise of serum prolactin levels in the human. Coupled with our findings indicating a role of endogenous opiates in the stress- and suckling-induced release of prolactin in the rat (Figs 4 and 5), the data obtained in the human give further support for a physiological role of endorphins in the control of prolactin secretion.

D. Role of dopamine in the opiate-induced stimulation of pro-lactin in the rat. Convincing evidence suggests that dopamine (DA) may be the main or even the only inhibitory substance of hypotha-lamic origin controlling prolactin secretion[28]. It thus appeared important to study the role of DA in the potent stimulatory effect of opiates on prolactin secretion. In order to minimize possible interference by changes of TRH secretion, adult male rats which show no or little prolactin response to TRH were used. The inte-rest of such study was strenghtened by the recent findings that intraventricular injection of met-enkephalin led to a marked inhibition of DA turnover in the tubero-infundibular neurons[29].

In order to avoid interference by stress or anesthesia, all stu-dies were performed in unanesthetized freely-moving rats bearing an intrajugular cannula inserted two days previously. That the

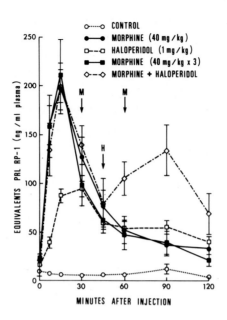

Fig. 6. Effect of a single injection of high doses of morphine, haloperidol, repeated injection of morphine or a combination of both drugs on plasma prolactin levels in the male rat. Morphine (40 mg/kg) was injected as a single dose (●——●) or given at times 0, 30 and 60 min (■——■). Haloperidol (1 mg/kg) was injected as a single dose (□--□) or 45 min after morphine (◇-◆-◇).

potent stimulatory effect of morphine on prolactin release is secondary to inhibition of dopaminergic activity is indicated by the observation that the acute response (up to 30 min) of plasma prolactin induced by a maximal dose of morphine (40 mg/kg) was not further increased by simultaneous administration of a high dose of haloperidol (1 mg/kg) (Fig. 6).

The present data clearly indicate that the acute release of prolactin induced by morphine can be accounted for by an inhibition of the inhibitory hypothalamic dopaminergic influence on prolactin secretion. This is well illustrated by the absence of further increase of prolactin by a high dose of haloperidol in animals already treated with morphine (Fig. 6). These data are in agreement with the findings of an inhibition of dopamine turnover in the medial palissade zone of the median eminence in rats

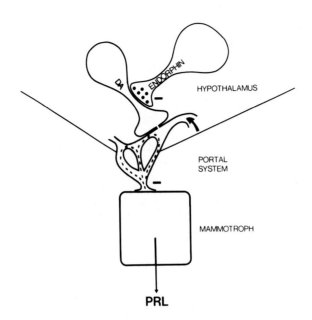

Fig.7. Schematic representation of the stimulatory effect of endorphins on prolactin release. This effect appears to be exerted, at
least partly, through inhibition of DA release.

injected intraventricularly with met-enkephalin[29].These effects are
probably due to the activation of presynaptic inhibitory opiate receptors located on tuberoinfundibular dopaminergic nerve endings
(Fig. 7).

REFERENCES

1. Kokka, N., Garcia, J.F., George, R. and Elliot, H.W. (1972) Endocrinology,
    90, 735-743.

2. Ferland, L., Labrie, F., Arimura, A. and Schally, A.V. (1976) Mol. Cell.
    Endocrinol. 2, 247-252.

3. Meites, J. (1966) in Neuroendocrinology, vol. 1, Martini, L. and Ganong,
    W.F. eds., Academic Press, New York, pp. 669-707.

4. Tolis, G., Hickey, J. and Guyda, H. (1975) J. Clin. Endocrinol. Metab., 41,
    797-800.

5. Chang, J.J., Fong, B.T.W., Pert, A. and Pert, C.B. (1976) Life Sci. 18,
    1473-1482.

6. Morin, O., Caron, M.G., De Léan, A. and Labrie, F. (1976) Biochem. Biophys.
    Res. Commun. 73, 940-946.

7. Loh, H.H., Tseng, I.F., Wei, I. and Li, C.H. (1976) Proc. Natl Acad. Sci.
    USA, 73, 2895-2898.

8. Belluzi, J.D., Grant, N., Garsky, V., Sarantakis, D., Wise, C.D. and Stein,
    L. (1976) Nature, 260, 625-626.

9. Pert, A. (1977) In Opiates and Opioid Peptides, Kosterlitz, H., Archer, S., Simon, E.J. and Goldstein, A. eds., Elsevier Publishing Co., Amsterdam, pp. 87-94.

10. Bloom, F., Segal, D., Ling, N. and Guillemin, R. (1976) Nature 194, 630-636.

11. Dupont, A., Cusan, L., Garon, M., Labrie, F. and Li, C.H. (1977) Proc. Natl. Acad. Sci. USA, 74, 358-359.

12. Dupont, A., Cusan, L., Labrie, F., Coy, D.H. and Li, C.H. (1977) Biochem. Biophys. Res. Commun. 75, 76-82.

13. Rivier, C., Vale, W., Ling, W., Brown, M. and Guillemin, R. (1977) Endocrinology 100, 238-241.

14. Labrie, F., Dupont, A., Morin, O., Kledzik, G.S., Coy, D.H. and Li, C.H. (1978) in Current Studies of Hypothalamic Functions, Part I, Hormones, Lederis, K. and Veale, W.L., eds., S. Karger, pp. 949-960.

15. Dupont, A., Cusan, L., Garon, M., Alvarado-U., G. and Labrie, F. (1977) Life Sci., 21, 907-914.

16. Cusan, L., Dupont, A., Kledzik, G.S., Labrie, F., Coy, D.H. and Schally, A.V. (1977) Nature, 268, 544-547.

17. Labrie, F., Dupont, A., Cusan, L., Lissitzky, J.C., Lepine, J., Raymond, V. and Coy, D.H. (1978) in Endorphins in Mental Health Research, Usdin, E., ed., in press.

18. Terkel, J., Blake, C.A. and Hoover, V. (1973) Proc. Soc. Exp. Biol. Med. 143, 1131-1135.

19. Neill, J.D. (1970) Endocrinology, 87, 1192-1197.

20. Blake, C.A. (1974) Endocrinology, 94, 503-508.

21. Jobin, M., Ferland, L., Côté, J. and Labrie, F. (1975) Neuroendocrinology, 18, 204-214.

22. Noel, G.L., Suh, H.F., Stone, G. and Frantz, A.G. (1972) J. Clin. Endocrinol. Metab. 35, 840-851.

23. Robyn, C., Delvoye, P., Nokin, J., Vekemans, M., Badawi, M., Perez-Lopez, F.R. and L'Hermite, M. (1973) in Human Prolactin, J.L. Pasteels and C. Robyn, eds., Excerpta Medica, Amsterdam 193, pp. 167-182.

24. Kordon, C., Blake, C.A., Terkel, J. and Sawyer, C.H. (1973/74) Neuroendocrinology 13, 213-223.

25. Marchlewska-Koy, A. and Krulich, L. (1975) Fed. Proc. 34, 352.

26. Parker, D.C., Rossman, L.G. and Vander Loan, E.F. (1973) J. Clin. Endocrinol. Metab. 36, 1119-1124.

27. Sassin, J.F., Frantz, A.G., Kapen, S. and Weitzman, E.D. (1973) J. Clin. Endocrinol. Metab. 37, 436-440.

28. Labrie, F., Beaulieu, M., Caron, M.G., and Raymond, V. (1978) In Progress in Prolactin Physiology and Pathology, Robyn, C. and Harter, M., eds., Elsevier-North Holland, pp. 121-136.

29. Ferland, L., Fuxe, K., Eneroth, P., Gustafsson, J.A. and Skett, P. (1977) Eur. J. Pharmacol. 43, 89-90.

EFFECTS OF MORPHINE, NALOXONE, NALTREXONE AND β-ENDORPHIN ON MONOAMINE SYNTHESIS IN RAT BRAIN

LIISA AHTEE[*], J.A. GARCIA-SEVILLA, T. MAGNUSSON AND A. CARLSSON

Department of Pharmacology, University of Göteborg, Fack S-40033 Göteborg 33 (Sweden)

ABSTRACT

Morphine and β-endorphin increased the accumulation of DOPA and 5-HTP in different brain regions of rats treated with an inhibitor aromatic amino acid decarboxylase, whereas naloxone and naltrexone clearly decreased the accumulation of DOPA and tended to decrease that of 5-HTP. Thus the opiate receptors and their endogenous ligands seem to be involved in the regulation of the synthesis of brain monoamines.

INTRODUCTION

Narcotic analgesics increase the turnover of dopamine and 5-HT in the brain and naloxone antagonizes these effects[1,2]. Therefore it can be anticipated that there is a functional connection between opiate receptors and monoaminergic systems.

RESULTS AND DISCUSSION

Morphine, naloxone and naltrexone were injected i.p. and β-endorphin i.c.v. to male Sprague-Dawley rats. The brain monoamine synthesis was studied by measuring accumulation of DOPA and 5-HTP following inhibition of the aromatic L-amino acid decarboxylase by a supramaximal dose of NSD 1015 (100 mg/kg)[3].

Morphine (3-30 mg/kg, 1-2 h) increased DOPA accumulation dose-dependently (25-80%) in dopamine-rich brain regions (limbic forebrain and corpus striatum). In noradrenaline-predominated part of the brain (containing hemispheres, diencephalon and lower brain stem) only the 30 mg/kg dose of morphine increased DOPA formation (47%). β-Endorphin (5-10 μg per rat) about doubled DOPA formation in limbic forebrain, corpus striatum and cerebral hemispheres.

[*]Permanent address: Dept. of Pharmacy, Div. of Pharmacology, Univ. of Helsinki, Kirkkokatu 20, SF-00170 Helsinki 17 (Finland)

10-20 μg of β-endorphin was needed to increase DOPA formation in diencephalon and lower brain stem. Naloxone antagonized the β-endorphin-induced increase of DOPA formation. Naloxone and naltrexone (10-100 mg/kg, 1 h) decreased DOPA formation in dopamine-rich but not in noradrenaline-predominated parts. Maximum decrease (20-25%) was caused already by 10 mg/kg. Morphine (30 mg/kg, 2 h) and β-endorphin (5 μg per rat, 1.5-2 h) increased 5-HTP formation by about 50% and the narcotic antagonists tended to decrease the formation of 5-HTP by 15-20%.

Our results show that the effects of β-endorphin on brain monoamine synthesis are remarkably similar to those of morphine. In addition to the results given above we found that both morphine and β-endorphin increase the cerebral concentrations of tyrosine and tryptophan[4]. Furthermore, the effects of pure narcotic antagonists, naloxone and naltrexone on the rate of formation of DOPA and 5-HTP are opposite to those of morphine and β-endorphin. Thus it is probable that the opiate receptors and their endogenous ligands are involved in the regulation of synthesis of dopamine and 5-HT. However, the efficacy of opiate receptors in mediating processes controlling dopamine synthesis seems to be less than that of dopamine receptors, because the narcotic antagonists decreased DOPA formation only by 20-25% but apomorphine does by 80%[5] and the narcotic agonists increased DOPA formation by 80% but haloperidol has been found to cause an increase of about 200%[5].

ACKNOWLEDGEMENTS
    We thank for gift of β-endorphin   Prof. C. H. Li (Univ. of Calif.) and of naloxone and naltrexone   Dr. M. J. Ferster (Endo Lab.).

REFERENCES
1. Kuschinsky, K. (1976) Arzneim.-Forsch., 26, 563-567.
2. Yarbrough, G.G., Buxbaum, D.M. and Sanders-Bush, E. (1973) J. Pharmac. Exp. Ther., 185, 328-335.
3. Carlsson, A., Davis, J.N., Kehr, W., Lindqvist, M. and Atack, C.V. (1972) Naunyn-Schmiedeberg's Arch. Pharmac., 275, 153-168.
4. Garcia-Sevilla, J.A., Ahtee, L., Magnusson, T. and Carlsson, A. (1978) J.Pharm. Pharmac., in press.
5. Carlsson, A., Kehr, W. and Lindqvist, M. (1977) J. Neural. Trans., 40, 99-113.

INTERACTION OF OPIOID PEPTIDES WITH MONOAMINERGIC NEURONS IN THE RAT CNS.

Sergio ALGERI, Gabriella CALDERINI, Adriana CONSOLAZIONE, Giuseppe LOMUSCIO
Istituto di Ricerche Farmacologiche 'Mario Negri' - Via Eritrea, 62
20157 Milan, Italy

INTRODUCTION

$/\overline{D}$-ALA$^2\overline{/}$ methionine enkephalinamide (DALA), a synthetic analog of the naturally occurring opioid pentapeptide methionine-enkephalin, has morphine-like pharmacological action. Morphine is known to increase dopamine (DA) and serotonin (5HT) in rat brain. Therefore it was of interest to establish whether the analogy between the alcaloid and the peptide extended to this biochemical action.

METHODS

DALA (25 µg/rat) was administered into the lateral cerebral ventricles of male Sprague Dawley rats through 2 permanently implanted polyenthylene cannulas. DA, its metabolites DOPAC and 3 methoxytyramine, and noradrenaline (NA) were determined spectrophotofluorimetrically and/or radiometrically after cerebroventricular administration of a tracer dose of $/^3H\overline{/}$ tyrosine (14 µg/rat 50C mmol). Accumulation of HVA and DOPAC and the 5HT metabolite 5HIAA was measured spectrophotofluorimetrically after their transport had been blocked with probenecid (400 mg/kg i.p.). All methods are described in details elsewhere (1).

RESULTS

Effect of DALA treatment on catecholaminergic neurons. Administration of DALA led to a dose dependent increase in HVA and DOPAC, maximum at the dose of 25 µg/rat. This increase is due to enhancement of DA turnover as shown by the increased formation of $/^3H\overline{/}$DA and $/^3H\overline{/}$DOPAC after $/^3H\overline{/}$tyrosine administration (Table 1) and by the increase in HVA and DOPAC accumulation after transport blockade (Fig. 1) in the striata and limbic region of rats treated with the peptide. This effect was completely reversed by treatment with Naloxone, indicating that it is due to DALA interaction with opiate receptors. In spite of the increased turnover 3MT, a metabolite reflecting released DA; was not modified (Table 1) suggesting that DA release is reduced.

These results, resembling those observed after stimulation of the gabergic system, suggest that the action of the opioid peptides may be mediated by gabergic stimulation. Preliminary results showing that some of the effects of DALA are inhibited by picrotoxin and potentiated by ethanolamine O sulfate are in line with this hypothesis. Unlike DA, NA metabolism in the cortex was not affected by DALA. Serotonin turnover was also increased by DALA treatment (Fig. 1); however this effect was significant in the limbic area but not in the striatum. Naloxone reversed the effect of DALA on the serotonergic system. These results show that the biochemical effects of opioid peptides closely resemble those of morphine and other narcotic drugs.

TABLE 1

DALA action on synthesis and metabolism of striatal dopamine

	Tyrosine μCi/nmol	DA μCi/g	DOPAC μCi/g	3MT μCi/g
Vehicle	26.5 $\pm$ 2.5	450 $\pm$ 44	104 $\pm$ 7.6	44 $\pm$ 3.6
DALA	29.4 $\pm$ 3	610 $\pm$ 23[+]	153 $\pm$ 5.8[++]	37 $\pm$ 3.3

$/^3$H$/$tyrosine (s.a. was injected 15 min after DALA and 15 min before killing.
[+]$p < 0.01$; [++]$p < 0.001$

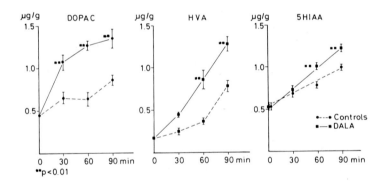

Fig. 1. Effect of DALA injection on probenecid induced accumulation of HVA DOPAC or 5HIAA in rat limbic area.

ACKNOWLEDGEMENTS

    This work is a part of research project sponsored and funded by Tecnofarmaci S.p.A., Pomezia, Italy

REFERENCES

1. Calderini G., Consolazione A., Garattini S. and Algeri S. (1978) Brain Res., 146, 393-399.

Characteristics and Function of Opioids, editors Van Ree and Terenius
© *1978 Elsevier/North-Holland Biomedical Press*

MORPHINE-INDUCED BEHAVIOUR OF MICE AND ITS RELATION TO BRAIN CATECHOLAMINES

İ. HAKKI AYHAN

Department of Pharmacology, Medical School of Ankara University, Ankara (TURKEY)

ABSTRACT

The influence of some drugs which effect the brain catecholamines on morphine-induced hyperactivity was studied in mice. Amphetamine, DOPA or apomorphine were found to antagonise the hyperactivity induced by 25 mg/kg of morphine. On the other hand, drugs which block noradrenaline receptors completely inhibit the stereotyped locomotion induced by high dose of morphine and mice became cataleptic. These results suggest that morphine-induced hyperactivity in mice may be due to the stimulation of NA systems. When this component is blocked, morphine may also produces catalepsy in mice as it does in rats, by a mechanism which probably related to DA systems in the brain.

INTRODUCTION

It is well known that morphine produces a dose-dependent behavioural excitation in mice and this excitation may be due to an action on brain catecholamines (CA), dopamine (DA) and noradrenaline (NA)[1].

In the present study, some relations and relative importances of brain DA and NA to the behavioural action of morphine have been investigated.

MATERIALS AND METHODS

The experiments were carried out on adult male mice weighing 20-28 g. The following drugs were used in the motor activity experiments: d-Amphetamine (AMPH), 1 mg/kg; L-DOPA Methylester (DOPA), 200 mg/kg 30 min after 50 mg/kg Ro 4-4602, a peripheral decarboxylase inhibitor; Apomorphine (APO), 1 mg/kg and Morphine (M), 25 mg/kg. M was given simultaneously with AMPH or APO and 30 min after DOPA. Immediately after the administration of M, mice were placed on Animex activitymeter and their activity were recorded for 75 minutes.

In the other series of experiments, cataleptic action of morphine (100 mg/kg) were tested in mice pretreated with drugs which blocks DA reseptors; Spiramide (SPD), 0.25 mg/kg and Pimozide (PIM), 0.5 mg/kg and NA receptors; Aceperone (ACP), 10 mg/kg and Phenoxybenzamine (PBZ), 10 mg/kg[2]. Catalepsy was scored on a 0-3 conventional rating scale by use of "Vertical Wire" test (for calculations see ref.3). In these experiments, M was given 150 min after the administrations of PBZ and PIM and 30 min after that of ACP and SPD.

RESULTS

Fig.1 shows that the hyperactivity of mice induced by M have significantly been antagonised when animals simultaneously injected with AMPH or APO or pretreated with DOPA. On the other hand, the behaviour of mice by 100 mg/kg of M was completely stereotyped, consisting only locomotion. This stimulation was inhibited by small doses of NA blockers, PBZ and ACP and mice became cataleptic. These

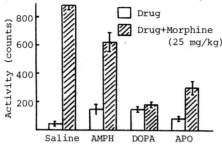
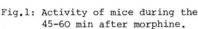
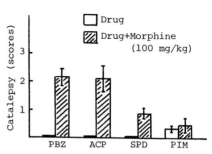

Fig.1: Activity of mice during the
45-60 min after morphine.

Fig.2: Catalepsy in mice 60 min
after morphine.

drugs alone did not produce catalepsy. The DA blockers also caused the appearance of catalepsy after M but they were less effective than NA blockers (Fig.2).

DISCUSSION

It has been reported that the depletion of CA from the brain could inhibits the hyperactivity of mice induced by M and this hyperactivity might be releated to the action of M on brain DA and/or NA[1,5]. If the stimulation of DA systems are responsible for the excitant effect of M, it is expected that drugs which already has a stimulant action on DA systems such as AMPH, DOPA and APO may potentiate this effect of M. This expectation was not confirmed by our experiments showing that by combined administrations all three drugs inhibited the hyperactivity induced by M, and so, it can be concluded that the stimulant effect of M in mice may be due to stimulation of NA rather than DA systems. Catalepsy experiments also supported this interpretation and showed that NA blockers strongly inhibited the stereotyped locomotion by high dose of M and led to the appearance of catalepsy in mice. Catalepsy is a well known action of M in rats and it has been suggested that this action may be releated to the blockade of DA systems[4]. M has also been shown to block DA systems in mice in a way similar to neuroleptics[5].

All these results suggest that, in mice M blocks DA as it does in rats (producing catalepsy), but in mice concurrent stimulation of NA (hyperactivity) is so strong that it overcome the cataleptic effect of DA blockade.

REFERENCES

1. Kuschinsky,K. (1976) Arzneim-Forsch. (Drug Res.), 26, 563-567.

2. Ayhan,I.H. & Randrup,A. (1973) Psychopharmacol. (Berl.), 29, 317-328.

3. Papeschi,R., Theiss,P. & Ayhan,H. (1976) Psychopharmacol.(Berl.),46, 149-157.

4. Kuschinsky,K. & Hornykiewicz,O. (1972) Europ.J.Pharmacol., 19, 119-122.

5. Eidelberg,E. & Erspamer,R. (1975) J.Pharmacol.exp.Ther., 192, 50-57.

Characteristics and Function of Opioids, editors Van Ree and Terenius
© *1978 Elsevier/North-Holland Biomedical Press*

THE EFFECTS OF OPIATES ON CALCIUM-STIMULATED PHOSPHORYLATION OF SYNAPTIC
MEMBRANE PROTEINS IN INTACT SYNAPTOSOMES FROM RAT STRIATUM

DORIS H. CLOUET, JAMES P. O'CALLAGHAN and NORMAN WILLIAMS
New York State Substance Abuse Services Laboratory, Brooklyn, N.Y. U.S.A.

ABSTRACT

The calcium ionophore, A23187, which increases the intrasynaptosomal levels
of calcium when added to intact synaptosomes[1], increases dose-dependently the
phosphorylation of synaptic membrane proteins by P_i. The increased phosphorylation induced in rat striatal synaptosomes by A23187 is inhibited in a dose-
dependent manner by methadone, and by morphine at higher drug concentrations.

INTRODUCTION

The biochemical signal generated by the binding of an opiate to a specific
opiate receptor in neuronal membranes is translated into biochemical actions
that alter neuronal function via mediator systems[2]. One such mediator system,
the cyclic nucleotide/cyclase system is associated in the synaptic plasma membranes (SPM) with protein kinases that are able to affect function by altering
the state of phosphorylation of proteins in the SPM[3]. We have shown that morphine has two effects on phosphorylation in isolated striatal (SPM): (1) the
chronic treatment of rats with morphine results in a depression of phosphorylation of specific proteins in SPM, and (2) calcium-stimulated phosphorylation
of SPM proteins is inhibited by adding morphine to the assay[4]. This report concerns the effect of opiates on phosphorylation in intact striatal synaptosomes.

METHODS

A purified synaptosomal preparation was obtained by centrifuging a crude
P_2 fraction from rat striatum through a discontinuous sucrose gradient. An
aliquot of synaptosomes (500 µg protein) was incubated with 7.5 µM P_i^{32} for 30
minutes. After synaptosomolysis the SPM proteins were separated by electrophoresis on slab gels in a 7-14% linear acrylamide gradient containing 0.1%
sodium dodecylsulfate. The gels were exposed to X-ray film for 3-5 days to
prepare autoradiographs.

RESULTS AND DISCUSSION

Krueger and his colleagues reported that the addition of A23187 to a synaptosomal preparation produced dose-related increases in intrasynaptosomal calcium

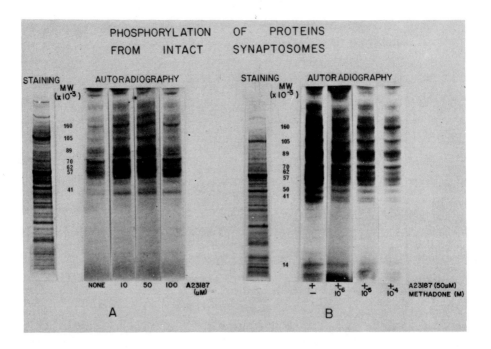

Fig.1. A. The calcium ionophore A23187 was added to the phosphorylation assay.
B. 50 μM A23187 and various concentrations of methadone were added to the assay.

ions and protein phosphorylation[1]. In this study, the ionophore increased the
phosphorylation of SPM proteins with a maximum at 50 μM (Fig.1A). The addition
of methadone to the assay inhibited dose-dependently the stimulation induced by
A23187 (Fig.1B). Morphine is inhibitory at higher concentrations (10^{-4}M).
Since naloxone also has little effect in the assay system, it is probable that
the lipophilicity of methadone enabled the drug to enter the synaptosomes.

In our experiments, the stimulation produced by calcium of endogenous protein kinase activity was much larger in intact synaptosomes than in isolated
membranes, possibly due to the enhancer effect of a calcium dependent regulator
found in synaptosomal cytoplasm[5]. These results suggest that cAMP-dependent
and calcium-dependent protein kinase activity in SPM may mediate some of the
effects of opiates on impulse transmission.

REFERENCES

1. Krueger,B.K., Forn,J. and Greengard,P. (1977) J. Biol. Chem. 252, 2764-2773.
2. Greengard, P. (1978) Science 199, 146-152.
3. Nathanson, J.A. (1977) Physiol. Rev. 57, 157-256.
4. O'Callaghan, J.P., Williams, N. and Clouet, D.H. (1977) Fed. Proc. 36, 968.
5. Schulman, H. and Greengard, P. (1978) Nature 271, 478-479.

Characteristics and Function of Opioids, editors Van Ree and Terenius
© *1978 Elsevier/North-Holland Biomedical Press*

ROLE OF DOPAMINE AND SEROTONIN IN THE STIMULATORY EFFECT OF OPIATES ON PROLACTIN SECRETION.

LOUISE FERLAND, PAUL-A. KELLY, FRANCINE DENIZEAU AND FERNAND LABRIE,
Medical Research Council Group in Molecular Endocrinology, Le Centre Hospitalier de l'Université Laval, Québec G1V 4G2, Canada.

We have previously found that endogenous opioid peptides β-endorphin and met-enkephalin can, like morphine, stimulate prolactin secretion in the rat (1). Morphine has also been found to stimulate prolactin release in the human (2). Convincing evidence suggests that dopamine (DA) may be the main or even the only inhibitory substance of hypothalamic origin controlling prolactin secretion (3,4). Evidence has also been obtained for a role of endorphins and serotonin in the rise of prolactin secretion induced by stress and suckling (5). Following this evidence of a role of DA and serotonin in spontaneous and induced prolactin secretion, it appeared important to study the role of DA and serotonin in the potent stimulatory effect of opiates on prolactin secretion.

A maximal stimulatory effect of morphine injected s.c. on plasma prolactin was obtained at a dose of 25 to 100 mg/kg B.W. Maximal plasma prolactin levels (100-200 ng/ml) were measured 15 to 20 min. after injection of the opiate. That the potent stimulatory effect of morphine on prolactin release is secondary to inhibition of dopaminergic activity was clearly indicated by the observation that the acute response of plasma prolactin induced by a maximal dose of morphine (40 mg/kg) was not further increased by simultaneous administration of a high dose of haloperidol.

Evidence for a role of endogenous serotonin in the stimulatory action of opiates on prolactin secretion was suggested by the finding that inhibition of serotonin biosynthesis by parachlorophenylalanine (PCPA) or blockage of serotonin receptors by methysergide led to a 40 and 95% inhibition of the stimulatory effect of morphine on plasma prolactin levels, respectively. Treatment with PCPA or methysergide alone had no significant effect on the already low plasma levels of prolactin in control animals.

The present data clearly suggest that the acute release of prolactin induced by morphine is mediated by an inhibition of the hypothalamic dopaminergic influence on prolactin secretion. These
data are in agreement with the findings of an inhibition of dopamine turnover in the medial palissade zone of the median eminence
in rats injected intraventricularly with met-enkephalin (6). Since
serotonergic agents have no direct effect on prolactin release at
the pituitary level (4), the present data also suggest that the
inhibitory effect of opiates on hypothalamic dopamine is partly
mediated by activation of serotonergic pathways.

The present observations suggest that presynaptic inhibitory
opiate receptors are present on dopaminergic neurons of the tuberoinfundibular system. Since the stimulatory effect of morphine
on prolactin secretion is partly inhibited after inhibition of
serotonin biosynthesis with PCPA or blockage of serotonin receptors by methysergide, it is also likely that presynaptic stimulatory opiate receptors are present on serotonergic nerve endings
which are in functional relationship with the tuberoinfundibular
dopaminergic system. It is however possible that the effect of
opiates on the dopaminergic and serotonergic systems are not direct but are, instead, mediated by other neurotransmitter(s).

REFERENCES
1. Dupont, A., Cusan, L., Garon, M., Labrie, F. and Li, C.H.(1977)
   Proc. Natl. Acad. Sci. USA 74, 358-359.

2. Tolis, G., Hickey, J. and Guyda, H. (1975) J. Clin. Endocrinol.
   Metab. 41, 797-800.

3. MacLeod, R.M. and J.E. Lehmeyer (1974) Endocrinology 94, 1077-
   1085.

4. Labrie, F., Beaulieu, M., Caron, M.G. and Raymond, V. in Progress in Prolactin Physiology and Pathology (C. Robyn and M.
   Harter eds.) Elsevier-North Holland, 121-136.

5. Ferland, L., Kledzik, G., Cusan, L. and F. Labrie (1978) Mol.
   & Cell. Endocrinol., in press.

6. Ferland, L., Fuxe, K., Eneroth, P., Gustafsson, J.A. and Skett,
   P. (1977) Eur. J. Pharmacol. 43, 89-90.

OPIATES INHIBIT PROSTAGLANDIN E_2-STIMULATED ADENYLCYCLASE IN SLICES OF CORPUS STRIATUM OF RATS

U. HAVEMANN, K. KUSCHINSKY

Max-Planck-Institut für experimentelle Medizin, Hermann-Rein-Str.3, D-3400 Göttingen, F.R.G.

In rat brain homogenates Collier and Roy[1] found a stimulation of adenylcyclase by prostaglandins E and an inhibition of this effect by opiates, whereas other groups did not observe similar effects in brain tissue. These different results led us to do own experiments on rat corpus striatum to find a possible explanation for these contradictory results.

For experiments, the striata were transversally cut into slices of 300 μm thickness, and, after a short pre-incubation, incubated for 5 minutes in fresh Krebs-Henseleit medium containing 1 mM of the phosphodiesterase inhibitor 3-isobutyl-1-methylxanthine (IBMX). During the incubation period, the striatum of one side was incubated in presence of PGE or of both, PGE and opiate, whereas the contralateral striatal tissue was incubated without agents as a control. The reaction was terminated by putting the slices together with the medium into boiling water for 3.5 minutes. The slices were homogenized in the medium and the cyclic AMP-content was measured.

In an other series of experiments, the striata were weighed and gently homogenized in a hypotonic medium. Aliquots of the homogenates were incubated for 5 minutes, as described by Seeber and Kuschinsky[2], in absence or in presence of dopamine or prostaglandins and/or of opiates. After terminating the reaction in boiling water, cyclic AMP-concentration was measured.

In striatal slices, morphine (2 μM) completely antagonized the prostaglandin E_2-induced elevation of cyclic AMP-synthesis. The effect of morphine was prevented by an equimolar concentration of naloxone, was mimicked by met-enkephalin (100 μM, in presence of 0.2 mM bacitracin) and by levorphanol (10 μM), but not by an equimolar concentration of its stereoisomer dextrorphan. Adenosin (1 mM) or an elevation of K^+-ions to 54 mM raised the cyclic AMP-concentration, and PGE_2 induced a further elevation, which however was not antagonized by morphine under these conditions. Evidently the presence of high concentrations of endogenous stimulators of cyclic AMP-synthesis could mask the inhibitory effect of morphine. In contrast, no stimulation by PGE_2 of cyclic AMP-synthesis could be observed in striatal homogenates, whereas morphine (20 - 50 μM) slightly lowered the concentration of cyclic AMP.

Further studies were performed to evaluate the localization of the PGE_2-sensitive adenylcyclase and of those opiate receptors mediating the antagonism against it. 6 days after injection of kainic acid (1 μg / 1 μl) into the head of the caudate nucleus, the stimulation by PGE_2 of cyclic AMP-synthesis was even enhanced, compared with slices of sham-operated rats. In contrast, the stimulation by dopamine of cyclic AMP-synthesis was lowered in homogenates of striata treated with kainic acid. This observation and own histological examinations support the assumption that kainic acid selectively destroys neurones, the cell bodies of which are located in the injection region including the neurites and dendrites but leaves terminals of nerves afferent from outside this region intact[3]. We therefore suggest that the PGE_2-stimulated adenylcyclase is mainly localized in nerve endings of afferent neurones, whose cell bodies are located outside the striatum. In striata lesioned by kainic acid, morphine did not significantly inhibit the PGE_2-induced stimulation. It seems that the opiate receptors involved are located on neurones, the cell bodies of which are within the striatum. They are clearly located differently from those, found on dopaminergic terminals in the striatum[4].

REFERENCES

1. Collier, H.O.J. and Roy, A. (1974) Nature (Lond.), 248, 24-27.
2. Seeber, U. and Kuschinsky, K. (1976) Arch. Tox., 35, 247-253.
3. Coyle, L.T. and Schwarcz, R. (1976) Nature (Lond.), 263, 244-246.
4. Pollard, H., Llorens, C., Bonnet, J.J., Costentin, J. and Schwartz, J.C. (1978) Neurosc. Letters, 7, 295-299.

INHIBITORY EFFECT OF MORPHINE ON THE RELEASE OF PRELOADED ^{3}H-GABA FROM RAT SUBSTANTIA NIGRA IN RESPONSE TO THE STIMULATION OF CAUDATE NUCLEUS AND GLOBUS PALLIDUS

KATSUYA IWATSUBO AND YASURO KONDO

Department of Pharmacology, Osaka University Dental School, Kitaku, Osaka 530, Japan

ABSTRACT

A push-pull cannula was placed in substantia nigra in lightly anesthetized, paralyzed rat. Morphine (i.v.) inhibited the release of preloaded ^{3}H-GABA from SN evoked by stimulation of caudate nucleus (CD) or globus pallidus (GP) and by K^+ depolarization in SN. Since morphine increases the firing rate of dopaminergic neurons in SN[1], morphine-induced decrease in the release of GABA may be one of the causes of the increased firing rate of SN neurons.

INTRODUCTION

Morphine alters GABA content of some areas of thalamus[2] and spinal cord[3]. Stimulation of GABA receptor by muscimol affects the morphine induced analgesia[4]. These observations suggested that central GABA system plays a role in morphine action. Spontaneous firing rate of dopaminergic neurons in SN is increased by administration of morphine[1]. Since GABAergic innervation from the anterior basal ganglia to SN has been suggested and we have found that stimulation of CD or GP enhanced release of preloaded ^{3}H-GABA from SN[5], the effects of morphine on the spontaneous and evoked release of ^{3}H-GABA from SN were investigated.

MATERIALS AND METHODS

Methods for perfusion of rat SN to observe ^{3}H-GABA release have been described[5]. In brief, tips of the cannulae were positioned in SN or GP. Bipolar stimulating electrods were positioned in CD or GP and square waves (40V, 0.7 msec, 50 Hz) were given. To stimulate locally small regions such as SN, 40 mM K^+ was added in perfusion fluid. The artificial cerebrospinal fluid contained aminooxyacetic acid to inhibit catabolism of ^{3}H-GABA and β-alanine to reduce preferential uptake of the labeled GABA by glia[6]. Cis-3-aminocyclohexanecarboxylic acid which inhibits the neuronal GABA uptake[7] was added in the perfusion fluid before stimulation. Using such inhibitors, considerable mount of enhanced release of ^{3}H-GABA could be detected following stimulations.

RESULTS AND DISCUSSION

Fig. 1. Effects of morphine and levallorphan on ^{3}H-GABA release from SN. Caudate nucleus
was stimulated for 9 min. Five mg/kg morphine
and 1 mg/kg levallorphan were injected intravenously. Ordinates; ^{3}H-GABA release expressed
as per cent deviation from the predicted baseline levels. Open circles; different from
control ($p < 0.05$). Filled circles; different
from values of morphine group ($p < 0.05$).

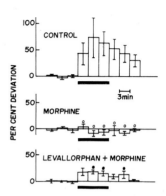

Thirty to 40 min after labeling of SN with [3]H-
GABA (1 μCi), electrical stimulation of CD caused
an increase in the levels of ^{3}H-GABA over the
baseline levels by 75 % (n=6). Morphine which
was administered 6 min before stimulation di-
minished the evoked release of GABA (Fig. 1). When levallorphan was given 5 min
before morphine administration, a partial recovery from the diminished response
was found. Both drugs did not change the basal release. On the other hand,
haloperidol (0.05 mg/kg, i.v.) which can also activate the spontaneous firing
of nigral neurons[1], failed to change ^{3}H-GABA release from nigra evoked by the
caudate stimulation. GP stimulation produced an increase in the GABA release
from SN by 40 to 70 %; the response was blocked by morphine administration.
Morphine administration also reduced the evoked release of the labeled amino
acid from SN following K^+ depolarization in SN and the release from GP following
local electric stimulation in GP.

These findings indicate that morphine reduces the release of GABA in the
caudato- and pallido-nigral neurons and one of the sites of morphine action is
the terminals of those neurons. Haloperidol may not affect those GABAergic
neurons. The above doses of morphine and haloperidol were both supramaximal
to increase the spontaneous firing rate of SN neurons[1]. Therefore, a possibility arises that the decreased GABA release from the terminals of those
neurons is one of the causes of the enhancement of the activity of SN neurons
produced by morphine.

REFERENCES
1. Iwatsubo, K. and Clouet, D.H. (1977) J. Pharmacol. exp. Ther. 202, 429-436.
2. Yoneda, Y., Kuriyama, K. and Kurihara, E. (1977) Brain Res. 124, 373-378.
3. Kuriyama, K. and Yoneda, Y. (1978) Brain Res. 148, 163-179.
4. Biggio, G., Della Bella, D., Frigeni, V. and Guidotti, A. (1977) Neuropharmacol. 16, 149-150. 5.Kondo, Y. and Iwatsubo, K. Brain Res.(to be published).
6. Neal, M.J. and Iversen, L.L. (1972) Nature New Biol. 235, 217-218.
7. Bowery, N.G., Jones, G.P. and Neal, M.J. (1976) Nature, 264, 281-284.

EFFECTS OF ENDOGENOUS AND EXOGENOUS ENKEPHALINS ON BRAIN ACETYLCHOLINE:
CROSS TOLERANCE BETWEEN MORPHINE AND ENKEPHALINS

KHEM JHAMANDAS and MAAJA SUTAK
Department of Pharmacology, Queen's University, Kingston, Ontario, Canada

We have shown previously that methionine (met) and leucine (leu) enkephalin
inhibit the release of acetylcholine (ACh) from the rat cerebral cortex.[1] In
this study we have compared the magnitude and duration of the anti-release
action of these agents with each other and with D-ala[2]-met-enkephalinamide
(DALA) in order to determine if significant differences exist between these
agents. To determine if there is a cross tolerance between morphine and
enkephalins, the effect of met- and leu-enkephalin has been investigated in the
morphine tolerant rats.

The methods used to measure the cortical release have been described previously.[1] Morphine treatment was administered to rats by a single injection
of a 'slow release' morphine suspension as described by Fredrickson and Smits.[2]

Leu-enkephalin and DALA depressed the release of ACh (Fig. 1A) and this
effect was antagonized by naloxone (0.2 mg/kg i.v.). DALA (5 µg) produced a
slightly greater effect than leu-enkephalin (20 µg) and its effect persisted
for a longer period. In morphine tolerant rats the anti-release action of
leu-enkephalin (20 µg) was reduced (Fig. 1A), but the difference between naive
and tolerant animals became apparent only 30 minutes after its injection. The
action of met-enkephalin (20 µg) was similar to that of leu-enkephalin and it
was also reduced in morphine tolerant rats (Fig. 1B). However, in this case
the reduced response of the tolerant animals to met-enkephalin became apparent
immediately after its injection.

These tests show that both met- and leu-enkephalin have a very similar anti-
release action on cortical ACh. Since the peptides are degraded rapidly by the
brain tissue[3] a difference between the potency of their action may not be
detectable until metabolism is prevented. DALA, which is resistant to
metabolism[4], is more potent than the endogenous enkephalins. The reduced
effect of met- and leu-enkephalin in morphine treated rats indicates a cross
tolerance between these enkephalins and the exogenous opiate. The reason for

360

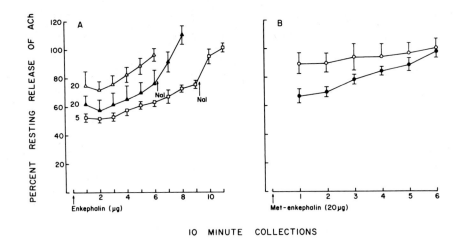

10 MINUTE COLLECTIONS

Fig. 1A.   Inhibition of spontaneous release of ACh by intraventricular leu-enkephalin in naive (▲) and morphine treated (△) rats, and DALA (□) in naive rats. B. Inhibition of release of ACh by met-enkephalin in naive (●) and morphine treated (○) rats. Morphine was administered 48 hours prior to the injection of enkephalins. Values are expressed as a percentage of the resting release obtained in two initial collections. (n=3-4).

the failure to observe this reduced effect immediately after leu-enkephalin injection, is not clear at present.

This work was supported by the Medical Research Council of Canada. We thank Endo Laboratories for the gift of naloxone.

1. Jhamandas, K., Sawynok, J. and Sutak, M. (1977) Nature, 269, 433-434.

2. Fredrickson, R.C.A. and Smits, S.E. (1973) Research Communications in Chemical Pathology and Pharmacology, 5, 867-870.

3. Hambrook, J.M., Morgan, B.A., Rance, M.J. and Smith, C.F.C. (1976) Nature, 262, 782-783.

4. Pert, C.B., Pert, A., Chang, J.K. and Fong, B.T.W. (1976) Science, 194, 330-332.

OPIATES, STEROIDS, Ca^{++} ANTAGONISTS: COMPARISON OF CENTRAL EXCITATORY EFFECTS

FRANK LABELLA, VIKTOR HAVLICEK, and CARL PINSKY

Department of Pharmacology and Therapeutics and Department of Physiology, University of Manitoba, Faculty of Medicine, Winnipeg, Manitoba, Canada, R3E 0W3

ABSTRACT

Morphine, steroid-0-sulfates, EGTA, Na_2SO_4 or Na_2HPO_4 given intracerebroventricularly (ICV) in rats elicits a syndrome characterized by behavioral and EEG activation, stereotypies, hyperresponsiveness, and analgesia. Naloxone antagonized the effects of androsterone sulfate (AS) but not those of cortisol-21-sulfate, Na_2SO_4 or EGTA.

INTRODUCTION

We have noted that the activation of motor and EEG activity by morphine given ICV is mimicked by certain steroid sulfates and by compounds known to form complexes with ionized calcium. Further work showed that analgesia was another similar effect of the non-opiates. However, naloxone had only limited effectiveness in antagonizing the non-opiates.

MATERIALS AND METHODS

Test substances in 10 μl of 10% ethanol in saline were infused over 5 min into the lateral ventricle of chronically cannulated, freely-moving Sprague-Dawley rats (150-250 g). The vehicle was inactive and did not alter the response to those compounds known to be active in saline. For each compound, mean motor responses and EEG spikes for 2-15 rats were scored over a 35 min period, the score comprising locomotor and body movements including wet dog shakes, spikes and epileptiform seizures on the EEG. Analgesia was estimated by a hot plate test at $44.5^{\circ}C$ with hindpaw licks recorded over 15 min. The Mann-Whitney analysis for nonparametric data was used to assess behavioral effects and unpaired t-test for results from the hot plate.

RESULTS

All of the steroid sulfates (ethereal-0-sulfates) tested, except for pregnenolone and allopregnanolone, elicited responses at 10-20 μg and were equivalent to those by 30-100 μg morphine sulfate (H_2SO_4 salt) (Table I). Behavioral and EEG effects of the steroids were indistinguishable from those elicited by morphine and were, for both compounds, dose-related, followed the same time course, and progressed to lethal convulsions. Steroid glucuronides, cortisol-21-phosphate, and non-steroid sulfates were inactive. Qualitatively similar

TABLE I. EXCITATORY EFFECTS OF SUBSTANCES GIVEN ICV TO FREELY MOVING RATS

Drug	Dose μg	Excit. Score	Drug	Dose μg	Excit. Score
Morphine	50	121	Testosterone gluc.	10	3
			Estradiol-3-gluc.	10	2
Sulfates			Estradiol-17β-gluc.	10	0
Androsterone	10	87	Nitrophenol Sulfate	10	0
Epiandrosterone	10	54	Umbelliferol Sulfate	10	0
Dehydroepiandrost.	10	63	Taurine	10	0
Etiocholanolone	10	34	Cortisol-21-PO_4	10	6
Testosterone	10	115	Na_2SO_4	200	28
Estradiol-3-	10	34	Na_2SO_4	400	212
Estradiol-3,17β-	10	138	Na_2HPO_4	400	173
Estrone-3-	10	43	NaCl	2000	0
Cortisol-21-	10	49	$NaNO_3$	360	0
Pregnenolone	10	11	NaOAc	576	4
Allopregnanolone	10	0	EGTA	50	149

responses were induced by 10-20 μg EGTA, 200-400 μg Na_2SO_4 and 200-400 μg Na_2HPO_4 (Table I). Naloxone pretreatment (10 mg/kg i.p.) profoundly and significantly diminished the motor and EEG changes induced by AS but not by cortisol-sulfate, Na_2SO_4, or EGTA. In two experiments AS significantly reduced the frequency of pawlicking. In a third experiment, Na_2SO_4 (200 μg) induced significant analgesia, and morphine sulfate (10 μg) diminished pawlicking but not significantly. This dose of morphine usually induces excellent analgesia. Naloxone antagonism of the chemical-induced analgesia has not yet been studied.

DISCUSSION

Similarities in central excitatory effects between steroid sulfates or calcium antagonists and those of morphine suggest a role for extracellular calcium in opiate action. Others have found that opiate analgesia is antagonized by calcium and mimicked by calcium antagonists[1,2]. Steroid sulfates may act by releasing free sulfate ion close to sites of bound calcium, because Na_2SO_4 is much less potent and certain steroid-sulfates and non-steroid sulfates are inactive. Naloxone antagonism of AS but not of other steroid sulfates, Na_2SO_4, or EGTA suggests a specific role for AS in activating opiate receptors. It should be noted that AS and related sulfates are present in blood in $\mu g/ml$ levels . Finally, the opiate abstinence syndrome in rats resembles the excitatory responses to ICV opiates and calcium antagonists, suggesting a role for calcium both in opiate action and in opiate dependence.

REFERENCES

1. Kaneto, H. (1971) Inorganic Ions: The Role of Calcium. Narcotic Drugs; Biochemical Pharmacology, Plenum Press, New York, p. 300.

2. Harris, R.A., Loh, H.H. and Way, E.L. (1975) J. Pharmacol. Exp. Ther., 195, 488-498.

Characteristics and Function of Opioids, editors Van Ree and Terenius
© 1978 Elsevier/North-Holland Biomedical Press

EFFECTS OF MORPHINE ON SERUM GONADOTROPIN AND PROLACTIN LEVELS IN RATS OF BOTH SEXES

TAKAMURA MURAKI, YUKIKO TOKUNAGA, EIKICHI HOSOYA AND RYUICHI KATO

Department of Pharmacology, School of Medicine, Keio University, Tokyo (Japan)

SUMMARY

Morphine increased the serum prolactin levels in normal male rats and decreased the serum LH levels in both normal and castrated male rats without affecting the serum FSH levels. Morphine abolished the proestrus surges of serum prolactin and gonadotropins in female rats. These effects of morphine were antagonized by naloxone. The changes of the hypothalamic content of LHRH by the administration of morphine were studied in relation to the changes of serum LH levels.

INTRODUCTION

Morphine-tolerant male rats showed decreased copulation rate, low fertilizing ability, decreased sperm content in the epididymis and low serum testosterone and LH levels[1]. Administration of morphine between 1200 and 1400 hr on the pro-estrous day prevented ovulation[2]. These findings suggest that morphine affects the secretion of gonadotropins in rats. We examined how morphine changes the serum gonadotropins and prolactin levels in rats of both sexes.

MATERIALS AND METHODS

Adult Wistar rats of both sexes were used. The castrated rats were used more than 3 days after castration. They were kept in an air-conditioned room (22°C) with controlled lighting(lights on from 0600 to 1800 hr). They were given drugs s.c. and were killed by decapitation. Gonadotropins and prolactin were determined by radioimmunoassay using NIAMDD kits. Hypothalamic LHRH was determined by radioimmunoassay[1,3].

RESULTS AND DISCUSSION

Effects of morphine on serum gonadotropins and prolactin levels and on the hypothalamic content of LHRH in male rats.

Morphine(100 mg/kg) increased the serum prolactin levels of normal male rats and this effect disappeared by 4 hr after the administration of morphine. The serum LH levels decreased gradually after the administration of morphine and were significantly lower than 0 hr levels between 12 and 24 hr after morphine. The duration of the stimulatory effect of morphine on serum prolactin levels was shorter than the inhibitory effect on serum LH levels in male rats. Morphine did not generally affect the serum FSH levels. Hypothalamic content of LHRH of normal male rats was not significantly changed by the administration of morphine except an increase at 8 hr. Morphine depressed the serum LH levels of the castrated male rats determined 4 hr after morphine, but it had no effect on the serum FSH levels again. The mechanism of the differential effect of morphine on the serum gonadotropins is not clear. Administration of morphine 4 hr before sacrifice had no effect on the hypothalmic content of LHRH in the castrated males. The stimulatory effect of morphine on the serum prolactin levels was antagonized by naloxone with 1/20 the dose of morphine, while the inhibitory effect of morphine on the serum LH levels was antagonized by naloxone with 1/4 the dose of morphine but not with 1/20.

Effects of morphine on the proestrus surges of serum gonadotropins and prolactin and on the hypothalamic content of LHRH in female rats.

In our lighting condition the serum gonadotropins and prolactin levels of female rats spontaneously increased in the afternoon of the proestrous day with the peak at 1800 hr(proestrus surge)[3]. When morphine(50 mg/kg) was administered to the proestrous female rats at 1200 or 1400 hr, the proestrus surges of the serum LH, FSH and prolactin at 1800 hr were abolished. The difference of these hormonal effects of morphine between male and female rats suggests that neural mechanism to provoke the proestrus surges is different from that controlling the basal levels of serum gonadotropins and prolactin in male rats. Naloxone with 1/20 the dose of morphine reversed the inhibition of the proestrus surges by morphine when naloxone was administered concurrently with or even 2 hr after morphine. Administration of morphine at 1400 hr increased the hypothalamic content of LHRH determined at 2000 hr. Since the correlation between the hypothalamic content of LHRH and its release is not established, it would be necessary to study the effect of morphine on the LHRH levels in the pituitary portal blood in order to clarify the mechanism of morphine to lower the serum LH levels.

REFERENCES
1. Tokunaga,Y., Muraki,T. and Hosoya,E.(1977) Japan J. Pharmacol., 27, 65.
2. Barraclough,C.A. and Sawyer,C.H.(1955) Endocrinology 57, 329.
3. Muraki,T., Tokunaga,Y. and Makino,T.(1977) Endocrinol. Japon. 24, 313.

Characteristics and Function of Opioids, editors Van Ree and Terenius
© 1978 Elsevier/North-Holland Biomedical Press

BEHAVIORAL AND CHEMICAL INTERACTIONS OF L-DOPA AND OPIATES

Lily C. Tang and George C. Cotzias

Sloan-Kettering Institute for Cancer Research, N.Y., N.Y.

ABSTRACT

Administration of morphine or endorphin to mice elicits certain neurological
behavioral responses similar to those induced by L-dopa. Giving morphine or
endorphin to mice in combination with L-dopa enhances the L-dopa effect. These
observations suggest opiates may act on dopaminergic neurons. Morphine stimulates the dopamine-sensitive adenylate cyclase in the caudate nucleus of mice as
does dopamine. This enzyme may be involved in the mechanism of pain regulation.

INTRODUCTION

The interaction between the dopaminergic system and opiates has been suggested by the enhanced sensitivity to the locomotor excitatory actions of L-dopa
exhibited by morphine-tolerant mice[1] and by the finding that morphine and other
narcotics induce a dose-dependent increase in dopamine turnover in the corpus
striatum.[2] The morphine-like polypeptides have affinities for the opiate receptors similar to morphine[3] and are analgesic.[4] L-dopa can relieve the bone
pain of advanced cancer patients.[5] These findings imply that dopamine and
opiates act on the same neurons and may have a common mechanism in regulating pain.

MATERIALS AND METHODS

Morphine (30μg or 250μg/gm body wt. intraperitoneally i.p.) or endorphin
(20μg intraventricularly) were administered alone or in combination with L-dopa
(0.4 mg/g body wt. i.p.) or apomorphine (1μg/gm body wt. i.p.) to 5-7 week old
male Swiss Albino Hale-Stoner mice. Dopamine-sensitive adenylate cyclase activity was measured by dissecting caudate nuclei in the cold and adding various
amounts of morphine to the caudate homogenates.[6] Animal behavioral scores were
obtained by observing mice for at least one hour following the last injection.[6]

RESULTS

Morphine (30μg/gm body wt.) injected into mice produces corkscrew tail,
ataxia, and light sedation. Higher doses (250μg/gm body wt.) produce hyperactivity, corkscrew tail, and circular running. The lower dose of morphine given in
combination with L-dopa yields a higher behavioral score than L-dopa alone (15.7
± 0.5 versus 12.4 ± 0.22; p<0.01). The same dose of morphine in combination
with apomorphine yields a similar result. Endorphin produces an effect similar
to that produced by L-dopa alone (Fig. 1). Endorphin and L-dopa (0.4 mg/gm body
wt.) administered in combination produced a neurological behavioral effect similar to the administration of a higher dose (0.8 mg/g body wt.) of L-dopa alone
(Fig. 2). Morphine at low concentrations (1-10μM) inhibits and at high concentrations (500μM-8 mM) stimulates the dopamine-sensitive adenylate cyclase of the
caudate nucleus.

+In all cases endorphin is β-endorphin

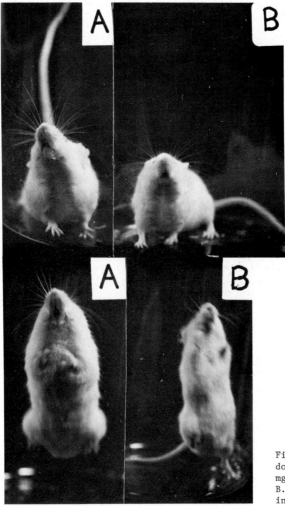

Fig.1. A. Mouse injected 20 μg intraventricularly endor-phin. B. Mouse injected 0.4 mg/g body wt. L-dopa.

Fig. 2. A. Mouse injected 20 μg en-dorphin intraventricularly and 0.4 mg/g L-dopa intraperitoneally B. Mouse injected 0.8 mg/g L-dopa intraperitoneally.

SUMMARY

These data show that morphine and endorphin produce effects similar to those of L-dopa when administered to mice and enhance the motor excitatory action of L-dopa. Morphine and dopamine also act on dopamine-sensitive adenylate cyclase. These data suggest that morphine and dopamine act on the same receptor and thus dopamine-sensitive adenyl cyclase may be involved in the regulation of pain.

REFERENCES

1. Eidelberg, E. & Erspamer, R. (1975) J. Pharm. 23, 274-276.
2. Dahlstrom, B. et al. (1975) Life Sci. 17,11-16.
3. Hughes, J. et al. (1975) Nature 258,577-579.
4. Bloom, F. et al. (1976) Science 194,630.
5. Minton, J.P. (1974) Cancer 33,358-363.
6. Tang, L.C. & Cotzias, G.C. (1977) PNAS 74,1242-1244.

Characteristics and Function of Opioids, editors Van Ree and Terenius
© *1978 Elsevier/North-Holland Biomedical Press*

THE ROLE OF ENDORPHINS IN BEHAVIOR

B. BOHUS and W.H. GISPEN

Rudolf Magnus Institute for Pharmacology, Medical Faculty, University of Utrecht, Utrecht (The Netherlands)

The discovery that some fragments of β-LPH were naturally occurring peptides with opiate-like activity (endorphins) immediately initiated research on the physiological role of such peptides. It appeared that only part of the CNS responses to endorphins can be blocked by classical selective opiate antagonists. Although present knowledge is far from complete this paper stresses the notion that there is a multiple interaction of endorphins with the central nervous system. The strong behavioral effects of fragments of β-LPH suggest that their preliminary physiological role involves the homeostasis of brain and behavior relationships.

Endorphin-induced excessive grooming: a behavior dependent on opiate receptors

Intracranial but not systemic injection of ACTH or N-terminal fragments of this hormone in mammals, produced a stretching and yawning syndrome[1,2]. At least in some species this syndrome is preceded by an enhanced display of grooming behavior[1,3,4]. In view of the short latency to the onset of the effect and its independence of endocrine activity, the induction of excessive grooming behavior seems the result of a direct effect of ACTH on the central nervous system[4,5]. The observation that peripheral administered opiate antagonists (naloxone, naltrexone) suppresses the peptide-induced grooming response[6], strengthened the notion that ACTH-like peptides and opiates have a common denominator in their interaction with the central nervous system[7,8]. If indeed the ACTH-induced grooming is mediated by opiate receptors or opiate sensitive structures in the brain, endogenous peptides with morphinomimetic properties (endorphins) should have similar, if not more pronounced activity in this respect.

Saline-treated rats, when placed in a novel glass box usually display exploratory and grooming behavior which may last for some 15-20 min after intraventricular injection but then invariably fall asleep provided the observation is carried out during daytime. Thus the exposure to novelty which is inherent to the experimental procedure used (preobservation transportation, intraventricular injection and novel glass observation box) enhanced the display of grooming behavior. As hypophysectomized rats also showed novelty-induced grooming, it was concluded that this behavioral response does not depend on the integrity of the pituitary adrenal system[9]. Evidence is available to suggest that the displayed

grooming primarily is related to the activating influence of environmental stimuli[9].

If, however, instead of saline low doses of β-endorphin |β-LPH$_{61-91}$| are in-
jected into the foramen interventriculare of conscious rats an enormous increase
in grooming activity is observed in a period of 15-60 min after the injection[10].
The grooming response can be elicited in a dose-dependent manner. A dose of as
little as 30 ng significantly induces excessive grooming and doses in the range
of 0.1 - 0.3 µg already elicit nearly maximal grooming behavior. Administration
of β-endorphin in low doses not only elicits grooming but also excitation in
some rats, typified by quick movements of body and head, jumping, gnawing and
body shakes. β-endorphin is about 10 times more potent than ACTH$_{1-24}$ or β-MSH
with respect to the induction of excessive grooming[10].

It has been reported that β-endorphin (30 µg into lateral ventricle; 4 µg
into periaquaductal grey) in rats elicits wet dog shaking behavior followed by
a marked prolonged muscular rigidity and immobility similar to a catatonic
state[11,12]. Also with such doses profound analgesia is induced[13,14,15]. Recently it has been reported that intraventricular administration of still high but
sub-cataleptic doses of β-endorphin (7.5 µg) in rats, results in wet dog
shaking behavior followed by copious salivation accompanied by a clonic,
seizure-like state[16].

All here reported behavioral responses to intracranial administration of β-
endorphin can be blocked by pre-or simultaneous treatment with the opiate antagonist naloxone. Such evidence is interpreted to indicate that the effects are
brought about by activation of opiate receptors. Indeed, intraventricular administration of morphine into rats in low doses is followed by the display of
excessive grooming[6] whereas high doses induce analgesia and immobility.

The biological significance of β-endorphin-induced grooming is not totally
understood. Some authors favor the view that as grooming in rodents may serve
thermoregulation, β-endorphin grooming would relate to β-endorphin-induced body
temperature changes[16]. However, we failed to find body temperature effects of
low doses β-endorphin sufficient to induce grooming behavior, although we did
see hyperthermia at higher doses when no grooming was observed.

We tend to explain the behavioral effect in quite a different way. As reported below, there is good evidence to suppose that ACTH and β-endorphin increase
the arousal state in midbrain limbic structures[17]. As was suggested for ACTH-
induced behaviors in pigeons and rats[18,9], we believe that the excessive grooming reflects a dearousal mechanism to reduce the arousal brought about by low
doses of β-endorphin.

β-LPH itself is devoid of grooming-inducing activity although is has been reported that intraventricular administration of 2.5 mg sheep β-LPH in the rat elicits some grooming[3]. Yet, it is conceivable that formation of β-endorphin from this enormous dose underlies the observed activity.

Sequences which are located N-terminal from the 61 amino acid residue and which upon intraventricular administration induce excessive grooming are LPH_{41-58} (β-MSH) and LPH_{48-51} ($ACTH_{4-7}$)[4,19].

The peptide with the highest activity and located C-terminal from the 61 residue is β-endorphin itself. Shortening the sequence to LPH_{61-77} (γ-endorphin) or LPH_{61-76} (α end) is accompanied by a dramatic reduction in activity. The sequence 61-69 is the shortest peptide beginning with the 61 residue which has notable activity. The sequence 61-65 (enkephalin) even in high doses is devoid of grooming inducing activity[10].

The fact that both sequences N-terminal and C-terminal from the 61st residue can induce the same behavior is not as uncommon as it seems. Also for the effects of ACTH on extinction of learned responses and for the MSH effects on the malanocyte, more than one active sequence seem to be present in one peptide molecule[20]. It may be that the stereoconformation of the molecule at the receptor favors the interaction with only one site. One should bear in mind, however, that structure-activity relations as discussed here, certainly not only involve peptide-receptor interactions but also concern metabolic fate, availability, transport, etc.

Recently it was observed that daily intraventricular administration of $ACTH_{1-24}$ did not result in a reduction of the observed grooming behavior[5]. However, a remarkable suppression of the grooming response was found when a second injection of $ACTH_{1-24}$ was given within 8 h after the first injection[21]. Subsequently, it was demonstrated that also with respect to β-endorphin grooming a single dose tolerance seems to occur without development of longer term tolerance[21]. Pretreatment with naloxone not only inhibited the grooming induced by the first injection of β-endorphin but also prevented the development of the acute tolerance as a second injection 4 h after the first was fully active again[21]. It may be that the observed single dose tolerance to endorphin grooming relates to the acute tolerance which is known to occur to temperature responses to morphine[22]. Thus, it was suggested that activation of opiate receptors is a prerequisite for the development of acute tolerance. Furthermore, at this acute level there is a cross tolerance between $ACTH_{1-24}$ and β-endorphin. Thus a first injection with $ACTH_{1-24}$ will reduce the effect of the subsequent injection with β-endorphin and vice versa[21]. It is likely therefore that the fragments of LPH and ACTH have a common neural substrate for part of their behavioral effects.

As is shown in the next section, however, other behavioral effects of these peptides may be elicited independently from brain opiate receptors.

Behavioral effects of endorphins independent from opiate receptors

The involvement of the pituitary gland in the modulation of adaptive behavior was indicated by the fact that the removal of the pituitary is followed by an impairment of active and passive avoidance behavior[23,24,25]. The behavioral abnormalities of the hypophysectomized rats can be corrected by the administration of ACTH[23,24], but also with MSH and fragments of ACTH which are practically devoid of classical endocrine target effects[26,27]. The hypothesis that the pituitary gland manufactures peptides, designated as neuropeptides, which are involved in learning, motivation and memory processes[27] received further support in the course of search for more potent neuropeptides from hog pituitary material than those related to ACTH[28]. Tryptic digestion of a purified peptide fraction which showed potent activity on the extinction of a pole-jumping avoidance response resulted in three oligopeptides[29]. Due to the insufficient quantity of the peptides the amino acid compositions but not the structures were determined. Two of them resembled the composition of β-LPH$_{61-69}$ and$_{70-79}$ The recognition that the C-terminal fragment of β-LPH possessed profound behavioral activities and that the peptides became available in pure form, stimulated us to determine whether endorphins are involved in the physiological modulation of adaptive behavior. Therefore, the influence of endorphins on active and passive avoidance behavior of the rat was investigated.

Subcutaneous administration of α- and β-endorphin and Met^5-enkephalin in a dose range of 0.1 to 3.0 µg increased resistance to extinction of a pole-jumping active avoidance response[17]. Met^5-enkephalin was almost as active as ACTH$_{4-10}$ which shares the amino acid sequence 47-53 of the N-terminal of β-LPH. Longer fragments of β-LPH appeared to be more potent. α-endorphin (αE, β-LPH$_{61-76}$) was the most active followed by β-endorphin (βE, β-LPH$_{61-91}$) and β-LPH$_{61-69}$. Metabolic degradation of the peptides, especially that of Met^5-enkephalin[30,31] may influence the behavioral potency of the various LPH fragments. Oxidation of methionine^5 residue of Met^5-enkephalin to the sulfoxide level which increases metabolic stability[32], profoundly potentiated the effect of this peptide. Differences in degradation in the periphery or different rate of uptake by the brain can not entirely explain the potency of the peptides. Administration of the peptides into a lateral ventricle in a dose range of 3 to 100 ng mimicked the effect of peripheral treatment - that is increased resistance to extinction. αE appeared to be the most active followed by ACTH$_{4-10}$,

β-LPH$_{61-69}$ and βE. Accordingly, the intrinsic behavioral activity of αE is the highest and ACTH$_{4-10}$ is almost as active. The potency of βE is substantially lower than that of αE.

Resistance to extinction of a pole-jumping avoidance response by endorphins was observed at dose levels much lower than those needed to induce analgesia or other behavioral effects[11,13,33,34,35,36,37,38]. This suggests that analgesia is not the primary physiological effect of endorphins. αE, the most potent peptide in the pole-jumping test facilitated the retention of a one-trial learning passive avoidance response when administered subcutaneously in a dose of 1.5 μg prior to the retention test. Comparable effect of ACTH$_{4-10}$ can be observed after subcutaneous administration of 15 μg of the peptide. Accordingly, αE similarly to ACTH$_{4-10}$ enhances retrieval processes[39,40].

The mechanism by which these behavioral effects are mediated may be similar for endorphins and ACTH$_{4-10}$. Electrophysiological observations showed that ACTH$_{4-10}$ causes a shift in the dominant frequency of the hippocampal theta activity towards higher frequencies both during the stimulation of the mesencephalic reticular formation and paradoxical sleep episodes[41,42]. βE and β-LPH$_{61-69}$ caused similar changes in the hippocampal theta rhythm during paradoxical sleep[17]. The changes in the hippocampal rhythmic activity by ACTH$_{4-10}$ were interpreted as signs of increased arousal state in midbrain-limbic structures. Accordingly, endorphins seem to affect the midbrain-limbic system in a similar way. It is, however, questionable whether the site of action of ACTH- and endorphin-like peptides is in the same location.

In contrast to the analgesic effect of endorphins, shortening of the peptide chain of βE increased the potency to delay extinction of active avoidance behavior. This may mean that the βE molecule contains more than one behavioral information and the behavioral effects depend upon the degradation of the peptide. Metabolic transformation of βE in the brain yields γ- and α-endorphin[43]. Therefore, the influence of two further fragments of βE, γ-endorphin (γE, β-LPH$_{61-77}$) and β-LPH$_{78-91}$ was compared with that of αE on extinction of a pole-jumping avoidance response[44]. γE markedly facilitated extinction of the avoidance response in rats which were made resistant to extinction. Subcutaneous administration of 30 ng of γE was sufficient to facilitate extinction behavior significantly. Similar effects were observed after intracerebroventricular administration of 300 pg of γE. β-LPH$_{78-91}$ showed some activity in delaying extinction but it was much less potent than αE. Passive avoidance behavior was also oppositely affected by α- and γ-endorphin injected immediately after the learning trial in a dose of 1.5 μg subcutaneously. Passive avoidance behavior was

markedly facilitated by αE and it was slightly attenuated by this dose of γE.
The effectiveness of postlearning administration of the peptides suggest that
endorphins, in contrast to $ACTH_{4-10}$[45], affect memory consolidation. Administration of the peptides 1 h prior to the first retention test gave somewhat different results. αE facilitated passive avoidance behavior but γE resulted in a
bimodal behavioral effect: facilitated passive avoidance behavior was observed
in a part of the population while attenuation occurred in the other. The bi-
directional effect of the peptide might be due to individual differences in the
breakdown of γE which may result in the formation of αE or shorter but behaviorally active fragments with an effect which is opposite to that of γE.

These observations suggest βE may be the source of behaviorally active fragments which influence adaptive behavior in various directions. Interestingly,
the presence or absence of a single amino acid residue in position 77 (leucine)
is of importance for opposite behavioral effects rather than the fragment
78-91. It is not clear yet whether βE has an intrinsic behavioral activity at
this dose level. Intraventricular administration of subanalgesic but comparatively high doses of βE (10 to 100 times higher amounts than the effective dose
in extinction behavior) disrupt male sexual behavior[37] and operant responding
for food reward[35]. It may therefore be that disruption of behavioral performance
by βE is due to the breakdown of the peptide and consequent formation of γE.
This suggestion may not be true. The half-life of βE in the brain tissue is
quite long[30]. Furthermore, high doses of Met^5-enkephalin or analogues are also
capable to disrupt operant responding for food or water reward when administered intracerebroventricularly[38,46].

The disruption of behavioral performances by βE obviously involves opiate
receptors. Pretreatment with an opiate antagonist such as naloxone or naltrexone
prevents the effect of βE on sexual behavior[37] and operant responding[35]. The
effects of endorphins on avoidance extinction are, however, independent from
opiate receptors. Pretreatment with naltrexone did not abolish the effect of
αE or $ACTH_{4-10}$. It was found that naltrexone itself facilitates the extinction
of a pole-jumping avoidance response in a dose-dependent manner. Subcutaneous
administration of αE or $ACTH_{4-10}$ normalizes extinction behavior of naltrexone
pretreated rats[17]. Behavioral effects of enkephalins which are independent from
opiate receptors were also observed. Met^5-enkephalin and Leu^5-enkephalin
administered peripherally in low doses appeared to alleviate Co_2-induced amnesia
in the rat. The opiate antagonist naloxone did not block the antiamnesic effect
of these peptides[47]. Met^5-enkephalin and $|D-Ala^2|-Met^5$-enkephalin administered
intraperitineally facilitated maze performance for food reward. $|D-Phe^4|-Met^5$ -

enkephalin which is practically devoid of opiate activity showed comparable effects[48].

The influence of γE on active avoidance extinction and passive avoidance behavior is also independent from opiate-like activity of this peptide. Removal of the N-terminal amino acid residue tyrosine which destroys opiate-like activity of Met[5]-enkephalin[49] resulted in a peptide (Des-Tyr[2]-γ-endorphin, DTγE) which was twice as active as γE in facilitating extinction of a pole-jumping avoidance response. Passive avoidance behavior was also markedly attenuated in a long term way whether the peptide was administered immediately after the learning trial or prior to the first retention test[44]. Opiate-like activity of the peptide was practically absent as determined by the guinea pig ileum method[44]. Oxidation of methionine[5] residue to the sulfoxide level further potentiated the activity of DTγE on extinction behavior.

Austen et al.[43] demonstrated that membrane-bound enzymes from rat brain and also striatal slices degrade βE in discrete stages. This process results in the formation of γ- and α-endorphin successively. At the same time, N-terminal degradation leads to the loss of amino acid residue tyrosine and a consequent loss of opiate activity. Our observations on the opposite effects of αE and γE and DTγE therefore strongly suggest that the generation of peptide fragments from βE is not simply a degradation process but a mechanism of physiological significance. Bloom et al.[11] suggested that subtle derangements in the physiological mechanisms regulating βE homeostasis could result in pathological changes in psychic functions. Jacquet and Marks[12] proposed that βE might be an endogenous neuroleptic. This assumption was not substantiated by Segal et al.[50], who showed that the pharmacological spectrum of the effects of βE resembles that of morphine and not of haloperidol. In view of the fact that γE and DTγE influence avoidance behavior similar to haloperidol, the pharmacological spectrum of these peptides was determined. γE but particularly DTγE show typical neuroleptic characteristics[44]. There is some preliminary evidence pointing to a connection between DTγE and brain dopamine systems. Previously it was demonstrated that local application of neuroleptics into DA projection regions (neostriatum, n.accumbens) interfere with ACTH-induced excessive grooming in the rat[51,52]. Similar implantation of naloxone was without effect. It was suggested that the activity of dopaminergic nigro-striatal and nigro-accumbens pathways was essential for the expression of ACTH and morphine induced excessive grooming[51,52]. Recently, we found that local application of as little as 30 ng DTγE into the n.accumbens is able to completely block the grooming response brought about by intraventricularly administered ACTH$_{1-24}$(0.3 μg). Further experiments are carried out to characterize this effect of DTγE in more detail (Gispen et al.,

in press). Moreover, low doses of these peptides which profoundly affect avoidance behavior unlike haloperidol failed to affect gross behavior in an open-
field test. Accordingly, it was proposed that DTγE or a closely related neuropeptide is an endogenous neuroleptic. The profile of such a peptide is more
specific than that of the current neuroleptic drugs[44].

Concluding remarks

Large amounts of informations collected during the last three years established a clear pharmacological profile of opioid peptides. The question of
physiological significance remained to be answered. Our observations may provide
a clue to understand the role of endorphins in the homeostasis of the brain
functions. Discrete changes in the generation of fragments of βE, depending on
the site of enzymatic cleavage, may assure a well-balanced modulation of behavioral adaptation to environmental events. On the other hand, an imbalance in
the generation of behaviorally powerful fragments may lead to disturbances in
adaptive processes and serves as an etiological basis of pathological changes
in brain functions. It was proposed that a reduced availability of DTγE may be
responsible for psychopathological states in which neuroleptic drugs are effective[53]. Pilot clinical observations suggest that DTγE treatment improves the
condition of schizophrenic patients[54].

REFERENCES

1. Ferrari,W.,Gessa,G.L. and Vargiu,L. (1963). Ann.New York Acad.Sci. 104,
   330-345.

2. Gessa,G.L., Pisano,M., Vargiu,L., Crabai,F. and Ferrari,W. (1967) Rev.Canad.
   Biol. 26, 229-236.

3. Izumi,K., Donaldson,J. and Barbeau,A. (1973) Life Sci. 12, 203-210.

4. Gispen,W.H., Wiegant,V.M., Greven,H.M. and de Wied,D. (1975) Life Sci. 17,
   645-652.

5. Colbern,D.L., Green,E., Isaacson, R.L. and Gispen,W.H. (1978) Behav.Biol.
   in press.

6. Gispen,W.H. and Wiegant,V.M. (1976) Neurosci.Lett. 2, 159-164.

7. Zimmermann,E. and Krivoy,W. (1973) In: Progress in Brain Research,Vol. 39.
   E.Zimmermann, W.H.Gispen, B.H.Marks and D. de Wied,eds. Elsevier,Amsterdam,
   pp. 383-394.

8. Wiegant,V.M., Gispen,W.H., Terenius,L. and de Wied,D. (1977) Psychoneuroen -
   docin. 2, 63-69.

9. Jolles,J., Rompa-Barendregt,J. and Gispen,W.H. (1978) Behav.Biol. in press.

10. Gispen,W.H., Wiegant,V.M., Bradbury,A.F., Hulme,E.C.Smyth,D.G., Snell,C.R. and de Wied,D. (1976). Nature 264, 794-795.

11. Bloom,F., Segal,D., Ling,N. and Guillemin,R. (1976) Science 194, 630-632.

12. Jacquet,Y.F. and Marks,N. (1976) Science 194, 632-634.

13. Van Ree,J.M., de Wied,D., Bradbury,A.F., Hulme,E.C., Smyth,D.G. and Snell, C.R. (1976) Nature (London) 264, 792-794.

14. Feldberg,W.S. and Smyth,D.G. (1976) J.Physiol. (London) 260, 30-31P.

15. Graf,L., Szekely,J.I., Ronai,A.Z., Dunai-Kovacs,Z. and Bajusz,S. (1976) Nature 263, 240-241.

16. Holaday,J.W., Loh, H.H. and Li, C.H. (1978) Life Sci. 22, 1525-1536.

17. de Wied,D., Bohus,B., Van Ree, J.M. and Urban,I. (1978) J.Pharm. exp.Ther. 204, 570-580.

18. Delius,J.D., Craig,B. and Chaudoir,C.(1976) Z.Tierpsychol. 40, 183-193.

19. Wiegant,V.M. and Gispen,W.H. (1977) Behav.Biol. 19, 554-558.

20. Gispen,W.H., Van Ree,J.M. and de Wied,D. (1977). Int.Rev.Neurobiol. 20, 209-250.

21. Wiegant,V.M., Jolles,J. and Gispen,W.H.(1978)This volume.

22. Lotti,V.J., Lomax,P. and George,R. (1966) Int.J.Neuropharmacol.5, 35-42.

23. de Wied,D. (1964) Amer.J.Physiol. 207, 255-259.

24. Gold,P.E., Rose,R.P., Spanis,C.W. and Hankins,L.L.(1977) Horm.Behav. 8, 363-371.

25. Lissak,K. and Bohus,B. (1972) Int.J.Psychobiol. 2, 103-115.

26. de Wied.D., (1969) In: Frontiers in Neuroendocrinology.W.F.Ganong and L. Martini,eds. Oxford Univ.Press,New York.pp.97-140.

27. Bohus,B., Gispen,W.H. and de Wied,D.(1973).Neuroendocrinol 11,137-143.

28. de Wied,D., Witter,A. and Lande,S. (1970) In:Pituitary, Adrenal and the Brain. D. de Wied and J.A.W.M., eds. Progress in Brain Research Vol.32, Elsevier, Amsterdam. pp 213-218.

29. Lande,S., de Wied,D. and Witter,A. (1973)In: Drug Effects on Neuroendocrine Regulation. E.Zimmermann, W.H.Gispen, B.H.Marks and D. de Wied, eds.Progress in Brain Research Vol.39. Elsevier, Amsterdam. pp. 421-427.

30. Marks,N., Greynbaum,A. and Neidle,A. (1977) Biochem.Biophys.Res.Commun. 74, 1552-1559.

31. Miller,R.J., Chang,K.J. and Cuatrecasas,P. (1977) Biochem.Biophys.Res.Commun 74, 1311-1317.

32. Witter,A., Greven,H.M. and de Wied,D. (1975) J.Pharmacol.exp.Ther. 193, 853-860.

33. Chrétein,M., Seidah,N.G., Benjannet,S., Dragon,N.,Routhier,R., Motomatsu,T., Crine,P. and Lis,M. (1977) Ann.N.Y.Acad.Sci. 297, 84-105.

34. Guillemin,R., Ling,N., Lazarus,L., Burgus,R., Minick,S., Bloom,F., Nicoll,R. Siggins,G. and Segal,D. (1977) Ann.N.Y.Acad.Sci. 297, 131-156.

35. Lichtblau,L., Fossom,L.H. and Sparber,S.B. (1977) Life Sci. 21, 927-932.

36. Loh,H.H. and Li, C.H. (1977) Ann.N.Y.Acad.Sci. 297, 115-128.

37. Meyerson,B.J. and Terenius,L. (1977) Eur.J.Pharmacol. 42, 191-192.

38. Carney,J.M. and Rosecrans, J.A. (1978) Pharmacol.Biochem.Behav. 8, 185-189.

39. de Wied,D. (1974) In:The Neurosciences, 3rd Study Program. F.O.Schmitt and F.G.Worden, eds. M.I.T.Press, Cambridge. pp. 653-666.

40. Rigter,H., van Riezen,H. and de Wied,D. (1974). Physiol.Behav. 13, 381-388.

41. Urban,I. and de Wied,D. (1976) Exp.Brain Res. 24, 325-334.

42. Urban,I. and de Wied,D. (1978) Pharmacol.Biochem.Behav. 8, 51-59.

43. Austen,B.M., Smyth,D.G. and Snell,C.R. (1977) Nature 269, 619-621.

44. de Wied,D., Kovacs,G.L., Bohus,B., Van Ree,J.M. and Greven,H.M. (1978) Eur.J.Pharmacol. in press.

45. Van Wimersma Greidanus,Tj.B. (1977) In:Frontiers in Hormone Research.Tj.B. van Wimersma Greidanus,Ed. Vol.4.Karger,Basel. pp.129-139.

46. Belluzzi,J.D. and Stein,L.(1977) Nature 266, 556-558.

47. Rigter,H.,Greven,H. and van Riezen,H.(1977) Neuropharmacol.16,545-547.

48. Kastin,A.J.,Scollan,E.L.,King,M.E.,Schally,A.V. and Coy,D.H. (1976) Pharmacol.Biochem.Behav. 5, 691-695.

49. Fredrickson,R.C.A.(1977) Life Sci. 21, 23-42.

50. Segal,D.S.,Bloom,F., Ling,N. and Guillemin,R. (1977) Science 198,411-414.

51. Wiegant,V.M.,Cools,A.R. and Gispen,W.H. (1977) Eur.J.Pharmacol. 41,343-345.

52. Cools,A.R., Gieles,L.C.M., Janssen,H.J. and Megens,A.A.P.H.(1978) Eur.J. Pharmacol. 48, 67-85.

53. De Wied,D., Bohus,B., van Ree,J.M., Kovacs,G.L. and Greven,H.M. (1978) Lancet i, 1046.

54. Verhoeven,W.M.A., van Praag,H.H., Botter,P.A., Sunier,A., van Ree,J.M. and de Wied,D (1978) Lancet i, 1046-1047.

Characteristics and Function of Opioids, editors Van Ree and Terenius
© 1978 Elsevier/North-Holland Biomedical Press

BEHAVIORAL EFFECTS OF β-ENDORPHIN

DAVID S. SEGAL, RONALD G. BROWNE, AMY ARNSTEN, AND DAVID C. DERRINGTON
Department of Psychiatry, School of Medicine, University of California,
San Diego, La Jolla, California 92093 (U.S.A.)

ABSTRACT

The endogenous opioid peptide, β-endorphin, produces a broad spectrum of dose- and time-related effects, ranging from behavioral activity to rigid immobility[1,2]. A similar response pattern is induced by the metabolically resistant enkephalin analogs, D-Met^2-Pro^5-enkephalinamide (D-Met^2-Pro^5·NH$_2$) and D-Ala^2-Met^5-enkephalinamide (D-Ala^2-Met^5·NH$_2$). These naloxone reversible effects closely resemble the response patterns which result from the central and systemic administration of opiates. Therefore, it appears that the β-endorphin-induced behaviors may be mediated through the activation of opiate receptors in the brain. Furthermore, these findings suggest that the endogenous opioid peptides may play an important role in the regulation of behavior.

CHARACTERISTICS OF β-ENDORPHIN-INDUCED IMMOBILITY

Introduction. β-Endorphin induces in rats a profound state of immobilization characterized by the absence of movement, loss of the righting response, and extreme generalized muscular rigidity[1-3]. A similar rigid immobility syndrome has also been observed by others[4-6]. Opiates also induce a state of immobility which, especially at higher doses, is accompanied by muscular rigidity and loss of the righting response[7-10]. Systemic administration of etonitazene at doses as low as 12.5 μg/kg produced extreme rigidity of the trunk and limb musculature[7]. Recently we found that the spectrum of effects seen after injection of methadone (5-10 mg/kg) closely resembled that induced by intraventricular injection of β-endorphin[2,3]. These studies were extended to include the characterization of the behavioral effects produced by the intraventricular administration of the human and porcine forms of β-endorphin as well as the the metabolically resistant enkephalin analogs, D-Met^2-Pro^5·NH$_2$ and D-Ala^2-Met^5·NH$_2$. The behavioral response profiles resulting from intraventricular and systemic injection of the opiates, morphine, methadone, and etonitazene were also assessed. Further, the neuroanatomical substrates mediating the various components of the immobility syndrome were examined by injection of opioid peptides and opiates into specific brain regions.

Materials and Methods. For these studies male Wistar rats (300-325 g; obtained from Hilltop Laboratories, Pittsburgh, PA) were maintained under standard laboratory conditions for at least one week prior to experimentation. Stainless steel guide cannulae (21 ga) were stereotaxically implanted above the right lateral ventricle, caudate, globus pallidus, amygdala or periaqueductal gray (PAG). Internal patency of the guide cannula was maintained by a stainless steel stylet which projected to the cannula tip. At least one week separated surgery and behavioral testing. A 27 ga infusion needle, connected to a Hamilton microliter syringe by polyethylene tubing, extended 1 mm beyond the tip of the guide cannula for intraventricular administration, and 2 mm beyond the tip for injection into discrete brain sites. Intraventricular and localized brain injections were made in unrestrained rats over a one-minute interval; injection volumes were 10 µl and 0.5-1.0 µl, respectively. Following infusion, an additional one minute was allowed for diffusion prior to removal of the needle and replacement of the stylet.

Animals were placed into observation chambers (54x32x15 cm) for at least 30 minutes prior to injection and were then tested for rigidity, immobility, and righting responses every 15-30 minutes for up to six hours. The rats were also regularly observed for the occurrence of wet-dog shakes, motility, and responsiveness to auditory and tactile stimulation.

Results. Intraventricular infusion of β-endorphin produced a dose-related increase in rigid immobility (Table 1). The immobilization was characterized by a number of features, including the complete absence of spontaneous movement, loss of righting response, and rigidity. During the rigidity phase which persisted for at least six hours at the highest dose tested (300 µg), animals remained motionless if left undisturbed or handled gently; however, they could be provoked into moving with the presentation of relatively mild auditory, visual or tactile stimulation. This effect was apparent particularly before and subsequent to the period of peak rigidity, and occurred at a time when the animals were not responsive to noxious stimuli. Furthermore, the intensity of the rigidity appeared to be reduced during tests at night, a time when rats are normally active. These results indicate that during the rigidity phase animals were capable of coordinated motor activity and that the behavioral immobility may have been partially due to an impaired ability to initiate voluntary movement.

All doses of β-endorphin tested produced wet-dog shaking behavior within 15 minutes after infusion. Initially these shaking episodes were followed by brief periods of activity, however, eventually most animals displayed a "trance-like" state, lasting for up to 15 minutes, during which time they remained motionless in a standing or rearing position. A 2.5 µg dose of β-endorphin which did not produce detectable rigidity did induce wet-dog shaking behavior as well as periods of the "trance-like" behavioral state. Rigid immobility was also induced by synthetic human β-endorphin (50 µg) and by the metabolically resistant enkephalin analogs, $D\text{-Met}^2\text{-Pro}^5\text{·NH}_2$ (25 µg) and $D\text{-Ala}^2\text{-Met}^5\text{·NH}_2$ (50 µg) (Table 1).

TABLE 1

OPIOID PEPTIDE-INDUCED IMMOBILITY

A minus righting response was designated when the rat stayed in a supine position for 10 seconds. The rigidity score represents a composite measure derived from three tests: (1) stiffness, assessed during handling (scored 0-3); (2) trunk rigidity, based on the time (up to 4 seconds) that the animal remained in an upright posture when held above the knee joints of the hind limbs (scored 0-4); and (3) bridge test, a positive score assigned when the animal remained self-supporting for 10 seconds after being placed across metal bookends. Values (expressed as mean ± S.E.M.) indicate peak effects after intraventricular injection; β_p, synthetic porcine β-endorphin, β_h, synthetic human β-endorphin.

TREATMENT	DOSE (µg/10 µl)	N	RIGHTING RESPONSE (10 Sec)	RIGIDITY (0-4)
Saline	10 µl	13	+	0
β_p-Endorphin	2.5	4	−	0
	5.0	19	−	2.0 ± 0.2
	10.0	12	−	2.8 ± 0.3
	25.0	4	−	3.5 ± 0.5
	50.0	43	−	3.7 ± 0.1
	100.0	4	−	4
	150.0	3	−	4
	300.0	5	−	4
β_h-Endorphin	50.0	3	−	3.6 ± 0.3
$D\text{-Met}^2\text{-Pro}^5\text{·NH}_2$	25.0	3	−	4
$D\text{-Ala}^2\text{-Met}^5\text{·NH}_2$	50.0	5	−	1.6 ± 0.2

Rats injected with β-endorphin or other opioid peptides would quickly climb off a vertical grid before and after the period of rigidity and typically would slide or fall off the grid during the rigidity phase. In contrast, rats that received haloperidol tightly grasped the grid and remained stationary for relatively long periods of time (Table 2). Furthermore, doses as high as 12 mg/kg of haloperidol did not produce rigidity or loss of the righting response. Instead, animals injected with haloperidol (0.5-12 mg/kg, s.c.) typically displayed a hunched posture, abducted limbs, and vocalized when handled. Rigidity resulting from injection of β-endorphin could be rapidly reversed by naloxone administered subcutaneously (0.1 mg/kg) or intraventricularly (0.5 µg/10 µl). In contrast, the effects of haloperidol were unaltered by doses of naloxone as high as 2 mg/kg. The immobility syndrome could also be produced by injection of β-endorphin into the ventromedial PAG, but not into the caudate, globus pallidus, amygdala or the dorsolateral PAG. Injection into the ventromedial PAG did not elicit wet-dog shaking behavior and the rigidity induced by a dose of 8 µg β-endorphin was relatively mild (2.2 ± 0.2). Therefore, although this region may be implicated in the behavioral response to β-endorphin, additional sites activated by intraventricular administration of this peptide may also be involved.

Like β-endorphin, the opiates, morphine, methadone, and etonitazene produced a dose-dependent increase in rigidity and loss of righting response (Table 3). Furthermore, opiate-treated rats were also selectively non-responsive to noxious stimuli. Intraventricular administration of morphine or etonitazene produced

TABLE 2

CHARACTERISTICS OF IMMOBILITY INDUCED BY HALOPERIODOL

The vertical grid test was scored on a 0-3 scale, based on the time (up to 60 seconds) that the rat remained immobile on the grid.

TREATMENT	DOSE (mg/kg)	N	RIGHTING RESPONSE (10 Sec)	RIGIDITY (0-4)	VERTICAL GRID (0-3)
Saline	1 ml/kg	10	+	0	0
Haloperidol	0.5	12	+	0	1.8 ± 0.3
	1.0	12	+	0	2.9 ± 0.1
	2.0	15	+	0	2.6 ± 0.2
	4.0	10	+	0	2.5 ± 0.2
	8.0	15	+	0	2.3 ± 0.2
	12.0	6	+	0	2.6 ± 0.2

a similar response profile (Table 4). Furthermore, naloxone (0.5-10 g) injected intraventricularly or into the caudate, globus pallidus, amygdala or PAG rapidly reversed the rigidity and immobility produced by 7.5 mg/kg (s.c.) of methadone.

TABLE 3

OPIATE-INDUCED IMMOBILITY: SUBCUTANEOUS ADMINISTRATION

Subcutaneous injection of morphine, methadone, and etonitazene resulted in rigidity and accompanying loss of righting (+-, rats remained supine for at least 5 seconds, but were capable of self-righting within 10 seconds).

TREATMENT	DOSE	N	RIGHTING RESPONSE (10 Sec)	RIGIDITY (0-4)
Saline	1 ml/kg	13	+	0
Morphine (mg/kg)	5.0	18	+	0
	7.5	11	+-	0.7 ± 0.2
	10.0	18	-	1.9 ± 0.3
	20.0	10	-	3.5 ± 0.2
Methadone (mg/kg)	1.0	10	+	0
	2.5	17	+	0
	5.0	21	-	2.5 ± 0.6
	7.5	20	-	3.6 ± 0.2
	10.0	11	-	3.9 ± 0.1
Etonitazene (μg/kg)	1.0	8	+	0
	5.0	11	+-	2.1 ± 0.4
	10.0	11	-	3.7 ± 0.2
	20.0	4	-	4

TABLE 4

OPIATE-INDUCED IMMOBILITY: INTRAVENTRICULAR ADMINISTRATION

TREATMENT	DOSE (μg/10 μl)	N	RIGHTING RESPONSE (10 Sec)	RIGIDITY (0-4)
Saline	10 μl	13	+	0
Morphine	25.0	3	+-	0
	50.0	4	-	1.2 ± 0.6
	100.0	5	-	2.4 ± 0.4
Etonitazene	0.5	2	+	0
	1.0	10	+-	1.5 ± 0.6
	2.0	2	-	3.5 ± 0.5
	5.0	10	-	3.2 ± 0.3
	10.0	6	-	4

β-ENDORPHIN-INDUCED BEHAVIORAL ACTIVATION

A prolonged period of hyperactivity follows the opioid peptide-induced immobility in rats[11]. We have found that a similar biphasic pattern results from intraventricular administration of β-endorphin and the enkephalin analogs, $D\text{-Met}^2\text{-Pro}^5\cdot\text{NH}_2$ and $D\text{-Ala}^2\text{-Met}^5\cdot\text{NH}_2$. For these studies adult, male Wistar rats (350-400 g) were habituated to the activity chambers[12-14] for at least 24 hours prior to administration of the opiates or opioid peptides. Locomotion in the form of crossovers and rearings was then monitored for at least four hours.

Results. Morphine at doses of 2.5 mg/kg or greater significantly reduced crossovers and rearings for the first hour after injection and stimulated locomotion during the subsequent three hours (Table 5). An initial depression and subsequent increase in locomotor activity were also exhibited by rats injected with doses as low as 1.0 mg/kg of methadone and 2.5 μg/kg of etonitazene. In agreement with the findings of Domino et al.[11] both the immobility and hyperactivity phases were antagonized by pretreatment with naloxone.

TABLE 5

OPIATE-INDUCED BIPHASIC ALTERATIONS IN LOCOMOTION

Values are mean + S.E.M. Significant differences from control values are indicated: *$P<0.05$, **$P<0.02$, ***$P<0.01$ (two-tailed t-test).

TREATMENT (s.c.)	DOSE	N	CROSSOVERS		REARINGS	
			HOUR 1	HOURS 2-4	HOUR 1	HOURS 2-4
Saline	1.0 ml/kg	15	22 + 2	9 + 2	14 + 1	2 + 1
Morphine (mg/kg)	1.0	5	17 + 5	26 + 6***	11 + 4	11 + 3***
	2.5	5	12 + 2***	42 + 5***	5 + 2***	7 + 2
	5.0	10	4 + 1***	38 + 8***	2 + 1***	3 + 1
	10.0	5	1***	62 + 9***	0***	6 + 1
Methadone (mg/kg)	0.25	5	28 + 9	9 + 3	18 + 5	3 + 1
	0.5	5	41 + 12	28 + 8***	17 + 3	6 + 2
	1.0	11	13 + 5	34 + 10***	7 + 2***	14 + 4***
	2.5	5	1 + 1***	45 + 10***	1 + 1***	15 + 4***
Etonitazene (μg/kg)	0.5	5	29 + 8	11 + 5	15 + 2	2 + 1
	1.0	5	38 + 13	10 + 5	14 + 3	3 + 1
	2.5	10	16 + 6	19 + 6**	7 + 2**	9 + 4*
	5.0	5	5 + 1***	39 + 13***	3 + 1***	14 + 6***

Intraventricular infusion of β-endorphin, $D\text{-}Ala^2\text{-}Met^5\cdot NH_2$ or $D\text{-}Met^2\text{-}Pro^5\cdot NH_2$ resulted in a similar biphasic pattern of locomotion (Table 6). β-Endorphin at doses up to 5 μg in 10 μl produced a dose-dependent reduction in locomotion (as reflected primarily in the rearing measure) during the first hour after infusion. A similar decrease in rearings was produced by 10 μg of $D\text{-}Ala^2\text{-}Met^5\cdot NH_2$ during this initial time period, and both measures of locomotion were markedly reduced by 1.0 μg of $D\text{-}Met^2\text{-}Pro^5\cdot NH_2$. During the period of reduced activity videotape monitoring revealed that the locomotion of most animals was interrupted by recurrent episodes of wet-dog shaking and the "trance-like" behavioral state. Animals injected with 50 μg of β-endorphin were completely immobile for up to four hours.

TABLE 6

OPIOID PEPTIDE-INDUCED BIPHASIC ALTERATIONS IN LOCOMOTION

Values are mean $\pm$ S.E.M. Significant differences from control values are indicated: $*P<0.05$, $**P<0.02$, $***P<0.01$ (two-tailed t-test).

TREATMENT (i.v.t.)	DOSE (μg/10 μl)	N	CROSSOVERS		REARINGS	
			HOUR 1	HOURS 2-4	HOUR 1	HOURS 2-4
Saline	10.0 1	12	55 ± 8	16 ± 5	27 ± 5	3 ± 1
β-Endorphin	1.0	5	46 ± 9	$53 \pm 8***$	14 ± 5	8 ± 4
	2.5	10	$27 \pm 9*$	$93 \pm 22***$	$6 \pm 2***$	$19 \pm 5***$
	5.0	13	36 ± 12	$140 \pm 26***$	$3 \pm 1***$	$32 \pm 11*$
$D\text{-}Met^2\text{-}Pro^5\cdot NH_2$	1.0	4	$10 \pm 2**$	$113 \pm 18***$	$0.5 \pm 03***$	8 ± 4
$D\text{-}Ala^2\text{-}Met^5\cdot NH_2$	10.0	4	67 ± 8	$63 \pm 15***$	$7 \pm 5*$	7 ± 4

During the second through fourth hours after infusion, all three opioid peptides significantly enhanced locomotion. $D\text{-}Met^2\text{-}Pro^5\cdot NH_2$ at doses as low as 2.5 mg/kg, s.c., also induced biphasic behavioral effects. The depression and stimulation of locomotion produced by intraventricular infusion of 2.5 mg/kg of β-endorphin was antagonized by pretreatment with naloxone (5 mg/kg, s.c.) (Table 7).

Oral stereotypy was a prominent feature of the behavioral activation produced by higher doses of the opiates or opioid peptides. Stereotypy as well as the locomotion produced by 7.5 mg/kg of methadone (s.c.) or by 50 μg of β-endorphin (intraventricularly) were antagonized by administration of either naloxone (0.05 mg/kg, s.c.) or haloperidol (0.5 mg/kg, s.c.). Furthermore, naloxone, when administered during the hyperactivity phase, was also effective

in reducing locomotion and stereotypy. This finding suggests that the hyperactivity phase does not simply reflect a rebound from immobilization and, in
fact, may be mediated through opiate receptor activation.

TABLE 7

NALOXONE REVERSAL OF β-ENDORPHIN-INDUCED ALTERATIONS IN LOCOMOTION

Values are mean ± S.E.M. Naloxone was subcutaneously (s.c.) injected 15 minutes
prior to intraventricular infusion of β-endorphin. Significant differences from
control values are indicated: * P<0.05, **P<0.02, ***P<0.01 (two-tailed t-test).

TREATMENT	N	CROSSOVERS		REARINGS	
		HOUR 1	HOURS 2-4	HOUR 1	HOURS 2-4
Saline	12	55 ± 8	16 ± 5	27 ± 5	3 ± 1
β-Endorphin (2.5 μg/10 μl)	10	27 ± 9*	93 ± 22***	6 ± 2***	19 ± 5***
Naloxone (5 mg/kg, s.c.) and β-Endorphin (2.5 μg/10 μl)	5	62 ± 18	26 ± 11	31 ± 12	4 ± 2

Many strains of mice respond to systemic administration of opiates with a
dose-related increase in stereotyped motility[15-17]. We have found a similar response pattern after intravenous injection of morphine, methadone or etonitazene
in male, Swiss-Webster mice (23-35 g) which were habituated to the experimental
chambers for one hour prior to injection (Table 8). In addition to the perseverative locomotor activity, mice responded to all three opiates with tail
elevations. Pretreatment with naloxone prevented both these actions (Table 9).

TABLE 8

PERSEVERATIVE LOCOMOTION INDUCED BY OPIATES

Values are mean crossovers ± S.E.M. during the first hour after intravenous
injection of saline or opiates in mice. Significant differences from control
values are indicated: ***P<0.01 (two-tailed t-test).

TREATMENT (i.v.)	DOSE	N	CROSSOVERS
Saline	2.5 mg/kg	26	150 ± 17
Morphine (mg/kg)	5.0	8	651 ± 96***
Methadone (mg/kg)	1.0	11	198 ± 13
	5.0	14	663 ± 39***
	7.5	8	969 ± 105***
Etonitazene (μg/kg)	5.0	4	180 ± 52
	10.0	7	356 ± 67***

As with the opiates, intravenous administration of D-Met^2-Pro^5·NH$_2$ elicited stereotyped locomotion and tail erections (Table 10). However, in contrast, β-endorphin did not induce behavioral activation. At the lower doses of β-endorphin (5 and 10 mg/kg), mice were indistinguishable from saline controls; in fact, with the highest dose tested, 20 mg/kg, locomotion was significantly reduced. It appears, therefore, that after systemic administration, β-endorphin may not accumulate in the brain in amounts sufficient to produce opiate-like changes in locomotion.

TABLE 9

NALOXONE ANTAGONISM OF OPIATE-INDUCED PERSEVERATIVE LOCOMOTION

Values are mean crossovers $\pm$ S.E.M. during the first hour after intravenous in-injection of either saline or methadone (5 mg/kg). Mice were previously injec-ted (2 min) with either naloxone (2 mg/kg, s.c.) or saline. Significant dif-ferences from control values are indicated: ***P<0.01 (two-tailed t-test).

TREATMENT (DOSE)	N	CROSSOVERS
Saline, 10 ml/kg, s.c.	6	68 $\pm$ 17
Naloxone, 2 mg/kg, s.c.	7	49 $\pm$ 12
Saline, 10 ml/kg, s.c. and Methadone, 5 mg/kg, i.v.	3	298 $\pm$ 43***
Naloxone, 2 mg/kg, s.c. and Methadone, 5 mg/kg, i.v.	4	39 $\pm$ 15

TABLE 10

PERSEVERATIVE LOCOMOTION INDUCED BY OPIOID PEPTIDES

Values are mean crossovers $\pm$ S.E.M. during the first hour after intravenous injection of either saline or opioid peptides in mice. Significant differences from control values are indicated: *P<0.05, ***P<0.01 (two-tailed t-test).

TREATMENT (i.v.)	DOSE (mg/kg)	N	CROSSOVERS
Saline	2.5 ml/kg	36	138 $\pm$ 15
D-Met^2-Pro^5.NH$_2$	5.0	6	222 $\pm$ 77
	10.0	7	325 $\pm$ 52***
	20.0	11	612 $\pm$ 57***
	40.0	4	1186 $\pm$ 108***
β-Endorphin	5.0	5	169 $\pm$ 31
	10.0	9	139 $\pm$ 21
	20.0	9	69 $\pm$ 7*

EFFECTS OF NALOXONE ON SPONTANEOUS AND STIMULANT-INDUCED LOCOMOTOR ACTIVITY

Introduction. Naloxone antagonizes many of the behavioral effects of the opioid peptides, therefore, this opiate antagonist may similarly influence behaviors mediated by endogenous opioid peptides. In fact, naloxone at doses of 3 mg/kg or greater has been reported to reduce locomotor activation produced by some doses of amphetamine in the rat[18]. We have found that doses of naloxone as low as 0.5 mg/kg antagonized locomotor activation produced by 0.5 mg/kg of d-amphetamine. However, whereas the locomotor activity induced by a higher dose of d-amphetamine (2.5 mg/kg) was also antagonized by naloxone, this opiate antagonist at doses as high as 20 mg/kg did not appear to alter the focused stereotypy significantly. A similar dose-response relationship was observed for naloxone and methylphenidate[3].

Naloxone at doses as low as 0.5 mg/kg also produced a significant reduction in spontaneous activity, and observations of these animals suggested that investigatory behaviors might be selectively altered by naloxone. Therefore, a multicompartment, experimental chamber (79x79x84 cm) was designed to further examine the behavioral mechanisms underlying these naloxone effects[3].

Materials and Methods. The experimental chamber consisted of nine interconnecting compartments, each of which contained two wire mesh stimuli, one recessed in the floor and the other suspended from the ceiling. Each animal was placed in the chamber 25 minutes after injection with either saline or naloxone (5 mg/kg), and then observed for 30 minutes by a behavioral rater who was unaware of the treatment conditions. Locomotion was monitored in the form of compartment entries and rearings and investigatory behavior in terms of frequency and duration of contact with the upper and lower stimuli.

Results. Both measures of locomotion declined at similar rates for the two groups; however, as we found previously, naloxone significantly reduced both the number of compartment entries and rearings throughout the duration of the observation period (Table 11). As with locomotor activity, the number of contacts with the lower stimulus also declined gradually although the two two groups were significantly different only during the last five-minute interval (Table 12). In contrast, time spent per stimulus contact (which progressively increased for both groups) was significantly enhanced by naloxone during most of the 30-minute test session. The response to the upper stimulus was similarly affected by naloxone. Therefore, the reduction in locomotor activity induced by naloxone may be due, at least in part, to a potentiated interaction with environmental stimuli.

TABLE 11

NALOXONE-INDUCED ALTERATIONS IN LOCOMOTION

Values are mean compartment entries $\pm$ S.E.M. and rearings $\pm$ S.E.M. during successive five-minute intervals; N = 10 animals in each group. Significant differences from control values are indicated: *P<0.05, **P<0.02, ***P<0.01 (two-tailed t-test).

TIME (MINUTES)	COMPARTMENT ENTRIES		REARINGS	
	SALINE	NALOXONE	SALINE	NALOXONE
0 - 5	63 + 5	39 + 3***	23 + 3	11 + 1***
6-10	52 + 4	36 + 4**	17 + 2	7 + 3***
11-15	38 + 3	24 + 2***	12 + 2	5 + 1***
16-20	27 + 3	15 + 1***	8 + 1	3 + 1*
21-25	22 + 3	12 + 2**	6 + 3	2 + 1***
26-30	21 + 3	5 + 2***	6 + 3	1 + 1

TABLE 12

NALOXONE-INDUCED ALTERATIONS IN LOWER STIMULUS CONTACT

Values are mean number of contacts $\pm$ S.E.M. and time spent per lower stimulus contacts $\pm$ S.E.M.; N = 7 animals in each group. Significant differences from control values are indicated: *P 0.05, **P 0.02, ***P 0.01 (two-tailed t-test).

TIME (MINUTES)	NUMBER OF CONTACTS		TIME(SEC)/CONTACT	
	SALINE	NALOXONE	SALINE	NALOXONE
0- 5	14 + 3	17 + 2	2 + 1	3 + 1***
6-10	13 + 2	16 + 2	2 + 1	3 + 1***
11-15	15 + 2	10 + 1	3 + 1	4 + 1
16-20	11 + 2	8 + 1	5 + 1	9 + 1***
21-25	10 + 1	8 + 2	5 + 1	10 + 2***
26-30	9 + 1	5 + 1	6 + 1	12 + 3

SUMMARY

In conclusion, β-endorphin and other opioid peptides produce a broad spectrum of behaviors ranging from locomotor excitation to extreme muscular rigidity. These effects, which are reversed by naloxone and closely resemble the behavioral actions of opiates, appear to be mediated through the activation of opiate receptors in the brain. These findings along

with the behavioral alterations produced by naloxone suggest that the
endogenous opioid peptides may play an important role in the regulation
of behavioral arousal and attention.

ACKNOWLEDGEMENTS
     This research was supported by USPHS Grants DA-01568-03 and DA-01994-01;
D.S.S. is the recipient of USPHS Research Scientist Award MH-70183-05; R.G.B.
is the recipient of a postdoctoral fellowship, USPHS AA-07129-02; A.A. is the
recipient of a predoctoral fellowship provided by the A.P. Sloan Foundation;
and, D.C.D. is the recipient of a predoctoral fellowship, USPHS GM-07198.

REFERENCES
1. Bloom, F., Segal, D.S., Ling, N. and Guillemin, R. (1976) Science, 194,
   630-632.
2. Segal, D.S., Browne, R.G., Bloom, F., Ling, N. and Guillemin, R. (1977)
   Science, 198, 411-414.
3. Segal, D.S., Browne, R.G., Arnsten, A. and Derrington, D.C. (1978) in
   Endorphins in Mental Health Research, Usdin, E., Bunney, W. and Kline,
   N., eds., MacMillan, London, pp. 307-324.
4. Izumi, K., Motomatsu, T., Chretien, M., Butterworth, R.F., Lis, M. and
   Seidah, A. (1977) Life Sci., 20, 1149-1156.
5. Tseng, L.F., Loh, H.H. and Li, C.H. (1977) Biochim. Biophys. Res. Commun.,
   74, 390-396.
6. Motomatsu, T., Lis, M., Seidah, A. and Chretien, M. (1977) Can. J. Neurol.
   Sci., 4, 49-52.
7. Barnett, A., Goldstein, J., Fiedler, E. and Taber, R. (1975) Eur. J.
   Pharmacol., 30, 23-38.
8. Wand, P., Kuschinsky, K. and Sontag, K.-H. (1973) Eur. J. Pharmacol.,
   24, 189-193.
9. Shizgal, P., Sklar, L.S., Brown, Z.W. and Amit, Z. (1977) Pharmacol.
   Biochem. Behav., 6, 17-20.
10.Ahtee, L., Kaariainen, I. and Paasonen, M.K. (1972) Ann. Med. Exp. Biol.
   Fenn., 50, 180-185.
11.Domino, E.F., Vasko, M.R. and Wilson, A.M. (1976) in Tissue Responses to
   Addictive Drugs, D.H. Ford and D.H. Clouet, eds., Spectrum, NY, pp. 143-167.
12.Segal, D.S. (1975) in Advances in Biochemical Psychopharmacology, V. 13,
   Mandell. A.J.. ed.. NY, Raven, pp. 247-266.
13.Segal, D.S. (1976) Brain Res., 116, 267-277.
14.Browne, R.G. and Segal, D.S. (1977) Pharmacol. Biochem. Behav., 6, 545-552.
15.Kuschinsky, K. and Hornykiewicz, O. (1974) Eur. J. Pharmacol., 26, 41-50.
16.Shuster, L., Webster, G.W., Yu, G. and Eleftheriou, B.E. (1975) Psychopharmacologia, Berl., 42, 249-254.
17.Brase, D.A., Loh, H.H. and Way, E.L. (1977) J. Pharmac. exp. Ther., 201,
   368-374.
18.Holtzman, S.G. (1974) J. Pharmac. exp. Ther., 189, 51-60.

Characteristics and Function of Opioids, editors Van Ree and Terenius
published by Elsevier/North-Holland Biomedical Press, 1978

THE EFFECTS OF OPIATES ON NIGROSTRIATAL DOPAMINERGIC ACTIVITY

AGU PERT

Section on Biochemistry and Pharmacology, Biological Psychiatry Branch, National
Institute of Mental Health, Bethesda, Maryland (U.S.A.)

SUMMARY

An attempt was made to evaluate a number of longstanding observations regarding the actions of opiates on dopaminergic nigrostriatal function and to inte-
grate these observations with new findings. Although opiates have been postulated to induce catatonia by inhibiting dopamine activity, recent findings make
this unlikely. In fact, the catatonic effects of opiates appear to be mediated
through structures outside of the extrapyramidal system. In addition, instead
of depressing dopaminergic activity, opiates appear to enhance dopamine nigrostriatal function through a number of mechanisms.

The extrapyramidal system is a grouping of neural structures that are
assumed to function as a unit to modulate some aspects of motor behavior. It
includes the corpus striatum (caudate nucleus and putamen), the subthalamic
nucleus, the substantia nigra, the red nucleus, and the brainstem reticular
formation. The striatum appears to receive afferents from every level of the
central nervous system (the cerebral cortex, intralaminar thalamic nuclei and
the substantia nigra). The substantia nigra and the striatum appear to be
reciprocally related. Nigrostriatal fibers appear to convey dopamine (DA) to
the striatum while striatonigral fibers convey GABA to the substantia nigra (SN).
The DA cell bodies of the SN are located in the zona compacta, a cell-rich
region composed of large pigmented cells. The zona reticulata of the SN, on the
other hand, is high in GAD (the enzyme utilized in the synthesis of GABA) and
is thought to receive the majority of GABAergic input. The SN may also receive
GABAergic afferents from the globus pallidus. The globus pallidus is also
reciprocally connected with the subthalamic nucleus and, in turn, receives
afferents from the caudate nucleus and putamen.

For the interest of the present analysis it is important to note that a number of extrapyramidal structures (especially the globus pallidus, caudate
nucleus and substantia nigra) are high in both opiate receptors[1,2,3], enkephalin
content[4] and enkephalinergic terminals[5]. The precise origin of these enkephalinergic neurons is not known at this time, and it is not clear whether they
are predominantly intrinsic interneurons or whether they represent afferents

from other structures. At least some enkephalinergic neurons associated with extrapyramidal structures are not interneurons. Cuello and Paxinas[6] and Uhl *et al.*[7] have recently demonstrated that some enkephalinergic neurons appear to project from the caudate nucleus to the globus pallidus. Other enkephalinergic neurons appear to synapse on DA terminals in the caudate nucleus[8]. Considering these relationships of enkephalinergic neurons and opiate receptors with the extrapyramidal structures it is not surprising that opiates and opiate peptides exert powerful effects on motor behaviors[9].

Small doses of morphine produce increases in spontaneous locomotor activity while large doses cause an initial depression and catatonia[10,11] which is followed by excitation[10]. These psychomotor as well as cataleptic effects of opiates have generally been ascribed to their actions on various components of the nigrostriatal DA system[12,13]. Specifically, it has been proposed that some of the motor effects of opiates like those of neuroleptics are due to their direct actions on striatal DA neurons[12].

Neuroleptics have been postulated to induce catalepsy by blocking the DA receptors in the striatum. This initial blockade of postsynaptic DA receptors has been thought to produce a compensatory increase in the activity of DA neurons via a feedback mechanism[14] which results in an apparent increase in release, synthesis and metabolism of DA in the striatum[15].

Several parallels seem to exist between the actions of opiates and neuroleptics on the DA systems. Opiate agonists, including morphine, have also been found to increase DA synthesis as measured by their ability to increase the conversion of radioactive tyrosine into DA in the striata, as well as the mesolimbic components of DA brain regions[16-20]. Likewise, opiates also accelerate depletion of brain DA after catecholamine synthesis inhibition[21-23] which has been interpreted as being due to increased activity within the ascending DA neurons. Opiates also increase striatal as well as mesolimbic levels of homovanillic acid (HVA), a major metabolite of DA[24-30]. Increased striatal HVA has also been recently observed after intraventricular injections of β-endorphin[31] and D-Ala^2-met-enkephalin[32], as well as after direct intranigral injections of D-Ala^2-met-enkephalin[33].

Considering these striking similarities between the actions of opiates and neuroleptics on the DA system, it is not surprising that several investigators have proposed that the cataleptic actions of opiates may likewise be related to an inhibition of DA transmission in the striatum[12,13,27]. Recently, however, several important differences have emerged between the actions of these two classes of drugs which makes this hypothesis less attractive. First, it appears certain that opiates do not inhibit DA transmission by interacting directly with postsynaptic DA receptors. Carenzi *et al.*[20] found that while both neuroleptics and morphine increased the turnover of DA in the striatum, there were clear differences in their actions on DA-stimulated adenylate cyclase. Haloperidol was found to block the *in vitro* activation of adenylate cyclase by DA, while morphine was entirely ineffective in this respect. More recently, Leysen *et al.*[34] have shown that opiate agonists do not have a significant affinity for the DA receptor as demonstrated by their inability to inhibit neuroleptic binding. While opiates do not block DA receptors directly, it is possible that an inhibition of DA transmission could be achieved through a different mechanism. Pollard *et al.*[8], for example, have recently demonstrated the presence of opiate receptors on DA terminals in the striatum and suggested that opiates may induce catatonia by inhibiting the release of DA. Arbilla and Langer[35], however, failed to find any inhibition of potassium-stimulated release of DA by either morphine or β-endorphin in striatal slices.

Kuschinsky and Hornykiewicz[29], on the other hand, have suggested that opiates may influence DA metabolism directly in the presynaptic neuron by diverting newly synthesized DA from storage sites to sites of catabolism by some unspecified mechanism. The increased breakdown of newly formed DA would then result in a deficiency of this amine at the receptor sites. Carenzi *et al.*[20] have also suggested that opiate-induced catatonia could be attributable to a defect in the stimulation of postsynaptic receptors in the striatum resulting from an impairment of the extraneuronal release of DA.

Although the effects of opiates on the disposition of DA in the striatum have been tied to their cataleptic actions in a correlative fashion, it seems that they may not be related to this opiate-induced behavior at all.

If both opiates and neuroleptics induce catalepsy by inhibiting DA transmission in the striatum, then lesions of this structure should have similar effects on the cataleptic actions of both classes of drugs. Costall and Naylor[11], however, found that while lesions of the caudate-putamen, as well as the globus pallidus, reduced or abolished haloperidol-induced catalepsy, morphine catatonia was enhanced by the same lesions. Nakamura *et al.*[36] have also found increases in morphine-induced catatonia after destruction of the DA terminals in the rat striatum with 6-hydroxydopamine (6-OHDA). Koffer *et al.*[37] have recently reported similar interactive effects between striatal lesions and opiate or neuroleptic catatonia. These authors concluded that while the striatum appears to be a primary site of action of neuroleptic drugs in the production of catalepsy, opiate-induced catatonic effects may be mediated through other structures.

More direct evidence concerning the brain sites which mediate neuroleptic and opiate cataleptic effects comes from studies in which these compounds have been

injected directly into brain. Costall *et al.*[38] have found that injections of
haloperidol into the caudate-putamen, as well as the globus pallidus, produce
catalepsy. Pert *et al.*[9] recently evaluated the catatonic as well as spontaneous
locomotor effects of opiates following injections into various brain sites.
Injections into the periaqueductal gray matter (PAG) were found to induce the
most profound catatonic actions while modest catatonic effects were elicited by
injections into the ventral tegmentum, hippocampus and globus pallidus. More
recently we have attempted to further analyze the differential actions of neuroleptics and opiates by comparing their cataleptic effects following injections
into the caudate nucleus or the PAG. Essentially, rats were implanted with
bilateral 23 gauge cannulae guides aimed for an area 2 mm dorsal to the caudate
nucleus (AP 7.5, LAT 2.5, DV 1.0[39]) or with unilateral cannulae guides aimed for
an area 2 mm dorsal to the PAG (AP 0.6, LAT 0.5, DV -0.5[39]). Following recovery
the rats were divided into groups and injected with either 1 μl saline, 50 μg
of chlorpromazine or 5 μg of morphine sulfate bilaterally in the caudate nucleus
or unilaterally with the same amounts of each substance in the PAG. A fourth
PAG group was pretreated with 5 mg/kg of naloxone prior to the intracerebral
injection of morphine. Injections were made through 30 gauge injectors which
protruded 2 mm past the guide cannula. Catalepsy was assessed 15 and 30 min.
after injection by placing the rat's front paws on a horizontal bar and measuring the time in seconds that they remained standing on it[9]. The results of this
study appear in Fig. 1. While chlorpromazine was found to produce catalepsy
following intracaudate injections, morphine was found to be ineffective. Injections of morphine into the PAG, on the other hand, produced profound catalepsy
while chlorpromazine did not. These findings clearly indicate that while the

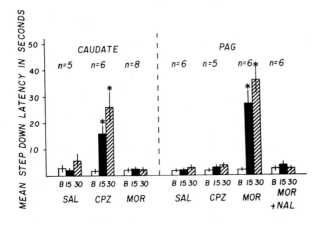

Fig. 1. The cataleptic actions of morphine and chlorpromazine following injections into the caudate nucleus or the PAG. The caudate injections were bilateral (total of 10 μg morphine and 100 μg chlorpromazine) and the PAG injections were uni-lateral (total of 5 μg morphine and 50 μg chlor-promazine). *p <0.05 for comparisons of postinjec-tion step-down latencies with saline controls.

cataleptic actions of chlorpromazine appear to be mediated through the striatum, the cataleptic actions of morphine are predominantly determined by its action in the PAG. Although the cataleptic actions of opiates do not appear to be determined by their actions in the striatum, it is still possible that the effects of opiates on striatal DA disposition are related to other motor effects of opiates.

The clearest evidence supporting the notion that opiate agonists do, in fact, exert functionally significant effects on the DA nigrostriatal system comes from recent behavioral studies. One behavioral situation that has been particularly useful in analyzing the actions of drugs on DA nigrostriatal activity is the rotational model first introduced by Andén et al.[40] and extended by Ungerstedt[41]. Essentially, this model is based on the principle that animals will rotate away from the striatum with the preponderance of dopaminergic activity. A dopaminergic imbalance is usually created by unilaterally lesioning the SN either electrolytically or by injections of 6-OHDA. Such lesions result in the degeneration of ascending DA neurons in the nigrostriatal pathway and the development of DA receptor supersensitivity in the ipsilateral striatum[42].

Since opiate agonists appear to induce at least part of their excitatory behavioral effects through catecholaminergic mechanisms[43-45], it was of interest to examine the effects of opiates on nigrostriatal function using the rotational model. Our early findings were somewhat disappointing. Although rats that had been lesioned unilaterally in the substantia nigra were found to rotate ipsilaterally to the lesion after amphetamine and contralaterally after apomorphine, acute administrations of morphine had no apparent effect on rotational behavior[9]. The lack of effect of morphine was surprising since Iwamoto et al.[46] had previously reported that rats do have a tendency to rotate toward the lesion after systemic morphine. Von Voightlander and Moore[47], on the other hand, had also failed to observe any effect of morphine on rotational behavior following 6-OHDA lesions to the striatum of mice.

Since a number of brain regions outside of the extrapyramidal system appear to mediate the motor depressant effects of opiates, it was possible that the actions of systemically administered morphine in these areas may attenuate the expression of rotational behavior. Since animals became tolerant rapidly to the motor depressant effects of morphine[10] but not the excitatory actions, it is possible that the effects of morphine on rotational behavior would be unmasked after chronic administration. This, in fact, proved to be the case. Fig. 2 illustrates the effects of daily morphine or saline injections over a period of 10 days on rotational behavior. Chronic administration of morphine was found to produce distinct ipsilateral rotations when measured 30 min. after injection. Interestingly, this behavior increased in intensity over the 10-day

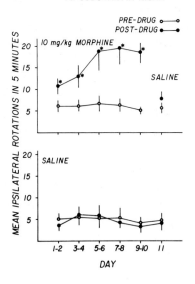

EFFECT OF CHRONIC MORPHINE ON ROTATIONAL BEHAVIOR FOLLOWING 6-OHDA LESIONS TO SUBSTANTIA NIGRA

Fig. 2. Effects of chronic intraperitoneal morphine (10 mg/kg) on rotational behavior following unilateral 6-OHDA lesions to substantia nigra. Animals in both groups were injected with saline on Day 11. *p <0.05 for comparisons of post-drug performance with pre-drug performance. (From Pert *et al.*[9])

injection period. The actions of morphine on rotational behavior appeared to be pharmacologically specific in that naloxone antagonized the effect. Furthermore, since haloperidol was also found to be an effective antagonist, it appeared that the morphine-induced rotations could be causally related to an activation of the ascending nigrostriatal DA pathways. Thus, these findings certainly do not offer support to the notion that opiate agonists block DA transmission in the striatum. Drugs which block DA receptors, e.g., haloperidol, have been found to induce contralateral rotations in rats with unilateral substantia nigra lesions[40]--precisely opposite to the opiate actions.

What is the precise mechanism of action of morphine in producing rotational behavior? It is clear that the effects of morphine were not similar to those of apomorphine (a direct DA receptor agonist) which produced contralateral rotations by its action on supersensitive DA receptors in the striatum ipsilateral to the SN lesion. This is not surprising since opiate agonists have little affinity for the DA receptor[34]. The effects of morphine, therefore, had to be related to an enhanced activation of DA nigrostriatal neurons. The precise locus of this action, however, was not clear. Was morphine acting in the striatum to enhance DA release (like amphetamine), was it activating SN dopamine neurons either directly or indirectly, or was it acting by some other mechanism to increase DA activity?

Another method of creating an imbalance of activity between the two ascending DA nigrostriatal pathways is to unilaterally stimulate the SN either electrically or with compounds which directly increase the activity of DA neurons. Such unilateral stimulation produces rotational behavior that is contralateral to the stimulation. Thus, unilateral injections of substance P (a neuropeptide which increases the activity of SN neurons after iontophoretic application) or electrical stimulation have been reported to produce contralateral rotations in rats[48,49]. Using this approach, there is now considerable evidence that at least part of the facilitatory effects of opiates on DA transmission are determined by their actions directly in the SN. Both Pert *et al.*[9] and Iwamoto and Way[50] have recently reported that morphine injections into the SN induce rotations contralateral to the injection. Fig. 3 illustrates the intensity and time course of rotational behavior following unilateral intranigral injections of either 5 μg of morphine, [D-Ala^2,Met^5]enkephalinamide[51], or β-endorphin. All of these compounds were found to induce rotations contralateral to the injection. The effects of β-endorphin and [D-Ala^2,Met^5]enkephalinamide decreased over the 3-hour observation period while the effects of morphine were actually enhanced.

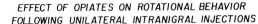

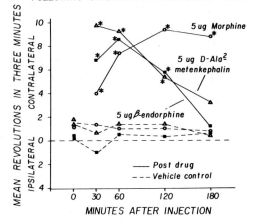

Fig. 3. Effects of 5 μg of morphine, β-endorphin and [D-Ala^2-met^5]enkephalinamide on rotational behavior following unilateral intranigral injections. *p <0.05 for comparisons of drug-induced behavior with the vehicle baseline[9]. (From Pert *et al.*[9])

Although intranigral injections of opiates induced rotational behavior contralateral to the injection, it was still not clear whether these effects were related to the activation of ascending DA pathways. To answer whether intranigral morphine activates ascending pathways, rats were prepared in which knife cuts were made either anterior or posterior to the SN injection cannula. In this study it was found that while caudal knife cuts had relatively little

effect on rotational behavior following intranigral morphine, rostral knife cuts
had relatively little effect on rotational behavior following intranigral morphine, and rostral knife cuts resulted in a clear inhibition. Thus, opiates in
the SN apparently do activate some ascending pathways. Are these pathways dopaminergic? We have recently answered this question by preparing 9 rats with
cannulae in both the SN and the ipsilateral caudate. Following recovery, the
rats were injected in the SN with 7.5 µg of morphine sulfate. The animals were
then tested for rotational behavior in a Plexiglas cylinder (28 cm in diameter
and 27 cm high). Rotational behavior was transmitted to an automated recording
apparatus through a flexible steel spring which was attached to a standard rat
harness fitted to the animal. When rotational behavior had stabilized, the rats
were quickly injected in the ipsilateral caudate nucleus with either 7.5 µg
haloperidol or 1.5 µl saline and tested for an additional hour. Seven days
later all the animals were again injected with morphine in the SN but with the
opposite compound (saline or haloperidol) in the caudate. The results of this
study appear in Fig. 4. In this experimental situation a 7.5 µg injection of
morphine into the SN produced contralateral rotations with an intensity of
approximately 2 rpm. Following injections of saline into the ipsilateral caudate nucleus, the rotational behavior continued to increase in intensity, while
following haloperidol the rotations decreased precipitously and remained at a
low level throughout the session. Thus, injections of a DA blocker into the
terminal region of the nigrostriatal pathway were effective in drastically
reducing the rotational behavior following injections of morphine into the SN--
the origin of the DA nigrostriatal pathway. Iwamato and Way[50] have also presented evidence to support the notion that opiates act in the SN to activate
ascending DA pathways. These investigators found that both systemically administered haloperidol and 6-OHDA lesions of the medical forebrain bundle (pathway

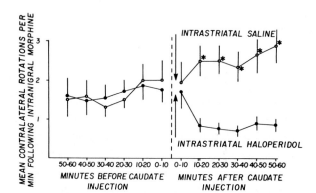

Fig. 4 Blockade of intra-
nigral morphine induced
rotational behavior (7.5
µg) following injections
of haloperidol into the
ipsilateral caudate
nucleus. *p <0.05 for
comparisons between rota-
tional behavior following
intrastriatal haloperidol
and intrastriatal saline.

of the nigrostriatal DA neurons) attenuated rotational behavior induced by unilateral intranigral injections of morphine.

In this context it is again important to note that the SN is quite high in
both opiate receptors[3] as well as enkephalin terminals[5]. It is not clear, however, whether the nigral opiate receptors are located directly on DA neurons or
whether they are on other neurons intrinsic to the SN or even on terminals of SN
afferents. The question is--Do opiates activate zona compacta DA neurons
directly or is this activation achieved by their primary action on neurons associated with DA cells?

Recent electrophysiological studies have also demonstrated that morphine
increases the basal activity of DA neurons in the SN[52,53]. We have also observed a modest (10-20%) increase in the firing rates of zona compacta DA cells
in the unanesthetized rat following intravenous injections of 2.5 mg/kg morphine
(Pert and Gallager, unpublished observation). This increased DA activity has
also been assumed to be caused by a mechanism similar to that of neuroleptics--
a compensatory increase in the activity of DA cells following inhibition of DA
transmission in the caudate nucleus[53]. Indeed, the notion that morphine may
activate DA cells in the SN by a feedback mechanism is strengthened by the
demonstration that injections of morphine directly into the caudate nucleus
were also effective in increasing the activity of zona compacta neurons[53].

Although opiates may increase the activity of DA cells in the SN via a feedback mechanism from the striatum, the behavioral evidence for a direct action
of morphine in the SN was overwhelming. For this reason we have recently initiated a series of electrophysiological studies aimed at further elucidating the
actions of opiates in the SN. Although the results are at the present somewhat
preliminary, they strongly suggest that opiates do not exert a direct effect on
DA neurons in the SN (Pert and Gallager, unpublished observations). While ion-
tophoretically applied DA was found to characteristically depress the basal
activity of identifiable DA cells in the zona compacta, morphine had little, if
any, apparent effect on the same neurons. In addition, when morphine and DA
were applied concurrently, morphine did not appear to prevent the depression
normally seen following DA. Thus, while opiates do appear to act in the SN to
activate ascending DA pathways, this effect is not achieved by a direct activation of DA cells in the SN or by a blockade of DA "autoreceptors" located on the
DA cell bodies.

While opiates do not appear to exert profound behavioral effects through the
caudate nucleus, the presence of enkephalinergic neurons and opiate receptors in
this structure makes it likely that some pharmacological effects of opiates are
mediated by it. Although we found unilateral injections of morphine into the

caudate nucleus to have relatively little effect on rotational behavior, it is possible that more subtle actions might be revealed while the DA system was simultaneously being activated by DA agonists.

In the following study 14 rats were implanted with bilateral intracerebral cannulae guides which were aimed for an area 2 mm dorsal to the caudate nucleus (AP 7.5, LAT 2.5, DV 1.0[39]). One week following surgery the rats were injected with the following drugs or drug combinations: unilateral intrastriatal morphine (10 µg) followed 20 min. later by either saline, apomorphine (1 mg/kg), or amphetamine (2.5 mg/kg) administered intraperitoneally or unilateral intrastriatal saline followed 20 min. later by either amphetamine or apomorphine. Rotational behavior was assessed both prior to and after drug injections in an automated recording apparatus. All rats received all five drug combinations spaced at least 5 days apart. Two weeks after the termination of the first study, all animals were again tested for rotational behavior after unilateral intrastriatal haloperidol (7.5 µg) followed by systemic amphetamine or saline 5 min. later or after intrastriatal saline followed by systemic amphetamine 5 min. later. Several predictions can be generated. If morphine somehow inhibits the release of DA in the striatum, then the rats should rotate ipsilateral to the striatal morphine injection following systemic injections of amphetamine and not be affected by apomorphine. On the other hand, if morphine somehow inhibits DA transmission postsynaptically (like haloperidol) then amphetamine and apomorphine should both induce ipsilatereal rotations. The other possibility is that morphine actually enhances DA transmission in the caudate. In this case, both amphetamine and apomorphine should induce contralateral rotations.

The results from this study appear in Fig. 5. True to expectations, amphetamine produced rotational behavior ipsilateral to the striatal haloperidol injection. This finding seems to suggest that morphine in the caudate nucleus actually enhances the effects of apomorphine and amphetamine on DA transmission. Interestingly, both opiates and DA have been found to exert inhibitory effects on striatal neurons[54-57] probably through different mechanisms.

CONCLUSION

The notion that opiates block DA receptors or DA functions in the striatum to induce catalepsy is no longer tenable. Opiates, in fact, appear to produce catalepsy through structures outside of the extrapyramidal system. While opiates do not induce their cataleptic effects through the striatum, it is apparent that these compounds still influence nigrostriatal activity. It is still to early, however, to make any definitive statements regarding the precise loci and mechanisms of action of opiates in modulating the DA nigrostriatal

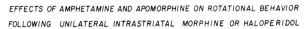

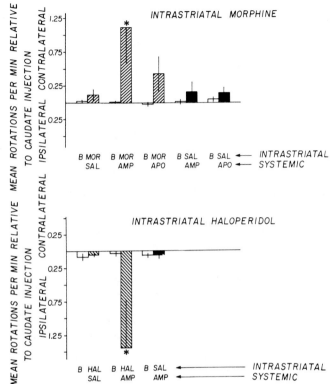

Fig. 5. Effects of amphetamine on rotational behavior following unilateral intrastriatal morphine or haloperidol. Ipsilateral or contralateral rotations are relative to the unilateral intrastriatal injection. *p <0.05 for comparison of amphetamine effects following intrastriatal morphine (or haloperidol) with amphetamine effects following intrastriatal saline.

system. There appear to be several anomalies regarding the effects of opiates on striatal DA neurons. In the caudate nucleus direct injections of morphine appear to both increase HVA and enhance the effects of DA agonists and at the same time increase the activity of DA neurons in the SN. Iontophoretic applications of morphine, on the other hand, appear to inhibit striatal neurons, just like DA. While opiates also clearly activate the nigrostriatal pathway by a direct action in the SN, the effects are not determined by a direct effect on the DA neurons of the zona compacta. The opiate effects in the nigra may be determined by their actions on intrinsic interneurons or on inhibitory afferent terminals to the zona compacta cells.

It seems that our inability to understand the complex actions of opiates on the nigrostriatal system is related directly to our lack of understanding and appreciation regarding its complex organization and interconnections.

REFERENCES

1. Kuhar, M.J., Pert, C.B. and Snyder, S.H. (1973) Nature, 245, 447-450.

2. Hiller, J.M., Pearson, J. and Simon, E.J. (1973) Res. Commun. Chem. Pathol. Pharmacol., 6, 1052-1062.

3. LaMotte, C., Snowman, A., Pert, C.B. and Snyder, S.H. (1978) Brain Res., in press.

4. Hong, J.S., Yang, H-Y.T., Fratta, W. and Costa, E. (1977) Brain Res., 134, 383-386.

5. Elde, E., Hökfelt, T., Johansson, O. and Terenius, L. (1976) Neuroscience, 1, 349-351.

6. Cuello, A.C. and Paxinas, G. (1978) Nature, 271, 178-180.

7. Uhl, G., Kuhar, M.J., Goodman, R.R. and Snyder, S.H. (1978) in Endorphins in Mental Health Research, Usdin, E., Bunney, W.E. Jr. and Kline, N.S. eds., Macmillan, London, in press.

8. Pollard, H., Lloreus-Cortes, C. and Schwartz, J.C. (1977) Nature, 268, 745-747.

9. Pert, A., DeWald, L., Liao, H. and Sivit, C. (1978) in Endorphins in Mental Health Research, Usdin, E., Bunney, W.E. Jr. and Kline, N.S. eds., Macmillan, London, in press.

10. Babbini, M. and Davis, W.M. (1972) Br. J. Pharmacol., 46, 213-224.

11. Costall, B. and Naylor, R.J. (1973) Arzneim-Forsch., 23, 674-683.

12. Kuschinsky, K. (1976) Arznium-Forsch., 26, 563-567.

13. Lal, H. (1975) Life Sci., 17, 483-496.

14. Carlsson, A. and Lindqvist, M. (1963) Acta Pharmacol. Toxicol., 20, 140-144.

15. Hornykiewicz, O. (1966) Pharmacol. Rev., 18, 925-964.

16. Clouet, D.H. and Ratner, M. (1970) Science, 168, 854-855.

17. Smith, C.B., Sheldon, M.I., Bednarczyk, J.H. and Villarreal, J.F. (1972) J. Pharmacol. Exp. Ther., 180, 547-557.

18. Bloom, A.S., Dewey, W.L., Harris, L.S. and Brasius, K.K. (1976) J. Pharmacol. Exp. Ther., 198, 33-41.

19. Gauchy, C., Agid, Y., Glowinski, J. and Cheramy, A. (1973) Eur. J. Pharmacol., 22, 311-319.

20. Carenzi, A., Guidotti, A., Resuelta, A. and Costa, E. (1975) J. Pharmacol. Exp. Ther., 194, 311-318.

21. Gunne, L-M. and Jansson, J. (1969) J. Eur. Pharmacol., 5, 338-342.

22. Sugrue, M.F. (1974) Br. J. Pharmacol., 52, 159-165.

23. Maleman, P. and Bruinvels, J. (1976) Prog. Neuropsychopharmacol., 1, 101-106.

24. Westerink, B.H.C. and Korf, J. (1975) Eur. J. Pharmacol., 33, 31-40.

25. Ahtee, L. (1973) J. Pharm. Pharmacol., 25, 649-651.

26. Laverty, R. and Sharmon, D.F. (1965) Br. J. Pharmacol., 24, 20-26.

27. Salame, H.A., Perez-Cruet, J., DiChiara, G., Tagliamonte, A., Tagliamonte, P. and Gessa, G.L. (1972) J. Neurochem., 19, 1953-1957.

28. Kuschinsky, K. and Hornykiewicz, O. (1972) Eur. J. Pharmacol., 19, 119-122.

29. Kuschinsky, K. and Hornykiewicz, O. (1973) Eur. J. Pharmacol., 26, 41-50.

30. Papeschi, R., Theiss, P. and Herz, A. (1975) Eur. J. Pharmacol., 34, 253-261.

31. Berney, S. and Hornykiewicz, O. (1977) Commun. Psychopharmacol., 1, 597-604.

32. Algeri, S., Calderini, G., Consalazione, A. and Garattini, S. (1977) Eur. J. Pharmacol., 45, 207-209.

33. Biggio, G., Casu, M., Corda, M.G., DiBello, C. and Gessa, G.L. (1978) Science, 200, 552-554.

34. Leysen, J., Tallenaere, J.P., Kach, M.H.J. and Laduron, P. (1977) Eur. J. Pharmacol., 43, 253-267.

35. Arbilla, S. and Langer, S.Z. (1978) Nature, 271, 559-561.

36. Nakamura, K., Kuntzman, R., Maggio, A. and Carmey, A.H. (1973) Neuro-pharmacol., 12, 1153-1160.

37. Kaffer, K., Berney, S. and Hornykiewicz, O. (1978) Eur. J. Pharmacol., 47, 81-86.

38. Costall, B., Naylor, R.J. and Olley, J.E. (1972) Neuropharmacol., 11, 645-663.

39. König, J.F.R. and Klippel, R.A. (1963) The Rat Brain, Krieger, New York.

40. Andén, N.E., Dahlstrom, A., Fuxe, K. and Larson, K. (1966) Acta Pharmacol. Toxicol., 24, 263-274.

41. Ungerstedt, U. (1971) Acta Physiol. Scand., 82 (suppl. 367), 69-93.

42. Creese, I., Burt, D.R. and Snyder, S.H. (1977) Science, 197, 596-599.

43. Ayhan, I.H. and Randrup, A. (1973) Psychopharmacologia, 29, 317-328.

44. Buxbaum, D.M., Yarbrough, G.G. and Carter, M.E. (1973) J. Pharmacol. Exp. Ther., 185, 317-327.

45. Davis, W.M., Babbini, M. and Khalsa, J.H. (1972) Res. Commun. Chem. Path. Pharmacol., 4, 267-278.

46. Iwamoto, E.T., Loh, H.H. and Way, E.L. (1976) J. Pharmacol. Exp. Ther., 197, 503-516.

47. Von Voightlander, P.F. and Moore, K.E. (1973) Neuropharmacology, 12, 451-462.

48. Olpe, H-R. and Koella, W. (1977) Brain Res., 126, 576-579.

49. Arbuthnott, G.W. and Crow, T.J. (1971) Exp. Neurol., 30, 484-491.

50. Iwamoto, E.T. and Way, E.L. (1977) J. Pharmacol. Exp. Ther., 203, 347-359.

51. Pert, C.B., Pert, A., Chang, J-K. and Fong, B.T.W. (1976) Science, 194, 330-332.

52. Nawycky, M.C. (1976) Ph.D. dissertation submitted to Yale University.

53. Iwatsubo, K. and Clouet, D.H. (1977) J. Pharmacol. Exp. Ther., 202, 429-436.

54. Nicoll, R., Siggins, G.R., Ling, N., Bloom, F.E. and Guillemin, R. (1977) Proc. Nat. Acad. Sci. USA, 74, 2584-2588.

55. Bradley, D.B. and Gayton, R.J. (1976) Br. J. Pharmacol., 57, 425-426P.

56. Frederickson, R.C.A. and Norris, F.H. (1976) Science, 194, 440-442.

57. Siggins, G.R. (1978) in Psychopharmacology: A Generation of Progress, Lipton, M.A., DiMascio, A. and Killam, K.F. eds., Raven Press, New York.

Characteristics and Function of Opioids, editors Van Ree and Terenius
© *1978 Elsevier/North-Holland Biomedical Press*

BEHAVIORAL ACTIONS OF SOME N-FURYL BENZOMORPHANS AND KETAZOCINES IN
RHESUS MONKEYS AND MICE

J. H. WOODS, C. L. FLY AND H. H. SWAIN

Department of Pharmacology, University of Michigan, Ann Arbor, Michigan 48109, U.S.A.

ABSTRACT

We have made a set of behavioral observations of ketazocine, ethylketazocine and some tetrahydrofurfuryl and methylfurfuryl N-substituted benzomorphans. They have been shown to produce analgesia in rodents and, in general, to be devoid of morphine antagonistic properties. In mice, these compounds increase locomotor activity; some of the compounds increase loco-motor activity to a lesser degree than metazocine or morphine. In large doses, some decrease locomotor activity. Chronic administration of ethylketazocine induces tolerance to its loco-motor depressant actions without decreasing the response to morphine. In rhesus monkeys, ketazocine decreases food-reinforced operant behavior; tolerance develops to this effect without decreasing the response to morphine. These compounds also produce a variety of directly observable effects in the monkey that differentiate them from morphine. They do not suppress narcotic abstinence signs when given to morphine-dependent monkeys. When administered chronically, they show signs during withdrawal that are different from those seen in morphine withdrawal. Neither of the ketazocines nor the N-furyl benzomorphans are self-injected by rhesus monkeys at rates comparable to codeine. The results suggest that similar behavioral actions may be obtained from the two different benzomorphan structures, and that the mode of action for these drugs may be different from those of morphine-like drugs.

INTRODUCTION

Over the last two decades, there have been three types of approaches towards development of dependence-free analgesics. One of these involves attempts to find analgesics that provide clinically significant pain relief by a non-narcotic biological mechanism. Examples of com-pounds of current interest which stem from this approach are clonidine and baclofen. The two other approaches follow the lead produced by the serendipitous finding that nalorphine induces analgesia in man, while producing significant reversal of the effects of morphine-like drugs. The possibility of developing an analgesic with antagonist properties suddenly seemed attainable. A problem with nalorphine was that at analgesic doses it also produced dysphoria sufficient to negate its clinical usefulness. Therefore, the challenge of this approach was that of developing an analgesic free of disturbing side effects, while retaining antagonist activity. The compounds that have developed from this approach that have received significant scientific and clinical attention are pentazocine and, more recently, buprenorphine. The third approach disregards the capacity of a drug to produce morphine-type antagonism and centers on reducing or eliminating undesirable effects (*e.g.* dysphoria, morphine-type dependence, and potential for abuse) from narcotic agonist analgesics. Because the approach investigates variations of narcotic agonist actions, it is presumed that most, if not all of the effects of these drugs will be reversed by a narcotic antagonist.

Our paper deals with the last approach mentioned above, *i.e.*, studies of narcotic agonist analgesics that differ from morphine in a variety of pharmacologically significant manners. The compounds of special interest are ketazocine, ethylketazocine, and four N-furyl benzomorphans (see Figure 1). These compounds have in common the ability to displace etorphine[1] or dihydromorphine[2] from binding sites in rat brain homogenates. In addition, each of the compounds interacts with sodium as an agonist in binding experiments.[1] Each of the compounds is relatively more potent in suppressing the electrically induced contractions of the vas deferens of the mouse compared to the similarly treated ileum of the guinea pig[1]; a situation

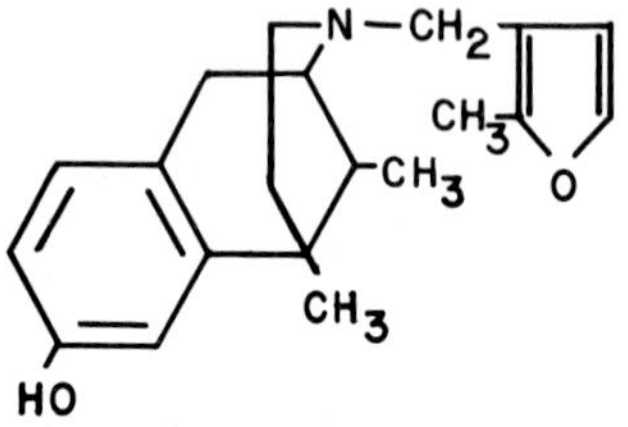

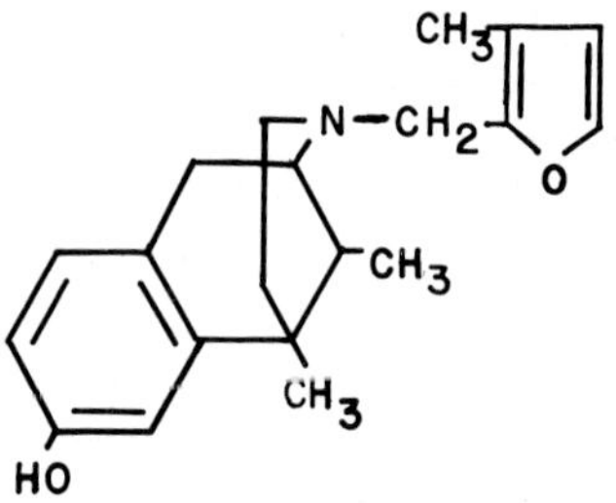

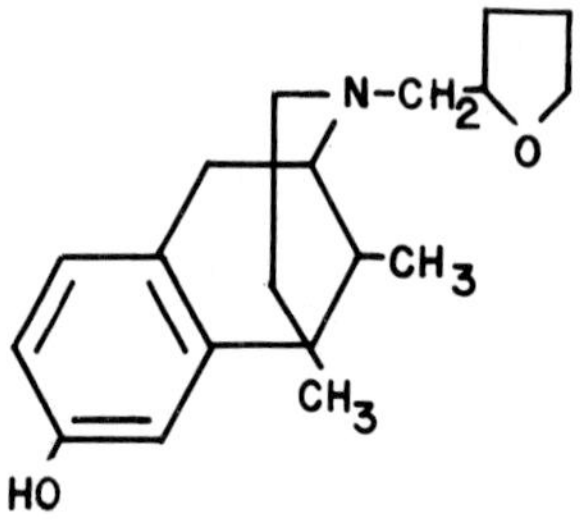

Fig. 1. The structural formulae of UM 909, 911, 1070, and 1072. UM 909 has also been labeled NIH 8735 and Mr 1268-MS: 2-(2-Methyl-3-furylmethyl)-2'-hydroxy-α-5,9 dimethyl-6,7-benzomorphan methanesulfonate. UM 911 has also been labeled NIH 8737 and Mr 1353-MS: 2-(3-Methylfurfuryl)-2'-hydroxy-α-5,9-dimethyl-6,7-benzomorphan methanesulfonate. UM 1070 has also been labeled MCV 4049, NIH 9100, Mr 2184-CL: (±)-(1R/S, 5R/S, 9S/R, 2" R/S)-5,9-Dimethyl-2'hydroxy-2-tetrahydrofurfuryl-6,7-benzomorphan hydrochloride. UM 1072 has also been labeled MCV 4051, NIH 9102, and Mr 2033-CL: (±)-(1R/S, 5R/S, 9R/S, 2" R/S)-5,9-Dimethyl-2'-hydroxy-2-tetrahydrofurfuryl-6,7-benzomorphan hydrochloride.

that, according to Lord *et al.*,[3] indicates action at a different set of receptors than morphine. The ketazocines have been studied also by Gilbert and Martin[4] in the chronic spinal dog, and their effects have been characterized as producing a spectrum of responses that differ significantly from morphine in both acute and chronic administration studies. We shall focus on the behavioral differentiation of a set of these drugs in mice and monkeys in situations where we have assessed the character of their acute actions, the patterns they provide in evaluation of tolerance and dependence, and their capacity as reinforcers of self-injection behavior.

ACUTE BEHAVIORAL EFFECTS

Observations in monkeys

The ketazocines and N-furyl benzomorphans have a number of directly observable behavioral effects in rhesus monkeys. They produced a dose-related motor incoordination which has components of both muscle weakness and ataxia. General activity seemed to be reduced, and there was a tendency for the monkeys to doze. When the monkeys were handled, a reduction in abdominal tone could be felt. There was a marked mydriasis; respiration rate appeared unchanged. There were no major differences among the drugs in their ability to produce these effects. The drugs may be arranged in order of potency in producing these effects in the following way: UM 1072 > UM 1070 > ethylketazocine ≥ ketazocine > UM 911 > UM 909. Although there were no quantitative measures or dose-effect determinations made, these direct effects appeared to be partially and transiently reversed by naloxone.

Locomotor activity in mice and correlated effects *in vivo* and *in vitro*

As described below, these six compounds produced an increase in mouse locomotor activity. In doses above those necessary to produce the maximal locomotor stimulation, mice showed ataxia and incoordination. In the case of ethylketazocine, periods of virtually complete immobility were observed at these doses; hyperventilation and splayed hind limbs accompanied this immobility. At no dose did any of the compounds produce the erect "Straub" tail that is pathognomonic of morphine administration in the mouse.

Morphine administration to mice also causes an increase in locomotor activity. Since the purpose of these investigations was to find behavioral techniques that differentiate test drugs from morphine, it was hoped that the compounds under investigation, that were known to be different from morphine in their acute effects, would produce less locomotor stimulation than morphine. Swiss Webster mice were studied in circular photocell chambers in which the number of interruptions of perpendicular photobeams was taken as a measure of locomotor activity over a 1-hr assessment. As can be seen in Figure 2 each of the compounds increased locomotor activity relative to controls.[5] The compounds differed in both their efficacy and their potency in increasing locomotor activity. Clearly , the hope that the locomotor stimulant properties of these drugs would differentiate them from morphine was not supported by the data. It may be possible, however, to differentially antagonize equivalent locomotor acitivity changes with

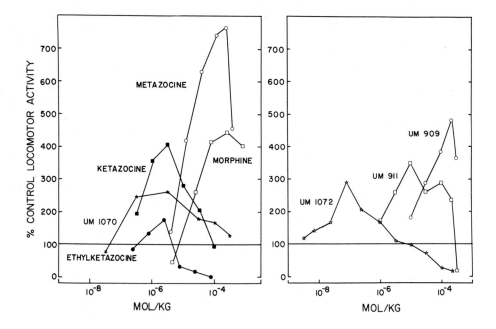

Fig. 2. Locomotor activity increasing effects of morphine, metazocine, the ketazocines, and four N-furyl benzomorphans. Counts/hr in control mice given saline varied from 300 to 500 in all groups except the ethylketazocine control group which was 1250.

various narcotic antagonists, thus revealing differences in mechanisms between morphine and these drugs. Holtzman,[6] for example, has found that in the rat, the increased locomotor activity produced by cyclazocine is more resistant to antagonism by naloxone than that of morphine.

The rank order potencies for a variety of effects of these drugs is shown in Table 1. In order to have a comparison to locomotor activity, we have ranked the compounds according to the lowest dose that produced a 50% or greater increase in locomotor activity. The rankings show considerable agreement, and the possible correlations between the various *in vitro* and *in vivo* behavioral effects is strong and suggestive of common properties. Despite the small number of ranks, all the possible correlations were significant statistically except for the correlation between analgesia and locomotor activity and the correlation of analgesia with etorphine binding.

CHRONIC EFFECTS

Tolerance studies in mice and monkeys

If these drugs operate through different pharmacological mechanisms, it may be possible to produce specific tolerance to their effects that will not generalize to morphine-like compounds.

TABLE 1

RANK ORDER POTENCIES OF SEVERAL NARCOTICS ON VARIOUS MEASURES OF ACTIVITY

	Etorphine Binding (-Na)[a]	Mouse Vas Deferens[b]	Mouse Analgesia[c]	Mouse Loco. Activity
UM 1070	2	1	1	2
UM 1072	1	3	2	1
EKC	3	2	3	5
Ketazocine	5	4[d]	4	3
UM 911	4	5	7	4
Morphine	6	6	5	7
UM 909	7	7	6	6

[a]From Woods et al.[1]
[b]From Smith (this volume)
[c]From Arthur Jacobson, personal communication
[d]Potency estimate from Lord et al.[3]

Tepper and Woods[5] administered ethylketazocine chronically to Swiss-Webster mice over a three day period. On the first day, 10 mg/kg was given every eight hours and on the second and third days, 32 mg/kg was given; on the fourth day, a series of doses was given in lieu of the maintenance dose and locomotor activity change was evaluated relative to a naive control group. There was a 6-10 fold loss in sensitivity to the drug; periods of immobility were shortened and ataxia was less severe in the chronically treated mice. These ethylketazocine-tolerant mice, however, continued to show a significant increase in running following either morphine or cocaine administration, demonstrating a lack of cross tolerance between ethylketazocine and morphine (Fig. 3).

Llewellyn[7] has extended the observations described above to situations involving food-reinforced operant behavior in rhesus monkeys. The experiment involved acute administration of morphine, ketazocine and cyclazocine in a series of doses. Following these determinations chronic administration of ketazocine was undertaken over a three month period. Ketazocine in a dose of 0.1 mg/kg was given three times daily for four weeks and then in a dose of 0.2 mg/kg, five times daily for the next eight weeks. A 3 to 10 fold decrease in potency of both ketazocine and cyclazocine was observed in the monkeys given chronic ketazocine. However, no consistent change in the potency of morphine was observed in these monkeys. Thus, the observation of a lack of cross-tolerance between morphine and ethylketazocine in the mice is supported by a similar lack of cross-tolerance between morphine and ketazocine in the monkey.

Dependence studies in mice and monkeys

In the non-withdrawn, morphine dependent monkey, neither the ketazocines nor the N-furyl benzomorphans elicited withdrawal signs. Indeed, the major effect in these monkeys was

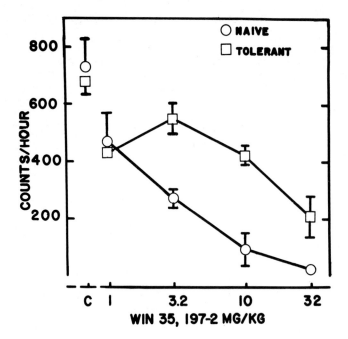

Fig. 3. Locomotor activity changes for 1 hr. immediately after the intraperitoneal administration of ethylketazocine (WIN 35, 197-2) to mice. Open circles: acute administration. Open squares: chronic administration of 10 to 32 mg/kg. Points at C on abscissa: vehicle controls for two drug conditions. Data points: average of 5 observations. Brackets: ± 1 S.E. [From (5)].

production of the direct effects mentioned earlier. In morphine-withdrawn, dependent monkeys, it was again the direct effects of these drugs that were most readily observed. The abdominal rigidity, the increased respiration rate, the increased irritability and the diarrhea produced by morphine withdrawal were not altered by administration of any of these drugs.

Two of these compounds—UM 1070 and UM 1072—have been studied in chronic administration paradigms for development of dependence. The initial dose was 0.05 mg/kg given subcutaneously at 6 hr intervals. This dose was increased over one month to 1.6 mg/kg in the case of UM 1070 and to 3.2 mg/kg in the case of UM 1072. The acute effects of administration were the same as noted earlier: dozing, muscle weakness, ataxia, pupil dilation, decreased activity and occasionally, retching and vomiting. These signs became less severe as a given dose was continued, allowing steady increments in dose every 4-5 days. The acute signs reappeared however, with each increment in dose. When administration of the drugs was abruptly discontinued, there was a gradual development of abstinence signs which peaked in the third day. During withdrawal, prominent signs were an increased irritability on handling, piloerection, and a tendency for the monkeys to hold their abdomens. These are also signs observed when morphine administration is abruptly discontinued. There was, however, no abdominal tenderness on handling, as is characteristic of morphine abstinence. Additionally, there was a complex response involving retching and yawning that was seen with both drugs, but is not seen with morphine withdrawal. Also, particularly with UM 1072, there was the assumption of peculiar postures and mannerisms including tongue rolling, licking, lip smacking, and grimacing, that are not seen with morphine withdrawal. These withdrawal signs were elicited as well by administration of naloxone or nalorphine.

In the study of chronic ketazocine administration described earlier, Llewellyn[7] found no evidence of a precipitated abstinence following naloxone administration in monkeys made tolerant to ketazocine. Neither was there evidence of withdrawal when ketazocine administration was abruptly discontinued. This lack of ketazocine dependence may be due to the short duration of action of this drug.

In the study of chronic ethylketazocine administration to mice discussed earlier, administration of naloxone to ethylketazocine-tolerant mice resulted in a jumping response.[5] This response, which is also found when naloxone is given to mice following chronic morphine administration, has been taken by many as one sign of physical dependence in rodents.

DRUG SELF-INJECTION STUDIES

It was possible that the ketazocines and N-furyl benzomorphans may be differentiated from morphine-type narcotics on the basis of their differences in capacity to maintain self-injection responding. In order to assess this behavioral property, we conditioned rhesus monkeys to self-inject codeine intravenously. After conditioning, and when stable performances were maintained on the final schedule of drug delivery, saline was occasionally substituted for codeine. The response rate maintained by saline was much lower than that maintained by codeine. When rates of responding were reliably different between these reinforcement conditions, another drug was introduced. It was studied at a variety of doses until a complete relationship had been obtained between dose and rate of drug-reinforced responding. The essential details of the procedure are described elsewhere.[8] When narcotic agonists from a variety of chemical families were substituted for codeine, each drug maintained rates of reinforced responding equivalent to or slightly lower than codeine. Some drugs such as nalbuphine and profadol, that have morphine-like effects but are also antagonists under some pharmacological conditions, also maintained significantly higher rates of responding than saline. Under these conditions, however, nalorphine, cyclazocine, ketazocine, and ethylketazocine were not self-injected at rates above those maintained by saline.[1] These findings led to the expectation that the N-furyl benzomorphans would not be self-injected at rates comparable to codeine. It can be seen in Figure 4 that this generalization holds. However, both UM 909 and UM 911 supported drug self-injection rates that were significantly greater than saline. UM 909 and UM 911 have large sodium response ratios in binding assays, and are relatively stronger locomotor stimulants in mice than UM 1070 and UM 1072. Otherwise, they appear, at present, indistinguishable from UM 1070 and UM 1072.

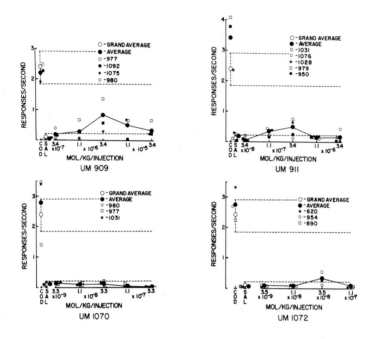

Fig. 4. The rates of fixed-ratio responding maintained by codeine, saline, and various doses of UM 909, 911, 1070, and 1072 (Fig. 1 for structural formulae). Duplicate observations on codeine (7.5 x 10^{-5} mol/kg/injection; 0.32 mg/kg/injection) and saline were obtained in each monkey. A saline substitution was conducted before and after the series of observations on one of the drugs; the rates of codeine-reinforced responding were obtained by randomly sampling two sessions of those between the drug substitution sessions. These data are represented in the graph with individual symbols for each of the monkeys at the points COD (codeine) and SAL (saline). In addition, using the same symbols, the mean of duplicate observations is given for the various doses of the different drugs studied in each monkey. There are two types of additional averaged data. The large closed circles indicate the averaged data for observations on the subset of monkeys used to study each drug. The large open circles indicate the codeine and saline rate of responding of 20 monkeys studied under the same conditions. The brackets indicate ± 3 standard errors of the mean.

DISCUSSION

The ketazocines and N-furyl benzomorphans described here have in common analgesic activity and the other effects noted in Table 1. They are, at present, most cleanly differentiated behaviorally from morphine-like drugs in the following ways: 1) the ketazocines induce tolerance that shows no cross-tolerance to morphine; 2) the drugs do not suppress morphine abstinence in the monkey; 3) the drugs induce a state of dependence that shows some signs of withdrawal not observed during morphine withdrawal; and 4) none of these drugs maintains rates of drug self-injection comparable to morphine-like agents. These drugs may induce a dysphoria similar to that of nalorphine. No direct investigation of this possibility has yet been made in animals, although some relevant experiments are planned.

It is premature to speculate about other properties that these drugs may have in common. Nevertheless, two obvious characteristics may be cross-tolerance among themselves, and, compared to morphine-like agents, greater resistance to antagonism by naloxone. The latter property holds in other experimental situations (e.g. Kosterlitz et al.[9]).

ACKNOWLEDGMENTS

Research was supported by Grants DA00154 and DA00254. Each of the following individuals contributed greatly to the research effort reported here. Some of the locomotor activity data were collected by M. A. Nemeth and E. Patterson; F. Adams and R. Storm made the observations on dependent monkeys; W. Pound collected the data on drug self-injection; the manuscript was prepared by I. Herling with careful help of G. Winger and S. Herling. We greatly appreciate the efforts of each and all.

REFERENCES

1. Woods, J. H., Smith, C. B., Medzihradsky, F., and Swain, H. H. (In press) in Mechanisms of Pain and Analgesic Drugs J. E. Villarreal, et al. eds., Raven Press, New York.
2. Hutchinson, M., Kosterlitz, H. W., Leslie, F. M., and Waterfield, A. A. (1975) Brit. J. Pharmacol. 55, 541-546.
3. Lord, J. A. H., Waterfield, A. A., Hughes, J. and Kosterlitz, H. W. (1977) Nature, 267, 495-499.
4. Gilbert, P. E. and Martin, W. R. (1976) J. Pharmacol. Exp. Therap. 198, 66-82.
5. Tepper, P. and Woods, J. H. (In press) Psychopharmacology.
6. Holtzman, S. G. (1973) in Narcotic Antagonists M. C. Braude et al. eds., Raven Press, New York, pp. 371-382. Adv. in Biochem. Psychopharmacol., Vol. 8.
7. Llewellyn, M. E. (1978) Fed. Proc. 37, 310.
8. Woods, J. H. (Submitted for publication).
9. Kosterlitz, H. W., Waterfield, A. A. and Berthould, V. (1973) in Narcotic Antagonists M. C. Braude et al. eds., Raven Press, New York, pp. 319-334. Adv. in Biochem. Psychopharmacol., Vol. 8.

β-ENDORPHIN- AND OPIATE-INDUCED IMMOBILITY: BEHAVIORAL CHARACTERIZATION AND
TOLERANCE DEVELOPMENT

RONALD G. BROWNE AND DAVID S. SEGAL
Department of Psychiatry, School of Medicine, University of California, San
Diego, La Jolla, California   92093 (U.S.A.)

ABSTRACT

Intraventricular administration of β-endorphin, enkephalin analogs, and
opiates results in an immobility syndrome in rats which could also be produced
by injection into the ventromedial periaqueductal gray (PAG). After long-term
pretreatment with opiates, β-endorphin produced less immobility and correspondingly greater locomotor activity.

INTRODUCTION

β-Endorphin administered intraventricularly in rats produces a profound
state of immobilization characterized by the absence of movement, loss of
righting response, and extreme generalized muscular rigidity[1,2]. Opiates
also induce a state of immobility[2-4] which is followed by a prolonged period
of hyperactivity. A similar biphasic pattern results from intraventricular
administration of β-endorphin and enkephalin analogs. With repeated administration of the opiates the behavioral depression progressively subsides
and the onset of the hyperactivity phase is correspondingly decreased. Continued treatment results in the appearance of hyperactivity shortly after
injection[5]. The present studies were designed to examine the effects of
chronic opiate pretreatment on the behavioral response to β-endorphin.

RESULTS

Within 15-30 minutes after intraventricular injection, male Wistar rats
(300-325 g) responded to doses of β-endorphin greater than 2.5 µg with generalized muscular rigidity accompanied by stiffness of the tail and loss of
the righting response. The rigid immobility syndrome was also produced by
synthetic human β-endorphin and by the enkephalin analogs, $D-Met^2-Pro^5$-
enkephalinamide ($D-Met^2-Pro^5 \cdot NH_2$) and $D-Ala^2-Met^5$-enkephalinamide ($D-Ala^2$-
$Met^5 \cdot NH_2$) as well as by subcutaneous administration of the opiates, morphine
(5-20 mg/kg), methadone (2.5-10 mg/kg), or etonitazene (1-10 µg). Intraventricular administration of morphine (25-100 µg) or etonitazene (1-10 µg)

resulted in behavioral effects comparable to those induced by their systemic injection.

Rats were also treated for 9 days with either saline or escalating doses of morphine (initially, 10 mg/kg, b.i.d. with subsequent 5 mg/kg/day increments) and 12 hours after the last injection (50 mg/kg), were administered either 15 mg/kg of morphine or 5 μg of β-endorphin. Saline pretreated rats responded to morphine and β-endorphin with a relatively prolonged decrease in activity; whereas, the morphine pretreated group exhibited enhanced locomotion shortly after injection.

SUMMARY

Opiates and β-endorphin produce a state of immobility which is accompanied by muscular rigidity. Pretreatment with escalating doses of morphine resulted in tolerance to opiate- and β-endorphin-induced immobility and hyperactivity. The resemblance between the behavioral profile produced by the opiates and β-endorphin suggests that their effects may be mediated through common mechanisms.

ACKNOWLEDGEMENTS

This research was supported in part by U.S.P.H.S. (N.I.D.A.) Research Grant DA-01994-01; D.S.S. is the recipient of U.S.P.H.S. (N.I.M.H.) Research Scientist Award MH-701893-05; R.G.B. was supported by a postdoctoral fellowship provided by U.S.P.H.S. Training Grant AA-07129-02.

REFERENCES

1. Bloom, F., Segal, D.S., Ling, N. and Guillemin, R. (1976) Science, 194, 630-632.

2. Segal, D.S., Browne, R.G., Bloom, F., Ling, N. and Guillemin, R. (1977) Science, 198, 411-414.

3. Browne, R.G., Derrington, D.C. and Segal, D.S. (1978), manuscript in preparation.

4. Barnett, A., Goldstein, J., Fiedler, E. and Taber, R. (1975) Eur. J. Pharmacol., 30, 23-30.

5. Domino, E.F., Vasko, M.R. and Wilson, A.E. (1976) in Tissue Responses to Addictive Drugs, Ford, D.H. and Clouet, D.H. eds., New York, Spectrum, pp. 143-167.

ANTINOCICEPTIVE ACTIVITIES OF BUPRENORPHINE, MORPHINE AND TILIDINE INJECTED
INTO THE MEDIAL RAPHE NUCLEUS OF THE CONSCIOUS RAT

R. M. BRYANT[*], J. E. OLLEY[*], M. B. TYERS[†] and A. S. MARRIOTT[†]

[*] School of studies in Pharmacology, University of Bradford, West Yorkshire,
England, [†]Pharmacology Department, Glaxo-Allenbury's Research (Ware), Ware,
Herts, England, This work was supported by an SRC CASE Award with Allen and
Hanbury's Ltd

INTRODUCTION

   Lesion[1] and electrophysiological[2] studies have indicated that the medial
raphe nucleus may be involved in the antinociceptive actions of morphine. In
the present study the antinociceptive and behavioural actions of buprenorphine,
morphine and tilidine, which may have different mechanisms of analgesic action,
were compared.

MATERIALS AND METHODS

   Sprague Dawley CFE male rats (200-350 g) were used throughout. Antinociceptive activity was measured using the hot plate, $55\pm2^{o}C$, (HP) and the paw
pressure (PP) tests, with cut off points at 60s and 500g, respectively.
Behavioural effects were assessed using a modified Irwin[3] procedure. Antinociceptive and behavioural properties of the analgesics were determined after
subcutaneous injection and after micro-injection (1 µl), via indwelling
cannulae, into the medial raphe nucleus. Antagonism studies using naloxone
pretreatment (1 mg/kg ip) served to indicate the nature of the activity
involved. Central injection sites were identified postmortem with the aid of a
stereotaxic atlas[4].

RESULTS

   The antinociceptive activity of the analgesics is presented, Figs 1-4. The
behavioural effects after s.c. injection at the time of peak antinociceptive
activity (30 m) were not considered significant enough to alter the capacity to
respond. However, the reduction in reflex and spontaneous activity, and
increase in muscle tone seen after m. raphe inj. may have influenced the maximum
response to noxious stimuli at 10 m although these were more marked later. The
vehicle control for m. raphe. inj. induced minimal effects persisting <2 m.
Naloxone was found to prevent all the antinociceptive effects except those of
tilidine in the paw pressure test. Histology revealed accurate placement of
cannulae tips with minimal damage to overlying structures.

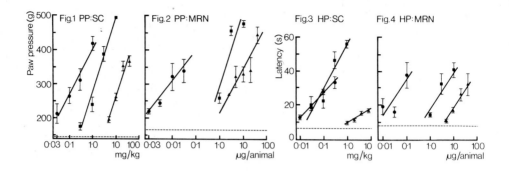

Figures 1-4 Antinociceptive activity in the paw pressure (PP) and hot plate (HP) tests after subcutaneous (SC) and medial raphe nucleus (MRN) injection of Buprenorphine ● ; morphine ■ ; and tilidine ▲ N = 18 SC; N = 5 MRN.
-------- basal levels

DISCUSSION

Parallel dose response lines are seen in Fig 4 only, therefore relative potency values are inappropriate. Comparison of the antinociceptive activity after s.c. inj. demonstrates the typical profiles of the analgesics, the slight changes in normal behaviour having no significant effect. The behavioural effects after m. raphe inj. probably contribute to the apparent antinociceptive activity. Differing extents of metabolism could be involved in the increased potency of buprenorphine relative to morphine after central injection. The The relative central activity of tilidine, Fig 4 indicates that the parent compound has opiate-like activity and that peripheral metabolism reduces this considerably, Fig 2. Naloxone confirmed the opiate-like activity of the drugs but tilidine also appears to have non-opiate activity demonstrated by its effectiveness after naloxone pretreatment, Fig 2, this property presumably being shared by its metabolite, Fig 1. These findings suggest that the m. raphe nucleus possesses both opiate and non-opiate receptor sites which may be involved in the activity of analgesic drugs.

REFERENCES

1. Adler, M. et al., (1975), Eur. J. Pharmac., 32, 39-44.

2. Oleson, T. D. et al., (1978), Pain, 4, 211-230.

3. Irwin, S. (1968), Psychopharmacologia (Berl.)., 13, 222-257.

4. Pellegrino, L. J. and Cushman, A. J., (1967), A stereotaxic atlas of the rat brain, Elliott, R. M. et al., eds.; Meredith, New York.

Characteristics and Function of Opioids, editors Van Ree and Terenius
© 1978 Elsevier/North-Holland Biomedical Press

NALOXONE REVERSIBLE ANALGESIA PRODUCED BY D-PHENYLALANINE IN MICE

S. EHRENPREIS, J. E. COMATY AND S. B. MYLES

Department of Pharmacology, The Chicago Medical School, 2020 W. Ogden Avenue, Chicago, IL 60612 (U.S.A.)

ABSTRACT

D-phenylalanine, an inhibitor of carboxypeptidase A, produces naloxone-reversible analgesia as tested by the hot-plate method. Analgesia is potentiated by indomethacin and other prostaglandin synthetase inhibotors. Tolerance to analgesia by D-phenylalanine does not develop and naloxone-induced withdrawal symptoms are not observed upon chronic administration of the amino acid.

INTRODUCTION

Two factors limit the usefulness of enkephalins as possible substitutes for the opiates as longterm analgesics in man. First, analgesia by the enkephalins is of short duration, attributable to rapid degradation mainly by carboxypeptidase A and leucine aminopeptidase[1]. Second, repeated administration of enkephalins has resulted in tolerance to the analgesic action as well as dependence, as demonstrated by naloxone-induced withdrawal symptoms[2]. In an attempt to obviate these problems, we have used a new approach, namely, to prolong and intensify the effects of endogenously produced enkephalins or other endorphins by inhibiting the metabolizing enzymes. Two inhibitors of carboxypeptidase A are D-phenylalanine (DPA) and hydrocinnamic acid[3]. Although these are weak inhibitors and probably have difficulty crossing the blood-brain barrier, we have succeeded in demonstrating that these compounds can produce naloxone-reversible analgesia in mice.

MATERIALS AND METHODS

Analgesia was determined by the hot-plate method (55° C $\pm$ 0.5° C) using mice weighing 25-30 g. DPA (Sigma or Aldrich) and hydrocinnamic acid (Aldrich) were dissolved in distilled water or Tyrode's solution and injected i.p. After testing at regular intervals for 2-3 hours, mice showing analgesia were administered naloxone, 0.5-20 mg/kg, and testing was continued for an additional 30 minutes. In another series of experiments, indomethacin, 10 mg/kg, was injected prior to the DPA. This dose produced only minimal increase in latency to jump.

For chronic experiments, DPA was administered at a dose of 250 mg/kg twice daily for 9 days. Analgesia was determined at the beginning and after the 9 days, and naloxone, 20 mg/kg, was administered on the 9th day.

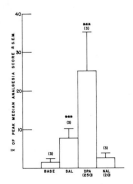

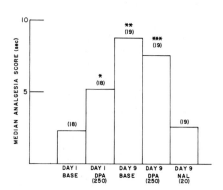

Fig. 1 Naloxone-reversible analgesia by DPA. Sal is saline control.

Fig. 2 Analgesia from chronic administration of DPA. *, p < 0.008, DPA day 1 vs.
base. **, p < 0.002, analgesia on day 9
vs. control (base) day 1. ***, p < 0.002,
DPA day 9 vs. control, day 1.

RESULTS

Fig. 1 shows that DPA, 250 mg/kg, causes significant analgesia and that this effect is abolished by naloxone, 20 mg/kg. 2 mg/kg naloxone also produces reversal. Similar results were obtained with hydrocinnamic acid.

Indomethacin, 10 mg/kg plus DPA, 125 mg/kg, gave analgesia which was significantly greater than that by each agent alone (p < 0.05). This analgesia, as well as that by other synthetase inhibitors, was reversed by naloxone.

Prolonged administration of large doses of DPA does not result in tolerance development to the analgesic action (Fig. 2). DPA analgesia after 9 days was even greater than that of the first day. Furthermore, naloxone produced no withdrawal symptoms on day 9.

ACKNOWLEDGEMENTS

This work was supported in part by a grant from Hoffman - La Roche.

REFERENCES

1. Hughes, J. (1975). Brain Res., 88, 295-306.

2. Wei, E., and Loh, H. (1976). Science, 193, 1262-1263.

3. Delange, R. J., and Smith, E. L. (1971) in The Enzymes, Boyer, P. D., ed., Academic Press, New York, pp. 81-118.

Characteristics and Function of Opioids, editors Van Ree and Terenius
© 1978 Elsevier/North-Holland Biomedical Press

BEHAVIORAL AND ELECTROPHYSIOLOGICAL EFFECTS OF ENDORPHINS AND ENKEPHALINS

F. R. ERVIN, R. M. PALMOUR, C. GUZMAN FLORES, J.-K. CHANG AND B. FONG

NPI, UCLA, Los Angeles (USA); Genetics, U. California, Berkeley (USA); Instituto
Biomedicas, U. Mexico (Mexico); Peninsula Laboratories, San Carlos (USA)

The behavioral effects of opioid peptides in experimental animals have stimulated intense interest in the role of endorphin in normal and abnormal behavior,
but few studies of the underlying brain physiology of these effects have been
pursued. Leibeskind and colleagues[1,2] have described cortical seizures and dramatic behavioral alterations following intraventricular (IVT) morphine or enkephalin, while Henriksen et al.[3] report limbic and hippocampal ictal spiking
episodes precipitated by D-ala^2-met enkephalinamide (DAME) or β-endorphin. We
report here the behavioral and electrophysiological effects of IVT DAME, D-ala^2-
leu enkephalinamide (DALE), met^5-β-endorphin (ME) and synthetic and isolated
leu^5-β-endorphin (LE) in the cat.

MATERIALS AND METHODS

Peptides were synthesized by solid state methods as described before[4,5] and
purified chromatographically. LE was isolated from human hemodialysate as previously described[5,6] in yields of 12.5-25 µg/L of fluid.

Cats were prepared with IVT cannula guides and semi-micro recording electrodes in the frontal cortex, reticular formation (RF), amygdala (Am) and hippocampal formation (HC). Baseline behavioral and EEG recordings (Grass polygraph)
were taken 1 week after surgery, before and after saline and peptide control
injections (10 µl in saline, 5 µl/15 sec). Doses of 100, 200 and 400 µg DAME
and DALE and 12.5, 25, 50 and 100 µg ME and LE were given in saline adjusted to
pH 6. Gross changes in behavior and autonomic function were recorded throughout.

RESULTS

The opioid peptides studied have behavioral effects which are similar to
those observed following morphine administration. The earliest effect (1-4 min)
is a tremorous shake, followed by hyperventilation, urination or defecation,
mydriasis and alert immobility. At 4-6 min, cats typically become restless,
lick or sniff, prowl the recording chamber, then begin periods of fixed, staring
immobility punctuated by repetitive grooming, persistent miaowing, motor stereotypies, crouching, backing and occasional violent attacks on the chamber.

The earliest EEG changes typically begin about 5 min (range 2-17) post injec-

420

tion. Cortical and limbic hypersynchronous bursts follow the first restless period and subsequent periodic paroxysms (3-4/30 sec) of high amplitude spiking activity in RF, Am and HC accompany staring immobility; behavioral and electrophysiological changes may be interrupted by sound or light. Alternating per- of motor activity are marked by a relatively normal EEG (Figure 1). Backing and staring behavior characteristically occurs with very high amplitude spiking (3/sec) and is frequently preceded by the buildup of HC slow waves. Myoclonic twitches often accompany EEG seizures. The duration of effect was dose dependent with ME and LE; at doses of 50 or 100 µg, some changes persisted >24 hr. Although naloxone generally suppressed EEG changes, it did not obliterate them; frequently a frenetic outburst of EEG and behavioral activity occurred 15-20 min post naloxone. DAME produced only moderate changes.

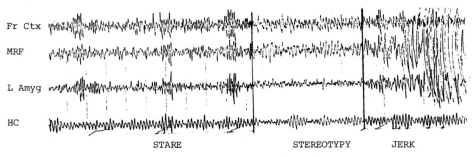

Fr Ctx

MRF

L Amyg

HC

STARE   STEREOTYPY   JERK

FIGURE 1. ELECTROPHYSIOLOGICAL EFFECTS OF IVT LEU^{5}ENDORPHIN (30 NMOLES)

These studies, in accord with those of other investigators[1,2,3] suggest that ME, LE and DALE may elicit long-lasting limbic seizures at doses which do not elicit profound behavioral or analgetic effects, and that seizure activity may underlie the fixed immobility ("catalepsy") observed by many. Whether these substances are psychotogens, euphoriants, hallucinogens or epileptogens will remain a topic of considerable speculation.

REFERENCES

1. Urca, G. et al. (1977) Science, 197, 83-86.
2. Frenk, H. et al. (1978) Science 200, 335-338.
3. Henriksen, S. J. et al. (1976) Neurosci. Soc., A 933.
4. Chang, J.-K. et al. (1976) Life Sci. 18, 1473-1482.
5. Palmour, R. et al. (1978) Intl. J. Prot. Pept. Res., in press.
6. Palmour, R. et al. (1978) in Endorphins in Mental Health Research, Usdin, E., ed., Macmillan Press.

Characteristics and Function of Opioids, editors Van Ree and Terenius
© *1978 Elsevier/North-Holland Biomedical Press*

INTRAVENOUS (IV) AND INTRAVENTRICULAR (IVT) ADMINISTRATION OF BETA ENDORPHIN (β_h-EP) IN MAN: SAFETY AND DISPOSITION.

K.M. FOLEY, C.E. INTURRISI, I.A. KOURIDES, R.F. KAIKO, J.B. POSNER, R.W. HOUDE
AND CHO HAO LI[*]

Memorial Sloan-Kettering Cancer Center, New York City (USA), and [*]Hormone
Research Laboratory, University of California, San Francisco, California (USA)

ABSTRACT

The disposition and certain pharmacologic effects of β_h-EP were evaluated in
3 cancer patients with pain after IV or IVT administration. No significant alteration in pain, mood, pupil size or vital signs was noted following doses up
to 10 mg IV in nontolerant patients. In a tolerant patient, 7.5 mg IVT produced
analgesia and drowsiness. Plasma prolactin levels increased following IV and
IVT administration of β_h-EP. The terminal plasma half-life ($t\frac{1}{2}$) of IV β_h-EP
ranged from 13 to 22 minutes with the apparent volume of distribution only one-
tenth that of morphine.

INTRODUCTION

Behavioral, hormonal and analgesic effects of β_h-EP[1,2] have been reported in
laboratory animals following IV and IVT administration. This study evaluates
the effects of both IV and IVT β_h-EP administered to cancer patients with pain.

MATERIALS AND METHODS

IV doses of 1, 5 or 10 mg of β_h-EP were administered single-blind to one male
and one female patient not tolerant to narcotics and compared to the effects of
a 10 mg IV dose of morphine sulfate. IVT doses from 100 ug to 7.5 mg were administered single-blind via an Ommaya reservoir to a male patient with meningeal
carcinomatosis chronically receiving narcotics. β_h-EP in plasma and CSF was determined using an homologous radioimmunoassay (RIA) developed in our laboratory.
Plasma morphine, prolactin (PRL), growth hormone (GH), and thyroid stimulating
hormone (TSH) were determined using previously reported RIAS[3,4].

RESULTS

In contrast to the response produced by a 10 mg dose of morphine, no significant change in pain, mood, pupil size or vital signs were noted following IV
doses of 1,5 or 10 mg of β_h-EP. Plasma PRL levels increased 3-fold without a
change in TSH or GH levels. The time course of plasma disappearance of 10 mg
IV β_h-EP and morphine are given in Figure 1. The $t\frac{1}{2}$ was 138 minutes for morphine

422

Fig. 1. Plasma β_h-EP (•————•) and morphine (o————o)
levels following IV administration of 10 mg of β_h-EP
and 3 days later 10 mg of morphine sulfate to the same
patient.

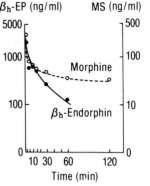

and 22 minutes for β_h-EP (after 5 mg IV, the t½ of
β_h-EP was 13 minutes). The apparent volume of distribution of β_h-EP was estimated to be one-tenth that
of morphine.

Following the 7.5 mg dose of β_h-EP, significant
changes in pain, mood and pupil size occurred and were
maximal at 2.5 hours. Marked drowsiness and mild con-
fusion lasted for 21 hours. The patient reported mild pain but required no narcotic analgesics. Scalp EEG recordings during this time revealed no evidence of
seizure activity. In this patient, β_h-EP could be measured in CSF for at least
21 hours while concurrent plasma samples demonstrated no detectable levels of
β_h-EP. Plasma PRL levels rose seven-fold following IVT β_h-EP administration
without a change in plasma GH or TSH.

SUMMARY

These studies suggest that large IV doses of β_h-EP may be necessary to produce analgesia in nontolerant patients. This may be related to the limited distribution from plasma of β_h-EP compared to morphine. The IVT administration of
7.5 mg to a tolerant patient produced significant analgesia and drowsiness lasting 21 hours without evidence of seizure activity. The IV to IVT potency ratio
cannot be determined from this study. The β_h-EP induced increase in plasma PRL
may precede the onset of analgesia and may be independent of the analgesic
effects.

ACKNOWLEDGEMENTS

This work was supported in part by NIDA Grant DA-01707, USPHS Grant CA-23185
and NIMH Grant MH-30245.

REFERENCES

1. Costa, E. and Trabucchi, M., eds. (1978) The Endorphins: Advances in
   Biochemical Psychopharmacology, Vol. 18, Raven Press, New York.

2. Rivier, C. et al. (1977) Endocrinology, 100, 238-241.

3. Spector, S. (1971) J. Pharmacol. Exp. Ther., 178, 253-258.

4. Kourides, I.A. et al. (1976) J. Clin. Endocrinol. & Metab. 43, 97-106.

Characteristics and Function of Opioids, editors Van Ree and Terenius
© *1978 Elsevier/North-Holland Biomedical Press*

BEHAVIORAL AND EEG RESPONSES TO β-ENDORPHIN INTRACEREBROVENTRICULARLY IN RATS.

V. Havlicek[+], F. LaBella[*], C. Pinsky[*], R. Childiaeva[+] and H. Friesen. Department of Physiology[+] and Department of Pharmacology[*] and Therapeutics, University of Manitoba, Faculty of Medicine, Winnipeg, Manitoba, Canada.

INTRODUCTION

An understanding of the role of brain peptides in CNS functions have derived from central administration of their synthetic forms. Whereas certain peptides promote integrated behaviors such as drinking[1] or mating[2], others, e.g. endogenous opioids tend to foster disorganization, inducing, at lower doses, withdrawal syndrome, and at higher doses, seizures[3,4] or akinesia (described as a catatonic-like[5] state). This report describes three behavioral syndromes induced by ICV administration of BE: a) insomnia; b) epileptic-like state and c) akinesia progressing to general anesthesia.

MATERIALS AND METHODS

Spraque-Dawley male rats (cca 250 g body weight) were implanted with platinum epidural electrodes in sensory-motor cortex and intracerebroventricular (ICV) cannula. Camel BE (Peninsula Labs. Inc.) was dissolved in sterile solution and injected in the volume 10 μl over 11 min. Controls were injected with vehicle. Animals were placed in a sound-proof and electrically shielded chamber (20x21x35 cm) having a grid floor. Our techniques for EEG recording of the sleep-waking cycle in rats[6] and the fast Fourier transform of the EEG[7] have been described elsewhere.

RESULTS AND DISCUSSION

a) <u>Insomnia</u> was observed with as little as 0.1 μg of BE (Table 1).

TABLE 1

GROOMING AND SLEEP AFTER 0.1 μg BE (IN MINUTES OVER 2 HRS POSTINFUSION)

Treatment	n	Grooming	Awake	Slow-wave sleep	Paradoxical sleep
Saline	6	3.5 ± 1.1	62.8 ± 12.2	47.9 ± 9.1	9.3 ± 3.2
BE	6	10.2[*] + 1.6	95.2[*] + 1.3	5.8[*] ± 1.5	0

[*] $p \leq 0.05$; ± S.E.

During the wakeful state BE treated animals showed normal desychronized or activated EEG. Increased grooming (Table 1) described by other authors[8], can be attributed to absence of sleep, since nonhabituated controls which remained awake most of the time also showed increased grooming (14.1 ± 1.5 min/2 hrs).

b) Effect of BE antiserum (AS) on sleep-waking cycle. Specific AS to synthetic camel BE[9] (10 μl of rabbit AS binds approximately 2.5 ng of BE) was infused twice over two hrs. Controls were infused with normal AS. There was a significant increase in duration of deep slow-wave sleep after the second infusion (Table 2).

TABLE 2

EFFECT OF β-ENDORPHIN ANTISERUM ON SLEEP-WAKING CYCLE

Duration of stages of sleep and wakefulness in min during the second postinfusion hr

Treatment	n	Slow-wave sleep (deep) ± S.E.	Slow-wave sleep (Shallow)± S.E.	Paradoxical sleep ± S.E.	Awake ± S.E.
Normal rabbit AS	8	23.4 ± 3.7	15.0 ± 3.4	9.0 ± 1.1	12.6 ± 3.2
Beta-endorphin AS	8	33.6* ± 2.7	11.7 ± 2.5	10.1 ± 0.7	4.6* ± 7.6

*$p \leq 0.05$

c) Pathological EEG, motor discoordination and opiate withdrawal signs were detected after 2 μg of BE and often occurred during infusion. EEG showed clusters of spikes increasing amplitude preceeding "wet-dog shakes" (Fig. 1A). The frequency of EEG spiking usually diminished gradually, converting to a regular spike-wave pattern resembling that of human pepit mal epilepsy (Fig. 1B) Epileptiform EEG usually persisted for 10 - 30 sec and was associated with "frozen stares", body and limb jerks, "wet-dog shakes", motor discoordination, hypermotility, or very prominent excessive grooming.

d) Akinesia progressing to general anesthesia developed after an initial stage of hyperactivity (10 - 15 min), epileptic-like EEG and opiate-withdrawal signs, with 50 μg BE.* EEG showed deactivation, even hypersynchrony, which, during the first 20 - 25 min - could be interrupted in response to stimulation (Fig. 2), but animals became unresponsive after 30 min. This latter stage is defined as general anesthesia with muscle rigidity[10]. Our findings underline

---

*Fresh solutions of BE never induced grand-mal type seizures. Older solutions with partially decomposed BE occasionally induced motor seizures with salivation.

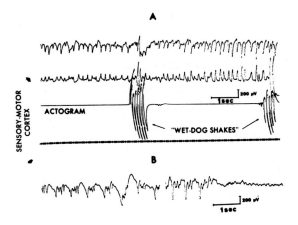

Fig. 1. A: Cluster of EEG discharges preceeds wet-dog shakes already during the ICV infusion of 2 µg of BE. B: Regular spike-wave discharges occur later.

the inappropriateness of the term "catatonia" for a state induced by BE[5]: in catatonic man consciousness is not affected and is characterized by an EEG with normal wakeful pattern; on the other hand BE promotes EEG deactivation. Analysis of the EEG spectra after BE shows significant dose-dependent increase in power in all tested frequencies (Fig. 3). Similar changes in the EEG power-spectrum can be detected with the use of other anesthetics.

    e) Naloxone completely reversed both EEG and behavioral effects of BE.

SUMMARY

    Synthetic camel beta-endorphin infused into the lateral ventricle of freely moving rats induces the following dose-dependent responses:

    (a) at 0.1 µg, insomnia,

    (b) at 2 µg, epileptiform EEG activity accompanied by excessive grooming, wet-dog shakes, frozen stares etc.

    (c) at 50 µg, general anesthesia with prominent EEG hypersynchrony.

    (d) BE antiserum significantly prolonged the slow-wave sleep.

    (e) Naloxone completely reversed both EEG and behavioral effects of BE.

ACKNOWLEDGEMENTS

    This research has been supported by MRC and NMUD/Health and Welfare Canada.

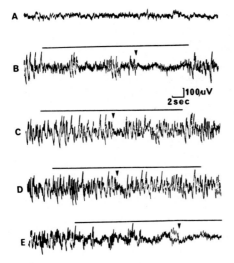

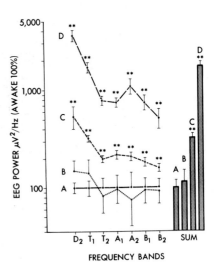

Fig. 2. EEG hypersynchrony after ICV infusion of 50 μg BE. A: Wakeful rat before
infusion. B: 15 min after BE infusion. EEG
arousal in response to the presence of the
man (horizontal bar) and strong arousal to
corneal stimulation (arrow). C: 30 min after infusion no response to the man and
minimal response to pain (ear piercing -
arrow). D: 53 min after infusion no response
to pain (arrow). E: 70 min after infusion
recovery of the EEG arousal to both man
and pain.

Fig. 3. Dose-response changes in
the EEG power spectrum after ICV
administration of BE. Presented
are percent changes of the averaged
values from 6-8 animals. A: During
awake state after ICV infusion of
vehicle. B: After 2 μg of BE. C:10
& D: 50 ug of BE. EEG segments
without epileptic activity were analysed. Frequency bands: D2=1.56-
3.51 Hz; T1=3.61-5.57 Hz; T2=5.66-
7.52 Hz; A1=7.62-9.47 Hz; A2=9.57-
12.5 Hz; B1=12.6-17.48 Hz;B2=17.58
-25Hz.Vertical lines indicate S.E.
** =p$\leq$0.01.

REFERENCES

1. Simpson, J.B. and Routtenberg, A. (1973) Science, 181, 1172-1175.

2. Foreman, M. and Moss, R.L. (1975) Neurosci. Abstr., 1, 435.

3. Havlicek, V., Rezek, M. et al. (1976) Neurosci. Abstr., 2, 568.

4. Urca, G., Erenk, H. et al. (1977) Science, 197, 83-86.

5. Bloom, F., Segal, D. et al. (1976) Science, 194, 630-632.

6. Havlicek, V. and Sklenovsky, A. (1967) Brain Research, 4, 345-357.

7. Havlicek, V., Childiaeva, R. et al. (1977) Neuropädiatrie, 8, 360-373.

8. Gispen, W.H., Wiegand, V.M. et al. (1976) Nature, 264, 794-795.

9. Ogawa, N., Panerai, A.E. et al. (1977) Neurosci. Abstr., 3, 354.

10. Havlicek, V., LaBella, F. et al. (1977) Physiologist, 20, #4, 41.

Characteristics and Function of Opioids, editors Van Ree and Terenius
© *1978 Elsevier/North-Holland Biomedical Press*

STEREOTYPED BEHAVIOR INDUCED BY INTRANIGRAL OPIATE MICROINJECTION IN RATS

EDGAR T. IWAMOTO and E. LEONG WAY
Department of Pharmacology, University of California, San Francisco, California

ABSTRACT

Bilateral stereotaxic microinjection of morphine or β-endorphin, but not naltrexone or naloxone, into the substantia nigra of rats induced profound stereotyped behavior characterized by continuous sniffing, licking, biting and gnawing. These data demonstrate that opiates may enhance nigrostriatal activities via interactions at the level of the substantia nigra.

INTRODUCTION

Small doses of morphine, 1-2 mg/kg s.c., induce an increase in activity of rats[1,2] that is dissimilar to the opiate-induced stimulation of locomotion observed in mice. The morphine-induced hyperactivity in rats is characterized by enhanced locomotion, rearing, grooming, or gentle chewing on extremities, cage or tail[3]. Since stereotyped behavior is associated with activation of dopamine-containing systems, the role of the nigrostriatal pathway in opiate-induced stereotypy was determined using the technique of subcortical microinjections.

MATERIALS AND METHODS

A 5 µl Hamilton microsyringe mounted on a Kopf stereotaxic carrier was used for delivery of drugs into the substantia nigra (2.2 mm anterior, 2 mm lateral, -2 mm vertical[4]) of Sprague-Dawley rats anesthetized with halothane-oxygen. Test drugs were administered in 1 µl of artificial CSF at a rate of 0.1 µl/15 sec. After withdrawing the syringe needle and closing the wound, the animals were placed in white plastic cages for behavioral observation. Stereotyped behavior was assessed and evaluated using rank scoring methods[5]. Catalepsy lasting greater than 1 min was taken as a positive response.

RESULTS

After delivery of either 16 nmol of morphine/1 µl CSF into both substantia nigrae (32 nmol total dose, N = 4), or 1 nmol of β-endorphin/ 1 µl (2 nmol total dose, N = 4), continuous sniffing was observed immediately after recovery from the injection procedure. After 15-20 min, severe biting, licking and gnawing were observed which lasted for 45-90 min. Lastly, discontinuous sniffing and forward locomotion were exhibited before the animals returned to control behavior. The stereotypy induced by morphine and β-endorphin was antagonized in separate groups of 3-4 rats within 5 min after the injection of 4 mg/kg s.c. naloxone. One hr pretreatment with 1 mg/kg i.p. haloperidol significantly diminished morphine- and β-endorphin-induced stereotypy (N = 5 each).

Like morphine and β-endorphin, bilateral intranigral ℓ-methadone injections (2 x 16 nmol) induced severe stereotyped behavior in rats; CSF injections were without effect[6]. In another group of intranigral CSF- or methadone-treated rats (Table 1), ℓ-methadone, given *parenterally* (2.3 mg/kg s.c., 45 min after the nigral injections), induced intense catalepsy in the CSF-pretreated group whereas *no* cataleptic behavior was observed in the nigral-methadone pretreated group. In fact, stereotyped sniffing, biting, and exploratory behaviors induced by prior bilateral intranigral methadone were *not* altered by subsequent parenterally administered opiate.

TABLE 1

EFFECT OF INTRANIGRAL METHADONE ON CATALEPSY INDUCED BY PARENTERAL METHADONE

Injection Group		Observations
2 x 1 µl CSF ▶	Administer 2.3 mg/kg s.c. methadone 45 min *after* intra-nigral CSF or methadone.	▶ Positive cataleptic response: Onset 10-15 min; Duration 1-2 hr.
2 x 16 nmol methadone ▶		▶ Continuation of ongoing sniffing, biting and exploratory behaviors.

ACKNOWLEDGEMENTS

This work was supported in part by grant DA 00037 from the National Institute on Drug Abuse. E.T.I. is a recipient of a research starter grant from the Pharmaceutical Manufacturers Association Foundation.

REFERENCES

1. Ayhan, I.H. and Randrup, A. (1972) Psychopharmacology, 27, 203-212.
2. Fog, R. (1970) Psychopharmacology, 16, 305-312.
3. Buxbaum, D.M., Yarbrough, G.G. and Carter, M.E. (1973) J. Pharmacol. Exp. 185, 317-327.
4. König, J.F.R. and Klippel, R.A. (1963) The Rat Brain, Williams and Wilkins, Baltimore.
5. Iwamoto, E.T., Loh, H.H. and Way, E.L. (1976) Eur. J. Pharmacol., 37,339-356.
6. Iwamoto, E.T. and Way, E.L. (1977) J. Pharmacol. Exp. Ther., 203, 347-359.

Characteristics and Function of Opioids, editors Van Ree and Terenius
© 1978 Elsevier/North-Holland Biomedical Press

"OPIOID" BEHAVIORAL EFFECTS FOLLOWING ACTH OR B-ENDORPHIN INJECTIONS
IN PERIAQUEDUCTAL GRAY OF DRUG-NAIVE RATS: A DUAL MECHANISM OF DRUG DEPENDENCE?

YASUKO JACQUET

NY State Research Institute for Neurochemistry, Ward's Island, New York 10035

ACTH(1-24) injected in the periaqueductal gray (PAG) of drug-naive rats resulted in an explosive motor behavior (EMB) characterized by repeated and rapid
high leaps ("flying") similar to the behavior seen in opiate-dependent rats undergoing precipitated abstinence. This was followed by a period during which
other "recessive" abstinence signs were manifested, i.e., wet-dog shakes, teeth
chatter, squeal on touch, etc. Shorter analogues resulted in attenuated forms
of the abstinence syndrome. Naloxone pretreatment failed to block these.

We previously reported[1] that a morphine injection in the PAG of drug-naive
rats resulted in 2 paradoxical effects: (a) analgesia/catatonia, and (b) EMB
characterized by rapid high leaps similar to those seen in opiate-dependent rats
undergoing precipitated abstinence. Pretreatment with naloxone (1 mg/kg) blocked (a) but not (b). B-endorphin injections in the PAG of rats resulted in a naloxone-reversible syndrome of analgesia/catatonia, but not in EMB, while injections in the PAG of the inactive stereoisomer, (+)-morphine, did not result in
(a) but in (b) which was not naloxone-reversible. Thus, morphine effects appeared to be mediated by 2 classes of receptors, one that had stereospecific recognition for opiates, was naloxone-reversible, and mediated the behavioral syndrome of (a) (the "endorphin" receptor), the other that had nonstereospecific
recognition for opiates, was naloxone-insensitive and mediated the behavioral
syndrome of EMB. The endogenous ligand of this receptor may be ACTH. Since
EMB is never seen following systemic administration of morphine, we hypothesize
that in systemic administrations, morphine is distributed to multiple neuronal
systems, activating endorphin receptors which exert an inhibitory influence on
the excitatory effects of morphine at the ACTH receptor sites in the PAG. Thus,

TABLE 1: EFFECTS OF PAG INJECTIONS OF MORPHINE, B-ENDORPHIN
OR ACTH FOLLOWING PRETREATMENT WITH I.P. NALOXONE OR MORPHINE

Pretreatment (i.p.)	Treatment (PAG)	(a) anal/cat.	(b) EMB
-----	morphine 10 ug	+	+
(a) naloxone 1 mg/kg 2' prior	morphine 10 ug	−	+
-----	B-endorphin 4 ug	+	−
(a) naloxone 1 mg/kg 2' prior	B-endorphin 4 ug	−	−
-----	ACTH 50 ug	−	+
(a) naloxone 1 mg/kg 2' prior	ACTH 50 ug	−	+
(b) morphine 30 mg/kg 30' prior	morphine 10 ug	+	−
(b) morphine 30 mg/kg 30' prior	ACTH 50 ug	+	−
(a) + (b)	morphine 10 ug	−	+
(a) + (b)	ACTH 50 ug	−	+

in morphine-treated rats, EMB is "precipitated" or unmasked following naloxone
blockade of, or following the selective development of tolerance to opiates of
the endorphin receptor (which normally acts to inhibit the behavioral expression
of the ACTH receptor). Opiate abstinence is thus seen as due to the residual
presence and not the absence of morphine at the ACTH receptor. The inverse
correlation between opiate dependence and naloxone dose required to precipitate
abstinence may be due to the selective increase in tolerance to opiates of the
endorphin receptor (but not of the ACTH receptor) which then requires increas-
ingly lower doses of naloxone for its blockade. Pretreatment of naive rats with
i.p. morphine followed by morphine or ACTH in the PAG resulted in (a) but not
(b); pretreatment with naloxone followed by morphine or ACTH in the PAG resulted in (b) but not (a). (Table 1). Thus, in the complex system of the living
brain, an important mechanism of opiate action may consist of the simultaneous
activation by opiates of receptors for endorphin and ACTH.

REFERENCES

1. Jacquet, Y. F. and Lajtha, A. (1974) Science 185, 1055-1057.

EFFECTS OF OPIATES AND OF NEUROLEPTICS ON ALPHA-MOTONEURONES IN
RAT SPINAL CORD: POSSIBLE CORRELATIONS WITH MUSCULAR RIGIDITY AND
AKINESIA

K. KUSCHINSKY, U. SEEBER, J. LANGER and K.-H. SONTAG
Max-Planck-Institute for Experimental Medicine, D-3400 Göttingen,
Fed. Rep. of Germany

In rats, opiates and opioid peptides can induce characteristic
alterations in motility, which might be described as "lead pipe
rigidity", characterized by an increase in EMG activity when
recorded from the gastrocnemius-soleus muscle which functions
mainly as an extensor muscle[1]. Neuroleptics (e.g. haloperidol), on
the other hand, induce akinesia and catalepsy, which are at a first
glance somewhat similar to opiate-induced effects, but are not
accompanied by a clear-cut muscular rigidity. Since alterations in
motility should be expected to reflect corresponding changes in
patterns of alpha-motoneurone activities, the actions of these
drugs on these parameters were studied.

Male Wistar rats of 200-350 g in halothane anesthesia were
laminectomized, the ventral roots of L_5-S_1 were cut (interrupting
the gamma-loop) and its proximal parts were split into functionally
single filaments, from which the discharges of alpha-motoneurones,
activated either by electrical tetanic stimulation of the ipsilateral gastrocnemius-soleus nerve ("extensor alpha-motoneurones")
or of the ipsilateral peroneal nerve ("flexor alpha-motoneurones"),
were recorded (for methodological details cf [2]). By the stimulation parameters used, only group I- and II-, but not nociceptive
fibres were stimulated.

Morphine enhanced the activation of extensor alpha-motoneurones, when given in the dose of 2 mg/kg, and even more pronounced after 4 mg/kg i.v. This effect was partly reduced by the
dopaminergic agonist apomorphine (1 mg/kg i.p.). In contrast, in
even slightly lower doses (0.5 or 1.5 mg/kg i.v.) morphine prevented the activation of flexor alpha-motoneurones. Hence morphine
induced a shift of the functional balance between flexor and extensor alpha-motoneurones in favour of the latter ones. Both

432

effects of morphine were mimicked by levorphanol, but not by dextrorphan, and were abolished by naloxone. After spinalization of
the rats, alpha-motoneurones still could be activated by the
stimulation parameters used, but the activating or inhibitory
actions of morphine, respectively, were completely abolished. Both
effects of morphine seem to reflect, at least in part, the increase in activity of extensor muscles characteristic for "lead
pipe rigidity".

Haloperidol, on the other hand, dose-dependently (0.15-0.60
mg/kg i.p.) reduced the activation of extensor as well as of
flexor alpha-motoneurones by the stimulation parameters used and
increased the threshold of the reflex activation of alpha-motoneurones. Apomorphine (2 mg/kg s.c.) antagonized the inhibitory
effects of haloperidol, suggesting that the blockade of dopamine
receptors was relevant for haloperidol's effect on alpha-motoneurones. It seems likely that haloperidol (and probably other
neuroleptics) reduces the activation of alpha-motoneurones by
proprioceptive stimuli, thus leading to akinesia and catalepsy.

Our results suggest that, at least in rats, opiates and haloperidol induce completely different patterns of effects on reflex
activation of alpha-motoneurones by proprioceptive stimuli, although the effects of both drug groups seem to be, at least partly,
due to a decreased dopaminergic neurotransmission.

A more detailed knowledge about the control of alpha-motoneurones seems to be of considerable relevance for the interpretation
not only of motility, but also of more complex behavioural parameters observed in rats after administration of these drugs.

ACKNOWLEDGEMENTS
These studies were supported by a grant (B-3) from the SFB-33
of the Deutsche Forschungsgemeinschaft.

REFERENCES
1. Wand, P., Kuschinsky, K. and Sontag, K.-H. (1973) Europ. J.
   Pharmacol. 24, 189-193.
2. Kuschinsky, K., Ropte, H., Meseke, R., Cremer, H. and Sontag,
   K.-H. (1977) Naunyn-Schmiedeberg's Arch. Pharmacol. 296, 249-
   254.

Characteristics and Function of Opioids, editors Van Ree and Terenius
© 1978 Elsevier/North-Holland Biomedical Press

NALOXONE ANTAGONISM OF SYMPATHOMIMETIC ANALGESIA

HILARY J LITTLE and J M H REES[*]

Department of Pharmacology, South Parks Road, University of Oxford, UK, and the Department of Pharmacology, University of Manchester, M13 9PT, UK. [*]

Physiological analgesia occurs during high sympathetic activity, and centrally acting sympathomimetic drugs are analgesic[1]. Since the neurotransmitter balance which favours sympathomimetic analgesia also favours that of opiates[2], a correlation between the two is proposed. There are also structural similarities between the two groups of drugs, and mice made tolerant to the analgesic action of opiates are tolerant to that of sympathomimetics[3].

The central stimulant action of amphetamine interferes with the end points of some analgesic testing methods. However its derivative 2-aminoindane retains analgesic activity, yet lacks the locomotor stimulant action of the parent molecule, and causes different behavioural effects[4].

METHODS

Groups of 12 female mice (ASH/XP Strain) weighing between 25 and 30 G were used. The experiments were done 'blind'.

Writing Test. Mice received subcutaneous injections of the test drug and naloxone, the test drug and saline, or saline. The writhing agent was 0.75% acetic acid injected intraperitoneally immediately following the s/c injections. The number of writhes observed in the following 20 min was then expressed as a percent of that observed in concurrent controls.

Hot Plate Test. Mice were placed individually on a metal plate maintained electrically at 55°. The end point was taken as any sign of discomfort in a hind limb. A maximum cut-off of 45 s was used. Results are expressed as the change (in s) compared with concurrent controls.

RESULTS

Writhing Test. At doses of 5 mg/kg and above naloxone inhibited writhing. A dose of 2 mg/kg abolished the inhibition of writhing caused by morphine (2 mg/kg ID100) but had no effect on that caused by mepyramine (5 mg/kg, ID70). 2-aminoindane inhibited writhing in doses above 0.5 mg/kg. In combination with naloxone (5 mg/kg) the log dose response line was shifted to the right, though the antagonism was only significant at one dose of 2-aminoindane.

Hot Plate Test. Naloxone (1 mg/kg) virtually abolished the analgesic action

of morphine (20 mg/kg). The effects of combinations of 2-aminoindane (10 and
20 mg/kg) and naloxone (2 and 5 mg/kg) were examined. In all instances naloxone
antagonised 2-aminoindane (Figure 1).

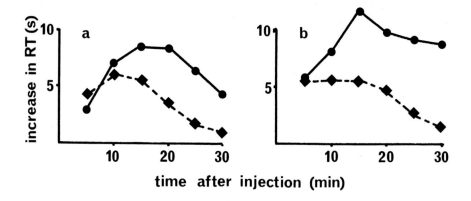

Fig. 1. The increase in hot plate reaction time (RT) caused by 2-aminoindane
10 mg/kg (a) and 20 mg/kg (b), alone (●), and in combination with naloxone
2 mg/kg (◆). In both cases the antagonism is statistically significant(P<0.05).

DISCUSSION

    Naloxone clearly antagonises the analgesic action of 2-aminoindane, though it
is stressed that the antagonism is not as impressive as that against opiates.
Naloxone, once assumed to lack pharmacological activity in the absence of opiate
agonists, is now known to have a variety of actions. In the context of our own
work its antagonism of stress-induced analgesia is of interest[5], as is its
antagonism of some behavioural actions of amphetamine[6].

REFERENCES

1. Colville, K.I. and Chaplin, E. (1964) Life Sciences, 3, 315-322.

2. Major, C.T. and Pleuvry,B.J. (1971) Br.J.Pharmac., 42, 512-521.

3. Little, H.J. and Rees, J.M.H. (1974) Experientia, 30, 930-931.

4. Witkin, L.B., Huebner, C.F., Galdi, F., O'Keefe, E., Spinaletta, P. and
   Plummer, A.J. (1961). J.Pharmac.exp.Ther., 133, 400-408.

5. Akil, H., Madden, J., Patrick, R.L. and Barchas, J.D. (1976) in Opiates and
   Endogenous Opioid Peptides, Kosterlitz, H.W. ed, Elsevier, Amsterdam, pp.63-70.

6. Dettmar, P.W., Cowan, A., and Walter, D.S., Neuropharmacology (in press).

Characteristics and Function of Opioids, editors Van Ree and Terenius
© *1978 Elsevier/North-Holland Biomedical Press*

EEG AND BEHAVIORAL EFFECTS OF ACUTE AND CHRONIC ADMINISTRATION OF OPIATE-LIKE PEPTIDES IN THE RAT

J. E. MORETON, F. C. TORTELLA AND N. KHAZAN
Department of Pharmacology and Toxicology, University of Maryland School of
Pharmacy, Baltimore, Maryland 21201 USA

ABSTRACT

The present study established dose-response relationships for i.vt. D-enkephalin[1], β-endorphin, and morphine using the direct and voltage integrated EEG and behavioral correlates in the rat. Moreover, the development of tolerance and cross-tolerance to these effects was demonstrated.

INTRODUCTION

The actions of opiates on the electroencephalogram (EEG) of the experimental animal have been well delineated. However, little data exist on the effects of opiate-like peptides on the EEG. This study characterized the pharmacology of centrally administered morphine and endogenous opiate-like peptides with respect to acute and chronic effects on the direct and voltage integrated EEG and overt behavior in the rat.

MATERIALS AND METHODS

Adult female Sprague-Dawley rats were prepared with chronic cortical and temporalis muscle electrodes and bilateral intraventricular (i.vt.) cannulae. The direct and voltage integrated EEG and integrated electromyogram (EMG) as well as gross behavior were monitored. The effects of acute i.vt. injection of morphine (2.5-40 µg), D-enkephalin (10-240 µg), β-endorphin (5-80 µg), naloxone (25-50 µg), or sterile water (10 µg) were assessed. Tolerance was assessed during repeated injection of 20 µg/4 hr of D-enkephalin or morphine. Cross-tolerance was determined with cross-challenges of morphine (20 µg) or D-enkephalin (20 and 40 µg).

RESULTS

EEG high-amplitude slow-frequency waves (EEG slow bursts) occurred after morphine, D-enkephalin, or β-endorphin and were associated with a behavioral stupor. The behavioral depressant phase was followed later by behavioral arousal and EEG activation. D-Enkephalin and β-endorphin characteristically

---

[1]In all cases D-Ala[2]-Met-enkephalinamide

produced wet-dog shakes associated with an initial epileptoid EEG which progressed to a high-voltage low-frequency EEG synchrony. Morphine did not produce
wet-dog shakes or epileptoid EEG at the doses used. Increasing doses of D-
enkephalin, β-endorphin, or morphine increased the EEG voltage output and duration of stupor in a dose-related manner. The order of potency on a molar basis
was β-endorphin > morphine > D-enkephalin. β-Endorphin and D-enkephalin
produced a greater maximal response, but morphine had a longer duration of
action. The i.vt. injection of naloxone alone or sterile water had no disrup-
tive effect on the EEG or behavior of the rat; however, the effects of morphine
and the peptides were antagonized by pretreatment with naloxone (10 mg/kg, s.c.).

During repeated injection of D-enkephalin, tolerance developed to its effects
on EEG and behavior within 48-72 hours. When these D-enkephalin-tolerant rats
were challenged with i.vt. morphine, cross-tolerance was evident. Similarly,
tolerance developed to morphine within 48-72 hours; and morphine-tolerant rats
were cross-tolerant to D-enkephalin. Physical dependence was also assessed in
the tolerant rats. While the morphine-tolerant rats demonstrated a marked
abstinence syndrome when challenged with naloxone (10 mg/kg, i.p.), no abstinence signs were observed in the D-enkephalin-tolerant rats. The lack of abstinence signs was likely due to the low maintenance dose of D-enkephalin.

SUMMARY AND CONCLUSIONS

Similarities between morphine and opiate-like peptides exist with respect to
production of EEG slow-wave activity, increase in EEG voltage output, production
of behavioral stupor, and production of tolerance and cross-tolerance. On the
other hand, differences exist with respect to the peptide-induced epileptoid
EEG, associated wet-dog shakes, and efficacy in increasing EEG voltage output
in the rat. These data further support the contention that heterogenous opiate
receptors mediate the actions of enkephalin and morphine.

ACKNOWLEDGEMENT

Supported by NIDA Grant DA01050.

Characteristics and Function of Opioids, editors Van Ree and Terenius
© *1978 Elsevier/North-Holland Biomedical Press*   437

AVERSIVE EFFECTS OF NARCOTIC ANTAGONISTS IN RATS

C.W.T. PILCHER[*], I.P. STOLERMAN AND G.D. D'MELLO
MRC Neuropharmacology Unit, The Medical School, Birmingham B15 2TJ.

Narcotic antagonists have behavioural and physiological effects in animals even in the absence of exogenous, narcotic agonists[2]. Conditioned taste aversion procedures have been used to show strongly aversive effects of naloxone in morphine-dependent rats, but when aversive effects were first reported in non-dependent rats, they were quite weak[3,5,6]. More extensive investigations have been carried out with procedures modified to maximise sensitivity, using several narcotic antagonists in addition to naloxone, and in circumstances more likely to involve endorphins.

Details of the methods have been given previously[1,7]. Briefly, water-deprived rats can learn to reduce their intakes of distinctively-flavoured but pharmacologically inert solutions if their consumption is followed by administration of certain drugs. The flavour stimulus becomes conditioned to the effects of the drugs, which are thereby defined as aversive. In the present experiments all drugs were given intraperitoneally, and a different group of at least eight rats was used for each dose.

After several conditioning sessions, the rats were given direct choice tests between drug-paired flavours and saline-paired flavours. The mean percentages of the total fluid intake consumed as the drug-paired flavours were 32.4%, 15.5% and 8.6% after conditioning with naloxone at 1.0, 3.2 or 10 mg/kg respectively; each of these dose-related scores was significantly below 50% ($p<0.01$), and thus met the criterion for aversion[1,7]. The mean score with naltrexone (3.2 mg/kg) was 32.1%, again showing significant aversion ($p<0.05$). Stereospecificity was tested with two antagonists in the benzomorphan series, Mr 1452 and BC-2860[7,8]. Significant taste aversions were induced only with the (-) isomers of these compounds, which were known to be active as narcotic antagonists[8].

Despite being dose-related and stereospecific, the aversive effects of narcotic antagonists were weaker than those of some other substances. Taste aversions were then conditioned with naloxone in the usual way, except that electric shocks were presented immediately after injections. Shock (0.8 mA for one second) was given through the grid-floor at unpredictable intervals averaging 30

[*]Present address: Department of Pharmacology, University of Kuwait.

438

seconds for 20 minutes. However, this type of stress failed to enhance the aversive effect of naloxone (3.2 mg/kg); the mean scores were 21.0% and 20.4% in the control and "stressed" rats respectively.

Finally, the reaction to naloxone (3mg/kg) was examined 28 days after terminating chronic administration of morphine (50 mg/kg twice daily). Dependence was shown by a mean loss in weight of 23 g at 48 hours after withdrawing morphine, from a baseline of 202g. Naloxone-induced taste aversion was not substantially enhanced in such post-dependent rats as compared with controls chronically treated with saline. The effects of intermittent administrations of morphine during taste aversion conditioning were then examined, since similar "priming" increased the reaction to naloxone in post-dependent mice[9]. Either saline or morphine (20 mg/kg) was administered on every alternate day, 15 hours before the next presentation of a flavoured solution. "Priming" with morphine enhanced (p<0.05) the aversive effect of naloxone; this was merely the known aversion due to precipitated morphine abstinence[4-6]. However, the effects of priming were not greater in 28-day post-dependent rats than in controls.

In conclusion, the consistency and stereospecificity of aversion with the antagonists tested so far lend some support to interpretations in terms of antagonist actions at receptors for endogenous opioids. Attempts to further implicate endorphin systems by means of environmental stress or by a previous history of morphine dependence have yielded negative results to date.

REFERENCES

1. Booth, D.A., D'Mello, G.D., Pilcher, C.W.T. and Stolerman, I.P. (1977) Br.J. Pharmac., 61, 669-677.
2. Frederickson, R.C.A. (1977) Life Sci., 23-42.
3. Le Blanc, A.E. and Cappell, H. (1975) Pharmac. Biochem. Behav., 3, 185-188.
4. Pilcher, C.W.T. (1976) Br. J. Pharmac., 57, 430-431P.
5. Pilcher, C.W.T. and Stolerman, I.P. (1976) Pharmac. Biochem. Behav., 4, 159-163.
6. Pilcher, C.W.T. and Stolerman, I.P. (1976) Opiates and Endogenous Opioid Peptides, North-Holland, Amsterdam, pp. 327-334.
7. Stolerman, I.P., Pilcher, C.W.T. and D'Mello, G.D. (1978) Life Sci., 22, 1755-1762.
8. Waterfield, A.A. and Kosterlitz, H.W. (1975) Life Sci., 16, 1787-1792.
9. Way, E.L., Brase, D.A., Iwamoto, E.T., Shen, J. and Loh, H.H. (1976) Opiates and Endogenous Opioid Peptides, North-Holland, Amsterdam, pp. 311-318.

APPARENT CENTRAL AGONIST ACTIONS OF NALOXONE IN THE UNRESTRAINED RAT**

CARL PINSKY, FRANK S. LABELLA, VIKTOR HAVLICEK AND ASHOK K. DUA*

Departments of Pharmacology and Therapeutics and of Physiology, University of Manitoba, Med. Faculty, 770 Bannatyne, Winnipeg, Manitoba, Canada, R3E 0W3

INTRODUCTION

Opioids exhibit considerable agonist and antagonist stereospecificity at very low concentrations[1]. At higher concentrations they exhibit "nonspecific" actions. These may be mediated by an opiate receptor which can distinguish between opioid and non-opioid chemical structure, but not as readily between opioid agonists and antagonists.

METHODS AND RESULTS

Electrocortical and motor behavioral responses to intracerebroventricular (ICV) infusion. Male Sprague-Dawley albino rats, 150-250 g at operation, were implanted with cannulas into the right lateral ventricle and with bipolar epidural electrodes on right and left sensorimotor cortices. Substances were infused in vehicle volumes of 10.0 μl over 5 min. ICV morphine sulphate (MS) in saline provoked electrocorticogram (ECoG) spikes, ECoG seizures and motor seizures. Severity and incidence of such responses were threshold at 30 μg and clearly related to dose (10,30,50,100 and 200 μg; tested in total of 13 rats). Naloxone.HCl (NLX) produced very similar results, but with a threshold dose of 100 μg. Infusion of 5000 μg NLX along with 400 μg calcium chloride (n = 3) resulted in activity almost identical to that observed in vehicle-infused controls (n = 10) as did dextrophan.HCl (DEX) at 3000 μg (n = 2) , DEX at 5000 μg (n = 1) and NaCl at 3000 μg (n = 3) and at 5000 μg (n = 3).

Effects of parenteral MS and NLX in rats tested on 44.5°C warmplate. Rats were injected with saline, MS or NLX, and tested 5 min later on a warmplate at 44.5°C. MS, 0.5-16.0 mg kg^{-1}, significantly diminished forepaw licking (FPL), hindpaw licking (HPL), exploratory rearing (ER) and leaping (L) in dose-related fashion. NLX, in the same dose range, increased the incidence of ER ($p < 0.05$ at 4.0 and 8.0 mg kg^{-1}) and of L ($p < 0.005$ at 4.0 mg kg^{-1}). Unexpectedly, NLX produced an apparent antinociceptive effect, showing significant suppression of FPL at 0.5, 1.0 and 16.0 mg kg^{-1}. NLX also diminished HPL activity, but not to a statistically significant level.

* Government of India Scholar
** Supported by NMUD (Health and Welfare Canada) and MRC (Canada)

440

DISCUSSION

The foregoing results suggest that MS and NLX exert a common excitant action
on nervous tissue accessible to substances infused into the rat lateral ventricle. With ICV infusion there was reversal of NLX-induced excitation by calcium ion, known to diminish many specific opiate actions[2,3]. Very large concentrations of DEX and of NaCl were inactive. Hence, at certain CNS sites responsible for electrocortical hypersynchrony in the rat, there may exist a
unique receptor for which MS is a full agonist with relatively low affinity
while NLX behaves as a weak or partial agonist with low intrinsic activity.
A peripheral model of such a receptor has already been demonstrated by Frank[4].
Whether this situation represents the existence of yet another class of CNS
opiate receptor or a specialized opiate-sensitive CNS excitant receptor[5,6] has
yet to be determined. The apparent antinociceptive effect of parenteral NLX
may be mediated at least in part by some mechanism other than that suggested
for our ICV results. A NLX blockade of the high-affinity stereospecific central opiate receptor might be involved in provoking an over-compensating release of endorphin, which could result in antinociception under the particular
conditions of our experiment. This latter possibility might explain the variable and sometimes seemingly contradictory results that have been reported for
the effects of NLX on nociception[7,8,9].

REFERENCES

1. Kosterlitz, H.W., Waterfield, A.A. and Berthoud, V. (1973) Adv. Biochem. Psychopharmacol., 8, 319-334.

2. Radouco, Thomas, S. (1971) Int. J. Clin. Pharmacol. Ther. Toxicol., 22, 271-277.

3. Sanfacon, G. and LaBrecque, G. (1977) Psychopharmacology, 55, 151-156.

4. Frank, G.B. (1975) J. Physiol. (Lond.), 252, 585-601.

5. Jacquet, Y.F., Klee, W.A., Rice, K.C., Iijima, I. and Minamikawa, J. (1977) Science, 198, 842-845.

6. LaBella, F.S., Pinsky, C. and Havlicek, V. (1978) Int. Congr. Pharmacology (Paris), abstract.

7. Grevert, P. and Goldstein, A. (1978) Science, 199, 1093-1095.

8. Jacob, J.J., Tremblay, E.C. and Colombel, M.C. (1974) Psychopharmacologia, 37, 217-223.

9. Pinsky, C., LaBella, F.S., Gigliotti, O. and Leybin, L. (1976) Proc. Can. Fed. Biol. Soc., 19, 169.

ACTIVITY OF NALOXONE AND NALTREXONE IN AN ANIMAL TEST PREDICTIVE OF CLINICAL ANTIPSYCHOTIC ACTIVITY

HENK RIGTER, HEMMIE BERENDSEN, JOHN C. CRABBE

CNS Pharmacology Department, Organon, Oss (The Netherlands)

Recent reports of elevated endorphin fraction levels in CSF of chronic schizophrenics have suggested that endogenous opiates may be involved in the pathogenesis of schizophrenia[1]. Naloxone has therefore been clinically tested for antipsychotic efficacy with equivocal results. Low doses of apomorphine induce stereotyped climbing in mice that may be blocked specifically by known antipsychotic agents. We report that naloxone and naltrexone are able to attenuate apomorphine-induced climbing, an effect predictive of clinical antipsychotic efficacy. We adapted the method of Protais[2], giving placebo or test compound s.c. 30 minutes before s.c. administration of doses between 0,5 and 1,0 mg/kg apomorphine (APO). APO induced stereotyped climbing (assessed 10 and 20 minutes later) in dose-dependent fashion, an effect blocked dose-dependently by haloperidol (0,022 - 0,22 mg/kg). The highest dose of haloperidol completely suppressed APO-induced climbing. Morphine (4,6 - 46,0 mg/kg) effectively potentiated APO-induced climbing. The lower doses of morphine potentiated 1,0 mg/kg APO, while the higher doses potentiated 0,5 mg/kg APO. In contrast to haloperidol, naloxone was effective only against the low (0,5 mg/kg) dose of apomorphine. All doses of naloxone tested (1,0 - 10,0 mg/kg) significantly inhibited APO-climbing (33 - 85% reduction from APO control values). Against the high (1,0 mg/kg) APO dose, however, naloxone was ineffective in doses between 2,2 and 22,0 mg/kg. Naltrexone (2,2 - 22,0 mg/kg) was tested against the low apomorphine dose and was also effective. The effect of naloxone was also demonstrable if given 45 min, but not 90 or 180 min before apomorphine.

To elucidate further naloxone's pattern of activity, we employed the acquired immobility test devised by Porsolt. In this test, antidepressant agents reduce immobility and neuroleptics tend to prolong it[3]. Amitriptyline (4,6; 10,0; or 22,0 mg/kg) reduced immobility at the two higher doses. Haloperidol (0,022;

0,046 and 0,100 mg/kg) increased immobility in the higher doses when given i.p. 1 hr before the test. Naloxone (4,6 - 22,0 mg/kg) tended to prolong immobility but statistical significance was not reached. The effect of naloxone was clearly not that of an antidepressant agent, in agreement with the failure of a clinical trial with naloxone[4].

In summary, naloxone and naltrexone responded positively in an animal test sensitive to antipsychotics and naloxone responded negatively in a test for anti-depressants. The dependency of naloxone's effects on the dose of APO may offer insight into the mechanism of its action. It is possible that naloxone's effects are weak and are thus only demonstrable against low APO doses. However, naloxone has been reported to antagonize APO stereotypies induced by 10,0 and 20,0 mg/kg doses[5,6]. A second possibility is that naloxone's mode of action differs from that of haloperidol. Support for this possibility may be inferred from the finding that naloxone and haloperidol were reported to have opposite effects on amphetamine toxicity: naloxone potentiated and haloperidol reduced toxicity[5]. The fact that naloxone's antagonism of APO-induced climbing is only demonstrable under limited conditions suggests that its predicted potency as an antipsychotic may be either weak or restricted in nature.

REFERENCES

1. Terenius, L., Wahlström, A., Lindstrom, L. and Widerlöv, E. (1976). Neurosci. Lett., 3, 157.

2. Protais, P., Constetin, J. and Schwartz, J. (1976), Psychopharmacol., 50, 1.

3. Porsolt, R.D., LePichon, M. and Jalfre, M. (1977), Nature, 266, 730.

4. Terenius, L., Wahlström, A. and Ågren, H. (1977), Psychopharmacol., 54, 31.

5. Malick, J.B., Billingsley, M.L., Kubena, R.K. and Goldstein, J.M. (1977), Commun. Psychopharmacol. 1, 475.

6. Cox, B., Ary, M., and Lomax, P. (1976). J. Pharmacol. Exp. Ther. 196, 637.

Characteristics and Function of Opioids, editors Van Ree and Terenius
© *1978 Elsevier/North-Holland Biomedical Press*   443

FOOTSHOCK MITIGATES THE SUPPRESSION OF OPERANT BEHAVIOR CAUSED BY NALOXONE
IN MORPHINE-NAIVE RATS

S.B. SPARBER AND B. COLELLI
Department of Pharmacology, University of Minnesota, Minneapolis,
Minn. 55455 (U.S.A.)

Naloxone (Nx) modifies unconditioned and conditioned behavior in morphine-
naive rats[1,2]. Footshock causes (partially Nx-reversible) analgesia[3] and Nx
causes hyperalgesia[4]. Therefore, tonic release of endorphins may be normal.
We report herein that footshock can antagonize Nx-suppression of operant
behavior.

Subjects (N = 6/group) were partially food deprived (80% free food wt)
mature male Long-Evans rats responding for food pellets on a fixed ratio 15
schedule in standard operant chambers[2]. A constant current (2mA) footshock
was delivered in different chambers. Shock duration was 0.5 sec and delivered
on a variable interval 1 min schedule. Shock sessions terminated after 60
shocks or 60 min. Controls were placed in shock chambers without shock.
Behavioral sessions were 36 min long, the first 5 min acting as a warm-up,
control period. Injections (i.p.) were made during the 6th min and behavior
monitored for the next 30 min.

Footshock 3 hr before behavioral sessions suppressed responding by 33%
(85 ± 6 vs 57 ± 7 responses/min, M ± SE, $p < .05$). Nx (10 or 25mg/kg) suppressed
responding about 60% ($p < .01$) in nonshocked rats while shocked rats showed
resistance to further suppression. Resistance to Nx in the shocked groups
could have been due to a rate-dependent effect, rather than a specific effect
related to shock. The control groups were used to test this possibility.
Three months later, the Nx-naive rats' behavior was restabilized. Response
rates of the nonshocked group were reduced by allowing free access to food
prior to behavioral sessions. The previously shocked control group was kept at
80% of their free feeding weight. This procedure would determine if the
previously shocked rats are affected by Nx, if they were not first shocked, and
if lowering response rates by other than footshock would mitigate Nx's
behavioral action.

Freer access to food lowered responding from 85 ± 6 to 61 ± 9 responses/min in the original nonshocked control group. The control group that was shocked 3 months earlier responded at a higher rate without shock (57 ± 7 to 73 ± 7 responses/min). Nx (10mg/kg) injection the next day lowered responding in the 80% deprived group from 73 ± 7 to 39 ± 10 responses/min (p<.01) and the free-feeding group from 61 ± 9 to 24 ± 8 responses/min (p<.01). Correlational analysis indicated that Nx suppressed responding, measured as % of prenaloxone rates, least in higher responders and most in rats with low rates of responding (r = 0.652, p<.05). These data argue against the possibility that Nx could not further lower response rates in shocked animals.

Stress releases β-endorphin (along with ACTH) into blood[5]. Whether it is released from central sites or it gains access to brain via some other means is problematic. β-endorphin is capable of suppressing fixed ratio behavior[6] in doses much lower than is necessary to produce rigidity[7], when injected into rats' ventricles.

It is concluded that excessive endorphinergic activity (e.g. stress-induced release) or too little activity (e.g. Nx injection) will result in a deficit in conditioned behavior in rats. Whether higher CNS activity can be affected in man by a similar imbalance is undoubtedly an area of fertile investigation.

ACKNOWLEDGEMENTS

Supported in part by USPHS grant DAO0532. Naloxone HCl was kindly supplied by Endo Laboratories, Garden City, N.Y.

REFERENCES

1. Holtzman, S.G. (1974) J. Pharmacol. Exp. Ther. 189, 51-60.

2. Gellert, V.F. and Sparber, S.B. (1977) J. Pharmacol. Exp. Ther. 201, 44-54.

3. Akil, H., Madden, J., Patrick, R. and Barchas, J.D. (1976) Opiates and Endogenous Opioid Peptides, H.W. Kosterlitz, ed. Elsevier-North Holland, Amsterdam, pp. 63-70.

4. Jacob, J.J., Tremblay, E.C. and Colombel, M.C. (1974) Psychopharmacologia 37, 217-223.

5. Guillemin, R., Vargo, T., Rossier, J., Minick, S., Ling, N., Rivier, C. and Bloom, F. (1977) Science 197, 1368-1369.

6. Lichtblau, L., Fossom, L. and Sparber, S.B. (1977) Life Sci 21, 927-932.

7. Bloom, F., Segal, D., Ling, N. and Guilleman, R. (1976) Science 194, 630-632.

Characteristics and Function of Opioids, editors Van Ree and Terenius
© *1978 Elsevier/North-Holland Biomedical Press*

ENKEPHALIN ANALOGS: CORRELATION OF POTENCIES FOR ANALGESIA AND PHYSICAL
DEPENDENCE

EDDIE WEI
School of Public Health, University of California, Berkeley, California, USA,
94720

INTRODUCTION

The idea that physical dependence and analgesia are inseparable actions of
pure opiate agonists is based on the investigations of Himmelsbach and
Isbell . They showed that the addictive potencies of narcotic analgesics in
human subjects generally paralleled analgesic potencies. This fundamental
property of pure opiate agonists, to produce analgesia and physical dependence
at similar potency ratios (dose for analgesia/dosage for a comparable degree
of physical dependence), may also be a characteristic of the enkephalin analogs,
a new class of peptide drugs with opiate-like activity. In this study, the
potential of enkephalin analogs for producing physical dependence and analgesia
are compared in an animal model.

MODEL OF PHYSICAL DEPENDENCE

The capacity of an agent for producing physical dependence may be directly
measured by continuous administration of the test substance at different dose
levels followed by quantification of the withdrawal syndrome after the drug is
withheld or after the administration of an opiate antagonist . The withdrawal
intensity is a function of the total dose of the narcotic and the dose-
response relationship indicates the potency of the compound for producing
physical dependence.

The methods used in this study were described in detail elsewhere.[1]
Enkephalin analogs were infused into the periaqueductal gray fourth-ventricular
spaces of the rat brain with osmotic minipumps, implantable devices that continuously deliver solutions at closely controlled rates (1 microliter/hour,
Alza Corp., Palo Alto, California). The withdrawal syndrome was precipitated
with the narcotic antagonist, naloxone hydrochloride, 4 mg/kg i.p. Withdrawal
intensity was quantified by counting the number of escape attempts made by the
animal from a one gallon glass jar in the 15 minute period after injection of
naloxone. This withdrawal sign is readily measured and is an objective index
of the withdrawal syndrome. The antinociceptive activities of the enkephalin

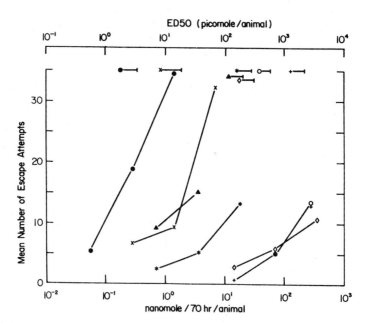

analogs were estimated by the median effective dose required to inhibit repetitive shaking movements, induced by immersion of anesthetized rats in ice water.

ENKEPHALIN ANALOGS AND PHYSICAL DEPENDENCE

The amino acid sequences, abbreviated names, symbol in Fig. 1, and source of the enkephalin analogs are given below. [D-Ala^2,D-Leu^5]enkephalin (BW 180C, symbol -o-), [NMeTyr^1,D-Ala^2]metenkephalin (BW 984C, symbol -*-) and [NMeTyr^1, D-Ala^2]metenkephalinamide (BW 985C, symbol -▲-) were gifts of S. Wilkinson. D. Roemer and S. Bajusz contributed [D-Ala^2, NMePhe^4, Met(O)^5-ol]enkephalin (FK 33-824, symbol -●-) and [D-Met^2, Pro^5]enkephalinamide (symbol -x-), respectively. J.K. Chang provided the [D-Ala^2,Leu^5]enkephalinamide (symbol -◊-) and [D-Ala^2]metenkephalinamide (symbol -+-).

The results (Fig. 1) obtained from the seven enkephalin analogs show there is a positive rank correlation between antinociceptive and physical dependence activities (Spearman rank correlation test, P<.05). The actual delivery rates of these peptides from the minipumps have not yet been measured, so the estimation of physical dependence potency may need adjustment. These preliminary data do seem sufficient, however, to predict that the enkephalin analog with the higher antinociceptive activity will also be one with a higher potential for producing physical dependence.

REFERENCES
1. Wei, E. and Loh, Horace (1976) Science, 193, 1262-1263.

Characteristics and Function of Opioids, editors Van Ree and Terenius
© *1978 Elsevier/North-Holland Biomedical Press*

β-ENDORPHIN GROOMING IN THE RAT: SINGLE DOSE TOLERANCE

V.M. WIEGANT, J. JOLLES and W.H. GISPEN
Division of Molecular Neurobiology, Rudolf Magnus Institute for Pharmacology,
Laboratory of Physiological Chemistry, Institute of Molecular Biology,
University of Utrecht, Utrecht (The Netherlands)

In rats, intraventricular administration of low doses of ACTH, MSH and fragments of LPH induces display of excessive grooming[3,4,5,7]. This peptide-induced behavior can be suppressed by peripheral administration of specific opiate antagonists (naloxone, naltrexone). As low doses of morphine also induce this behavioral response, it was suggested that part of the behavioral effects of these peptides and morphine may be mediated by a common substrate, presumably involving dopaminergic pathways[12,13]. Recently, it was observed that daily intraventricular administration of $ACTH_{1-24}$ for 10 days did not result in a reduction of the observed grooming behavior[2]. However, a remarkable suppression of the grooming response was observed when a second injection of $ACTH_{1-24}$ was given within 8 h after the first injection[9]. This single dose-induced tolerance was not the result of corticosteroid feedback and could be eliminated by pretreatment with the opiate antagonist naloxone. At this acute level, a cross tolerance of $ACTH_{1-24}$ with β-endorphin, $|D-Phe^7|ACTH_{4-10}$ or morphine was demonstrated[9]. The present study was undertaken to investigate whether there is a similar acute tolerance to β-endorphin grooming.

Male rats of an inbred Wistar strain (140-160 g body weight) received into their foramen interventriculare a plastic canula one week prior to the experimental session. The behavioral procedure consisting of a 15th sec grooming behavior sampling technique has been described previously[4,9]. After intraventricular injection by free hand into the conscious rats, the subjects were placed individually into glass observation boxes and recording of the behavior commenced 15 min thereafter and lasted another 50 min. The maximal possible grooming score therefore is 200. As can be seen in Fig. 1, a single dose of β-endorphin, dissolved in 3 μl saline, induces excessive grooming in the rat. In the figure the amount of saline-induced grooming (30) is subtracted from the value obtained after the peptide injection. The standard error of the mean of saline-induced grooming is represented by the hatched bar. The grooming response is dose-dependent and doses in the range of 100-300 ng already elicit nearly maximal grooming behavior. As was noted before, administration of low doses of β-endorphin not only elicits grooming but also excitation[5]. If higher doses are

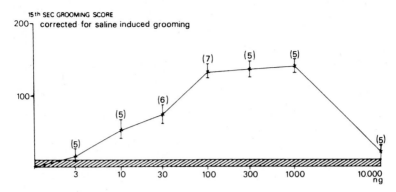

Fig. 1. β-endorphin-induced excessive grooming: dose response curve.
( ) = number of rats

used, grooming is hardly displayed (Fig. 1) but then wet-dog shake behavior followed by a cataleptic state is observed[1,6,8].

If rats first treated with 0.3 μg receive a second injection of β-endorphin (0.3 μg) 24 or 48 or 72 h later, the second injection is as effective as the first one (Fig. 2). However, the response to a second injection is greatly reduced if the interval between the two injections is relatively short. For, 2 and 4 h after the first injection hardly any excessive grooming can be elicited by a second injection with the same dose of β-endorphin. As the interval between the two injections increases, the effect of the first injection slowly dissipates.

In subsequent experiments on the nature of this phenomenon, a 4 h interval

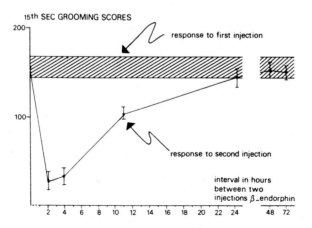

Fig. 2. Single dose tolerance to β-endorphin grooming (0.3 μg/3 μl).

between first and second injection was used. As can be seen in Fig. 3A, it is
unlikely that the observed reduction in grooming activity after the second injection can be explained in terms of habituation to the experimental situation
as saline/β-endorphin treated rats display a normal grooming response. It could
be argued that the interval between the two injections is short enough to allow
accumulation of the peptide to a dose sufficient to result in the cataleptic
state known to occur when higher doses of morphine or β-endorphin are used[1,8].
However, the data in Fig. 3B indicate that a single dose of 0.6 µg β-endorphin
per se is effective in inducing excessive grooming. Furthermore, as was reported
for $ACTH_{1-24}$, increasing the dose of β-endorphin used in the second injection
overcomes in part the reduction in grooming (Fig. 3B). Thus it seems unlikely
that β-endorphin still present from the first injection, can be responsible for
the observed loss of effectiveness of the second injection. The results from the
last experiments reported here imply that activation of opiate receptors may
underly the development of insensitivity of the rats to the second injection
with β-endorphin. As Fig. 3C shows, pretreatment with naloxone (1 mg/kg s.c.,
5 min prior to the first injection of β-endorphin, 0.3 µg) not only inhibits
grooming in the first injection as expected[5], but also prevents the development
of acute tolerance to β-endorphin.

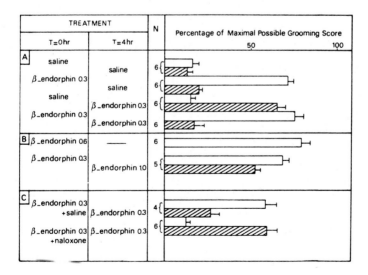

Fig. 3.   Naloxone blockade of acute tolerance to β-endorphin grooming.
Open bar : response to first injection ; doses in µg.
Closed bar: response to second injection; doses in µg.

450

The data presented here are in complete agreement with similar studies on ACTH-induced grooming[9] and once more underscore the notion that fragments of LPH and ACTH, and morphine have a common neural substrate for part of their behavioral effects[12,13]. It is tempting to speculate that the observed reduction of effectiveness of the second injection relates to the acute tolerance which is known to occur to temperature responses to morphine. The time course of both processes seems remarkably similar[10,11]. Since no apparent long term tolerance to β-endorphin (this study) or $ACTH_{1-24}$[2,9] grooming seems to develop, the grooming model may be extremely useful to study the phenomenon of acute tolerance to CNS effects of opiates and opioids.

ACKNOWLEDGEMENTS

The authors greatly acknowledge the assistence of J.H. Brakkee, R.J. Teunisse and C. Wirasantosa. Synthetic β-endorphin was obtained from Dr H.M.Greven, Organon Int.B.V., Oss (The Netherlands).

REFERENCES

1. Bloom, F., Segal, H., Ling, N. and Guillemin, R. (1976) Science, 194, 630-634.

2. Colbern,D.L.,Green,E.,Isaacson,R.L.and Gispen,W.H.(1978)Behav.biol.,in press

3. Ferrari, W., Gessa, G.L. and Vargiu, L. (1963) Ann. N.Y. Acad. Sci., 104, 330-345.

4. Gispen, W.H., Wiegant, V.M., Greven, H.M. and de Wied, D. (1975) Life Sci., 17, 645-652.

5. Gispen, W.H., Wiegant, V.M., Bradbury, A.F., Hulme, E.C., Smyth, D.G., Snell, C.R. and de Wied, D. (1976) Nature, 264, 794-795.

6. Holaday, J.W., Loh, H.H. and Li, C.H. (1978) Life Sci., 22, 1525-1536.

7. Izumi, K., Donaldson, J. and Barbeau, A. (1973) Life Sci., 12, 203-210.

8. Jacquet, Y.F. and Marks, N. (1976) Science, 194, 632-635.

9. Jolles, J., Wiegant, V.M. and Gispen, W.H. (1978) Neurosci. Lett., in press.

10. Lotti, V.J., Lomax, P. and George, R. (1966) Int. J. Neuropharmacol., 5, 35-42.

11. Rosenfeld, G.C. and Burks, T.R. (1977) J. Pharmacol. Exp. Ther., 202, 654-659.

12. Wiegant, V.M., Gispen, W.H., Terenius, L. and de Wied, D. (1977) Psychoneuroendocrinol., 2, 63-69.

13. Wiegant, V.M., Cools, A.R. and Gispen, W.H. (1977) Eur. J. Pharmacol., 41, 343-345.

Characteristics and Function of Opioids, editors Van Ree and Terenius
© 1978 Elsevier/North-Holland Biomedical Press

OPIATE RECEPTOR AUTORADIOGRAPHY: IN VITRO LABELING OF TISSUE SLICES

W. Scott Young, III and Michael J. Kuhar

Department of Pharmacology, Johns Hopkins University School of Medicine, Balto.,
Maryland 21205, USA.

INTRODUCTION

The demonstration of specific binding of opiates to a physiologically relevant receptor[1-3] stimulated efforts to localize the receptor in the central
nervous system[4-5]. The regional distribution of the opiate receptor as measured
by these biochemical assays often correlated with known or suspected sites of
opiate actions. However, the resolution provided by in vivo autoradiographic
techniques[6-8] revealed much more information and furthered our understanding of
several opiate actions. The use of an in vitro method should allow further
advances in our knowledge, especially if it is applied to the study of humans
through the use of tritiated opioid peptides.

MATERIALS AND METHODS

Male rats are perfused with ice-cold 0.5% formaldehyde in phosphate-buffered
saline. 10 μ-thick sections are cut in a Harris cryostat and thaw-mounted on
gelatine-coated slides.

The slides are then incubated in solutions containing ^{3}H-diprenorphine or
^{3}H-leucine-enkephalin. The sections are then rinsed for 20 min at 0° and
dipped in Kodak nuclear emulsion NTB 3. The slides are hung for 20 min, placed
at 4° for 3-4 weeks and subsequently developed and stained. Control sections
are incubated in the presence of 1 μM naloxone. Slides are also exposed to
light for assessment of negative chemography.

RESULTS

Figure 1 demonstrates light and dark-field photomicrographs of rat striatum
incubated in tritiated diprenorphine. There is a paucity of grains in the
white matter of the corpus callosum and the typical high grain density subcal-
losal streak seen previously in in vitro studies[8]. Similar results have been
obtained with ^{3}H-leucine-enkephalin. No binding is seen in the presence of
naloxone.

SUMMARY

A method for demonstrating in vitro regional distribution of the opiate receptor in tissue slices is described. Work is currently in progress to adapt
this technique to the study of the human central nervous system

This work was supported by NIMH Grant DA 00266. MJK is the recipient of
RCDA Award, Type II MH 00053.

452

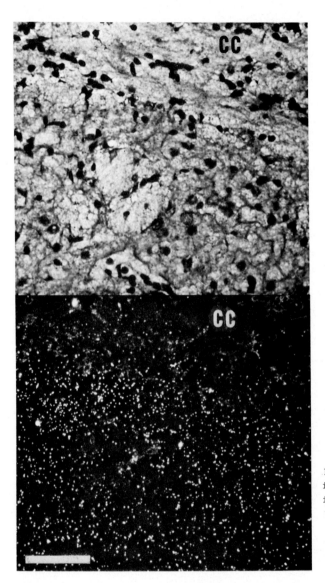

Fig. 1. Photomicrographs show
ing ^{3}H-diprenorphine binding
in the striatum (notice streak
below corpus callosum, CC).
Bar represents 50 μ.

REFERENCES

1. Simon, E.J., Hiller, J.M. and Edelman, I. (1973) Proc. Natl. Acad. Sci., 70,
    1947-1949.
2. Pert, C.B. and Snyder, S.H. (1973) Science 179, 1011-1014.
3. Terenius, L. (1973) Acta Pharmacol. Toxicol., 32, 317-320.
4. Kuhar, M.J., Pert, C.B. and Snyder, S.H. (1973) Nature, 245, 447-450.
5. Hiller, J.M., Pearson, J. and Simon, E.J. (1973) Res. Comm. Chem. Pathol.
    Pharmacol., 6, 1052-1062.
6. Atweh, S.F. and Kuhar, M.J. (1977) Brain Res., 124, 53-67.
7. Atweh, S.F. and Kuhar, M.J. (1977) Brain Res., 129, 1-12.
8. Atweh, S.F. and Kuhar, M.J. (1977) Brain Res., 134, 393-405.

Characteristics and Function of Opioids, editors Van Ree and Terenius
© 1978 Elsevier/North-Holland Biomedical Press

MULTIPLE OPIATE RECEPTORS REFLECTED IN REGION-SPECIFIC ALTERATIONS IN
BRAIN CYCLIC NUCLEOTIDES

K.A.BONNET, S.A.GUSIK and A.G.SUNSHINE
Department of Psychiatry, New York University School of Medicine,
550 First Avenue, New York, New York 10016

ABSTRACT

Opiate mediated brain region-specific changes in cyclic nucleotides are
interpreted to reflect localization of different opiate receptor types.
Morphine displaces calcium from thalamic membranes, blocking norepinephrine-
stimulation of adenylate cyclase.

INTRODUCTION

The wide range of pharmacological effects of opiate agonists has
prompted differentiation between classes of opioid agonists, antagonists and mixed agonist-antagonists. It has been reasoned that
opiate receptors with different affinities for specific opioid agonists
may mediate different pharmacological actions, and those with higher
specific affinities may not be of more importance than those with
lower affinity for a specific agonist[1,2]. Considerable work by Martin
and coworkers in the spinal dog preparation has led to the proposal
that three differentiable classes of opiate receptors are functionally
discriminable: μ-(morphine like; produces euphoria), κ-(benzomorphan
like; produces sedation), and σ-(mediates hallucinatory effects of
some opioid agonists such as cyclazocine and SKF 10,047)[3]. Generally,
morphine is a high affinity μ-agonist with some κ-receptor agonist
activity as well. Ketocyclazocine, cyclazocine and WIN35,197-2 are
high affinity κ-agonists, and cyclazocine is also a μ-antagonist.
Finally, cyclazocine is a partial σ-agonist that effects some apo-
morphine-like effects suggestive of an interaction with the dopamine
system. Tolerance develops to all three agonist-receptor types, and
all are blocked by naloxone or naltrexone but with greatest effect in
the order μ<κ<σ. The localization of these putative receptor types
and their functional interaction with neurotransmitter systems in
the nervous system remains unknown.

Kosterlitz has referred to multiple opiate receptor types as well,
based on resistance to naloxone reversability of opioid effects in
in vitro studies, and based on differential affinities of mouse vas
deferens, guinea pig ileum and rat brain for a given set of opiate
narcotics and peptides[4]. The enkephalins were most active in the

mouse vas deferens, β—endorphin and morphine were equipotent in vas
deferens and in guinea pig ileum, and the benzomorphans were markedly
more potent in the guinea pig ileum. β—Endorphin has recently been
shown to exhibit in vitro receptor binding characteristics more like
a benzomorphan than like morphine, and the peptide exert κ—agonist
effects in the guinea pig ileum.[5]

Coupling of the opiate receptor has remained a difficult area of
study. Two areas have proven fruitful, cyclic nucleotide metabolism
and neuronal calcium displacement. Collier and Roy[6] demonstrated
stereospecific inhibition of rat brain adenylate cyclase stimulation
by PGE with no apparent effect on the activity of the basal enzyme
or the NaF stimulated enzyme. The inhibitory effects were dose related
and correlated well with analgesic potency. Subsequently, a very fine
correlation with opiate receptor agonist inhibition of basal and PGE
or adenosine—stimulated adenylate cyclase was reported for NG108-15
cells containing opiate receptors[7,8]. The enkephalins also have a
potent inhibitory effect in these cells. However, these direct
biochemical studies applied to rat brain preparations remain contro-
versial, and several laboratories have reported opiate agonist—stimulated adenylate cyclase[9-10]. Incubation of the cells in the presence
of endorphins or narcotic agonist for more than twelve hours results
in elevation of adenylate cyclase activity, and removal of the opioid
results in sudden dramatic increases in 3',5'AMP levels[11]. We, and
others, have reported that some brain regions show decreased adenylate
cyclase activity and lowered 3',5'AMP levels with acute morphine and
that during tolerance there is increased adenylate cyclase activity
and 3',5'AMP levels[12-13]. However, on withdrawal the massive increases
in 3',5'AMP levels in brain that are predicted in theory,and from
the studies of the neuroblastoma—glioma cells, were reported by few
investigators and were not detected by several others[14-16]. It is
likely that such an event in brain may occur only in select brain
regions at very specific times after naloxone challenge such as we
report here for the rat thalamus.

The role of calcium in membrane stabilization and in the functioning
of neuronal membranes is well established. Early studies by Kaneto[17]
showed calcium infusion to attenuate opiate effects. Others have
shown recently that opiates precipitously deplete brain regions of Ca^{++}
and in vitro opiates stereospecifically displace calcium binding in

synaptic membranes in a naloxone-reversible manner[18,19]. Stimulation-
coupled release of neurotransmitters requires calcium influx, and the
activation of dopamine-sensitive adenylate cyclase, β-adrenergic-sen-
sitive adenylate cyclase, the regulation of high Km phosphodiesterase
and of guanylate cyclase are all calcium dependent[20-23]. We report
here a summary of some early studies of opiate modulation of calcium-
dependent activation of neurotransmitter-stimulated adenylate cyclase.

Our intention was to systematically differentiate between the effect
of morphine(a μ- and κ-agonist) and 1-cyclazocine(a κ- and σ-agoinst
and a μ-antagonist) on 3',5'AMP and 3',5'GMP levels in seven discrete
rat brain regions simultaneously and at time of peak pharmacological
effect. We summarize subsequent studies of one promising region, the
thalamus, with in vitro adenylate cyclase studies and with precipitated withdrawal from dependence in vivo.

MATERIALS AND METHODS

Sixty day old male Sprague-Dawley rats were injected s.c.with
morphine sulfate(10 mg/Kg), 1-cyclazocine (15 mg/Kg), naloxone (2 mg/
Kg) or saline. Dose ranging studies for effects on pain sensitivity
were followed by systematic time course determination for each drug.
Peak time of pharmacological effect was chosen as optimal sacrifice
time for biochemical study. Rats were sacrificed by a specialized
rapid freezing technique for cyclic nucleotide level determinations
and parallel experiments with microwave fixation gave excellent agreement between the methods (2.5kW,3sec.). Frozen brains were removed
to a freezing microtome stage and sectioned. Discrete brain regions
were punched out with specially made punches for each structure.
Frozen tissue plugs were homogenized and prepared for cyclic nucleotide
determiation by the procedures described elsewhere[12]. Dependence
was produced in vivo by routine implantation of a pellet containing
75mg morphine base, and animals were challenged at 72 hours by inject-
2mg/Kg naloxone-HCl. Withdrawal signs were clearly evident a four minutes postchallenge and animals were sacrificed at that point for biochemical study as outlined above. In vitro studies with thalamus
membranes were carried out with the preparation described by Gnegy,
et al.[24]. Membrane preparations were incubated at 37˚C with drugs,
precipitated at 50,000xg,20 minutes and the pellet resuspended for
adenylate cyclase assay. The 50,000xg supernatant was utilized to
determine the concentration of calcium released from the membranes

as a result of drug treatment. Calcium was determined by atomic absorption spectrometry.

RESULTS AND DISCUSSION

Systemic injection of either morphine or l-cyclazocine produced
increases in 3',5'AMP levels in thalamus and the cortex that corresponded to peak analgesic time (Table 1). This effect was blocked by
prior adminstration of systemic naloxone. According to the classification scheme of Martin and coworkers, this elevation of 3',5'AMP
levels could suggest a predominance of κ-receptor sites in these two
structures. This confirms our earlier report of morphine-induced
elevations in thalamic 3',5'AMP.[12] Neither morphine nor cyclazocine
affected 3',5'GMP levels in these structures. However, both drugs
effected significant elevations in cerebellar 3',5'GMP levels. This
effect substantiates an earlier report by others [25], but it is not
certain if the effect is the result of direct action at the cerebellum
or the result of neurotransmitter-related opiate effects in the mid-
brain cell bodies that project to the cerebellum.

Morphine produced effects that were distinct from cyclazocine and
that may be attributable to action at a μ-type of receptor site.
Effects of this type are most evident in the periaqueductal gray and
in the substantia nigra(Table 2). The 3',5'AMP levels and the 3',5'-
GMP levels were both significantly depressed by morphine in these two
structures. Naloxone given prior to morphine prevented most of these
effects. The depression of 3',5'AMP and 3',5'GMP levels in these areas
is in agreement with our earlier reports, and is analogous to the
effects of opioids on the neuroblastoma-glioma hybrid cell adenylate
cyclase activity.

l-Cyclazocine exerts effects that are distinct from morphine and
are attributed to pharmacological action through a σ-type receptor[3].
l-Cyclazocine elevated 3',5'AMP levels in the periaqueductal gray and
in the substantia nigra(Table 2). These effects were somewhat surprising since they appeared in the same structures as the μ-type of
effects of morphine. The effect of cyclazocine on 3',5'AMP levels was
opposite in direction of that of morphine but cannot be attributed
directly to the μ-antagonist activity since the 3',5'AMP levels were
not affected by the pure antagonist naloxone.

Changes in region-specific cyclic nucleotide levels are seen to
occur with cyclazocine or naloxone and might be interpreted to be due

Table 1

Narcotic effects attributable to the "kappa"-type receptors in rat brain regions. These effects are selectively those significant changes in cyclic nucleotide levels reliably seen following systemic administration of morphine or cyclazocine that are prevented by prior administration of naloxone.

Structure		Drug Treatment			
		Saline	Morphine	Cyclazocine	Nal/Morph
Thalamus	3',5'AMP[†]	3.7 + 0.4	4.7 + 0.1*	4.7 + 0.1*	4.0 + 0.1
Cortex	3',5'AMP[†]	5.7 + 0.2	6.5 + 0.1*	7.1 + 0.1*	5.2 + 0.1
Cerebellum	3',5'GMP[††]	671 + 12	924 + 30*	818 + 9*	698 + 49

[†]Figures are picomoles 3',5'AMP per milligram protein (mean + SEM)
[††]Figures are femtomoles 3',5'GMP per milligram protein (mean + SEM)

Table 2

Contrasting effects of morphine and cyclazocine on cyclic nucleotide levels in the rat brain periventricular gray and the substantia nigra. Effects unique to morphine may reflect action at putative "mu"-type receptors, whereas effects unique to cyclazocine may reflect action at "sigma"-type receptors. Prior naloxone treatment must attenuate "mu"-type effects.

Drug Treatment	Structure			
	Periventricular Gray		Substantia Nigra	
	3',5'AMP[†]	3',5'GMP[††]	3',5'AMP[†]	3',5'GMP[††]
Saline	7.9 + 0.2	361 + 5	9.0 + 0.4	572 + 21
Morphine Sulfate	3.1 + 0.1*	195 + 3*	5.4 + 0.4*	424 + 28*
Morphine + Naloxone	5.9 + 0.1	320 + 15	9.3 + 0.3	391 + 8*
1-Cyclazocine	11.7 + 0.4*	484 + 12*	9.9 + 0.7	562 + 14

[†]Figures are picomoles of 3',5'AMP per milligram protein (mean + SEM)
[††]Figures are femtomoles of 3',5'GMP per milligram protein (mean + SEM)
* p <.05

Table 3

Narcotic antagonist effects in three rat brain regions. These changes in cyclic nucleotide levels were seen after either naloxone or cyclazocine injection and were not seen in the case of naloxone when followed by an injection of morphine sulfate.

Structure		Drug Treatment		
		Saline	Naloxone	Cyclazocine
Thalamus	3',5'GMP	205 + 5	164 + 11*	150 + 13*
Periventricular Gray	3',5'GMP	361 + 16	676 + 21*	484 + 12*
Cerebellum	3',5'AMP	5.1 +0.1	3.8 + 0.1*	4.2 +0.1*

Figures are as in previous tables.
*p <.05

Table 4

"Nonspecific" effects of narcotic agonists and
antagonists on cyclic nucleotide levels in striata
of rats sacrificed at peak pharmacological effect
time for each drug treatment.

Drug	Time	3',5'AMP	3',5'GMP
Saline	30 min.	4.76	156
Morphine	30 min.	4.52(95%)	174(111%)
Naloxone	5 min.	5.94(125%)	172(110%)
Naloxone	50 min.	11.20(235%)	---
Nal + Morphine	50/30min.	7.73(162%)	157(101%)
Cyclazocine	5 min.	7.94(167%)	175(112%)

Table 5

PREINCUBATION	REINCUBATION	CALCIUM LOSS*	β-ADRENERGIC STIMULATION OF ADENYLATE CYCLASE
BUFFER	BUFFER	2.6	+ 65%
	NALOXONE	1.5	+ 55%
LEVORPHANOL	BUFFER	3.8	- 33%
	NALOXONE	2.3	+ 28%
DEXTRORPHAN	BUFFER	1.6	+ 55%
	NALOXONE	1.7	+ 33%

* Figures are nanograms of calcium released from 400μg
of thalamus membrane protein.

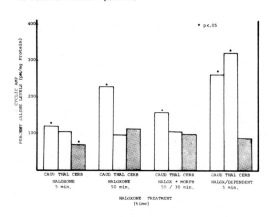

The effects of naloxone treatment on brain region cyclic AMP levels.

Figure 1

μ–type antagonist action. These effects are presented in Table 3. Narcotic antagonist activity of this type appears to significantly elevate 3',5'AMP levels in the hypothalamus, the 3',5'GMP levels in the thalamus and in the periventricular gray. This is particularly interesting in that morphine lowered both cyclic nucleotides in periventricular gray. It is possible that this action of μ-type antagonists on 3',5'GMP levels in the periventricular gray might contribute to their ability to precipitate abstinence signs when injected into this region in the morphine dependent rat[26].

In all the drug effects reported here, few specific effects could be attributed to cyclic nucleotide changes in the striatum. Naloxone and cyclazocine elevated 3',5'AMP levels significantly, and naloxone plus morphine partially attenuated that elevation (Table 4). It is likely that changes in the striatum are more readily detectable at different postinjection times with various of the drugs used here[12] and that the richness of interacting opiate receptor, biogenic amine and cholinergic systems impinging on cyclic nucleotide regulation via various pathways renders discrimination of specific effects difficult in in vivo studies.

These data are generally suggestive of multiple opiate receptor-mediated changes in cyclic nucleotide regulation in particular brain regions containing high densities of opiate receptors. It appears that κ–agonist effects might account for elevations in thalamic 3',5'-AMP , μ–agonist effects might result in depression of 3',5'AMP and of 3',5'GMP levels in periventricular gray and substantia nigra. Recently a very similar distinction has been made based on enkephalin-induced epileptogenesis in thalamus and periventricular gray[27]. We would suggest that a crude analogy might be drawn between the pharmacological sensitivities of the rat thalamus and the guinea pig ileum on the one hand, and between the rat periventricular gray and the neuroblastoma-glioma on the other hand.

We have further investigated the response of the thalamus adenylate cyclase system to morphine, benzomorphans and enkephalins in vitro. These data will be reported elsewhere, but generally there is a good correspondence between κ–receptor agonists and adenylate cyclase stimulation in thalamic membranes. Met- and leu-enkephalin both stimulate, but with quite differing potencies. It seemed important to distinguish between the immediate effects of opioids on adenylate cyclase regulation and the subsequent effects on neurotransmitter systems that are in close proximity and depend upon membrane calcium for their postreceptor activation of adenylate cyclase. Thalamic membranes were incubated for five minutes in the presence of buffer, levorphanol or dextrorphan. Each was then further incubated for five minutes in buffer or naloxone. The supernatants were then used to measure calcium loss from membranes (400 μg protein in each sample), and the membranes washed for use in subsequent adenylate cyclase assay. Basal and norepinepherine-stimulated incorporation of ^{14}C-ATP into ^{14}C-3',5'AMP were determined using aminophylline as phosphodiesterase inhibitor in all cases. Results are summarized in Table 5. Levorphanol ($10^{-6}M$) significantly increases calcium loss from thalamic membranes, and this was reversed by subsequent incubation with naloxone at the same concentration. Dextrorphan stabilized membrane calcium and naloxone had no subsequent effect. In direct correlation with calcium membrane loss in these same samples, the ability to stimulate adenylate cyclase by 10^{-4} M norepinepherine was completely lost with levorphanol. The subsequent naloxone treatment reversed this to allow some recovery of stimulation. Dextrorphan alone or in combination with subsequent naloxone treatment had no significant effect on norepinepherine-stimluation of adenylate cyclase.

It is apparent that the sequence of events in a specific brain region encountering acute opioid flux may be quite individual in that one must take into account the initial consequences of opioid receptor binding, such as region-specific cyclic nucleotide changes and calcium displacement, and the secondary consequences that develop a very short time later, such as attenuated neurotransmitter release[28] and attenuated biogenic amine receptor-mediated adenylate cyclase stimulation.

Several years ago Collier proposed that during the state of opiate dependence there develops a supersensitivity in neurohormonal systems such that displacement or withdrawal of the opiate results in exaggerated responses in these systems as reflected in withdrawal symptoms[29]. This has been difficult to demonstrate in the brain. Neuroblastoma-glioma hybrid cells grown in presence of opiate agonists for several hours clearly exhibit the predicted "release" phenomenon[11]. Klee, et al. have developed a model to account for the exaggerated 3',5'AMP formation on abrupt withdrawal from opiate dependence that suggests hyper-

trophic development of factors regulating adenylate cyclase[30] This is
thought to occur in response to opiate agonists or other substances
that effect inhibitory modulation of adenylate cyclase activity. Yet,
it has been difficult to substantiate this effect in brain tissues of
opiate-dependent animals[16] Considerable pharmacological evidence has
shown that previously drug-naive rats exhibit a quasi-abstinence syndrome when treated with drugs that inhibit phosphodiesterase degradation of 3',5'AMP[31] This effect is enhanced by narcotic antagonists
and is suppressed by opioid agonists. Further, treatment with these
phosphodiesterase inhibitors increases withdrawal intensity in heroin-
dependent animals challenged with naloxone   .

   We have examined cyclic nucleotide levels in several discrete brain
regions of morphine-dependent animals at four minutes following a
challenge with naloxone when signs of withdrawal are clearly evident.
Two particularly interesting phenomena are shown in Figure 1. Naloxone
injected into opiate-naive rats produced increases in 3',5'AMP levels
in striatum that were evident at 5 minutes and much larger at 50 minutes postinjection. Challenge of the morphine-dependent rat with
naloxone elevated striatal 3',5'AMP levels much like the 50 minute
effect in the naive rat. It is difficult to interpret the increase
in the dependent animal striatum as being central to overt signs of
narcotic withdrawal. Naloxone had no effect on thalamic 3',5'AMP
levels in the opiate-naive rat at any postinjection time studied.
However, in the dependent rat thalamus there occurred a very large
increase in 3',5'AMP levels much like that seen in the dependent
neuroblastoma-glioma hybrid cells. This effect seems to be specific
to withdrawal from opiate-dependence, then. A small increase in
the periaqueductal gray 3',5'AMP levels was also evident(50%) and
this was seen only in the withdrawing dependent animal brain, as well.
No significant changes were seen in 3',5'AMP levels in substantia
nigra or in the cerebellum or cortex of these withdrawal-state animals.
It is uncertain at this point whether the naloxone-induced elevations
in 3',5'AMP levels in dependent animal striatum, thalamus and periaqueductal gray directly involve the opiate receptor coupling to the
affected adenylate cyclases or if the changes in levels are the result
of release of nourotransmitter receptor-coupled adenylate cyclases from
opiate receptor controlled modulation. Nonetheless, turther study of
the thalamus in the naive and dependent states may prove fruitful in

specifying the locus of adaptation to chronic opioid agonist encounter
that results in substantial alterations in the regulation of adenylate
cyclase. Similar studies in the periaqueductal gray of the dependent
rat may prove to be very analogous to the neuroblastoma-glioma hybrid
cell model system for dependence. The results reported here give
substantial biochemical support to the theoretical and pharmacological
models currently subscribed to concerning opiate dependence and the
factors mediating withdrawal phenomena.

The studies we have summarized here indicate that the biochemical
differentiation of opiate receptor types and their relative regional
localization in the brain may be essential to the understanding of the
coupling of those receptors to factors regulating cyclic nucleotide
metabolism. Moreover, the effects seen in the thalamus contrast with
those in the periventricular gray in terms of the direction of effect
on cyclic nucleotide levels and possibly metabolism. Since we have
postulated a μ-type of receptor system in the periventricular gray
that lowers cyclic nucleotide levels it may be possible that in vitro
studies currently in progress can provide an analogy to the neuroblastoma-glioma hybrid. We have postulated a κ-type opiate receptor
system in thalamus that elevates cyclic nucleotide levels in vivo
and in vitro. Yet the analogy to a κ-system may be less satisfactory
than to specify a non-μ system. Nonetheless the differentiation between these regions,and the agonists and cyclic nucleotides operative
in each,can provide a highly specific preparation in which to study
the in vitro regulation of adenylate cyclase by opiate receptor-mediated changes in calcium flux and protein factors mediating adenylate
cyclase activation[20,30] Finally, the role of protein kinases in the
phosphorylation of specific neuronal membrane proteins is known to
relate to adenylate cyclase sensitivity and to the activity of the
protein factors mediating the stimulation of some adenylate cyclases[24].
We recently demonstrated that the phosphorylation of select membrane
proteins is attenuated in chronically dependent animal brain[32-34].The
use of highly specific opioid agonists in selected brain regions can
permit the direct study of adenylate cyclase regulation, and guanylate
cyclase activity, at the levels of coupling through membrane calcium,
activator proteins and membrane phosphorylating enzymes.

SUMMARY

The opiate regulation of cyclic nucleotide metabolism in rat brain regions has been studied in acute and chronic states.

(a) Thalamus 3',5'AMP is increased in vivo and in vitro by morphine or cyclazocine;

(b) Periventricular gray 3',5'AMP and 3',5'GMP are lowered by morphine;

(c) These contrasting effects suggest differing opiate receptor types in the two regions, and that the consequences of agonist binding to the opiate receptor has different consequences on cyclic nucleotide metabolism in each region;

(d) Opiate agonist stimulation of thalamus adenylate cyclase is accompanied by measureable displacement of calcium;

(e) Displacement of thalamic membrane calcium prevents subsequent stimulation of adenylate cyclase by norepinepherine;

(f) Naloxone challenge of morphine dependent animals results in 220% increases in thalamus 3',5'AMP levels at the time of withdrawal symptom appearence.

Supported by Grant DA 1113 from National Institute on Drug Abuse.

REFERENCES

1. Martin, W.R. (1967)Pharmacol. Rev.,19, 463.

2. Martin, W.R. (1976)J. Pharm. Exp.Ther.,197, 517.

3. Gilbert,P.E. and Martin, W.R. (1976) J. Pharm.Exp.Ther.,198, 66.

4. Lord, J.,Waterfield,A.,Hughes,J. and Kosterlitz,H.(1977) Nature, 267, 495.

5. Birdsall, N. (1976)Opiates and Endogenous Opioid Peptides, H.W. Kosterlitz,ed. North Holland, Amsterdam,pp19-26.

6. Collier,H.O.J. and Roy,A.C.(1974) Nature, 248, 24.

7. Sharma,S.K.,Klee,W. and Nirenberg,M.(1975) Proc.Nat.Acad.Sci.72,590.

8. Traber,J.,Fischer,K. and Hamprecht,B.(1975)Nature, 253, 120.

9. Puri,S., Cochin,J.and Volicer,P.(1976)J.Neurochem., 27, 1551.

10. Katz, J.B. and Catravas, G.(1977) Brain Res.,120, 263.

11. Lambert,A., Klee, W. and Nirenberg,M.(1976)Proc.Nat.Acad.Sci., 73, 3165.

12. Bonnet, K.A. (1975) Life Sci.,16, 1877.

13. Iwatsubo,M. and Clouet,D.H.(1975)Bioch. Pharmacol.,24,1499

14. Mehta,C., and Johnson, W.(1974) Fed. Proc. 33, 493.

15. VonVoigtlander,P. and Losey,E.(1977) Brain Res.,128,275.

464

16. Katz,J. and Catravas, G.(1977) Brain Res.,120, 263.

17. Kaneto, H. (1971) in Narcotic Drugs, Plenum Press, New York.pp.300.

18. Ross,D.H. and Cardenas, H.(1977) Life Sci.,20, 1455.

19. Yamamoto,H., Harris,R.A.,Loh,H.H. and Way,E.L.(1978),J.Pharm.Exp. Ther. 205, 255.

20. Gnegy,M., Uzunov, P. and Costa,E.(1976) Proc.Nat.Acad.Sci. 73,3887.

21. Schwabe,U. and Daly,J.(1977) J.Pharm.Exp.Ther. 202, 134.

22. Brostrom, C.O. and Wolff,D. (1976) Arch.Bioch.Biophys. 172, 301.

23. Goldberg,N. and Haddox,M.(1977) Ann. Rev.Biochem. 46, 823.

24. Gnegy,M., Uzunov,P. and Costa, E.(1976)Proc.Nat.Acad.Sci. 73, 352.

25. Askew,K.D. and Charalampous,W.(1976) Experientia, 32, 1454.

26. Young, R., Levitt,R. and Weyant,M.(1977) Neurosci.Abst. 3,980.

27. Frenk,H., McCarty,B. and Liebeskind,J.(1978)Science, 200, 335.

28. Loh,H.H.,Brase,D., Sampath-Kanna,S.,Mar,J. and Way,E.L.(1976) Nature, 264, 567.

29. Collier,H.O.J.(1966) Adv.Drug Res.,3, 171.

30. Sharma,S.K.,Klee,W. and Nirenberg,M.(1977) Proc.Nat.Acad.Sci., 74, 3365.

31. Francis,D.L.,Cuthbert,N.J.,Dineen,L.,Schneider,C. and Collier,H.O. (1976) in Opiates and Endogenous Opioid Peptides, Kosterlitz,H.W. ed., North Holland, Amsterdam.pp. 169.

32. Ehrlich,Y.,Brunngraber,E.,and Bonnet,K.(1977)Trans.Amer.Soc.Neuro- chem., 8, 82.

33. Bonnet,K., Branchey,L.,Friedhoff,A. and Ehrlich,Y.(1978) Life Sci. 22, 2003.

34. Ehrlich,Y.,Bonnet,K.,Davis,L.and Brunngraber,E.(1978) Life Sci. (in press).

Characteristics and Function of Opioids, editors Van Ree and Terenius
© *1978 Elsevier/North-Holland Biomedical Press*

FURTHER STUDIES ON THE LOCALIZATION AND FUNCTION OF OPIATE RECEPTORS ON
STRIATAL NEURONS OF RAT

CASACCI F., CARENZI A. and DELLA BELLA D.

ZAMBON S.p.A. Research Laboratories, Bresso-Milan, Italy.

ABSTRACT
    Evidence is reported that the lesion of the nigro-striatal pathway of rat
leads to a decrease of striatal opiate receptors that affects particularly the
high affinity binding sites. The block of dopamine (DA) synthesis by α-metilty-
rosine (α-MT) does not produce any change in both the number or the affinity
of striatal receptors for morphine. It is likely that the decrease of morphine
binding sites after 6-hydroxydopamine (6-OHDA) lesion is not due to the decrea
se of DA content in striatum. The destruction of intrinsic neurons by intra
striatal injection of kainic acid produces a fall in striatal opiate receptors
that affects in the same extent both high or low affinity binding sites.

INTRODUCTION
    It has been reported that both the lesion of the nigrostriatal pathway[1,2]
or the elimination of cortico-striatal afferents by cortical ablation reduce
the opiate receptor content of rat striatum. In agreement with a number of
biochemical studies[4,5,6], these observations are consistent with the view that
opiate receptors are localized to nerve terminals or axons. However, also the
destruction of intrinsic neurons by intrastriatal injection of kainic acid[7]
leads to a decrease of binding sites for opiates[2,8]. All these findings indica
te that in striatum opiate receptors may be associated not only with nerve
ending terminals of neurons projecting axons from substantia nigra or from
cerebral cortex, but also with axodendritic or axosomatic synapsis. Since two
populations of opiate receptors are present in striatum[9], we decided to investi
gate the effects of selective lesions on the kinetic of ^{3}H-dihydromorphine
(^{3}H-DHM) stereospecific binding (SSB) to striatal membrane preparations.
Furthermore, to exclude a possible conformational change of opiate receptors
due to a decrease of striatal DA following 6-OHDA lesion of the nigro-striatal
pathway, we studied the effect of α-MT wich impairs DA synthesis without
affecting nerve terminals, on the ^{3}H-DHM SSB.

MATERIALS AND METHODS
    Male Wistar rats were injected stereotaxically with 6-OHDA (8 μg/4 μl/5 min)
into left substantia nigra as described by Ungerstedt[10]. Animals were selected
8 days after 6-OHDA lesion by injecting apomorphine (0.4 mg/kg/s.c.). Only rats
showing positive response to apomorphine were used (at least 6 days later) to
perform opiate binding determinations. Membranes from rat striata were prepared
and assayed as described by Pastornak et al.[11] using different concentrations
of ^{3}H-DHM (88 Ci/mmol) as ligand. Opiate SSB is defined as the difference in
^{3}H-DHM binding in presence of either 1 μM dextrorphan or 1 μM levallorphan.
Kainic acid (2 μg/1 μl/1 min) was injected stereotaxically into the left

striatum as described by McGeer et al.[7]. DA dependent adenylate cyclase activity was used as an index of striatal intrinsic neurons degeneration. The enzyme activity was measured as described by Carenzi et al.[12]. Proteins were assayed following the procedure of Lowry et al.[13].

RESULTS

The ^{3}H-DHM SSB to membranes from 6-OHDA lesioned striata is about 30% lower than that of unlesioned side. The Scatchard analysis of ^{3}H-DHM SSB shows the presence in the normal striatum of two populations of opiate receptors as previously described by Pasternak and Snyder[9](fig. 1). In membrane preparations from striata of rats with 6-OHDA lesion of the nigrostriatal pathway the high affinity binding sites were clearly decreased (left panel, fig. 1). On the contrary, kainic acid degeneration of striatal intrinsic neurons seems to affect in the same extent (-40%) both the high or the low affinity binding sites for morphine (right panel, fig. 1). Basal and DA stimulated adenylate cyclase activity in homogenates of kainic acid injected striata was 60% lower than that of the controlateral unlesioned side. A treatment with α-MT (250 mg/kg i.p., 4 hrs before killing the animals) decreases by about 70% the content of DA in striatum[14] but does not affect the ^{3}H-DHM binding to striatal membrane preparations.

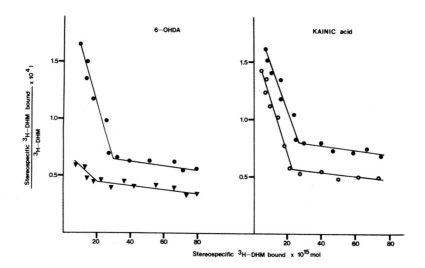

Fig. 1. Scatchard plots of ^{3}H-DHM SSB to membrane preparations from normal (●——●), 6-OHDA (▼——▼) or kainic acid (✪——✪) lesioned striata.

DISCUSSION

The presence of two populations of opiate receptors in striatum may suggest different functions or different localizations of the binding sites for morphine.

The fact that 6-OHDA lesion results in an extensive decrease of the high affini ty binding sites indicates that these receptors are highly concentrated on nerve ending terminals. On the contrary, kainic acid lesion affects in the same manner both high and low affinity receptors suggesting that morphine binding sites may be equally distributed on soma, dendritis and terminals of the striatal intrin sic neurons. Since morphine can modulate the sensitivity of striatal adenylate cyclase to DA[15] and some butyrophenones appear to possess both opiate receptor affinity as well as DA antagonistic properties[16], it was of interest to investi gate a possible conformational change of opiate receptors due to the decrease of striatal DA content. The results obtained after an acute treatment with α -MT seem to exclude a direct influence of DA on the striatal binding sites for morphine

REFERENCES

1. Pollard, H., Llorens-Cortes, C. and Schwartz, J.C. (1977) Nature, 268, 745-747.

2. Carenzi, A., Frigeni, V. and Della Bella D. (1978) in Advances in Biochemi cal Psychopharmacology, vol. 18, Costa, E. and Trabucchi, M. eds., Raven Press, New York, pp. 265-270

3. Guidotti, A. and Moroni, F. (1978) in The Proceeding of International Sympo sium on Biochemestry and Physiology of Glutamic acid, 29-31 May 1978, Milan.

4. Lamotte, C., Pert, C.B. and Snyder, S.H. (1976) Brian Res., 112, 407-412.

5. Atweh, S.F., Murrin, L.C. and Kuhar, M.J. (1978) Neuropharmacology, 17,65-71

6. Atweh, S.F. and Kuhar, M.J. (1977) Brian Res., 124, 53-67.

7. McGeer, E.G., Innanen, V.T. and McGeer, P.L. (1976) Brian Res., 118,356-358.

8. Schwartz, J.C., Pollard, H.,Llorens, C., Malfroy, B., Gros, C., Pradelles, P. and Dray, F. (1978) in Advances in Biochemical Psychopharmacology, vol. 18, Costa, E. and Trabucchi, M. eds., Raven Press, New York, pp. 245-264.

9. Pasternak, G.W. and Snyder, S.H. (1975) Nature, 253, 563-565.

10. Ungerstedt, U. (1971) Acta Physiol. Scan., 367, 69-93.

11. Pasternak, G.W., Wilson, H.A. and Snyder, S.H. (1975) Mol. Pharmacol., 11, 340-351.

12. Carenzi, A., Gillin, J.C., Guidotti, A., Schwartz, M.A., Trabucchi, M. and Waytt, R.T. (1975) Arch. Gen. Psychiatry, 32, 1056-1059.

13. Lowry, O.H., Rosenbrough, N.J., Farr, A.L. and Randall, R.J. (1951) J. Biol. Chem., 193, 265-275.

14. Gerhards, H.J., Carenzi, A. and Costa, E. (1974) Naunyn-Schmiedeberg's Arch. Pharmacol., 286, 49-63.

15. Tang,L.C. and Cotzias,G.C. (1978) Proc. Nath. Acad. Sci., USA, 75,1546-1548.

16. Creese,I., Feindberg,A.P. and Snyder, S.H. (1976) Europ.J.Pharmacol., 36, 231-235.

CHARACTERISTICS OF RECEPTORS MEDIATING THE PRO- AND ANTI-CONVULSANT EFFECTS OF OPIATES IN RATS

ALAN COWAN, ELLEN B. GELLER and MARTIN W. ADLER

Dept. of Pharmacology, Temple Univ. School of Medicine, Philadelphia, U.S.A.

INTRODUCTION

Although it is known that acute doses of morphine produce anticonvulsant effects in rats[1], the influence of other analgesic agents on seizure threshold (S.T.) has not been reported. In the present paper, we show that a) opiates and related compounds can be subdivided into 4 classes based on results obtained from the rat flurothyl test and b) the (presumed) receptors mediating the pro- and anti-convulsant effects of analgesics can be characterized by using the conventional approach of stereospecificity, naloxone-sensitivity, and development of tolerance/cross tolerance.

METHOD

Male S.D. rats (300-350 g; n=10-20) each received one of at least 3 doses of test compound s.c. 30 min prior to being exposed to the convulsant inhalant, flurothyl. The convulsant was given as a 10% solution in 95% ethanol to rats placed individually in one-gallon glass jars. The time interval between the start of the infusion and the onset of the clonic convulsion with loss of posture was considered the convulsive threshold.

RESULTS

1. Subdivision of test compounds

  A. *Compounds giving dose-related anticonvulsant effects*

    a) The σ receptor agonists[2] cyclazocine (1-5 mg/kg) and SK & F 10,047 (N-allylnorphenazocine) (10-40 mg/kg) caused *behavioral excitation* and raised the S.T. by 27% and 42%, respectively. A high dose of naloxone (30 mg/kg, s.c.) was required to antagonize the anticonvulsant effects.

    b) The μ receptor agonists[2] etorphine (0.005-0.02 mg/kg), levorphanol (2.5-20 mg/kg), ℓ-methadone (0.5-5 mg/kg), morphine (12.5-50 mg/kg), and phenazocine (0.5-5 mg/kg) caused *behavioral depression* and raised the S.T. by 16-30%. Low doses of naloxone (0.01 or 0.10 mg/kg) antagonized the anticonvulsant effects of these analgesics. Interestingly, in the presence of 30 mg/kg of naloxone, ℓ-methadone (2.5 mg/kg) markedly *lowered* S.T.

  B. *Compounds without dose-related effects*

    The κ receptor agonists[2] ethylketocyclazocine (0.5-12.5 mg/kg), ketazocine

470

(0.5-5 mg/kg), and nalorphine (25-100 mg/kg) raised the S.T. slightly (4-5%). Nalbuphine (5-20 mg/kg), naloxone (0.01-30 mg/kg), norcyclazocine (6.25-25 mg/kg), and normorphine (50-100 mg/kg) also produced no clear dose-related effects.

   C. *Compounds giving dose-related proconvulsant effects*
      Meperidine (6.25-25 mg/kg), normeperidine (6.25-25 mg/kg), and pentazocine (12.5-50 mg/kg) lowered the S.T. by 15%, 21%, and 32%, respectively. Naloxone (10 mg/kg) *potentiated* the proconvulsant effects of meperidine, normeperidine, and *ℓ*-pentazocine (but not *d*-pentazocine).

2. Comparison of enantiomers
   Anticonvulsant activity was more closely associated with the *levo*- enantiomers of cyclazocine and methadone. Thus, the S.T. was increased by 42% with *ℓ*-cyclazocine (5 mg/kg) and by 30% with *ℓ*-methadone (2.5 mg/kg). The corresponding values with the *d*-enantiomers were +20% and -3%, respectively. *d*-Pentazocine (50 mg/kg) (-39%) was a more effective proconvulsant than *ℓ*-pentazocine (-13%).

3. Tolerance/cross-tolerance studies
   Tolerance developed to the anticonvulsant effects of levorphanol (20 mg/kg) after rats had received twice daily injections of levorphanol (2.5-20 mg/kg) for 11 days. Rats from this study were also cross-tolerant to the anticonvulsant effect of morphine (50 mg/kg). Tolerance did not develop over 11 days to either the anticonvulsant effect of cyclazocine (1.25-5 mg/kg) or to the proconvulsant effect of pentazocine (6.25-25 mg/kg).

CONCLUSIONS

a) At least 3 different receptors mediate the effects of opiates in the rat flurothyl test. b) Certain analgesics may possess both pro- and anti-convulsant properties in rats. The proconvulsant effect can be unmasked or accentuated in the presence of high doses of naloxone. c) The rat flurothyl test is a simple and valuable addition to those procedures that are currently used for characterizing new analgesics *in vivo*.

REFERENCES

1. Adler, M.W., Lin, C., Smith, K.P., Tresky, R. and Gildenberg, P.L. (1974) Psychopharmacologia, 35, 243-247.
2. Martin, W.R., Eades, C.G., Thompson, J.A., Huppler, R.E. and Gilbert, R.E. (1976) J. Pharmac. exp. Ther., 197, 517-532.
(Supported by Grant DA 00376 from N.I.D.A.).

Characteristics and Function of Opioids, editors Van Ree and Terenius
© 1978 Elsevier/North-Holland Biomedical Press

2'-ACYLTHIO-6,7-BENZOMORPHANS AS POTENT ALLOSTERIC EFFECTOR ON THE
OPIATE RECEPTOR SITE(S)

HAJIME FUJIMURA, MASAKATSU NOZAKI, MASAYUKI NIWA, MIKIO HORI*, EIJI
IMAI* AND MASATOSHI BAN*
Department of Pharmacology, School of Medicine Gifu University,
*Department of Organic Chemistry, Gifu College of Pharmacy, Gifu,
500, (Japan)

It suggests that there is at least one allosteric site on the
opiate receptor and phenolic hydroxy group on A ring of morphine
plays an important part for interaction with the receptor. The present report deals with some aspects in the effect of thiol compounds on the stereospecific binding of opiate, and in the title
compounds.

The stereospecific binding of opiate to a crude membrane preparation (P_2-fraction) from rat brain without cerebellum were analyzed by Scatchard plot in the presence of a constant concentration
of thiol compounds. Curvilinear plots, concave upwards, were obtained. We make the assumption that this concave indicates negative
cooperativity. The maximum concentration of binding sites of opiate
(RT) and level of maximum occupancy (Ym) based on De Meyts plot
were calculated with curve fitting program. As shown in table 1,
RT of morphine and naloxone did not alter when adding sodium ions
to the incubation medium. Sodium ions lead to an increase Ym for
antagonist, and decrease it for agonist. Cysteine and methionine
enhanced RT of morphine by the modification of membrane structure.
But the specific binding of naloxone was blocked by these thiol
compounds.

TABLE 1   STEREOSPECIFIC BINDING OF MORPHINE AND NALOXONE

		RT $\times 10^{-10}$ M	Ym
Morphine		2.30	0.36
+ NaCl	100mM	2.30	0.20
+ cysteine	1mM	2.92	0.30
+ methionine	10mM	2.58	0.34
Naloxone		2.25	0.36
+ NaCl	100mM	2.25	0.49
+ cystein	1mM	1.10	0.50
+ methionine	10mM	0.49	0.61

Under the above results, a series of 2'-acylthio-6,7-benzomor-
phans was synthesized in order to develop allosteric effecting
analgesics for opiate receptor site. Typical compounds are 2'-ben-
zoylthio derivatives of metazocine and pentazocine.

Analgesic activity and inhibitory effect of those agonists on
the stereospecific binding of 5×10^{-9}M of ^{3}H-naloxone or ^{3}H-morphine
to the P_2-fraction of rat brain are summarized in table 2. Substitution of 2'-hydrox group to benzoylthio group generally decreased
analgesic potency. However, N-methyl derivative of benzoylthio-
benzomorphan showed analgesic activity as potent as morphine with
no Straub tail in mice. This activity was potentiated by morphine
and not antagonized by naloxone.

The receptor affinity of benzoylthiobenzomorphans on the inhibition of the stereospecific binding of ^{3}H-naloxone was very weak
but the affinity in the case of that of ^{3}H-morphine was significantly potent. The electrically induced contractions of the longitudinal muscle of guinea pig ileum were inhibited by the benzoylthio compounds. The onset of this action was slow and the inhibitory effect developed gradually. This inhibition was not restored
by naloxone or washing.

It is conceivable that the title compounds show allosteric effect or alteration of autoplasticity to opiate receptor site(s).

TABLE 2 ANALGESIC ACTIVITY AND STEREOSPECIFIC OPIATE RECEPTOR
BINDING OF 2'-BENZOYLTHIO-6,7-BENZOMORPHANS

	Analgesic Act. AcOH writhing[a]	Inhibit. of Specific Binding (IC50;nM)		
	ED50 (mg/kg)	^{3}H-Naloxone	Na-Index	^{3}H-Morphine
2'-Benzoylthio				
N-methyl	0.76 (0.44-1.22)	652	6	156
N-prenyl	3.11 (1.55-6.21)	312000	0.01	2710
2'-Benzoyloxy				
N-methyl	1.27 (0.62-2.60)[b]	107	8	241
N-prenyl	2.00 (1.25-3.20)	217	4	370
Metazocine	0.33 (0.21-0.64)	96	8	72
Pentazocine	1.25 (0.79-1.97)	380	5	420
Morphine	0.46 (0.29-0.74)	5.5	26	10

a) s.c., b) p.o.

Characteristics and Function of Opioids, editors Van Ree and Terenius
© 1978 Elsevier/North-Holland Biomedical Press

473

MODEL OF THE OPIATE RECEPTOR

ALEXANDER GERO

Hahnemann Medical College, Philadelphia, Pennsylvania 19102, USA

ABSTRACT

It is proposed that the opiate receptor is an oligomer associated with sodium-binding ionophores and attaches agonists with, antagonists without distortion of the receptor.

Five years ago this writer proposed a model of the opiate receptor[1] with binding sites for a benzene ring and for a hydrophobic cationic area so placed that a molecule with these two groups at 6-6$\frac{1}{2}$Å from each other can attach the receptor easily, but with the same groups rigidly held at 4$\frac{1}{2}$Å from each other the molecule can be bound only by deforming the receptor:

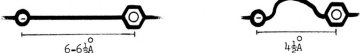

$$6\text{-}6\tfrac{1}{2}\overset{\circ}{\text{A}} \qquad\qquad 4\tfrac{1}{2}\overset{\circ}{\text{A}}$$

The increase in free energy caused by the distortion of bond angles and distances opposes the drug-receptor association;[2] it also causes an observable physiological change, thus defining the drug-binding site as a receptor. Hence drugs which deform the receptor are agonists, those which bind without deformation competitive antagonists, and agonists as a group must have lower affinity than antagonists, a generalization well documented for various opiate receptors.[1,3]

A defect of this model is that it does not provide for the "sodium effect" (Na[+]-induced decrease of agonist affinity and increase of antagonist affinity) which was not known at the time. To remedy this, Snyder[4] adds a Na[+]-binding site to the features of Gero's model, along with subsidiary drug-binding sites. He also assumes that the receptor exists natively as an equilibrium mixture of active and inactive conformations, a drug being an agonist or antagonist depending on which conformation it associates with, and Na[+] ion biasing affinities in favor of the inactive conformation. Why one conformation is active when the other is not, is not explained.

Simon[5] modified this model to account for his discovery that the opiate receptor binds both agonists and antagonists with positive cooperativity. His receptor is an oligomer with subunits essentially similar to Snyder's model. Interestingly, Simon found that in a brain homogenate the oligomer can dissociate and that isolated subunits do not show the sodium effect. This throws doubt on the view that a Na^+-binding site is an integral part of the receptor proper.

Therefore this writer has undertaken to propose a model which should account for all known facts. To this end, he retains his model with the two binding sites mentioned above, having a single, inactive, native conformation which is only a binding site for antagonists but is distorted and activated by agonists. This explains both agonistic behavior and the observed difference between affinities of agonists and antagonists - an explanation which the other models cannot provide. Now, however, the model describes the subunits of the receptor, held together by hydrogen bonds, etc., to form an oligomer, as in Simon's model. Distortion of one subunit is transmitted to other subunits in the receptor by the inter-subunit forces:

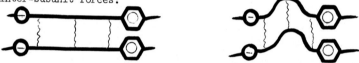

Conversely, the attachment of a (non-deforming) antagonist molecule to one subunit adds the binding energy of its attachment to the conformational stability of the receptor and thus helps further binding of antagonists but not of agonists. Thus cooperativity of both agonist and antagonist binding follows from the model. Further, while neither the subunits nor therefore the oligomer contain Na^+-binding sites, Na^+-binding ionophores are assumed in the cell membrane, not part of but associated with the opiate receptor. Coulombic repulsion of the positive charges or coordinative crosslinking of ionophores holds the oligomer-ionophore system rather rigidly in its native conformation. Removal of Na^+ ions removes this restraint and allows the oligomer a measure of conformational mobility: then attachment of antagonists becomes less easy but distortion by agonists easier. Thus the model postulates the sodium effect in the membrane-bound oligomer but not in subunits broken off from it.

ACKNOWLEDGMENT

The author is grateful to Dr.J.Baggott for helpful discussion and suggestions.

REFERENCES

1. Gero, A. (1973) Arch.int.Pharmacodyn., 206, 41-46.
2. See any textbook of physical chemistry.
3. Pert, C.B., Pasternak, G.W. and Snyder, S.H. (1973) Science, 182, 1359-1361.
4. Feinberg, A.P., Creese, I. and Snyder, S.H. (1976) Proc.Natl.Acad.Sci.USA, 73, 4215-4219.
5. Simon, E.J. (1976) Neurochemical Research, 1. 3-28.

Characteristics and Function of Opioids, editors Van Ree and Terenius
© *1978 Elsevier/North-Holland Biomedical Press*

FURTHER SUPPORT FOR THE HYPOTHESIS OF MULTIPLE OPIATE RECEPTORS

M.G.C. GILLAN, S.J. PATERSON and H.W. KOSTERLITZ

Unit for Research on Addictive Drugs, University of Aberdeen, Aberdeen, U.K.

INTRODUCTION

Recently Martin and colleagues[1,2] have proposed from behavioural and pharmacological studies in the chronic spinal dog that there are at least three different opiate receptors in the central nervous system.   Evidence for the view
that more than one receptor is required to explain the actions of opiates and
opioid peptides, has been reported by Lord et al.[3], who conducted parallel
assays in different in vitro models.   In this paper, we have tried to provide
more direct evidence for multiple opiate receptors from studies of the interaction of a number of primary ligands with the opiate receptors.

MATERIALS AND METHODS

Guinea-pig brains were divided into six regions as described by Glowinski
and Iversen[4].   The tissue was homogenised in 50 mM Tris buffer (pH 7.4, 0°C),
centrifuged at 49,000 g for 10 min; the pellet resuspended in Tris buffer (pH
7.4, 37°C) and incubated at 37°C for 45 min.   The homogenate was then centrifuged again and the pellet resuspended in the original buffer to give a final
concentration of 1 g tissue/100 ml.   Receptor binding was studied in the
absence of added Na^+, using 1.9 ml of homogenate made up to 2 ml with primary
ligand.   The primary ligands and the concentrations used were: 0.86 nM {^{3}H}-
leucine-enkephalin (30-40 Ci/mmol), 0.86 nM {^{3}H}-methionine-enkephalin (34.6
Ci/mmol), 1 nM {^{3}H}-dihydromorphine (81 Ci/mmol), 2 nM {^{3}H}-morphine (28 Ci/
mmol) and 0.4 nM {^{3}H}-naltrexone (10.8 Ci/mmol).   The samples were incubated
for 150 min at 0°C, then filtered and counted as previously described[3].
Specific binding was the difference in counts obtained in the absence and
presence of 50 nM of the antagonist, (-)-2-(3-furylmethyl)-5,9-diethyl-2'-
hydroxy-6,7-benzomorphan (Mr 2266).

In other experiments, guinea-pig and mouse brains minus cerebellum were
prepared as above.   The final homogenate was prepared in Tris buffer (pH 7.4
at either 25° or 0°C).   The homogenate was incubated with various concentrations of {^{3}H}-dihydromorphine, {^{3}H}-D-Ala^2-leucine-enkephalin amide (17.6 Ci/
mmol) or {^{3}H}-D-Ala^2-methionine-enkephalin amide (15 Ci/mmol) at either 25° for
40 min or 0° for 150 min; the kinetic parameters were determined by Scatchard

476

analysis.

RESULTS

The regional binding of the various primary ligands at $0°C$ showed no clear-cut differences. In all cases, the highest binding was found in the striatum and cortex, with intermediate binding in the hypothalamus, medulla and mid brain and low binding in the cerebellum.

There is apparently only one binding site for D-Ala^2-leucine-enkephalin amide in guinea-pig brain homogenate. At this site, the ligand has a K_D of 3.14 ± 0.53 nM (n = 3) and the maximum number of binding sites corresponds to 11.7 ± 1.3 pmol/g wet wt (n = 3) at $25°C$. Similar values were obtained with D-Ala^2-methionine-enkephalin amide (K_D 1.96 ± 0.16 nM; total binding sites 13.0 ± 1.5 pmol/g wet wt (n = 5). However for dihydromorphine, the total number of sites corresponds to 4.25 ± 0.36 pmol/g wet wt (n = 3). When the numbers of binding sites for D-Ala^2-leucine-enkephalin amide and dihydromor-phine were compared in the same homogenate, the difference of 8.96 ± 1.59 pmol/g wet wt (n = 4) was significant (P < 0.01). A similar significant difference was found between the two ligands in each of two strains of mice.

When the binding of the two ligands was compared in the same homogenate at $0°$ and $25°C$, it was found that the number of D-Ala^2-leucine-enkephalin amide sites was not influenced by differences in incubation temperature, but the number of dihydromorphine sites was reduced from 4.25 pmol/g wet wt at $25°C$ to 2.68 ± 0.67 pmol/g wet wt (n = 4) at $0°C$ (P < .01).

CONCLUSIONS

The findings, that the binding sites for D-Ala^2-leucine-enkephalin amide are more numerous than those for dihydromorphine and the differences in sensitivity to changes in incubation temperature, support the hypothesis of multiple opiate receptors[1-3].

Supported by grants from the Medical Research Council, the U.S. National Institute on Drug Abuse and the U.S. Committee on Problems of Drug Dependence.

REFERENCES

1. Martin, W.R., Eades, C.G., Thompson, J.A., Huppler, R.E. and Gilbert, P.E. (1976) J. Pharmac. exp. Ther., 197, 517-532.

2. Gilbert, P.E. and Martin, W.R. (1976) J. Pharmac. exp. Ther., 198, 66-82.

3. Lord, J.A.H., Waterfield, A.A., Hughes, J. and Kosterlitz, H.W. (1976) in Opiates and Endogenous Opioid Peptides, Kosterlitz, H.W. ed., North-Holland, Amsterdam, pp. 275-280.

4. Glowinski, J. and Iversen, L.L. (1966) J. Neurochem., 13, 655-669.

Characteristics and Function of Opioids, editors Van Ree and Terenius
© *1978 Elsevier/North-Holland Biomedical Press*

OPIATE RECEPTOR DISTRIBUTION IN ORGANIZED CULTURES OF FETAL MOUSE SPINAL CORD AND DORSAL ROOT GANGLIA

J.M. HILLER, E.J. SIMON, S.M. CRAIN AND E.R. PETERSON
Department of Medicine, New York University School of Medicine, New York, N.Y.
10016, and Department of Neuroscience, Albert Einstein College of Medicine,
Bronx, N.Y. 10461

In recent studies we have reported that the bioelectric activities of organotypic cultures of specific CNS tissues are sensitive to opiates[1]. These cultures consist of spinal cord explants with attached dorsal root ganglia (DRG), derived from 14-day-old fetal mice[2]. The characteristic sensory-evoked synaptic network discharges in the dorsal cord regions[2,3] can be selectively depressed by the introduction, into the fluid bathing the cultures, of analgesic concentrations of morphine (10^{-7}-10^{-6}M), levorphanol (10^{-7}M), or etorphine (10^{-8}-10^{-7}M). Dextrorphan is ineffective at 10^{-6}M. This depression is antagonized by naloxone (10^{-8}-10^{-6}M). More recently we have shown that the electrical response of the dorsal cord is also inhibited by a variety of enkephalins, enkephalin analogues and endorphins, and that their depressant potencies correlate very closely with their analgetic potencies in rodents[4].

The electrophysiological effectiveness of opiates and endorphins induced us to study opiate receptor levels and localization in these cultures[5]. Measurements of opiate receptor binding levels in these spinal cord-DRG cultures, as well as in cultures of isolated DRGs and deafferented cord explants, were made. Receptor binding was assayed[6] using the potent opiate antagonist ^{3}H-diprenorphine labeled at high specific activity (22.3 Ci/mmole). In these cultures, profuse neuritic outgrowth develops, primarily as a result of the stimulation of DRG neurons by added nerve growth factor, and extends for several millimeters beyond the explant zone. In some experiments separate determinations of opiate binding were made on explant and outgrowth zones. Homogenates of these cultures were found to exhibit stereospecific opiate binding. Fresh explants had little or no opiate binding but receptor levels increased with time in culture and reached maximum levels at 11 to 14 days after explantation. The greatest amount of binding was present in the neuritic outgrowth of both isolated dorsal root ganglion cultures (40-300 fM/mg protein) and cord-ganglion cultures. Since the central branches of DRG neurons have been shown to establish synaptic connections within the dorsal horn of co-cultured spinal cord explants,

478

the presence of high levels of opiate receptors on the neuritic outgrowth from DRG explants suggests a location on the presynaptic primary afferent fibers in the spinal cord.

Further binding studies in cord-DRG explants confirmed earlier evidence in adult mammals[7,8] that binding in the dorsal region of the spinal cord is greater than that seen in the ventral cord. Levels in DRG-innervated dorsal cord reached 22 to 57 fmoles/mg protein, whereas levels in deafferented dorsal cord were 9 to 19 fmoles/mg protein.

These data add further evidence suggesting a location of opiate receptors on the presynaptic primary afferent fibers in the spinal cord. Presynaptic location of opiate receptors was initially suggested by the finding that the receptor level in the dorsal horn of adult monkey spinal cord was reduced to about 50% of control values after rhizotomy[8]. These authors attributed this decrease to degeneration of opiate receptor-bearing afferent terminals, but they pointed out that their data could also be explained by transynaptic effects on opiate receptors located on post-synaptic cord neurons. However, taken together with the results from our cord-DRG cultures, these data strongly favor the presence of opiate receptors on the primary afferents that originate in DRG neurons. Such a presynaptic location is in agreement with current theories suggesting that opiates and enkephalins act by regulating the release of neurotransmitters.

This work was supported by research grants to E.J.S.: DA 00017 from NIDA: and to S.M.C.: NS 06545 and NS 12405 from NINCDS, DMS 75-03728 from NSF, and a grant from the Alfred P. Sloan Foundation.

REFERENCES

1. Crain, S.H., Peterson, E.R., Crain, B. and Simon, E.J. (1977) Brain Research, 133, 162-166.
2. Crain, S.M., Peterson, E.R. (1974) Brain Research, 79, 145-152.
3. Crain, S.M., Peterson, E.R. (1975) Science, 188, 275-278.
4. Crain, S.M., Crain, B., Peterson, E.R. and Simon, E.J. (1978) Brain Research, in press.
5. Hiller, J.M., Simon, E.J., Crain, S.M. and Peterson, E.R. (1978) Brain Research, 145, 396-400.
6. Simon, E.J., Hiller, J.M. and Edelman, I. (1973) Proc. Nat. Acad. Sci. (Wash.) 70, 1947-1949.
7. Lamotte, C., Pert, C.B. and Snyder, S.H. (1976) Brain Research, 112, 407-412.
8. Atweh, S.F. and Kuhar, M.J. (1977) Brain Research, 124, 53-67.

Characteristics and Function of Opioids, editors Van Ree and Terenius
© *1978 Elsevier/North-Holland Biomedical Press*479

RECEPTOR BINDING PROPERTIES *IN VITRO* AND *IN VIVO* OF NEW LONG ACTING NARCOTIC
ANALGESICS

JOSEE E. LEYSEN, PIERRE M. LADURON and CARLOS J.E. NIEMEGEERS
Department of Biochemical Pharmacology, Janssen Pharmaceutica, B-2340 Beerse,
Belgium

3-Methyl piperidine and 3-methyl 4-piperidine carboxylate derivatives of fentanyl are extremely potent narcotic analgesics (> 5 000 x morphine)[1] with pronounced stereospecific activity. The active enantiomer of the carboxylate derivative appeared to be extremely long-acting (> 24 hrs), both in pharmacological
and clinical tests. We now report on a detailed investigation of the *in vitro*
and *in vivo* opiate receptor binding of the compounds. For the first time, antagonistic properties of a fentanyl derivative are described.

MATERIALS AND METHODS

In vitro opiate receptor (O.R.) binding is measured in a cytoplasmic fraction
of rat forebrain using ^{3}H-fentanyl (2 nM, spec.act. 9 Ci/mmole; IRE, Belgium) or
^{3}H-naloxone (2 nM, spec.act. 19 Ci/mmole, NEN, Germany) in combination with levo-
and dextromoramide as previously described[2,3].

Dissociation of binding of non-labelled drugs is measured with an originally
developed dilution method. The cold drug is incubated with an enriched membrane
preparation (microsomal fraction) in a mixture of reduced volume (0.5 ml). At
binding equilibrium, the dissociation reaction is initiated by 80-fold dilution
with buffer and further incubated. After different time-intervals the reaction
is stopped by cooling in ice-water and membranes are rapidly precipitated by
centrifugation. The pellet is reconstituted in 4 ml of buffer and assayed for
^{3}H-fentanyl binding.

In vivo O.R. binding is determined after intravenous administration of the
compound and assessment *in vitro* of receptor occupancy in the brain of the treated animal using ^{3}H-fentanyl[4].

Analgesic potency of the drugs is measured in the tail-withdrawal reflex
(TWR) test in rats[5]. Antagonistic activity of compounds is evaluated by checking
their ability for releaving the respiratory depression induced with fentanyl
(0.63 mg.kg^{-1}, s.c.) in rats.

RESULTS AND DISCUSSION

Table 1 shows that there is a very good correlation between the O.R. binding
affinity and the analgesic potency of the compounds and between the dissociation

TABLE 1

In vitro inhibitory potency (IC_{50}) of stereospecific binding of ^{3}H-fentanyl (a) or ^{3}H-naloxone (b) in rat forebrain[3] and *in vivo* activity in the TWR-test in rats[5].

R-no	Piperidine substituent	O.R. BINDING IC_{50} (nM) − NaCl (a)	+ NaCl (b)	Diss. rate $t_{1/2}$	ED_{50} mg.kg^{-1}	TWR-TEST RAT Time at n x ED_{50} n = 1	n = 2
4263		2.5	35.5	< 2'	0.011	6'	30'
26 800	Cis+, 3-CH$_3$	0.21		~ 120'	0.0006	10'	65'
25 830	Cis−, 3-CH$_3$	18			0.052	4'	> 60'
18 140	Trans±, 3-CH$_3$	1.6			0.009	4'	> 30'
34 995	Cis−, 3-CH$_3$, 4-COOCH$_3$	0.2	0.15	> 180'	0.0006	12'	> 420'
34 994*	Cis+, 3-CH$_3$, 4-COOCH$_3$	10	28	< 2'	2.2	~ 7.5'	~ 30'
32 812	Trans±, 3-CH$_3$, 4-COOCH$_3$	1.6			0.008	~ 7.5'	

* *In vivo* antagonism of respiratory depression induced with fentanyl (0.63 mpk, s.c.) in rats : ED_{50} = 0.45 mg.kg^{-1}, duration < 5'.

rate of the receptor-drug complex and the duration of action *in vivo*.

R 34 995, the cis(-)-enantiomer of fentanyl-3-methyl 4-piperidine carboxylate is the most active compound of the series with an extremely long duration of action in both the O.R. binding and TWR-test. The cis(+)-enantiomer, R 34 994, is far less potent. However, it is the only pair of enantiomers for which there is a marked discrepancy between the ratio in binding affinity (50) and the ratio in analgesic potency (4 000).

When testing the compounds for antagonistic properties, only R 34 994 displayed a short lasting (< 5') antagonism of fentanyl-induced respiratory depression with an ED_{50} = 0.45 mg.kg^{-1}. In the same test the ED_{50} of naloxone was 0.03 mg.kg^{-1} and its IC_{50}'s for O.R. binding is 3.98 nM. Hence O.R. binding affinities of R 34 994 and naloxone is proportional to their antagonistic potency. Although, according to previous reports[6] antagonists should be detectable in *in vitro* binding assays by the ratio between binding affinity in the presence and absence of NaCl, this appeared not to apply to the compounds tested in this investigation; in contrast table 1 shows that the pure agonist, R 34 995, display higher affinity for the 'antagonist-state' than for the 'agonist-state' of the receptor whereas the reverse is observed for the partial antagonist, R 34 994.

In the *in vivo* receptor binding test, R 34 995 produced total O.R. blockage in rat forebrain after intravenous administration of 5 µg.kg^{-1}. At a dosage of 7.5 µg.kg^{-1}, maximal occupancy was reached after 5 mins and 24 hrs later 45 % of the receptors were still occupied. The time course of elevation of homovanillic acid levels in rat forebrain and receptor occupancy was completely parallel. *In vivo* as well as *in vitro*, R 34 995 showed a similar binding affinity and rate of dissociation from opiate receptors in rat striatum, thalamus, hypothalamus, mid-brain, cortex, hippocampus and medulla oblongata.

It can be concluded that there is a good correlation between *in vitro* O.R. binding affinity and *in vivo* analgesic or antagonistic potency of compounds. The cis stereoisomers of 3-methyl, 4-piperidine carboxylate fentanyl are the first pair of optic enantiomers of which one form is a potent agonist and the optic antipoole a partial antagonist. The long duration of action of R 34 995 appeared to be due to the long lasting fixation of the compound to the specific receptor sites, more than to pharmacokinetic or storage reasons. The use of the new compound may contribute to the study of the mechanism of opiate action.

ACKNOWLEDGEMENT

Part of this work was supported by a grant from I.W.O.N.L.

REFERENCES

1. Van Bever, W.F.M., Niemegeers, C.J.E. and Janssen,P.A.J. (1974) J. med. Chem., 17, 1047-1051.

2. Leysen, J. and Laduron, P. (1977) Life Sci., 20, 281.

3. Leysen, J., Tollenaere, J.P., Koch, M.H.J. and Laduron, P. (1977) Eur. J. Pharmacol., 43, 253-267.

4. Laduron, P.M. (1978) Biochem. Pharmacol., 27, 317-321.

5. Janssen, P.A.J., Niemegeers, C.J.E. and Dony, J.G.H. (1963) Arzneimittelforsch., 13, 502-507.

6. Pert, C.B. and Snyder, S.H. (1974) Mol. Pharmacol., 10, 868.

Characteristics and Function of Opioids, editors Van Ree and Terenius
© *1978 Elsevier/North-Holland Biomedical Press*

REVERSAL BY BOVINE SERUM ALBUMIN OF PHOSPHOLIPASE A INHIBITION OF OPIATE
RECEPTOR BINDING

HUNG-KUANG LIN AND ERIC J. SIMON

Department of Medicine, New York University School of Medicine, New York,
New York, 10016.

Opiate receptors in animal and human brain have been shown to be integrally
associated with cell membranes [1, 2, 3]. Opiate receptor binding activity has
been demonstrated to be sensitive to the action of phospholipase A (PL-A) from
Vipera russeli venom [4]. We have reported that inhibition of opiate binding by
PL-A can be reversed almost completely by incubation of the enzyme-treated
membranes with bovine serum albumin (BSA) [5]. The reversibility of this inhibition by BSA may provide a useful tool with which to define the role of
phospholipids in the stereospecific binding of opiates and endorphins.

Recovery of opiate receptor binding is a function of BSA concentration and
is dependent on the length of incubation with BSA. Optimum recovery of opiate
binding activity is obtained by incubation of the PL-A treated membranes with
1% BSA for sixty minutes at 0° C. The extent of recovery of binding activity
by BSA is inversely proportional to the length of exposure to PL-A. Opiate
binding activity of the PL-A treated membranes does not decrease significantly
after the enzyme is removed and binding levels are examined up to three hours
later. Similar results are obtained when ^{3}H-naltrexone or ^{3}H-etorphine is
used as ligand. Rat brain membranes treated with trypsin or pronase, whose
action inhibits opiate binding, were incubated with BSA, however, restoration
of receptor binding activity could not be demonstrated. This suggests that
the restorative effect of BSA is probably specific for PL-A treated membranes.
Sonicated suspensions of phospholipid hydrolysis products, lysolecithin and
linoleic acid, inhibit opiate binding only at much higher concentrations

484

(0.5 mM) than are present in PL-A membrane preparations. Exposure to BSA does not reverse this inhibition.

Results presented here seem to indicate that phospholipids play an important role in maintaining the integrity of the opiate receptor. The observation that BSA can reverse the effects of PL-A even three hours after removal of this enzyme, at which time binding is still greatly depressed, indicates that the perturbation of the receptor did not result in permanent damage. This indicates that inhibition is not due to the detergent properties of the hydrolysis products, since the receptor is damaged irreversibly by small concentratrations of detergents.

The following scheme is presented as a possible mechanism for the reversal, by BSA, of the effects of PL-A. The low concentrations of PL-A used, along with the short incubation periods were sufficient to hydrolyze a number of phospholipids at or near opiate binding sites. These hydrolysis products remain in place in the membrane. The interaction between phospholipids or between phospholipids and receptor protein is thereby altered in such a way that the tertiary structure of the binding site was altered, so as to reduce its ability to bind opiates. Addition of BSA results in the removal of lyso-compounds and free fatty acids which permits membrane components to resume their normal configuration and culminates in the reactivation of the opiate receptor.

This work was supported by Grant DA00017 from the National Institute of Drug Abuse.

1. Simon, E.J., Hiller, J.M., and Edelman, I. (1973) Proc. Natl. Acad. Sci. (Wash.) 70, 1947-1949.
2. Pert, C.B. and Snyder, S.H. (1973) Science, 179, 1011-1014.
3. Terenius, L. (1973) Acta Pharmac. Toxicol., 32, 317-320.
4. Pasternak, G.W. and Snyder, S.H. (1975) Molec. Pharmacol., 11, 478-484.
5. Lin, H.K. and Simon, E.J. (1978) Nature, 271, 383-384.

Characteristics and Function of Opioids, editors Van Ree and Terenius
© 1978 Elsevier/North-Holland Biomedical Press

BINDING SITES OF ^{3}H-ENKEPHALINS IN MOUSE BRAIN : PHARMACOLOGICAL CHARACTERIZA-
TION, LOCALIZATION AND EFFECTS OF CHRONIC TREATMENT WITH MORPHINE

BERNARD MALFROY, JEAN-PAUL SWERTS, JEAN-CHARLES SCHWARTZ, GILLES GACEL[+], MARIE-
CLAUDE FOURNIE-ZALUSKI[+] AND BERNARD ROQUES[+]
Unité 109 de Neurobiologie, Centre Paul Broca de l'INSERM, 2ter rue d'Alésia
75014 Paris (France)
[+]U.E.R. des Sciences Pharmaceutiques, Université René Descartes, 4 avenue de
l'Observatoire 75270 Paris (France).

ABSTRACT

Enkephalins bind to two classes of sites in mouse striatum : the opiate receptor and the second, not recognized by morphine. Both classes have a similar
regional distribution. Chronic morphine treatment increases selectively the
capacity of the second class. ^{3}H-compounds bound to each class are identified
as intact ENK on the first one, and degradated ENK on the second, which might
therefore be related to a membrane peptidase.

INTRODUCTION

Enkephalins (ENK) and endorphins recognize not only the opiate receptor but
also, with a somewhat lower affinity, a second class of binding sites in rat
brain which functions are not yet established[1,2].

MATERIALS AND METHODS

Binding experiments were performed on a striatal particulate fraction from
male swiss mice[2]. Incubations (15 min, 30°C) in the presence of 25μM bacitracine and non-saturable binding determined in the presence of 5μM non-radioacti-
ve ligand.

RESULTS AND DISCUSSION

[3]H-Leu-ENK and ^{3}H-Met-ENK bind in a similar manner to two distinct classes of
sites in mouse striatal membranes (Fig. 1 and 2) with apparent Kd of about
5nM and 50nM. Only the 1st is recognized by morphine or (D-Ala)$_2$ Met-ENK.

The regional distribution of the two classes between cerebral regions is
parallel (r = 0.96).

After selective interruptions of the dopaminergic nigro-striatal pathway, the

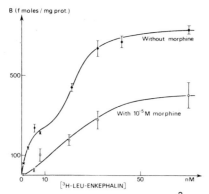

Fig. 1. Saturable binding of ^{3}H-Met-ENK to mouse striatal membranes.

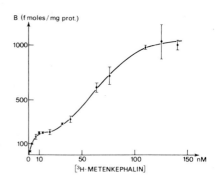

Fig. 2. Saturable binding of ^{3}H-Leu-ENK and partial inhibition by morphine.

two classes decrease similarly, suggesting that both are associated on the same cells.

Interestingly, after a chronic treatment with morphine, whereas ^{3}H-Leu-ENK binding to the 1st class is unchanged, as previously reported for ^{3}H-opiates[4,5] the capacity of the 2nd class is markedly increased (p<0.005).

Among a series of compounds tested, bacitracine selectively inhibits ^{3}H-Leu-ENK binding to the 2nd class (Ki = 20μM). Chromatographic isolation of bound ^{3}H-compounds[3] shows the 1st class occupied by unaltered ^{3}H-Leu-ENK whereas the 2nd class is occupied by a ^{3}H-fragment (probably ^{3}H-Tyr).

Taken together these data suggest that binding sites belonging to the 2nd class are related to a peptidase activity associated with opiate receptors.

REFERENCES

1. Audigier, Y., Malfroy, B., and Schwartz, J.C. (1977) Eur. J. Pharmacol., 41, 247-248.

2. Schwartz, J.C., Pollard, H., Llorens, C., Malfroy, B., Gros, C., Pradelles, Ph., and Dray, F. (1978) in Advances in Biochemical Psychopharmacology, Costa, E., and Trabucchi, M. eds, Raven Press, New York, pp. 245-264.

3. Vogel, Z., and Altstein, M. (1977) FEBS Letters, 80, 332-336.

4. Klee, W.A., and Streaty, F.A. (1974) Nature, 248, 549-551.

5. Pert, C.B., Pasternak, G.W., and Snyder, S.H. (1974) Science, 182, 1359-1361.

Characteristics and Function of Opioids, editors Van Ree and Terenius
© 1978 Elsevier/North-Holland Biomedical Press

REVERSIBLE INHIBITION OF OPIATE RECEPTORS BY AN ENDOGENOUS COPPER-GLUTATHIONE COMPLEX AND ANALGESIC EFFECTS OF INTRAVENTRICULARLY ADMINISTERED CUPRIC ION

GIOVANNI MARZULLO, BROMFIELD HINE and ARNOLD J. FRIEDHOFF

Millhauser Laboratories of the Department of Psychiatry, New York University School of Medicine, New York, N.Y. 10016 (USA)

ABSTRACT

The copper ion was identified as the active principle in an opiate receptor binding inhibitor extractable from brain and other tissues. This and other transition metals inhibit opiate binding with the same rank order as their affinity for SH groups. The etorphine binding activity of membranes inhibited by pretreatment with Cu^{++} is completely restored following incubation with SH reductants. This is consistent with a mechanism involving the reversible oxidation of essential SH groups at the active site. The EC_{50} for the Cu^{++} inhibition of receptors in vitro is lower than the concentration of this metal in brain tissue.

Intraventricular injections of cupric ion in mice produces analgesia with an ED_{50} of about 5 nmoles/mouse. Pretreatment with naloxone produced a parallel sixfold increase in the dose curve. It is possible that opiate receptor activity may be influenced in vivo, as well as in vitro, through the redox state of essential SH groups.

INTRODUCTION

In our laboratory a dialysable "peptide-like" factor from rabbit brain was first observed to inhibit the enzyme N-methyltransferase[1] and later also found to block the stereospecific binding of opiates to their receptors[2]. Recently we have identified this factor as a complex of oxidized glutathione and copper[3]. The cupric ion fully accounted for the inhibitory activity of the complex, while the peptide itself was inactive. Other transition metals were also found to be inhibitory with rank order Hg>Ag>Cu>Zn>Pb. We pointed out that this order of potency is the same as the order of affinity of these metals for protein SH groups. In this report we demonstrate reversal of the Cu^{++} inhibition by SH reductants. Moreover, here we report analgesic effects of intraventricular injections of cupric ion.

RESULTS

Table I shows that various SH reductants can reverse the action of Cu^{++} on opiate receptors. Brain membranes pretreated with sufficient concentrations of the cation to cause complete inhibition, followed by removal of the metal, were fully reactivated by preincubation with 3mM dithiothreitol prior to addition of the labelled opiate. Mercapto ethanol and reduced glutathione were also effective at this concentration, but to a lesser extent. Cysteine and ascorbic acid had little or no effect. Some degree of stimulation of untreated membranes also occurred with dithiothreitol.

Using rat brain membranes homogenized and washed in 100 volumes of buffer, the EC_{50} for the Cu^{++} inhibition of H^3-etorphine binding in the presence of 0.1 NaCl is 12 μM. The concentration of copper in brain tissue is of this order or higher: rat 17, mouse 105, rabbit 119, human cortex 470 nmoles/gm[4]. This renders possible an influence of the copper cation on the activity of opiate receptors in vivo.

Using the tail-flick response in mice we tested for pain sensitivity in mice after intraventricular injections containing $CuSO_4$. Conscious animals were injected by the procedure of Haley and McCormick[5] and tested by the method of D'Amour and Smith[6]. Percent analgesia was calculated by the method of Harris and Pierson[7] using a 10-second cut off time. Analgesia was observed immediately after the injections. As is shown in Fig. 1, at low doses the effect dissipated rapidly. At the higher doses, however, analgesic effects lasted more than one hour.

Normal recovery occurred in all animals with no visible toxic effects. In animals pretreated with naloxone the analgesia was reduced in degree and duration. Fig. 2 shows the dose-response curve analyzed according to Litchfield and Wilcoxon[8]. The ED_{50} was 4.8 with 95% Confidence Limits 2.7-9.0. In animals pretreated with 10 mg/kg naloxone there was a parallel shift of the curve to ED_{50} 30.2 (95% C.L. 18-48) giving a potency ratio of 6.3. Pretreatment studies with lower doses of naloxone have not been performed at this time.

The in vitro results suggest that opiate receptor activity may be influenced by the redox state of essential SH groups. The analgesia data support the idea that such a mechanism may occur in vivo.

TABLE I

REACTIVATION OF Cu^{++} -TREATED MEMBRANES BY SH REDUCTANTS

Homogenates (1:10) of rat membranes minus cerebellum were incubated with and without 90 μM $CuSO_4$ for 10 min. at 36 °C, followed by two 100-volume washes with standard buffer. Membranes were then preincubated with 3mM SH reductant, prior to addition of H^3-etorphine and assay[3].

Membranes	Add'n	% Activity
Control	---	100
"	DTT	119.2
Cu-treated	---	0
"	DTT	104
"	2ME	75.5
"	GSH	64.3
"	Cys	8.2
"	AA	0

DTT, dithiothretol; 2ME, 2-mercapto ethanol; Cys, cysteine; AA, ascorbic acid.

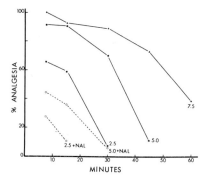

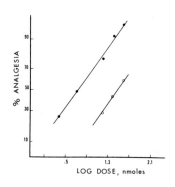

Fig. 1. Time course of tail-flick analgesia produced by Cu^{++} in mice. Numbers show concentrations injected.

Fig. 2. Dose-response curve in control mice (●) and in mice treated with 10 mg/kg naloxone injected intraperitoneally 20 min. prior to injection (○).

REFERENCES

1. Marzullo, G., Rosengarten, H. and Friedhoff, A.J. (1977) Life Sci., 20, 775-84.
2. Rosengarten, H., Marzullo, G. and Friedhoff, A.J. (1977) Phar. Bio. Beh. 5, 147.
3. Marzullo, G. and Friedhoff, A.J. (1977) Life Sci., 21, 1559-1568.
4. Hui, K.S., Davis, B.A. and Boulton, A.A. (1977) Neuroch. Res. 2, 495-506.
5. Haley, T.J. and McCormick, W. (1957) Brit. J. Pharm., 12, 12-15.
6. D'Amour, F.E. and Smith, D.L. (1941) J. Pharm. Exp. Ther. 72, 74-79.
7. Harris, L.S. and Pierson, A.K. (1964) J. Pharm. Exp. Ther. 143, 141-148.
8. Litchfield, J.T. and Wilcoxon, F. (1948) J. Pharm. Exp. Ther. 96, 99-113.

Characteristics and Function of Opioids, editors Van Ree and Terenius
© *1978 Elsevier/North-Holland Biomedical Press*

RECEPTOR BINDING AND INTERACTION OF NARCOTIC DRUGS IN CEREBRAL MEMBRANES, NEURONS AND GLIA

Fedor Medzihradsky, Patricia J. Dahlstrom, Steven V. Fischel and Michael A. Roberts
Departments of Biological Chemistry and Pharmacology, The University of Michigan
Medical School, Ann Arbor, Michigan 48109 (U.S.A.)

ABSTRACT

Stereospecific binding of various new narcotic drugs was investigated and related
to corresponding data of pure narcotic agonists and antagonists. The binding of
radiolabeled naltrexone, etorphine, met- and leu-enkephalin was characterized by
Scatchard analysis and Hill plots. Binding of these ligands was investigated in the
presence of competitor drugs, including the new narcotics, to detect heterogeneity of
binding sites. The binding properties of the above listed compounds was studied in
neurons and glia, bulk isolated from rat brain by different procedures.

INTRODUCTION

Within a cooperative project in which multiple approaches, including behavioral
aspects and bioassay methodology, are being utilized to evaluate new narcotic drugs[1],
we are investigating the receptor binding of these compounds, providing data on their affinity and agonist/antagonistic properties. In addition, we are focusing on
drugs which display overall characteristics suggestive of stereospecific binding to a
receptor site different than that for morphine. The binding of such narcotics, in the
absence and presence of competitor drugs, is then analyzed by kinetic plots, e.g.,
Scatchard, Hill and Klotz.

We have previously reported opiate receptor binding in neurons and glia, bulk
isolated from rat brain [2]. To further characterize the properties of opiate receptor
in these two cell types, we are isolating them by several different procedures and
are investigating the binding of narcotic drugs by the approach outlined above.

MATERIALS AND METHODS

The membrane preparation was obtained from the cerebrum of 200 g male Sprague-
Dawley rats. The membranes were isolated at 20^3x g for 15 minutes and kept at -70°
until use. The preparation exhibited 70% sterospecific binding at 3×10^{-9}M ^{3}H-
etorphine. For the determination of EC50 values, the final concentrations of protein,
dextrorphan (D), levorphanol (L) and ^{3}H-etorphine were 385 μg/ml, 6×10^{-7}M,
6×10^{-7}M and 3×10^{-9}M, respectively. Details of the assay have been published
earlier [2,1]. To determine the sodium response ratio [3], the receptor assay was
carried out in the presence and absence of 150 mM NaCl.

In experiments on characterization of opiate receptor sites, the binding of each
concentration of the radiolabeled ligand was investigated at exactly 100-fold excess
of D and L. Neuronal and glial cell fractions were isolated from 180 g male rats

according to two different procedures [4,5] which utilize mechanical disruption of the
tissue without the use of proteolytic enzymes which abolish stereospecific binding of
narcotics [6]. The isolation of cellular membranes and the other steps of the assay
were as described above.

RESULTS

The binding properties of over 40 narcotic drugs were determined. The potency of
the new experimental narcotics, e.g., UM911, UM1070, UM1072, in displacing ^{3}H-etor-
phine binding correlated well with that exhibited in the guinea-pig and mouse vas
deferens bioassays [1]. Futhermore, strong analgesic property correlated with a high
sodium response ratio [1]. While l-pentazocine had high affinity and sodium response
ratio (morphine-like), the d-isomer was 90-fold less potent and displayed a sodium
response ratio similar to that of ethylketocyclazocine.

In general, the Scatchard plots for the binding of naltrexone, etorphine, met- and
leu-enkephalin resembled those reported for the first two drugs by Simon et al [7].
However, at maintained 100-fold excess of D and L, at low concentrations of the
radiolabeled ligands a markedly potentiated bell-shape of the plots was obtained.
This was not observed at fixed concentrations of D and L. Despite these different
shaped Scatchard plots, the Hill coefficients were in all cases very close to 1.0.
The number of binding sites for naltrexone and etorphine was 0.5 pmoles/mg protein,
and for met- and leu-enkephalin, assayed at 25° in the presence of 30 μg/ml bacitracin, was 0.3 pmoles/mg. The Kd values for naltrexone and etorphine were 1.02 nM
and 0.62 nM, while for met- and leucine-enkephalin they were 0.11 nM and 0.06 nM,
respectively.

In initial experiments characterizing opiate receptor binding sites, Klotz plots of
^{3}H-naltrexone binding in the presence of morphine and UM1072, suggested competitive
interaction of these drugs at the same site.

Initial results on the characterization of opiate receptor in neurons and glia,
freshly isolated in bulk from rat brain by two different procedures, were similar,
showing significant stereospecific binding of ^{3}H-etorphine and ^{3}H-naltrexone in glia.

DISCUSSION

This publication represents a progress report on ongoing work aiming at the 3 ob-
jectives outlined under INTRODUCTION. The determination of EC50 values and of sodium
response ratios was undertaken within a cooperative project directed toward the testing of new narcotic drugs utilizing several methodologies [1]. The multitrack approach
in evaluating new narcotics offers the opportunity to identify compounds with unusual
i.e., morphine-unlike, narcotic properties. These drugs then become valuable tools
in attempts to characterize the molecular events underlying their exhibited gross
properties. To provide a frame-work within which to investigate interaction of such
'unusual' drugs with their receptor sites, we kinetically characterized the stereo-

specific binding of narcotic drugs and of endogenous opiates in our membrane preparation from brain. Scatchard analysis revealed identical number of binding sites for naltrexone and etorphine on one hand, and for met- and leu-enkephalin on the other. The Kd values for the peptides were by one magnitude lower than those for the narcotic drugs. At this place the value should be emphasized of providing for many narcotic ligands binding data obtained under identical experimental conditions (see under METHODOLOGY).

Initial competition experiments did not identify heterogeneity in the binding of naltrexone, morphine and UM1072, a tetrahydrofurfuryl derivative with 'unusual',morphine unlike properties [1].

Possible contamination of the bulk-isolated glial cell fraction by neuronal processes, and the different morphology of the isolated neurons and glia can lead to misinterpretations in studies of opiate receptor in these preparations[2]. Therefore, neurons and glia were isolated by two different methods. The previously reported presence of opiate receptor in both the neuronal and glial cell fraction was confirmed. Further characterization of stereospecific narcotic drug binding these two cell types is ongoing. Progress in this work is slowed by the low cellular yields, particularly in the isolation of glia.

REFERENCES

1. Woods, J.H., Smith, C.B., Medzihradsky, F. and Swain, H.H. (1978) in Mechanisms of Pain and Analgesic Drugs, J.E. Villarreal, ed., Raven Press, New York.
2. Medzihradsky, F. (1976) Brain Res., 108:212-219
3. Pert, C.B. and Snyder, S.H. (1974) Mol. Pharmacol., 10:868-879.
4. Sellinger, O.Z., Azcurra, J.M., Johnson, D.E., Ohlsson, W.G. and Lodin, Z. (1971) Nature (London), 230:253-256.
5. Iqbal, K. and Tellez-Nagel, J. (1972) Brain Res., 45:296-299
6. Guarnieri, M., Krell, L.S., McKhann, G.M., Pasternak, G.W. and Yamamura, H.L. (1975) Brain Res., 93:337-342.
7. Simon, E.J., Hiller, J.M., Edelman, I., Groth, J. and Stahl, K.D. (1975) Life Sci., 16:1795-1800.

Characteristics and Function of Opioids, editors Van Ree and Terenius
© *1978 Elsevier/North-Holland Biomedical Press*

THE EFFECTS OF SYNTHETIC AND NATURAL OPIOID PEPTIDES IN ISOLATED ORGANS

A. Z. Rónai, I. Berzétei, J. I. Székely and S. Bajusz
Institute for Drug Research, H-1325 Budapest P.O. Box 82. Hungary

ABSTRACT

The kinetics of inhibitory effect of opioid peptides was studied in electrically stimulated longitudinal muscle strip of guinea-pig ileum /GPI/, mouse vas deferens /MVD/, cat's nictitating membrane /CNM/ and rabbit's ear artery /REA/ preparation. The receptor effects were characterized using opiate and dopamine antagonists. It was found that the systems, where atypical opiate receptors are present, also contain dopamine receptors.

INTRODUCTION

Lord et al.[1] introduced a new class of opiate receptors /δ/, binding preferentially certain opioid peptides. This type of receptor could be distinguished from either classical μ or the recently postulated κ and σ receptors. Our aim was to obtain some more informations on the receptor effects of synthetic enkephalin analogs and natural opioid peptides. To characterize the ligand-receptor interaction, we determined the rank order of inhibitory potencies of selected compounds in electrically stimulated GPI, MVD, CNM and REA. The interaction was further characterized using dopamine or opiate antagonists.

MATERIALS AND METHODS

Peptides: β-endorphin was kindly supplied by L. Gráf. The synthesis of enkephalin analogs was the same as described previously[2]. Enkephalin analogs are specified by giving the position of the substituent amino acids. All the other compounds used were commercial ones.

Isolated organ preparations: The experimental conditions for GPI and MVD were the same as used previously[3]. The rabbit's ear artery was prepared according to De la Lande and Harvey[4]. The medial muscle of cat's nictitating membrane was prepared as described by Thompson[5]. Low-frequency field electrical stimulation was applied in each preparations.

Kinetics: The K_e values of antagonists were determined either from complete dose-response curves of agonists or by the single dose method[1].

RESULTS:

Normorphine, β-endorphin and the enkephalin analogs containing Pro or D-Met-ethylamide in position 5, were equipotent as opiate agonists in GPI and MVD, whilst short-chain endorphins, and the enkephalin analogs bearing Met or Nle in position 5 were 20 to 60 times more potent in MVD than in GPI. In MVD, where the proposed δ receptors are present, the K_e values of naltrexone are considerably higher against the opioid peptides than against normorphine; they vary from 1.9 ± 0.2 /n=8/, to 9.2 ± 0.8 /n=7/. The K_e changes rather independently from the MVD/GPI potency ratios of respective peptides. In GPI enkephalins and also β-endorphin are as readily antagonized by naltrexone, as is morphine. The rank order of inhibitory potencies of opioid peptides of different character is similar in GPI and CNM on the one hand, and in MVD and REA on the other /Table 1/.

TABLE 1

THE RELATIVE POTENCIES OF OPIOID PEPTIDES IN DIFFERENT ISOLATED ORGANS

Compound	Potency relative to Met^5 - enkephalin			
	GPI	CNM	MVD	REA
Met^5- enkephalin[a]	1.00	1.00	1.00	1.00
$D\text{-}Met^2,Nle^5$- enk.	5.6 ± 1.0 /6/[b]	8.5 ± 2.7 /5/	12.7 ± 1.0 /4/	16.7 ± 0.3 /3/
$D\text{-}Met^2,Pro^5\text{-}NH_2$-enk.	9.3 ± 1.8 /4/	23.8 ± 1.8 /4/	0.33 ± 0.05 /4/	0.06 ± 0.02/4/
β-endorphin	2.2 ± 0.3 /4/	0.9 ± 0.03 /3/	0.13 ± 0.03 /8/	~ 0.11 /5/[c]
Normorphine	1.3 ± 0.07 /56/	1.4 ± 0.2 /7/	0.04 ± 0.004/9/	$0.003 >$

[a] The ID_{50} values of Met^5-enkephalin were as follows: 183.5 ± 33.0 nM /n=8/ in GPI 863.9 ± 175.7 nM /n=12/ in CNM, 7.0 ± 0.6 nM /n=41/ in MVD and 105.0 ± 9.26 nM /n=4/ in REA.

[b] Mean $\pm$ SEM values are listed, the number of experiments is in parenthesis

[c] The relative potency was estimated from single doses /1000 nM/ given in 5 independent experiments

Whilst in CNM naltrexone antagonizes the effect of peptides in similar manner to that found in MVD, in REA extremely high concentrations /500-1000 nM/ of naloxone are required to reverse the inhibitory effect of compounds. However, the dopamine antagonist sulpiride /400 nM/ was able to antagonize the action of Met^5-enkephalin in this preparation, but not that of other peptides. The presence of presynaptic inhibitory dopamine receptors in REA has already been established. We found that dopamine receptors are present also in MVD and CNM.

REFERENCES

1. Lord et al. /1977/ Nature, 267, 495-499.
2. Bajusz et al. /1977/ FEBS Lett. 76, 91-92.
3. Rónai et al. /1977/ FEBS Lett. 74, 182-184.
4. De la Lande, I.S. and Harvey, J.A. /1965/ J. Pharm. Pharmac. 17, 589.
5. Thompson, J.W. /1958/ J. Physiol. /Lond/, 141, 46-72.

Characteristics and Function of Opioids, editors Van Ree and Terenius
© *1978 Elsevier/North-Holland Biomedical Press*

PHARMACOLOGICAL CHARACTERIZATION OF NARCOTIC RECEPTORS FOR HYPERTHERMIA IN RATS

F. CANKAT TULUNAY

Department of Pharmacology, Medical School of Ankara University, Ankara (TURKEY)

ABSTRACT

Receptor mechanisms of morphine and butorphanol-induced hyperthermia were compared by apparent pA2 values of morphine-naloxone and butorphanol-naloxone. The significant difference between pA2's of morphine-naloxone and butorphanol-naloxone for hyperthermia suggest, as previously shown for analgesia that narcotic and narcotic antagonist analgesics appear to interact with receptors in different manners.

INTRODUCTION

Narcotic analgesics produce a varriety of actions which are mediated by receptors in the central nervous system, including analgesia, respiratory depression, lethal effect and thermoregulatory changes in various species[1,2,3].

In the present investigation, butorphanol (BUT), a new synthetic antagonist type analgesic was used to study the nature of narcotic receptor interactions involved in body temperature by estimating the apparent pA2's of morphine (M)-naloxone (NLX) and BUT-NLX for hyperthermia.

MATERIAL AND METHODS

Male, white rats weighing 150-200 g were used for this study. Each animal was used only once. Rectal temperature was measured by a ten-channel electric thermometer at room temperature ($21-24^\circ$C). At least 10 rats were used for each dose. Control rectal temperature was $38.0 \pm 0.1 \ ^\circ$C (mean±SEM).

Changes in rectal temperature were made quantal by establishing an end point at the mean peak effect which represented an increase in the rectal temperature of an individual animal greater than 3 standard deviation of the control mean rectal temperature for all animals used in the group. The data were analyzed by parallel line assay with the aid of a computer program[1].

RESULTS

Peak hyperthermic effects were found 1 hr after M and 30 min after BUT injections (i.p.) and peak antagonism of these effects were seen when NLX was given together with BUT and 30 min after M injections. Data were shown on Table 1.

DISCUSSION

Schild's[4] concept has been used succesfully to characterize narcotic receptors for various narcotic effects *in vivo*[1,2,3]. A comparison of the apparent pA2 values of M-NLX and BUT-NLX with regards to hyperthermia has shown that the two

TABLE 1

Quantitative antagonism of morphine and butorphanol by naloxone.

TREATMENT	NALOXONE mg/kg	ED50 (95%confidence limits) mg/kg	pA2 (95% confidence limits)	SLOPE of pAx (± SEM)
M	none	4.7 (4.1- 5.4)		
M	0.125	10.3 (9.0-11.8)	6.57 (6.44-6.70)	-1.37±0.01
M	0.250	20.0 (17.5-22.8)		
M	0.500	41.2 (36.1-47.1)		
BUT	none	0.58(0.47-0.71)		
BUT	0.125	3.8 (3.1- 4.7)	7.35 (7.28-7.42)	-0.89±0.02
BUT	0.250	7.0 (5.7- 8.8)		
BUT	0.500	11.5 (9.4-14.1)		

apparent pA2 values significantly different from each other, suggesting, as previously reported for analgesic receptors[3,5],that the two analgesics interact with receptors in a different manner. McGilliard et al.[3] have reported that apparent pA2 values of M-NLX for analgesia, respiratory depression and hyperthermia were significartly different from each other, suggesting that the three effects of morphine are mediated by different receptors or different receptor interactions.

According to the present data, the apparent pA2 of M-NLX for hyperthermia of 6.57 was significantly different from apparent pA2 values for either analgesia[1] or respiratory depression in mice[3]. This value also appears significantly different from apparent pA2 for analgesia in rat of 6.8 reported by Hölt et al.[6]. There are good evidences that the comparison of apparent pA2 values between species is justified since a large number of apparent pA2 values for M-NLX in various analgesic assays have been ebtimated by various investigators in mice, rats and monkeys and all pA2 values have similar at about seven[2,3].

Present study suggests that the hyperthermic effects of M and BUT may be mediated by yet another type narcotic receptor interaction.

REFERENCES

1. Tulunay, F.C. & Takemori, A.E. (1974) J.Pharmacol.Exp.Ther., 190, 401-407.

2. Takemori,A.E. (1974) in Narcotic Antagonists, Braude,M.C.,Harris,L.S.,May,E.L. Smith,J.P. & Villarreal,J.E.,eds., Raven Press, New York, pp. 335-344.

3. McGilliard,K.L., Tulunay,F.C.,Takemori,A.E. (1976)in Opiates and Endogenous Opioid Peptides, Kosterlitz, H.W. ed., Elsevier, Amsterdam, pp. 281-288.

4. Schild, H.O. (1947) Brit. J. Pharmacol., 2, 251-258.

5. Smits, S.E. & Takemori, A.E. (1970) Brit. J. Pharmacol., 39, 627-638.

6. Hölt, V.,Dum,J.,Blässig,P,Schubert,P. & Herz,A. (1975) Life Sci., 16, 1823-1828.

Characteristics and Function of Opioids, editors Van Ree and Terenius
© *1978 Elsevier/North-Holland Biomedical Press*

EFFECTS OF PROPOSED μ, κ AND σ AGONISTS IN RODENTS

Susan J. Ward, G. Metcalf*, J.M.H. Rees. Department of Pharmacology, University of Manchester, M13 9PT, UK, and Reckitt and Colman, Dansom Lane, Kingston upon Hull, UK .

Three types of opiate receptor have been proposed following experiments in the chronic spinal dog[1]. We have examined some pharmacological actions of three pairs of drugs which may act as selective agonists at the proposed μ, κ and σ receptors using rodents. The drugs used, their classification and their dose ranges (mg/kg) were morphine (μ, 5-40), methadone (μ, 1.25-20), ketocyclazocine (κ, 1.25-80), ethylketocyclazocine (κ, 1.25-20), SKF 10,047 (σ, 5-80) and apomorphine (σ, 1.25-5).

METHODS

The parameters measured in mice included hot plate reaction time, oesophageal temperature, respiratory rate, and locomotor activity (Animex). In rats, tail flick reaction time, rectal temperature, locomotor activity (Animex) and ataxia (rotating rod) were measured. Susceptibility to naloxone (1 and 5 mg/kg) was also examined, and behavioural observations made.

RESULTS

These are summarised in Fig. 1. The proposed μ and κ agonists all produced analgesia, respiratory depression and ataxia. These actions were antagonised by naloxone. The two pairs of drugs differed in their effects on body temperature, locomotor activity and behaviour. In the case of body temperature, morphine had a biphasic effect in mice, in rats the direction of change depended on dose. In all cases the κ-agonists caused hypothermia. On the Animex, both morphine and methadone had biphasic actions, whilst the κ agonists decreased activity. The μ agonists caused characteristic stilted locomotion, Straub tail, and indifference to their surroundings. The κ agonists caused sedation.

The proposed σ agonists differed markedly. No evidence of analgesia was found, locomotion was increased, and the animals were agitated. None of the actions of SKF 10,047 or apomorphine were antagonised by naloxone.

Test		μ		κ		σ	
		morph	meth	keto	etketo	SKF	apo
analgesia (reaction time)	M	↑	↑	↑	↑	0	0
	R	↑	↑	↑	↑	–	0
respiratory rate	M	↓	↓	↓	↓	↓	↓
ataxia (falling time)	R	↓	↓	↓	↓	↓	↓
body temperature	M	↓↑	↓	↓	↓	0	↓
	R	↓or↑	↓	↓	↓	–	↓
locomotor activity	M	↓↑	↓↑	↓	↓	↑	0
	R	↓↑	↓↑	↓	↓	↑	0
behaviour		indifference		sedation		agitation	

Fig. 1. Summary of the qualitative effects of proposed μ, κ and σ agonists in tests in mice (M) and rats (R). Key: arrows indicate the directions of change (some are biphasic); 0 = no effect, – = not tested.

Whilst the three types of drug proposed to act at μ, κ and σ receptors are clearly distinguishable from one another in rodents, this alone is not sufficient evidence to classify three different receptor populations.

Other workers (using different tests) have shown SKF 10,047 to be analgesic, and there is in vitro evidence for the opiate nature of this compound. However the lack of analgesic activity in the standard methods used here, and the inability of naloxone to antagonise the other effects of the proposed σ agonists, questions the validity of classifying them as "opiate" in character.

ACKNOWLEDGEMENTS

We are grateful to Endo, S K + F and Winthrop Laboratories for donations of drugs.

REFERENCES

1. Martin, W.R. et al. (1976) J. Pharmac. exp. Ther., 197, 517-533.

Characteristics and Function of Opioids, editors Van Ree and Terenius
© 1978 Elsevier/North-Holland Biomedical Press

COVALENT LABELLING OF THE ENKEPHALIN RECEPTOR FROM RAT BRAIN

R. SUZANNE ZUKIN

Department of Biochemistry, Albert Einstein College of Medicine, New York, N.Y. 10461

ABSTRACT

A covalently bound [^{3}H]-enkephalin receptor complex has been prepared by cross-linking of the solubilized non-covalent complex. The complex has a molecular weight of about 380,000 daltons and has been purified 20-fold by molecular exclusion chromatography. Native gel electrophoresis shows a single major radioactive band.

INTRODUCTION

The stereospecific binding of opiates has been widely used to determine optimal binding re-quirements and distribution of opiate receptors within the nervous system. However, there is little information as to the nature of the opiate binding site apart from the fact that it is an integral membrane protein or proteolipid. In 1975 Simon and coworkers reported the solubil-ization of a non-covalent [^{3}H]-etorphine-macromolecular complex[1]. The present report describes the preparation of a covalently-bound [^{3}H]-enkephalin receptor complex.

MATERIALS AND METHODS

Mitochondrial-synaptosomal membranes[2] from the brains (without cerebella) of Sprague-Dawley rats were incubated (25° C, 30 min) with [^{3}H]-D-ala^2-met^5-enkephalinamide (DALA) (10 nM), in the presence of either levorphanol (10 μM) or dextrorphan (10 μM). Following incubation, membranes were solubilized with Brij 36T detergent as described elsewhere (R. S. Zukin, unpublished).

RESULTS AND DISCUSSION

Brij 36T extracts were fractionated by gel filtration on Sephadex G-25. In experiments in which dextrorphan was present in the incubation, about 25% of the applied radioactivity co-chromatographed with the protein void peak; when levorphanol was used instead, less than 1% cochromatographed (Fig. 1). The ratio of the radioactivity of dextrorphan to that of levor-phanol samples applied to the column was 3:1, the ratio of void peak radioactivities following their elutions was 20:1. Exposure of the solubilized extracts to trypsin (1 mg/ml, 25° C) or heat (50° C) for 10 min decreased ligand binding 50%. Thus, [^{3}H]-enkephalin is binding to a protein macromolecular site from which it can be much more readily displaced by

500

levorphanol than by dextrorphan. The labelled ligand was cross-linked to the receptor by reacting the protein void fractions with dimethyl suberimidate (0.2 mg/ml, pH 9.0, 22° C).
The resulting mixture was boiled 20 min, redissolved in 1% sodium dodecyl sulphate (SDS) and
again fractionated on G-25; on this column 20% of the applied radioactivity cochromatographed with the protein void peak (Fig. 2). Thus, a stereospecifically, covalently-bound
[³H]-enkephalin-protein complex has been obtained in soluble form.

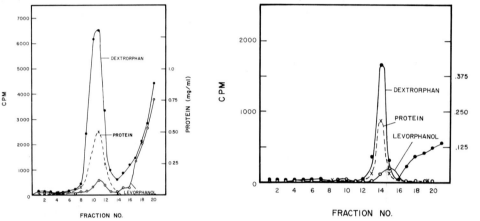

Fig. 1. Sephadex G-25 elution profile of Brij
extract of membranes bound with DALA
(42.3 Ci/mmol).

Fig. 2. Sephadex G-25 elution profile of
Brij extract after cross-linking and heat-
treatment.

The molecular weight of the enkephalin complex was determined by gel filtration on Seph-
arose 6B. Radioactivity from covalent [³H]-enkephalin complex and non-covalent [³H]-
etorphine coeluted at a position corresponding to a MW of ca. 380,000 daltons. The covalently bound enkephalin complex was purified 20-fold on a Sephadex G-150 column eluted
with 0.05 M Tris-HCl buffer, pH 7.4, 4° C. Native gel electrophoresis of the single radioactive peak from this column showed a major radioactive band; in preliminary studies, SDS
polyacrylamide gel electrophoresis of this band or of the entire peak demonstrated a major
radioactive species of MW ca. 90,000. Cross-linking with a radiolabelled marker thus provides a useful assay for the receptor and should enable its further purification.

REFERENCES
1. Simon, E. J., Hiller, J. M. and Edelman, I. Science 190, 389-390 (1975).
2. Simon, E. J., Hiller, J. M., Groth, J. and Edelman, I. J. Pharmacol. Exptl. Therap.
   192, 531-537 (1975).

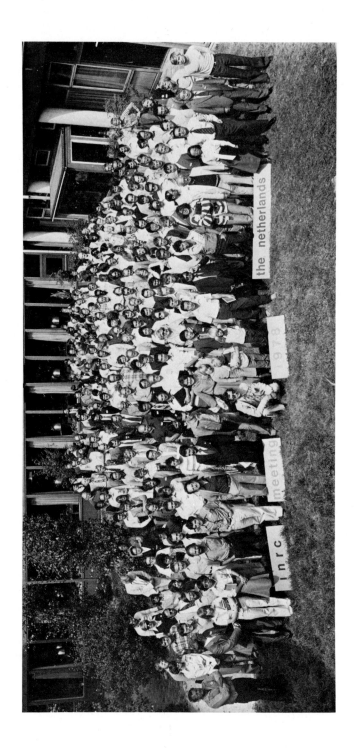

LIST OF PARTICIPANTS

L. AEPPLI	Basle, Switzerland
M. ADLER	Philadelphia, Pa., U.S.A.
G. AHNERT	Giessen, F.R.G.
L. AHTEE	Helsinki, Finland
H. AKIL	Palo Alto, Ca., U.S.A.
S. ALGERI	Milano, Italy
V. ALOYO	Memphis, Tn., U.S.A.
S. ARCHER	New York, N.Y., U.S.A.
M. ATTILA	Helsinki, Finland
I.H. AYHAN	Ankara, Turkey
M. BAN	Gifu, Japan
J.D. BARCHAS	Stanford, Ca., U.S.A.
J.L. BARKER	Bethesda, Md., U.S.A.
M.G. BAXTER	Beckenham, England
R.M.S. BELL	Wilmington, De., U.S.A.
H.N. BHARGAVA	Chicago, Ill., U.S.A.
M. BOARDER	Stanford, Ca., U.S.A.
B. BOHUS	Utrecht, The Netherlands
K.A. BONNET	New York, N.Y., U.S.A.
J. BÖRGER	Den Haag, The Netherlands
A.L.A. BOURA	Clayton, Australia
T.. BREIDENBACH	Giessen, F.R.G.
I. BRIGGS	Beckenham, England
R.M. BROWNE	San Diego, Ca., U.S.A.
R.M. BRYANT	Bradford, England
W.R. BUCKETT	Strasbourg, France
J.P.H. BURBACH	Utrecht, The Netherlands
T.F. BURKS	Tucson, Az., U.S.A.
E. BUURMAN	Apeldoorn, The Netherlands
W.L. BYRNE	Memphis, Tn., U.S.A.
A. CARENZI	Milano, Italy
F. CASACCI	Milano, Italy
J.K. CHANG	San Carlos, Ca., U.S.A.
G. CHAPPUIS	Bubendorf, Switzerland

R. CHILDAVEL	Manitoba, Canada
M. CHRÉTIEN	Montréal, Canada
S. CLARK	Beckenham, England
D.H. CLOUET	Brooklyn, N.Y., U.S.A.
J. COCHIN	Boston, Ma., U.S.A.
E. CODD	Memphis, Tn., U.S.A.
H.O.J. COLLIER	Slough, England
J. COLLINS	London, England
F.C. COLPAERT	Beerse, Belgium
A. COWAN	Philadelphia, Pa., U.S.A.
B.M. COX	Palo Alto, Ca., U.S.A.
J.C. CRABBE	Oss, The Netherlands
T. DE BOER	Amsterdam, The Netherlands
S. DE LA BAUME	Paris, France
W.S. DE LOOS	Utrecht, The Netherlands
D. DELLA BELLA	Milano, Italy
W.L. DEWEY	Richmond, Va., U.S.A.
D. DE WIED	Utrecht, The Netherlands
D.M. DORSA	Utrecht, The Netherlands
D. DUKA	München, F.R.G.
S. EHRENPREIS	Chicago, Ill., U.S.A.
L. FERLAND	STE-Foy, Quebec, Canada
S. FERRI	Catania, Italy
J. FLOREZ	Santander, Spain
C. FLY	Ann Arbor, Mi., U.S.A.
K. FOLEY	New York, N.Y., U.S.A.
R. FOLLENFANT	Beckenham, England
D.L. FRANCIS	Slough, England
R.C.A. FREDERICKSON	Indianapolis, In., U.S.A.
J.P. FRY	München, F.R.G.
H. FUJIMURA	Gifu, Japan
G. GACEL	Paris, France
Y. GELDERS	Leuven, Belgium
P. GENT	Leeds, England
A. GERO	Philadelphia, Pa., U.S.A.
M.G.C. GILLAN	Aberdeen, Scotland
W.H. GISPEN	Utrecht, The Netherlands
A. GOLDSTEIN	Palo Alto, Ca., U.S.A.

CHR. GRAMSCH	München, F.R.G.
H.M. GREVEN	Oss, The Netherlands
F. GUERRERO	San Francisco, Ca., U.S.A.
B.R. HAMPRECHT	Martinsried, F.R.G.
B.G. HANLON	Palo Alto, Ca., U.S.A.
S.L. HART	London, England
U. HAVEMANN	Göttingen, F.R.G.
V. HAVLICEK	Winnipeg, Manitoba, Canada
P.M. HEADLEY	Paris, France
G. HENDERSON	Maywood, Ill., U.S.A.
J.L. HENRY	Montreal, Quebec, Canada
A. HERZ	München, F.R.G.
R.C. HILL	Basel, Switzerland
R.G. HILL	Bristol, England
J. HILLER	New York, N.Y., U.S.A.
V. HÖLLT	München, F.R.G.
M. HORI	Gifu, Japan
E. HOSOYA	Tokyo, Japan
CHR.M.T.L. HUMBLET	Namur, Belgium
E. IMAI	Gifu, Japan
R. INOKI	Osaka, Japan
C. INTURRISI	New York, N.Y., U.S.A.
E.I. IWAMOTO	San Francisco, Ca., U.S.A.
K. IWATSUBO	Osaka, Japan
J.J.C. JACOB	Paris, France
Y. JACQUET	New York, N.Y., U.S.A.
K. JHAMANDAS	Kingston, Ontario, Canada
J. JOLLES	Utrecht, The Netherlands
L.L. JUDD	San Diego, Ca., U.S.A.
R.F. KAIKO	New York, N.Y., U.S.A.
S. KAIM	McLean, Va., U.S.A.
H. KANETO	Nagasaki, Japan
Y. KATAYAMA	Maywood, Ill., U.S.A.
I. KHAN	Genève, Switzerland
I. KITCHEN	London, England
W.A. KLEE	Bethesda, Md., U.S.A.
R.J. KOBYLECKI	Hull, England
I.A. KOURIDES	New York, N.Y., U.S.A.
H.W. KOSTERLITZ	Aberdeen, Scotland

G.L. KOVACS	Utrecht, The Netherlands
W. KROMER	München, F.R.G.
K. KUSCHINSKY	Göttingen, F.R.G.
F.S. LA BELLA	Winnipeg, Manitoba, Canada
F. LABRIE	Quebec, Canada
R.A. LAHTI	Kalamazoo, Mi., U.S.A.
L.A. LAMBERT	Birmingham, England
J.M. LECOMTE	Paris, France
R.L. LEE	Cardiff, Wales
E. LEONG WAY	San Francisco, Ca., U.S.A.
J.E. LEYSEN	Beerse, Belgium
J.J. LIPMAN	Cardiff, Wales
J.C. LISSITZKY	Marseille, France
J.G. LOEBER	Utrecht, The Netherlands
G.H. LOEW	Stanford, Ca., U.S.A.
J. LORD	Hull, England
A. LUINI	Milan, Italy
R.A.A. MAES	Utrecht, The Netherlands
B. MALFROY	Paris, France
L. MANARA	Milan, Italy
D. MARGULES	Philadelphia, Pa., U.S.A.
G. MARZULLO	New York, N.Y., U.S.A.
A. MAURSET	Oslo, Norway
A.T. MCKNIGHT	Aberdeen, Scotland
F. MEDZIHRADSKY	Ann Arbor, Mi., U.S.A.,
H. MERZ	Ingelheim, F.R.G.
G. METCALF	Hull, England
J.C. MEUNIER	Toulouse, France
W.F. MICHNE	New York, N.Y., U.S.A.
A.A. MILLER	Kent, England
B. MILLER	Memphis, Tn., U.S.A.
K. MILLS	Ware, England
G. MILNE	Groton, Ct., U.S.A.
J.E. MORETON	Baltimore, Md., U.S.A.
B.A. MORGAN	Hull, England
T. MURAKI	Tokyo, Japan
J. MUSACCHIO	New York, N.Y., U.S.A.
M. NIWA	Gifu, Japan
W.A. NOLEN	Den Haag, The Netherlands

A. NORTH	Maywood, Ill., U.S.A.
M. NOZAKI	Gifu, Japan
F.P. NIJKAMP	Utrecht, The Netherlands
J.E. OLLEY	Bradford, England
O. OMER	Berlin, F.R.G.
F. OPMEER	Utrecht, The Netherlands
K. ORNSTEIN	Düsseldorf, F.R.G.
H. OSBORNE	München, F.R.G.
R.M. PALMOUR	Berkeley, Ca., U.S.A.
G. PARRA	Madrid, Spain
S.J. PATERSON	Aberdeen, Scotland
G. PATEY	Paris, France
A.L. PELTENBURG	Utrecht, The Netherlands
A. PERT	Bethesda, Md., U.S.A.
C. PERT	Bethesda, Md., U.S.A.
CHR.M. PEPPER	Bristol, England
C.W.T. PILCHER	Kuwait
C. PINSKY	Winnipeg, Manitoba, Canada
J. PLESS	Basel, Switzerland
G.J.J. PLOMP	Utrecht, The Netherlands
B. POMERANZ	Toronto, Ontario, Canada
R. PRZEWLOCKI	München, F.R.G.
M. PUIG	New York, N.Y., U.S.A.
RABADAN PEINADO	Madrid, Spain
M.M. RANCE	Hull, England
K. RAVER	Giessen, F.R.G.
J.M.H. REES	Manchester, England
J.A. RICHTER	Indianapolis, In., U.S.A.
R.A. RIESE	Palo Alto, Ca., U.S.A.
F.M. ROBINSON	West Point, Pa., U.S.A.
L.E. ROBSON	Aberdeen, Scotland
D. RÖMER	Basel, Switzerland
A.Z. RONAI	Budapest, Hungary
B. ROQUES	Paris, France
P. SAINIO	Helsinki, Finland
J.R. SANCHEZ RAMES	Chicago, Ill., U.S.A.
C. SCHNEIDER	Beckenham, England
P. SCHOTMAN	Utrecht, The Netherlands
R. SCHULZ	Munchen, F.R.G.

J.CH. SCHWARTZ	Paris, France
N.G. SEIDAH	Montreal, Canada
R.D.E. SEWELL	Cardiff, Wales
N.N. SHARE	Dorval, Quebec, Canada
K. SHARIFI HOSSAINI	Shiraz, Iran
J.S. SHAW	Macclesfield, England
G. SIGGINS	San Diego, Ca., U.S.A.
E.J. SIMON	New York, N.Y., U.S.A.
C. SMITH	Hull, England
C.B. SMITH	Ann Arbor, Mi., U.S.A.
T.W. SMITH	Beckenham, England
D.G. SMYTH	London, England
A. SOLLES	Nevilly sur Seine, France
R.P. SOSA	Aberdeen, Scotland
S.B. SPARBER	Bath, England
S. SPAMPINATO	Catania, Italy
W.J. STEELE	Iowa City, Ia., U.S.A.
J.M. STEWART	Denver, Co., U.S.A.
K. STOCKHAUS	Engelbeim/Rhein, F.R.G.
I.P. STOLERMAN	Birmingham, England
H. SWAIN	Ann Arbor, Mi., U.S.A.
J.P. SWERTS	Paris, France
H.H. SZETO	Burlington, Vt., U.S.A.
E. TAGASHIRA	Tokyo, Japan
H. TAKAGI	Kyoto, Japan
A.E. TAKEMORI	Minneapolis, Mn., U.S.A.
L. TANG	New York, N.Y., U.S.A.
L. TERENIUS	Uppsala, Sweden
H. TESCHEMACHER	München, F.R.G.
J.H. TRABER	Koln, F.R.G.
F.C. TULUNAY	Ankara, Turkey
M.B. TYERS	Ware, England
K.R. UNNA	Rockville, Md., U.S.A.
DR. VAN DOORN	Arnhem, The Netherlands
TJ. B. VAN WIMERSMA GREIDANUS	Utrecht, The Netherlands
J.M. VAN REE	Utrecht, The Netherlands
J.W. VAN DER LAAN	Rotterdam, The Netherlands
H. VAUDRY	Mont-Saint-Aignan, France

K. VERHOEF	Utrecht, The Netherlands
W.M.A. VERHOEVEN	Utrecht, The Netherlands
D.H.G. VERSTEEG	Utrecht, The Netherlands
V. VON BRUCHHAUSEN	Ingelheim/Rhein, F.R.G.
B. VON GRAFFENRIED	Basle, Switzerland
K.M. VOIGT	Ulm, F.R.G.
H. WAGEMAKER	Louisville, Ky., U.S.A.
I. WAJDA	Ward's Island, N.Y., U.S.A.
S.L. WALLENSTEIN	New York, N.Y., U.S.A.
S. WARD	Manchester, England
A.A. WATERFIELD	London, England
S. WATSON	Palo Alto, Ca., U.S.A.
E.T. WEI	Berkeley, Ca., U.S.A.
B.A. WEISSMAN	Ness Ziona, Israel
H.B.A. WELLE	Maarssen, The Netherlands
D.L. WESCHE	Indianapolis, In., U.S.A.
DR. WESTERBERG	Utrecht, The Netherlands
J. WEIJERS	Amsterdam, The Netherlands
P. WEYLING	Den Haag, The Netherlands
J. WIDEMAN	Warszawa, Poland
V. WIEGANT	Utrecht, The Netherlands
S. WILKINSON	Beckenham, England
A. WITTER	Utrecht, The Netherlands
J.H. WOLSTENCROFT	Birmingham, England
J.H. WOODS	Ann Arbor, Mi., U.S.A.
W. WOUTERS	Utrecht, The Netherlands
K. YAMATSU	Tokyo, Japan
W.S. YOUNG	Baltimore, Md., U.S.A.
W. ZIEGLGÄNSBERGER	München, F.R.G.
E. ZIMMERMAN	Los Angeles, Ca., U.S.A.
CHR. ZIOUDROU	Bethesda, Md., U.S.A.
R.S. ZUKIN	New York, N.Y., U.S.A.

SUBJECT INDEX